Geriatrics Models of Care

Michael L. Malone

Elizabeth A. Capezuti • Robert M. Palmer

Editors

Geriatrics Models of Care

Bringing 'Best Practice' to an Aging America

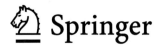 Springer

Editors
Michael L. Malone
Senior Services–Aurora Health Care/University
  of Wisconsin School of Medicine
  & Public Health
Milwaukee, WI, USA

Elizabeth A. Capezuti
Hunter-Bellevue School of Nursing
Hunter College of the City University
  of New York
New York, NY, USA

Robert M. Palmer
Eastern Virginia Medical School
Norfolk, VA, USA

ISBN 978-3-319-16067-2   ISBN 978-3-319-16068-9   (eBook)
DOI 10.1007/978-3-319-16068-9

Library of Congress Control Number: 2015938154

Springer Cham Heidelberg New York Dordrecht London

Printed on acid-free paper

Springer International Publishing AG Switzerland is part of Springer Science+Business Media (www.springer.com)

Foreword

We are living through an upheaval in health service delivery in the USA, driven by demographic, political, economic, and technological megatrends. The US population is aging rapidly, and with it the burden of chronic illness. Healthcare reform in the wake of the Affordable Care Act, and realignment of economic incentives towards a (theoretically) market-driven healthcare system that pays for the value of care provided, rather the volume of care provided appears ascendant. Technological advances in various forms, from remote monitoring to nanotechnology, genomics, health information technology, and personalized medicine will continue to put pressure on the current system.

In the midst of such change, the field of geriatrics has much of value to offer in the way of innovative, evidence-based, health service delivery models that improve quality and, in some cases, reduce the costs of care of vulnerable older adults with multiple chronic conditions who drive the use of technological advances and healthcare costs. In 1999, Calkins et al., in the book *New Ways to Care for Older Adults: Building Systems Based on Evidence*, described a number of early-stage innovative care delivery models [1]. In 2009, Boult et al. published an evidence review of 15 successful models of comprehensive care for older adults with chronic conditions for the Institute of Medicine's "Retooling for an Aging America" report [2].

This volume builds on those previous efforts and extends them. This book has chapters devoted to 30 or so healthcare models that span the gamut of the continuum, including the community, home, primary care, emergency department, and hospital. Some models are consultative, some demonstrate new approaches to co-management, while others focus on providing ongoing care to patients. Some models are "band-aid"-type, providing intense care to or monitoring patients at vulnerable junctures in the care continuum, such as immediately after discharge from an acute care hospital, while others focus on providing ongoing care to patients. Different models come with different provider types—some models have a full and robust interdisciplinary team, including physicians, nurses, nurse practitioners, social workers, pharmacists, aides, and mental health providers. Other models rely on trained volunteer lay persons. A number of models are focused on specific conditions, while others accommodate patients with any medical condition.

Many of the models described in this volume have a strong underlying evidence base, yet few have been widely disseminated and implemented. In our own work on dissemination of such models, we are continually struck by the fact that relatively few health systems have developed strategic initiatives around the care of older adults. Given that hospital beds are occupied to a great extent by older adults, and that achieving success in a population health and value-focused healthcare system will require addressing the needs of these people, rather than simply the needs of their specific organs or diseases, this volume provides timely and practical examples which can anchor new strategic priorities.

Bringing together into one volume robust and up-to-date descriptions of these care models will serve the cause of healthcare delivery improvement. We hope this book finds its way into the hands and hearts of the inhabitants of the C-suites in American health care—Chief Executive Officers, Chief Innovation Officers, Chief Financial Officers, and managers of clinical services who live close to or in the trenches of service delivery. Such readers will find many useful examples of improvements that impact the service delivery jigsaw puzzle.

For some time, we have advocated that clustering together multiple models into geriatric service lines would best serve the business interests of organizations and the health needs of older adults and their caregivers [3]. All healthcare delivery systems are unique—each with its own clinical, economic, and cultural drivers and imperatives. Mixing and matching and adapting models described in these pages will look different in different systems. A hospital-based accountable care organization (ACO) or health system that consists mostly of hospitals at financial risk for hospital readmissions, with employed hospitalist physicians and few outpatient assets, will benefit from implementing different models from an outpatient physician-owned ACO that seeks to prevent any hospital admission. A self-insured integrated delivery system that covers the inpatient, outpatient, and post-acute spheres may benefit from combinations of several models across the entire continuum of care. Advantages of such a service line approach include the ability to serve more patients, use shared screening processes and measures, and create greater economic and health benefits, and to leverage the possibilities of creating synergies across models [4].

The above discussion suggests that implementation of such models is an easy feat. It is not. Significant stumbling blocks exist for many—for a number of these models there is a lack of technical assistance capability and/or capacity. Another stumbling block is vocabulary. The term "geriatrics" may carry significant negative baggage in the marketplace. In one of our institutions a "geriatrics center" had its name changed to "care center," in part, because geriatrics was simply viewed as bad marketing. We submit that many of these models are appropriate for younger populations with significant burden of chronic illness and functional impairment.

This book is a major advance for the field. It is edited by world-class practitioners and champions of the field of geriatric health service delivery innovation, and they have selected authors who are experts in their areas. We look forward to a future when all hospitals and health systems will employ the models described in this volume.

Baltimore, MD   Bruce Leff
New York, NY   Al Siu
Durham, NC   Lynn Spragens

References

1. Calkins E, Boult C, Wagner EH, Pacala JT, editors. New ways to care for older people: building systems based on evidence. New York, NY: Springer Publishing Company; 1999.
2. Boult C, Green AF, Boult LB, Pacala JT, Snyder C, Leff B. Successful models of comprehensive care for older adults with chronic conditions: evidence for the institute of medicine's "Retooling for an Aging America" report. J Am Geriatr Soc. 2009;57(12):2328–37.
3. Siu AL, Spragens LH, Inouye SK, Morrison RS, Leff B. The ironic business case for chronic care in the acute care setting. Health Aff (Millwood). 2009;28(1):113–25.
4. Leff B, Spragens LH, Morano B, Powell J, Bickert T, Bond C, et al. Rapid reengineering of acute medical care for medicare beneficiaries: the medicare innovations collaborative. Health Aff (Millwood). 2012;31(6):1204–15.

Preface: The Adoption of Geriatric Practice Models

"I just figured I'd let the neighbors try it first." This account jumped off the page at me. It is a notation of a farmer from Bruce Ryan and Neal Gross in their report on the "Acceptance and Diffusion of Hybrid Corn Seed in Two Iowa Communities" [1]. The report describes the spread of "best practice" among farmers in the 1930s. We will describe the key points they learned and then link these concepts to the scaling of geriatrics models in America's healthcare system.

First let's go to Ames, Iowa. We will set the context of the farmer's challenges in the 1930s. Most farms were a family business. Most farming practices took the seed from one year and used a portion to provide for the following year's crop. The corn plants were generally good; however, many of the stalks of corn may not have stood up straight or were unable to withstand weather conditions. The yields were usually good and there were no major problems or crises for farmers in that part of the country at the time. Farmers used pollination strategies to assure their crops produced adequately.

Researchers at the University of Iowa had developed a hybrid corn seed in the 1920s. Cross-pollinated plants produced this new seed. The new plants yielded larger crops of corn for those who planted them. Farmers, however, needed to pay for the hybrid seed each year. The initial rate of adoption of this new practice between 1927 and 1933 was slow. Less than 10 % of the farmers in two small Iowa counties had begun to use the new seeds. These were the "early adopters."

Between 1933 and 1939, the practice of Iowa corn farmers changed dramatically. There was a rapid rise in the adoption of hybrid seed. Over the subsequent 2 or 3 years, from 1939 to 1941, nearly 95 % of the farm operators accepted the new seed. These folks who were last to change their practice were "the late adopters."

So what factors seemed to influence the adoption of new ideas in the counties near and including Ames, Iowa? It turns out that Ryan and Gross observed that there was a considerable period of 5–7 years between the time that the farmers had heard of the new hybrid seed and the time of accepting the seed in their practice. Most adopters of the hybrid seed used a trial approach before fully committing to the practice. A local seed salesman provided the initial information about the hybrid seed. This salesman had a major influence on the acceptance of the hybrid seed early (between 1933 and 1937). Later, it turned out that the most influential source for farmers accepting hybrid corn seed was their neighbors. Farmers in Iowa talk to each other. (They apparently listen to each other as well.)

During the years between 1933 and 1939, there was a rapid rate of adoption of hybrid corn seed among the Iowa farmers. They had hit an inflection point. This means that if you graph out the rate of acceptance of the hybrid seed over time, there is a point on the curve at which that line changes from convex to concave. Factors which influenced the early adoption of hybrid corn seed included youthfulness of the farmer, the size of the farm, the education of the farmer, and the social participation of the farmer.

What can we learn from a study of the diffusion of hybrid corn seed? Can any of these points help us to adopt new ideas in geriatrics? It turns out that several themes that hold true for the diffusion of innovations from 1930 are relevant today. We will transition from corn seed to the diffusion of geriatrics practice models. First, models of best practice in geriatrics must have intuitive appeal. The model must fit with the values of the organization and it must solve a problem which is important. Second, there must be a strong evidence base demonstrating benefit for patients. Third, there must be a cost savings for the organization which is sponsoring the practice change. Fourth, there must be a patient dissatisfaction with current care. Lastly, there must be a broad recognition of the importance of the new practice.

As you read this book about geriatrics models of care, we encourage you to consider how you will adopt the new ideas presented. These principles may help with the diffusion of innovations in geriatrics. Look for the relative advantage of the model when you compare to current practice. Next, determine if the model is compatible with your values, experiences, and needs. Also, look for the complexity of the model. This means the degree to which the innovation is perceived as difficult to understand or use. Further, define if the innovation can be tested, before full investment. And finally, define the degree to which the results of the innovation are visible to others. These approaches may help the reader to prioritize among multiple "best practice" models for seniors.

What are some themes that can help you to proceed with adopting best practices?

1. Focus on what is most important. There are many projects and priorities that come and go over the course of one's professional career. Choose and embrace the model that fits the best with what you are deeply passionate about. This focus helps you to address what your organization stands for and why it exists. Developing models, which you and your team care deeply about, will help you to articulate these values to folks whom you serve and to folks at the future dissemination sites. You will note multiple model descriptions in this book depicting areas of care that are vital to vulnerable elders. We encourage you to study these models and learn about the meaning of this work from the geriatrics leaders who have developed the models.

2. We would encourage you to develop your conceptual model for "what success looks like" at your program. This process helps to guide your direction during good and bad economic times. This helps funders understand where their contribution will lead. This process also helps to focus how your organization can uniquely contribute to the patients it touches.

3. Next, have a strong commitment to excellence. This will be required when you develop, manage, and guide your geriatrics practice model. This commitment will help you as you hire professionals who become team members of your model. Your program's commitment to excellence will make sure that the vulnerable older individuals whom you serve receive care that is safe and effective. As you read this book, you will see evidence of such commitment among the models described.

4. Provide a culture that supports the adoption of best practices. This means that you support innovation and tinkering with models, as you better understand the needs of your patients. The culture—which provides for adoption of new ideas—looks outward to find good ideas outside of their own hospital and outside of their own state/country. We would encourage you to do as the farmers in Iowa had done, that is, talk to your neighbors.

5. Measure your outcomes so that you have a clear understanding of your current clinical performance. This is particularly challenging because it is difficult to both provide the care and measure the care which you are delivering. In order to get buy in from the hospital leadership, you will need to be able to demonstrate their return on investment. No organization will allow you to broadly adopt a new model or program without showing outcomes pointing to excellent care. The reader should watch for key outcomes measures of each model, which is described in this book.

6. Finally, build momentum towards "better." You will not end up with perfect care for all individuals. It's just not possible. Instead take a humble, but disciplined approach to improving care in our complex health system. Use systems-based approaches to improving practice over a long period of time and you will be effective in providing safe care for large populations of older persons. You will read about multiple examples in this book demonstrating models that improve care for patients, but not all the patients served achieve the optimal outcomes. This work is difficult and our patients are vulnerable. This book is intended to guide the reader to lead models, which provide better care.

We would like to express our appreciation to the multiple chapter authors who have contributed to this book. We further express our thanks to Simone Katz, the developmental editor of this book, and to Patricia Maloney who helped to coordinate this project. Finally, we thank our families who have encouraged us throughout our careers.

Milwaukee, WI, USA   Michael L. Malone
New York, NY, USA   Elizabeth A Capezuti
Norfolk, VA, USA   Robert M. Palmer

Reference

1. Ryan B, Gross N. Acceptance and diffusion of hybrid corn seed in two Iowa communities. Research Bulletin. 1950;320:663–708.

Contributors

SangNam Ahn, Ph.D. Department of Health Systems Management and Policy, The University of Memphis School of Public Health, Memphis, TN, USA

Saima T. Akbar, M.D. University of Wisconsin School of Medicine and Public Health, Aurora St. Luke's Medical Center, Milwaukee, WI, USA

Catherine A. Alder, J.D., M.S.W. Eskenazi Health, Indianapolis, IN, USA

Tena M. Alonzo, M.A. Department of Education and Research, Beatitudes Campus, Phoenix, AZ, USA

Mary Guerriero Austrom, Ph.D. Department of Psychiatry, Indiana University School of Medicine, Indianapolis, IN, USA

Peter A. Boling, M.D. Department of Internal Medicine, Virginia Commonwealth University, Richmond, VA, USA

Marie Boltz, Ph.D., C.R.N.P., F.A.A.N. Connell School of Nursing, Boston College, Chestnut Hill, MA, USA

Katrina Booth, M.D. Division of Gerontology, Geriatrics, and Palliative Care, University of Alabama at Birmingham, Birmingham, AL, USA

Chad Boult, M.D., M.P.H., M.B.A. Independent Consultant, Boise, ID, USA

Malaz A. Boustani, M.D., M.P.H. Indiana University Center for Aging Research and Regenstrief Institute, Indianapolis, IN, USA

Ella Harvey Bowman, M.D., Ph.D. Department of Medicine, Sidney & Lois Eskenazi Hospital, Indiana University School of Medicine, Indianapolis, IN, USA

Sally Brooks, M.D. Kindred Healthcare, Louisville, KY, USA

Linda Bub, M.S.N.,R.N. NICHE Nurses Improving Care of Healthsystem Elders, NYU College of Nursing, New York, NY, USA

Dawn E. Butler, M.S.W., J.D. IU Geriatrics and Division of General Internal Medicine, Department of Medicine, Indiana University School of Medicine, Indianapolis, IN, USA

Angela Georgia Catic, M.D. Division Geriatrics Section, Department of Internal Medicine, Huffington Center on Aging and the Michael E. DeBakey VAMC, Baylor College of Medicine, Houston, TX, USA

Lindy Clemson, Ph.D. Faculty of Health Sciences, University of Sydney, Lidcombe, NSW, Australia

Steven R. Counsell, M.D. IU Geriatrics and Division of General Internal Medicine, Department of Medicine, Indiana University School of Medicine and Indiana University Center for Aging Research, Indianapolis, IN, USA

Benjamin F. Crabtree, Ph.D. Department of Family Medicine & Community Health, Rutgers, Robert Wood Johnson Medical School, Rutgers, The State University of New Jersey, Somerset, NJ, USA

Ellen S. Danto-Nocton, M.D. Aurora Sinai Medical Center and University of Wisconsin School of Medicine & Public Health, Milwaukee, WI, USA

Scott M. Dresden, M.D., M.S. Department of Emergency Medicine, Center for Healthcare Studies--Institute for Public Health and Medicine, Northwestern University Feinberg School of Medicine, Chicago, IL, USA

Leslie Chang Evertson, M.S.N. Division of Geriatrics, UCLA, Los Angeles, CA, USA

Joseph H. Flaherty, M.D. Department of Internal Medicine, Division of Geriatrics, Saint Louis University School of Medicine & Geriatric Research, Education and Clinical Center (GRECC), St. Louis VA Medical Center, St. Louis, MO, USA

Kathleen Fletcher, R.N., D.N.P.-B.C. Riverside Health System, Newport News, VA, USA

Kellie L. Flood, M.D. Division of Gerontology, Geriatrics, and Palliative Care, University of Alabama at Birmingham, Birmingham, AL, USA

Kathryn I. Frank, R.N., Ph.D. IU Geriatrics and Division of General Internal Medicine, Department of Medicine, Indiana University School of Medicine, Indianapolis, IN, USA

Thomas L. Frazier, B.A., M.P.A. Coalition of Wisconsin Aging Groups (Retired), Verona, WI, USA

Laura R. Holtz, B.S. IU Center for Aging Research, Regenstrief Institute, Indianapolis, IN, USA

Mary L. Hook, Ph.D., R.N.-B.C. Department of Knowledge-Based Nursing (KBN), Aurora Health Care, Milwaukee, WI, USA

Thomas R. Hornick, M.D. Geriatric Research Education and Clinical Centers, Louis Stokes Cleveland VAMC, Cleveland, OH, USA

Timothy Howell, M.D., M.A. Geriatrics Research, Education, and Clinical Center, Madison VA Hospital, Madison, WI, USA

Geriatrics Division, Department of Medicine, University of Wisconsin School of Medicine and Public Health, Madison, WI, USA

Tammy T. Hshieh, M.D. Division of Aging, Brigham and Women's Hospital, and Institute for Aging Research, Hebrew SeniorLife, Boston, MA, USA

William W. Hung, M.D., M.P.H. Brookdale Department of Geriatrics and Palliative Medicine, James J Peters VA Medical Center, Geriatric Research, Education and Clinical Center, Icahn School of Medicine at Mount Sinai, New York, NY, USA

Ula Hwang, M.D., M.P.H. Department of Emergency Medicine, Icahn School of Medicine at Mount Sinai, New York, NY, USA

Brookdale Department of Geriatrics and Palliative Medicine, Icahn School of Medicine at Mount Sinai, New York, NY, USA

Geriatric Research, Education and Clinical Center, James J. Peters Veterans Affairs Medical Center, New York, NY, USA

Sharon K. Inouye, M.D., M.P.H. Department of Medicine, Beth Israel Deaconess Medical Center and Institute for Aging Research, Hebrew SeniorLife, Harvard Medical School, Boston, MA, USA

Carlos Roberto Jaén, M.D., Ph.D. Department of Family and Community Medicine, University of Texas Health Science Center at San Antonio, San Antonio, TX, USA

Lee A. Jennings, M.D., M.S.H.S. Division of Geriatrics, UCLA, Los Angeles, CA, USA

Mihae Kim, M.S.N. Division of Geriatrics, UCLA, Los Angeles, CA, USA

Ariba Khan, M.D., M.P.H. Department of Geriatrics, Aurora Sinai Medical Center, Milwaukee, WI, USA

Cheryl E. Knupp, B.S. Beatitudes Campus, Phoenix, AZ, USA

Denise M. Kresevic, Ph.D., R.N. Louis Stokes VA Medical Center and Adult Medical Surgical Nursing Department, University Hospitals of Cleveland, Cleveland, OH, USA

Eileen M. Kunz, M.P.H. On Lok Senior Health Services, San Francisco, CA, USA

Michael A. LaMantia, M.D., M.P.H. Indiana University Center for Aging Research and Regenstrief Institute, Indianapolis, IN, USA

Bruce Leff, M.D. Division of Geriatric Medicine and Gerontology, Department of Medicine, Johns Hopkins Bayview Medical Center, Baltimore, MD, USA

Jing Li, M.D., M.S. Center for Health Services Research, University of Kentucky, Lexington, KY, USA

Meryl Lovarini, Ph.D., M.H.Sc. Discipline of Occupational Therapy, Ageing, Work and Health Research Unit, The University of Sydney, Lidcombe, NSW, Australia

Jane Mahoney, M.D. University of Wisconsin School of Medicine and Public Health, Madison, WI, USA

Laurie Mallery, M.D. Department of Medicine, Faculty of Medicine, Dalhousie University, Halifax, NS, Canada

Michael L. Malone, M.D. Senior Services – Aurora Health Care/University of Wisconsin School of Medicine & Public Health, Milwaukee, WI, USA

University of Wisconsin School of Medicine and Public Health, Milwaukee, WI, USA

Aaron Malsch, M.S.N., R.N. Department of Senior Services, Aurora Health Care, Milwaukee, WI, USA

Helen Maurer, M.A., C.H.E.S. IU Center for Aging Research, Regenstrief Institute, Indianapolis, IN, USA

Diane E. Meier, M.D. Department of Geriatrics and Palliative Medicine, Icahn School of Medicine at Mount Sinai, New York, NY, USA

Karen M. Mitchell, B.S.N. Health Care Center, Beatitudes Campus, Phoenix, AZ, USA

William L. Miller, M.D., M.A. Department of Family Medicine, Lehigh Valley Health Network, School of Nursing, Allentown, PA, USA

Paige Moorhouse, M.D., M.P.H. Faculty of Medicine, Dalhousie University, Halifax, NS, Canada

Jeanine Moreno, M.S. Division of Geriatrics, UCLA, Los Angeles, CA, USA

Lynne Morishita, G.N.P., M.S.N. Geriatric Health Care, Minneapolis, MN, USA

Arif Nazir, M.D. Division of General Internal Medicine and Geriatrics, Indiana University School of Medicine, Indianapolis, IN, USA

Paul Nutting, M.D., M.S.P.H. Center for Research Strategies, University of Colorado Health Sciences Center, Denver, CO, USA

Marcia G. Ory, Ph.D., M.P.H. Health Promotion and Community Health Sciences, School of Public Health at Texas A&M Health Science Center, College Station, TX, USA

Joseph G. Ouslander, M.D. Department of Integrated Medical Sciences, Charles E. Schmidt College of Medicine, Florida Atlantic University, Boca Raton, FL, USA

Robert M. Palmer, M.D., M.P.H. Glennan Center for Geriatrics and Gerontology, Norfolk, VA, USA

Eastern Virginia Medical School, Norfolk, VA, USA

Michelle Panlilio, M.S.N. Division of Geriatrics, UCLA, Los Angeles, CA, USA

Neela K. Patel, M.D., M.P.H. Division of Community Geriatrics, Department of Family and Community Medicine, University of Texas Health Science Center at San Antonio, San Antonio, TX, USA

Edgar Pierluissi, M.D. Division of Hospital Medicine and Geriatrics, San Francisco General Hospital, University of California, San Francisco, CA, USA

David B. Reuben, M.D. Division of Geriatrics, David Geffen School of Medicine at UCLA, Los Angeles, CA, USA

Mark S. Rosenberg, D.O., M.B.A. Department of Emergency Medicine, St. Joseph's Healthcare System, Paterson, NJ, USA

Laurence Rubenstein, M.D., M.P.H. Reynolds Department of Geriatric Medicine, University of Oklahoma Health Sciences Center, Oklahoma City, OK, USA

Greg A. Sachs, M.D. Division of General Internal Medicine and Geriatrics, Indiana University School of Medicine, Indianapolis, IN, USA

Bethann Scarborough, M.D. Brookdale Department of Geriatrics and Palliative Medicine, Mount Sinai Hospital, New York, NY, USA

Katherine Serrano, B.A. Division of Geriatrics, UCLA, Los Angeles, CA, USA

Manish N. Shah, M.D., M.P.H. Departments of Emergency Medicine, Public Health Sciences, and Geriatrics, University of Rochester School of Medicine and Dentistry, Rochester, NY, USA

Ronald J. Shumacher, M.D., F.A.C.P., C.M.D. Complex Population Management, Optum, Rockville, MD, USA

Jill Shutes, M.S.N. Department of Integrated Medical Sciences, Charles E. Schmidt College of Medicine, Florida Atlantic University, Boca Raton, FL, USA

Michelle R. Simpson, Ph.D., R.N. Center for Nursing Research and Practice, Aurora Health Care, Milwaukee, WI, USA

Matthew Lee Smith, Ph.D., M.P.H., C.H.E.S. Department of Health Promotion and Behavior, The University of Georgia College of Public Health, Athens, GA, USA

Soryal Soryal, M.D. Aurora West Allis Medical Center and University of Wisconsin School of Medicine and Public Health, Milwaukee, WI, USA

Kurt C. Stange, M.D., Ph.D. Department of Family Medicine and Community Health, Case Western Reserve University, Cleveland, OH, USA

Stephanie Sue Stein, M.A.P.S. Milwaukee County Department on Aging, Milwaukee, WI, USA

Zaldy S. Tan, M.D., M.P.H. Division of Geriatrics, UCLA, Los Angeles, CA, USA

Jonny A. Macias Tejada, M.D. University of Wisconsin School of Medicine and Public Health, Milwaukee, WI, USA

Samuel D. Towne Jr., Ph.D., M.P.H., C.P.H. Health Promotion and Community Health Sciences, Texas A&M Health Science Center, College Station, TX, USA

Kathleen T. Unroe, M.D., M.H.A. Division of General Internal Medicine and Geriatrics, Indiana University School of Medicine, Indianapolis, IN, USA

Marsha Vollbrecht, M.S., C.S.W., N.H.A. Department of Senior Services, Aurora Health Care, Plymouth, WI, USA

Lauren Williams, B.A., M.A. Kindred Healthcare, Louisville, KY, USA

Mark V. Williams, M.D. Center for Health Services Research, University of Kentucky, Lexington, KY, USA

Jennifer Wolff, Ph.D. Department of Health Policy and Management, Johns Hopkins Bloomberg School of Public Health, Baltimore, MD, USA

Division of Geriatric Medicine and Gerontology, Johns Hopkins University School of Medicine, Baltimore, MD, USA

Nancy E. Wood, M.S. Department of Emergency Medicine, University of Rochester Medical Center, Rochester, NY, USA

Robert S. Young, M.D., M.S. Department of Internal Medicine, University of Kentucky, Lexington, KY, USA

Jean Yudin, G.N.P.-B.C. Division of Geriatric Medicine, Department of Medicine, University of Pennsylvania Health System, Philadelphia, PA, USA

Jirong Yue, M.D. The Center of Gerontology and Geriatrics, West China Hospital, Sichuan University, Chengdu, Sichuan, China

Michael L. Malone is the Medical Director of Aurora Health
ra at Home. He is a Clinical Adjunct Professor of Medicine at
1ool of Medicine and Public Health. He also serves as the
ship Program at Aurora Health Care. Dr. Malone received his
es from Texas Tech University in Lubbock, Texas; he com-
dency and geriatric fellowship training at Mt. Sinai Medical
Health Care practice is to treat homebound older persons in

of the Public Policy Committee for the American Geriatrics
lodels of Geriatric Care, Quality Improvement, and Program
Dissemination for the *Journal of the American Geriatrics Society*. He led the development of
the first Acute Care for Elders (ACE) unit in Wisconsin. He and his colleagues have developed
innovative strategies to disseminate geriatrics models of care including the ACE Tracker software to identify vulnerable hospitalized elders, and the e-Geriatrician telemedicine program to
bring geriatrics expertise to rural hospitals with no geriatrician on staff. Dr. Malone has developed innovative teaching tools including ACE pocket cards and the Geriatrics Fellows' Most
Difficult Case conference. He has joined his colleagues at the Medical College of Wisconsin
to implement "Geriatric Fast Facts" on mobile devices and tablets. In August, 2014, he released
a book with Elizabeth A. Capezuti and Robert M. Palmer, MD, entitled *Acute Care for Elders –
A Model for Interdisciplinary Care*, Springer Business and Science.

Elizabeth A. Capezuti, Ph.D., R.N., F.A.A.N. Elizabeth A. Capezuti, Ph.D., R.N., F.A.A.N.,
is the William Randolph Hearst Chair in Gerontology and Professor at Hunter College of the
City University of New York (CUNY), where she serves as the Assistant Dean for Research and
Director of the Center for Nursing Research. She also serves as a Professor in the PhD Program
in Nursing at the CUNY Graduate Center. Dr. Capezuti is known for her work in improving the
care of older adults by interventions and models that positively influence healthcare provider's
knowledge and work environment. Dr. Capezuti has published extensively in the areas of fall
prevention, restraint and side rail elimination, geriatric syndromes, and models of care.
Dr. Capezuti is the recipient of the American Geriatrics Society Outstanding Scientific
Achievement for Clinical Investigation Award and the American Academy of Nursing Nurse
Leader in Aging Award. She is a Fellow of the American Academy of Nursing, the Gerontological
Society of America, and the New York Academy of Medicine.

Robert M. Palmer, M.D., M.P.H. Robert M. Palmer, M.D., M.P.H., is the John Franklin
Chair of Geriatrics and the Director of the Glennan Center for Geriatrics and Gerontology at
Eastern Virginia Medical School, where he is also Professor of Internal Medicine and Division
Chief of Geriatric Medicine. Dr. Palmer has attained international attention for his research
focused on improving the functional outcomes of hospitalization, patient safety, and quality of
care. Dr. Palmer was Principal Investigator of a grant from the John A. Hartford Foundation

that established the effectiveness of a medical unit for acute care of elders (ACE Unit). He is the author of numerous publications including research articles, geriatric textbooks, book chapters, and scientific reviews. Dr. Palmer is Associate Editor of the *Journal of the American Geriatrics Society* (JAGS). He is the Chair of the AGS Special Interest Group, Acute Hospital Care. In May, 2015, he will receive the Edward Henderson Award from the AGS.

Part I

Hospital Based Models of Care

Acute Care for Elders

Kellie L. Flood, Katrina Booth, Edgar Pierluissi,
Ellen S. Danto-Nocton, Denise M. Kresevic,
and Robert M. Palmer

Introduction

The aging tsunami has resulted in a significantly greater number of older adults with multiple chronic conditions. This phenomenon poses a unique challenge to clinicians from all disciplines, as well as health care systems, to provide evidence-based, cost-effective care to a greater number of vulnerable patients than seen in decades past. Currently, most health care organizations struggle to consistently provide this complex care across the care continuum. However, these challenges lead to opportunities for new models of care that offer holistic, coordinated care for complex patients that simultaneously improve care efficiency across a health system.

A hospitalization is an especially significant event in the health care journey of an older adult. All too often, despite proper treatment for the reason for hospital admission, older adults are discharged with new disability that was not present before the onset of illness [1]. In a 2008 study by Boyd et al., about 1/3 of hospitalized older adults experienced a decline from baseline function at hospital discharge, and over 20 % developed a new disability in the year following hospital discharge [2]. In addition to this hospitalization-associated disability (HAD), hospitalized older adults are vulnerable to other complications with serious consequences. These include delirium, falls, pressure ulcers, urinary and bowel dysfunction, and malnutrition. Apart from functional decline, these complications are significant in terms of patient suffering and added costs of care. When the aging population and the high rate of hospitalization amongst older adults are taken into account, the risks to older adults take on even greater significance for patients, health care systems, and policymakers. Older adults make up 13 % of the US population, but account for 36 % of hospital admissions and 44 % of hospital charges [3]. The consequences and cost of these hazards of hospitalization, coupled with an increasing number of hospitalized older adults, form the rationale for adopting a new model of acute care.

K.L. Flood, M.D. (✉) • K. Booth, M.D.
Division of Gerontology, Geriatrics, and Palliative Care,
University of Alabama at Birmingham,
1720 2nd Ave South, CH-19, Room 201 Birmingham,
AL 35294-2041, USA
e-mail: kflood@uabmc.edu

E. Pierluissi, M.D.
Division of Hospital Medicine and Geriatrics,
San Francisco General Hospital, University of California,
San Francisco, CA, USA

E.S. Danto-Nocton, M.D.
Aurora Sinai Medical Center and University of Wisconsin
School of Medicine & Public Health, Milwaukee, WI, USA

D.M. Kresevic, Ph.D., R.N.
Louis Stokes VA Medical Center and Adult Medical Surgical
Nursing Department, University Hospitals of Cleveland,
Cleveland, OH, USA

R.M. Palmer, M.D., M.P.H.
Glennan Center for Geriatrics and Gerontology, Norfolk, VA, USA

Eastern Virginia Medical School, Norfolk, VA, USA

Hospitalization-Associated Disability

Over the past 30 years, studies have documented the importance of new or worsening disability in hospitalized older adults. Many of these studies of HAD measure function using the Katz Index of Activities of Daily Living (ADLs) [4]. The ADLs used in most studies are bathing, dressing, transferring, toileting, and eating, while some include walking. A patient is considered dependent in an ADL if s/he cannot accomplish the activity or requires the assistance of another person to accomplish the activity. An elder who needs help with ADLs will require the assistance of a caregiver in the home or in an assisted living or long term care setting, depending on the level of ADL dependence and extent of psychosocial support in the home setting. In the 1980s, studies of HAD documented high rates of new disability among older adults. In one study of patients functionally independent at baseline, 81 % were dependent in at least four of seven functional domains (mobility,

M.L. Malone et al. (eds.), *Geriatrics Models of Care: Bringing 'Best Practice' to an Aging America*,
DOI 10.1007/978-3-319-16068-9_1, © Springer International Publishing Switzerland 2015

Fig. 1.1 Hospitalization-associated disability (From Covinsky KE, Palmer RM, Fortinsky RH, Counsell SR, Stewart AL, Kresevic D, Burant CJ, Landefeld CS. Loss of independence in activities of daily living in older adults hospitalized with medical illnesses: increased vulnerability with age. J Am Geriatr Soc. 2003;51(4):451–458 with permission.)

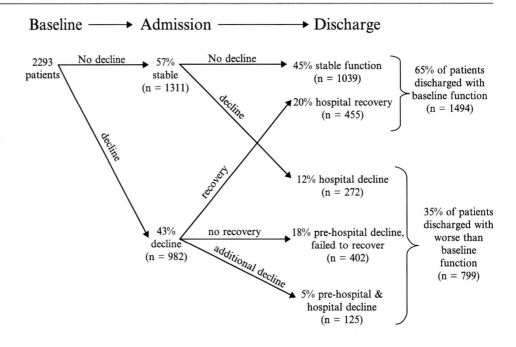

transferring, toileting, feeding, grooming, continence, and mental state) by day two of hospitalization [5]. Larger studies, conducted in the 1990s, examined functional decline from baseline (2 weeks prior to admission as assessed at the time of hospital admission) to hospital discharge. The largest of these documented that in people over 70 years old, 35 % developed HAD (Fig. 1.1). Even among those patients without disability at baseline, 31 % were dependent in one or more ADL at discharge [6]. In the 2000s, studies confirmed and extended the significance of functional decline in hospitalized older adults. The PROgetto DImissioni in GEriatria (PRODIGE) Study, conducted in Italy, demonstrated that among 1,048 hospitalized patients, approximately 30 % suffered new disability from baseline to hospital discharge [7]. The Support from Hospital to Home (SHHE) study demonstrated that even in adults 55 and older, 28 % developed new disability from baseline to 30 days after hospital discharge [8]. Thus, studies of hospitalized older adults are remarkably consistent in documenting high rates of HAD.

A separate stream of research, focusing on community-dwelling older adults, highlights the role of hospitalization in development of new disability. The Precipitating Events Project (PEP) investigators followed 754 persons aged 70 years and older who were not disabled to examine risk factors for new onset disability and found that half of new onset disability in community-dwelling elders was attributable to hospitalization [9]. A similar finding was observed using the University of Alabama at Birmingham (UAB) Study of Aging Life-Space Assessment (LSA). The LSA is a validated tool that measures mobility by accounting

for the frequency and ease with which a person moves to increasing distances ranging from their bedroom to beyond their community. In a study of 167 patients hospitalized on a medicine service, the mean pre-admission LSA corresponded to someone who needs no assistance to go into the neighborhood daily and to town 1–3 times a week and declined after hospital discharge to a mean LSA score corresponding to someone who needs a cane to go into town less than once a week. Those with restricted mobility often failed to recover baseline mobility [10]. This suggests that disability associated with hospitalization has long-term consequences and is of particular concern for patients admitted on a medicine service.

Consequences of Hospitalization-Associated Disability

HAD portends many deleterious outcomes including sustained disability, nursing home placement, and mortality. In the Boyd et al. study, only 1/3 of those with HAD recovered their baseline function in the year after hospital discharge. Even more striking, 41 % of patients discharged with new or additional ADL disability died in the year after discharge [2]. Recovery of function in the first month after discharge forecasts a better functional outcome and highlights the importance of exercise both during and after hospital discharge. On the other hand, patients not recovering function in the first month after discharge face a particularly grim prognosis, and care should include assessing functional capacity, helping patients and families discuss goals of care, and facilitating arrangements for durable powers of attorney for finances and health care. Not surprisingly, HAD is a strong risk factor for discharge to a nursing home. Nationally, 3/4 of all new nursing home placements are precipitated by hospitalization, and approximately 16 % of hospitalized Medicare beneficiaries over 65 years are discharged directly to a skilled nursing facility [11].

In addition to adverse health outcomes, the costs associated with HAD are significant for patients, their families, and society. Medicare Part A mean expenditure costs are twice as high for those who transition to dependence in mobility, and almost ten times as high for those who transition to dependence in mobility and one or more ADLs compared to those who maintain independence in mobility and ADLs [12]. In a cohort of 843 community-dwelling older adults, 20 % were dependent in ADLs at baseline or became dependent over 2 years, but accounted for 46 % of hospital, outpatient, home health care, and nursing home Medicare-reimbursed expenditures. Expenditures over a 2-year period for these groups were $10,000 more than those who maintained independence [13]. These costs do not take into consideration the financial, physical, and emotional burden of caregiving on patients and families. Custodial care costs are considered out of pocket expenses and can quickly deplete savings. This is in addition to the significant physical and emotional cost of caring for an older loved one who is becoming increasingly more dependent.

Risk Factors for Hospitalization-Associated Disability

Both patient- and hospital-level risk factors contribute to HAD. Patient factors most closely associated with HAD reflect a patient's vulnerabilities and capacity to recover from functional decline associated with an illness. These include preexisting disability, cognitive impairment, illness severity, and social isolation. The hospital factor most strongly associated with HAD is low mobility. Using the bedside nurses' reporting of patient mobility in the preceding 24 h, Brown et al. demonstrated that, among 498 hospitalized older adults, low and intermediate mobility (average mobility of ambulation one or two times with total assistance or less) was strongly associated with HAD when compared to patients with high mobility (average mobility of ambulation two or more times with partial or no assistance). These results remained even after adjusting for ADL performance, demographics, severity of illness, comorbidity, and intensive care unit/coronary care unit stay. In addition, low mobility was strongly associated with new institutionalization and death [14]. This work has been replicated. Other hospital factors such as iatrogenesis, inappropriate prescribing, and undernutrition may play a role in HAD but are less well studied. Nonetheless, coupled with low mobility, these hospital-level risk factors for HAD are modifiable and provide a map for components of an effective intervention, such as an Acute Care for Elders (ACE) Unit.

Other Serious Complications in Older Adults Associated with Hospitalization

HAD is not the only serious hospitalization-associated complication that older adults face. Delirium, urinary and bowel dysfunction, falls, pressure ulcers, and malnutrition are other common complications that impart significant suffering and burdens to patients and their families.

Delirium

Delirium is present in approximately 20 % of patients over age 70 admitted to a medicine service and develops in another 15–29 % during the course of hospitalization [15]. Unfortunately, even a single episode of delirium may result in increased nursing home placement, permanent decrease in baseline cognitive function, and increased morbidity. Like HAD, risk factors for delirium include both patient- and hospital-level factors. At the patient-level, cognitive impairment, visual impairment, disability, severity of illness, and dehydration (measured as elevated BUN/Cr) are associated with delirium. At the hospital-level, use of restraints, an indwelling bladder catheter, more than three new medications, a decline in albumin to less than 3 g/dL, and iatrogenesis are associated with delirium [16]. Additional hospital-level risk factors for delirium include low mobility, multiple room changes, lack of proper day–night orientation cues such as large clocks or windows, not providing eyeglasses or hearing aids, inadequate pain management, urinary retention and fecal impaction, sleep disruption, and inappropriate prescribing such as using diphenhydramine or a benzodiazepine as a sleeping aid. Hospitals have control over and can eliminate or significantly reduce these factors. Eliminating these harmful hospital practices and replacing them with evidence-based practices that promote patient function and recovery reduces delirium [17] and is another basis of the ACE model of care.

Urinary Incontinence

New urinary incontinence occurs in one of six hospitalized older adults and is another iatrogenic event with both patient- and hospital-level risk factors [18]. Patient factors include older age, high body-mass index, cognitive deficits, and functional impairment. Hospital factors include low mobility, use of restraints, use of diapers or urinary catheters, and treatment modalities such as diuretics. The use of an in-dwelling bladder catheter without a specific medical indication is particularly pernicious, as it is associated with greater risk of death and longer hospital stay [19]. Incontinence is associated with other complications, including pressure ulcers and falls. The phenomenon of one complication predisposing to another is known as cascade iatrogenesis and highlights the importance of addressing underlying risk factors.

Falls

Approximately 4 % of older adults admitted to a hospital with an acute illness will fall during their hospital stay [20]. Risk factors associated with falls include prior history of falls, functional/mobility impairment or low activity level, use of a walking aid or assistive device, cognitive impairment, receiving high-risk medications, and abnormal balance. Patients who fall in the hospital have longer lengths of stay (LOS) and higher costs associated with their hospitalization. The evidence on reducing the rate of falls in the hospital is strongest for risk assessment and targeted interventions including exercise, patient and family education, medication review, environmental review, medical examination, and eyesight correction [21]. A randomized trial demonstrated the effectiveness of a patient-specific fall prevention tool kit that included bed posters composed of brief text with an accompanying icon, patient education handouts, and plans of care, all communicating patient-specific alerts to key stakeholders [22]. This intervention mirrors components found in ACE Unit care processes.

Pressure Ulcers

Approximately 4.5 % of hospitalized Medicare beneficiaries develop a pressure ulcer at a price of $2.41 billion in excess health care costs [23]. The development of pressure ulcers can interfere with functional recovery, may be complicated by pain and infection, and contributes to higher in-hospital mortality, longer hospital LOS, and higher 30-day hospital readmission rates. In addition to incontinence, risk factors for pressure ulcers include older age, undernutrition, cognitive and functional impairment, and low mobility. Pressure ulcers can be prevented through the use of pressure redistribution support surfaces on beds, chairs, gurneys and operating tables, rigorous turning and repositioning interventions, and attention to mobility, continence, and nutrition. While repositioning is a mainstay in pressure ulcer prevention efforts, data to support specific turning regimens for patients with impaired mobility is lacking. For patients with nutritional deficits,

dietary consultation and supplements may be beneficial. As of October 1, 2008, the Centers for Medicare and Medicaid Services (CMS) no longer reimburses hospitals for the ancillary cost of a hospital-acquired pressure ulcer.

Malnutrition

Depending on the measure used to assess malnutrition, protein–energy malnutrition is present in 1/4 to 1/2 of hospitalized older adults. Malnutrition present on admission is associated with functional decline at 3 months after hospital discharge, and nursing home placement and increased mortality in the year after hospital discharge [24]. Undernutrition (intake of less than 50 % of calculated energy requirements) during a hospital stay occurs in 21 % of older adults and is associated with increased in-hospital mortality and 90-day mortality compared to patients who have higher levels of caloric intake [25]. Poor intake is due to a variety of factors including inappropriate nothing-by-mouth orders; lack of appetizing or culturally appropriate food; inappropriate food consistency or systems in place to have patients use their dentures (without losing them); lack of nutritional supplements; and presence of nausea. Many of these are factors that hospitals have control over and can modify.

Thus, HAD and other hospital acquired geriatric syndromes result in the "dysfunctional syndrome" for hospitalized elders (Fig. 1.2). This, in turn, increases morbidity and mortality for older adults, increases family caregiver burden, and increases health care expenditures. These adverse outcomes provide the rationale for the vital need to fundamentally redesign hospital care for elders. One model proven to improve outcomes for hospitalized older adults is the ACE Unit model of care.

ACE Unit Care Model, Setting, and Patient Population

ACE Unit Precursors

Prior to the first ACE study published in 1995 from the nation's first designated ACE Unit, early innovators began to address the hazards of hospitalization both in the acute and post-acute periods of illness in ways that foreshadowed the interdisciplinary team (IDT) model of care known today as the ACE Unit. As early as the 1980s, these first signs of geriatric care delivery redesign began to appear in descriptive reports from community hospitals [26] as well as in Geriatric Evaluation and Management (GEM) Units that were formed within the Veterans Affairs Medical Centers [27]. GEM Units were different than current day ACE Units

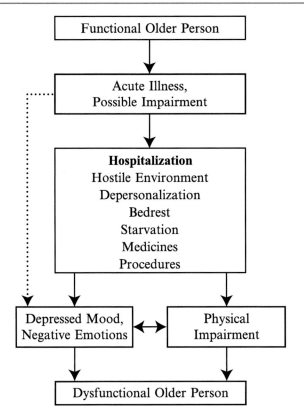

┌─────────────────────────────┐
│   Functional Older Person │
└─────────────────────────────┘
              ↓
┌─────────────────────────────┐
│   Acute Illness,   │
│   Possible Impairment   │
└─────────────────────────────┘
              ↓
┌─────────────────────────────┐
│   **Hospitalization**   │
│   Hostile Environment   │
│   Depersonalization   │
│   Bedrest   │
│   Starvation   │
│   Medicines   │
│   Procedures   │
└─────────────────────────────┘

Fig. 1.2 The dysfunctional syndrome (From Palmer RM, Counsell S, Landefeld CS. Clinical intervention trials: the ACE Unit. Clin Geriatr Med. 1998;14(4):831–849 with permission.)

in that patients were transferred from acute care units following stabilization of the acute illness to the GEM Unit to receive prolonged rehabilitative post-acute care. However, GEM Units resembled and informed the ACE model in that they were geographically distinct units staffed by an IDT that provided comprehensive geriatric assessment and met regularly to individualize treatment plans. The core of the GEM Unit IDT consisted of a geriatric provider, social worker, nurse, and unit director; this team typically assumed the primary responsibility of all aspects of patient care. This core team could be expanded to include additional members from rehabilitation, pharmacy, psychology, nutrition, and optometry [28].

Another geriatric inpatient model, the Geriatric Assessment Units (GAUs), first appeared in Quebec in the 1970s; as of 2004, there were 71 known GAUs in Quebec hospitals. Most GAUs also resemble a GEM Unit in that most patients were transferred from an acute care unit for post-acute rehabilitation; however, some GAUs manage acute care as well. As of 2004, the average LOS on a GAU was 23 days. Unlike ACE Units, most GAUs do not incorporate environmental changes, nursing leadership, or frequent IDT rounds; however, like ACE Units, GAU care includes an

interdisciplinary approach and incorporates standardized assessments and early care transition planning [29].

Core Components of the ACE Model of Care

The first ACE Unit was established at University Hospitals of Cleveland in the early 1990s. This new model of inpatient geriatric care incorporated principles from the GEMU and GAU models including comprehensive geriatric assessment coupled with continuous quality improvement to redesign care delivery for older adults admitted to acute care units. The ACE Unit care delivery redesign utilizes the concept of a "prehab" program from the day of hospital admission, with the primary goal to "help patients maintain or achieve independence in basic activities of daily living" [30]. The core components of the ACE Unit model of care are: (1) patient-centered IDT geriatric care, (2) nurse-driven geriatric care processes, (3) medical care review with a focus on preventing iatrogenesis, (4) early care transition planning, and (5) a prepared environment promoting safe mobility and cognitive stimulation, all with the aim to prevent HAD (Table 1.1) [30–32].

The first distinguishing component of ACE Units that differs from usual acute care units is the use of an IDT as opposed to a multidisciplinary model in which providers from all disciplines deliver care but practice predominantly independently, or in "silos." In an interdisciplinary model, disciplines collaboratively develop the patient-centered care plan, usually with face-to-face communication. Members of the team typically include a geriatrician medical director and/or a gerontological clinical nurse specialist (GCNS) or geriatric nurse practitioner (GNP), the unit nurse manager and the bedside nurses, a pharmacist, a social worker and case manager, members of the rehabilitation team (physical, occupational, and speech therapists), a dietitian, and chaplain. This team meets frequently (usually daily Monday–Friday) to discuss the patients on the unit and help to guide the daily care with an emphasis on maintaining function and mobility, preventing and managing geriatric syndromes including cognitive and functional impairment, and coordinating early care transition planning. The goal is to provide holistic, patient-centered rather than disease-centered care, in order to prevent HAD.

The second component of the ACE model of care is the use of nurse-driven care processes and protocols. ACE Units train and empower the unit nurse leaders in addition to bedside nurses to assess for geriatric syndromes and enact evidence-based nurse-driven care processes and protocols to prevent and manage syndromes (i.e., functional decline, delirium, falls, malnutrition; Table 1.2). This improves care efficiency and effectiveness and allows nurses to utilize their

Table 1.1 Core components of the ACE Unit model of care

Patient-centered geriatric care by an IDT with a focus on early rehabilitation/"prehab"	• Led by a geriatric trained provider (usually a physician or advanced practice nurse)
	• Proactive geriatric assessment with a focus on function and cognition
	• Manage existing geriatric syndromes
	• Mitigate risk factors for incident geriatric syndromes (i.e., delirium, falls, pressure ulcers, malnutrition, etc.)
	• Frequent (usually daily) IDT rounds for ongoing geriatric assessment and management
	• Prevent functional decline via early mobility
	• Assess need for physical and occupational therapy
	• Provide adaptive equipment and assistive devices during hospitalization
Nurse-driven geriatric care processes and protocols	• Preserve or prevent declines in mobility and ADL function, cognition, nutritional status and bowel management, and skin integrity
Medical care review	• Review for high-risk medications
	• Provide only interventions or treatments that align with patient/family goals of care
	• Avoid high-risk interventions or treatments that are not likely to provide benefit
	• Incorporate patient cognitive and functional status into medical decision-making
	• Prevent iatrogenesis
	• Discontinue intravenous medications and tethers as soon as possible
Early care transition planning	• Begin care transition planning from day of admission
	• Incorporate patient functional and cognitive status, psychosocial support, and goals into care transition planning and referrals
	• Liaising with community services and outpatient providers
Prepared environment promoting safe mobility and cognitive stimulation	• Hospital unit environment that promotes safe mobility and cognitive stimulation (see Table 1.3)

Data from Landefeld CS, Palmer RM, Kresevic DM, Fortinsky RH, Kowal J. A randomized trial of care in a hospital medical unit especially designed to improve the functional outcomes of acutely ill older patients. N Engl J Med 1995;332:1338–1344 and Fox MT, Sidani S, Persaud M, Tregunno D, Maimets I, Brooks, D, O'Brien K. Acute care for elders components of acute geriatric unit care: systematic descriptive review. J Am Geriatr Soc. 2013;61:939–946

IDT interdisciplinary team, *ADL* activities of daily living

Table 1.2 Nurse-driven care protocols

Mobility	*Preventive*
Purpose is to return patient's mobility or prevent functional decline during hospitalization	• Out of bed for meals unless contraindicated
	• Avoid bedrest
	• Ambulate TID in hallway unless contraindicated
Mobility goals:	• Shoes to be worn for activities (transfer, ambulation, etc.)
– Maintain safety	• Assess fall risk—implement fall prevention plan of care
– Patient/family aware of safety needs	• Teach patient/family: Active range of motion (ROM) exercises
– Maintain/restore independent ADLs	• Teach patient/family: Safe ambulation
– Skin integrity maintained	• Check postural blood pressure, head of bed up every shift
– No signs of postural hypotension	• Teach patient/family: Antipostural hypotensive exercises
– No signs of infection	*Restorative*
– All the above individualized	• ROM, Passive, TID
Preventive criteria: Patient ambulatory	• Shoes to be worn for activities (transfer, ambulation, etc)
Restorative criteria: Patient nonambulatory	• Assess fall risk—implement fall prevention plan of care
	• Assess for adaptive equipment
	• RN to recommend PT consult
	• Discharge Planning consult to SW for home care needs, Discharge anticipated: __/__/__ __
Function/ADL	*Preventive*
Purpose is to maintain function and encourage patients to be independent in ADLs	• Provide ADL supplies as needed (grooming, toothbrush, dentures, sensory aids, shoes)
	• Encourage family to bring in ADL supplies
	• Teach patient: Rationale for self-care
ADL goals:	*Restorative*
– Maintain safety	• Assist with setup for meals and/or feeding
– Self-care maintained/restored	• Encourage self AM care and provide assistance as needed
– No signs of infection	• Mouth care, assist TID
– Adequate nutrition	• Assist with individualized toileting schedule
– Continence maintained/restored	• Assess need for home ADL assist
– All the above individualized	• Review recommendations of PT and OT
Preventive criteria: Patient independent in bathing, dressing, toileting, eating	
Restorative criteria: Patient needs assistance	

(continued)

Table 1.2 (continued)

Continence	Preventive
Purpose is to maintain continence, independent toileting and prevent UTI *ADL goals*: – Maintain/restore continence – Patient/family knowledgeable about risk factors for UTI – Patient/family knowledgeable about all the above prevention for UTI (toileting schedules, Kegel exercises) – All the above individualized *Preventive criteria*: Independent with toileting, normal or minimal cognitive impairment *Restorative criteria*: Needs assistance with toileting, baseline or new incontinence with or without cognitive impairment	• Encourage patient to maintain normal voiding schedule (Q 2–4 h) • Teach patient: Risk factors for incontinence during hospitalization (IV fluids, diuretics, opioids, urinary catheter) • Teach patient: Kegel exercises *Restorative* • Order adaptive equipment as needed (urinal, bedpan, BS commode w/out wheels, elevated toilet seat) • Bladder, encourage: Assist with individualized toileting schedule; record results even if no void • Use UTI bundle (stat lock, discuss removal of urinary catheter daily) • Assess for UTI • Ensure adequate hydration of >1,000 cc • Encourage non-caffeinated beverages • Teach patient: Kegel exercises • Assess for urinary retention (bladder scan)
Nutrition	*Preventive*
Purpose is to maintain adequate caloric and fluid intake and to prevent dehydration and weight loss during stay *Nutrition goals*: – Maintain weight – Maintain fluid/electrolyte balance – Provide adequate cal/day – Provide 1,000 cc of fluid/day – Maintain skin integrity – Patient/family knowledgeable about caloric needs, dietary restrictions – All the above individualized *Preventive criteria*: Patient is consuming >50% of ordered diet (>1,000 cc >1,000 cal) *Restorative criteria*: Patient is consuming <50% of ordered diet (<1,000 cc <1,000 cal)	• Identify patient's food preferences • Maintain ideal weight and electrolyte balance • Maintain adequate nutritional and fluid intake • Promote environment conducive to eating: Out of bed for meals if able, minimize interruptions *Restorative* • Monitor weight • Monitor I & O • Oral assessment (dentures, pain, dry mouth, lesions, infection/plaque) including swallow assessment • Assess for constipation • Consider interdisciplinary meeting to discuss alternative nutrition (supplements, tube feeding, parenteral) • Validate NPO status with MD if >24 h • Assess need for IVF if NPO >8 h • Consider liberalizing diet if appropriate • Snacks: Dietary and family to supply • Dietary consult and calorie counts
Cognition	*Preventive*
Purpose is to promptly identify those patients at risk for acute confusion or those presently confused *Cognitive goals*: – Maintain safety – Decrease anxiety – Maintain/restore independent ADL – Maintain/restore normal wake and sleep cycles – All the above individualized *Preventive criteria*: No acute confusion, may have baseline chronic cognitive impairment *Restorative criteria*: Acute confusion, off of baseline cognition	• Review meds to ensure appropriate med and dose (opioids, antianxiety, antipsychotic; avoid meds with anticholinergic side effects) • Assess cognitive function using brief memory screen and brief delirium screen • Assure availability of sensory devices (glasses, hearing aids) and ensure in working condition • Facilitate normal sleep schedule • Foster orientation—frequently reassure and reorient patient, calendar/clocks, caregiver identification, communicate clearly, explain all activities, consistent caregivers *Restorative* • Review meds to ensure appropriate med and dose (opioids, antianxiety, antipsychotic, sleeping medication; avoid meds with anticholinergic side effects) • Assess for causes of acute confusion (e.g., infection, dehydration, electrolyte imbalance, hypoxia, pain, urinary retention, constipation) and consult with health-care team to treat underlying pathology • Avoid restraints • Foster orientation–frequently reassure and reorient patient, calendar/clocks, caregiver identification, communicate clearly, explain all activities, consistent caregivers • Noise reduction • Provide meaningful daytime activities • Facilitate normal sleep schedule • Complete family teaching regarding: Etiology, management, and anticipated needs at discharge

Modified from Palmer, RM and Kresevic, DM. The Acute Care for Elders Unit. In Acute Care for Elders. Malone, ML, Capezuti, EA and Palmer, RM. New York: Springer, 2014 with permission

Table 1.3 Environmental modifications employed by ACE Units

Flooring	• Non-slip, no wax vinyl floor that has a wood-look pattern and texture, providing a low/no-glare floor
	• Avoiding flooring designs to prevent patients with depth perception disturbances from confusing the designs for objects or holes
Lighting	• Direct/indirect lighting fixtures to provide an optimum mix of directional and diffuse reflected light and minimize shadows
Furniture	• Adequate numbers of chairs in patient rooms for patient and family
	• Chairs with arms and adequate firmness and straight back to ease transfers
	• Sleeper chair/sofa for family to stay overnight comfortably
	• Furniture with rounded edges instead of corners
Orientation	• Large print clocks
	• Whiteboard with updated date and care providers listed
Safe mobility	• Handrails in hallways
	• Dark colors for door frames and handrails in contrast to light colors for walls
	• Clutter free hallways
	• Raised toilet seats
	• Easy grip door levers
	• Grab bars in rooms and bathrooms
Cognitive stimulation	• Congregate room for activities (e.g., group meals, music/art therapy)
	• Sensory aids (hearing amplifiers, magnifying/reading glasses, headphones and large print remote control for TV)
Family support	• Family room/area with galley/snacks
	• Resource library/Internet access for review of caregiver educational materials and videos
	• Accommodations for family to stay with patients (comfortable sleeping, showers, meals)

skills at the highest level to prevent adverse outcomes and HAD. These care protocols often include appropriate and timely referrals to the other disciplines on the ACE team such as rehabilitation therapists, dieticians, and pharmacists.

The third ACE care model component is daily review of the hospital medical care with a geriatric lens. While this review can be done by any geriatric trained provider, this role is typically performed by a physician who is also the ACE Unit medical director and with the assistance of the nurse leader and the daily IDT rounds. In hospitals without a geriatrician on staff, a GCNS or GNP can fulfill this role. This provider performing the medical review should be trained in geriatrics, have excellent communication skills, and be well respected among the medical staff. The goal is to review the daily medical care plan and help to identify risk for iatrogenesis and adverse events, such as use of inappropriate medications or invasive procedures with high burden and little benefit. In some ACE Units the medical director also serves as a primary attending for patients admitted to the ACE Unit, while in other ACE Units the medical director role is more consultative, reviewing cases during the daily IDT rounds and providing recommendations to the patient's primary physician or care teams.

The fourth key component of the ACE model of care is early care transition planning. While today this is emphasized for hospital patients of all ages, this practice was not common in the early 1990s when the average LOS in the first ACE Unit study was 8 days and no penalties existed for unplanned readmissions. This practice represents one of several ACE innovations that now benefit hospital patients of all ages. Typically the ACE Unit social worker and/or case manager assesses the patient within the first 24 h of admission and, collaboratively with the IDT, begin care transition planning from day 1 of hospitalization, incorporating patient function, cognitive, and psychosocial support status into the planning. The goal is patient discharge to the least restrictive environment and aligning post-discharge support with patient/family goals. For most patients the goal is to return home.

Finally, the fifth component of the ACE model of care is a unit design that promotes safe patient mobility and improved cognition. This means that hallways are cleared of clutter and have handrails to assist patients with ambulation. Floors are usually covered with a non-glare surface. Many units have a common dining or social area to give patients a destination to walk to as they ambulate on the unit. Rooms should have prominent clocks and whiteboards with the date to help reorient patients, and bathrooms should have raised toilet seats to help facilitate toileting. See Table 1.3 for more examples of environmental modifications utilized by some ACE Units.

Roles of ACE Unit Interdisciplinary Team Members

Upon admission to the hospital, the bedside nurse performs a full physical assessment of each ACE patient, evaluating the acute medical needs based on the admitting diagnosis, as would occur on any hospital unit. On an ACE Unit, however, the nurse also evaluates the patient's functional status (ability to perform ADLs), mobility, cognition, and psychosocial status including living situation and social support system. The means and degree to which each of these domains are formally screened and documented by the bedside nurse versus another team member such as an ACE Unit coordinator varies amongst ACE Units nationwide. Findings from these nursing assessments are brought to the daily IDT rounds as this information is critical in guiding the daily geriatric care and making appropriate formal referrals to other disciplines such as rehabilitation therapists, dieticians, and chaplains. The social worker and/or case manager on the team further explores the patients' current living situation and social support network (e.g., family or other informal caregivers, formal caregivers and agencies, community resources), as well as patient financial and insurance status. The pharmacist reviews the patient's medications daily, monitoring for any potentially inappropriate (Beers' Criteria) or other high-risk medications or potential drug interactions. The nurse leader for an ACE Unit may be a GCNS, GNP, or unit nurse manager or other nurse designated as the lead nurse or ACE Unit Coordinator. The ACE medical director, nurse leader, or both contributes the daily review of the medical care to the overall geriatric care planning, identifying potential risk for iatrogenesis and helping the team to focus on specific geriatric syndromes identified during the team rounds. These leaders are also responsible for helping to develop the geriatric practice of the other nurses and providers on the unit via ongoing formal training and continuing education and reviews of current practice and policies.

In this interdisciplinary model, each team member contributes to the daily geriatric care planning that occurs via his/her participation in the IDT rounds as well as care protocols. This information then supports and informs the patient's primary physician (with or without residents, nurse practitioners, or physician assistants) who is managing the patient's acute medical problems, whether the attending is a geriatrician or non-geriatric provider. Each ACE Unit needs to develop a standard process for communicating any IDT recommendations or issues identified that require physician involvement back to the patient's primary physician team. For some ACE Units in teaching hospitals, the medical student, intern, or resident from the primary team may attend ACE rounds. For an ACE Unit in a nonteaching hospital, another representative such as a nurse practitioner or care coordinator from the admitting service may attend IDT rounds. For ACE Units without a representative from the attending team present during ACE rounds, alternative methods of coordinating care between the ACE IDT and the primary services is required. An integrated electronic health record (EHR) may provide means to enhance communication to all team members in a timely fashion. For hospitals without an EHR, team recommendations are often recorded on a well-labeled communication form that is placed in the patient's paper medical chart in a predetermined location that is easily accessed by the physicians. This communication sheet is not a permanent part of the hospital record and is labeled as such, so the physicians do not feel required to enact all recommendations if an aspect of the patient's acute medical illness precludes enacting a certain recommendation. Other ACE Units utilize a designated team member to communicate key information and recommendations to a designated representative from the admitting team. One of the many benefits of the ACE model is the empowerment of non-physician providers to advocate for evidence-based geriatric care; this includes having a non-physician team member such as a nurse leader or care manager communicate team recommendations to an attending physician. The propensity for an older adult's clinical and functional status to change acutely and rapidly and the short hospital LOS seen today are just two reasons for the ACE team rounds to occur daily if possible.

The geriatrician/medical director plays an important role on the unit during IDT rounds. In addition, this physician also serves an important administrative role as the champion for the ACE Unit within the hospital and in the midst of multiple competing priorities health care administrators face today. The medical director/geriatrician needs to educate his/her colleagues and hospital leaders about the benefits of ACE as well as best practice geriatrics in terms that align with hospital strategic priorities and goals. S/he also needs to highlight all ACE Unit successes, whether the outcome is one of process improvement, quality improvement, satisfaction amongst patients and staff, or professional development benefits. This is critical in ensuring continued support for the ACE Unit (see section "Leveraging ACE in the Current Health Care Environment").

What Does the ACE Model Mean for the Individual Patient Experience?

How does the ACE model described above look different for the individual patient and his/her family? Let us use an 80-year-old male admitted with community acquired pneumonia as a case example. In the traditional, multidisciplinary and disease-centered model of hospital care, this patient would receive admission assessments by a nurse and physician that are centered on his signs and symptoms and the evidence-based evaluation and treatment of community acquired pneumonia. The primary focus of care planning during his hospitalization would likely be the choice and duration of antibiotics (intravenous and by mouth), need for oxygen in hospital and at home, if required, and any other relevant medical comorbidities, such as concomitant diabetes or renal insufficiency. The patient's home medication list, which might include use of a sedative at night, would be continued. On hospital day 2 the patient may become mildly delirious, and this would likely be attributed to the underlying infection. Due to his need for oxygen he spends the first 48 h of his hospital stay in bed. Because he is bedbound, a urinary catheter is placed. Care transition planning would likely include arranging home health nursing for blood pressure and oxygenation monitoring but may not begin to be planned and coordinated until the day of or day before discharge. However, with bed confinement, the patient's new hospitalization-associated disability is unrecognized by the medical team. On the day of discharge, the patient's wife realizes that the patient is very unsteady and would not be safe to go home with her. Rehabilitation services are consulted and the patient spends an additional day in the hospital awaiting a room at a subacute rehabilitation facility.

If this same patient were admitted to an ACE Unit utilizing all five core components of the ACE model of care, all of the above evidenced-based pneumonia care regarding evaluation and antibiotic treatment would occur. However, in addition, upon admission the patient's functional and cognitive status would also be screened via brief, validated assessment tools and incorporated into the daily plan of care developed by the ACE IDT. This additional ACE model of care would have uncovered that the patient has mild cognitive impairment at baseline that limits his ability to recall instructions about his health care. The ACE team would recognize caregiver stress in his wife and provide her with education and counseling regarding memory loss and delirium prevention as well as referrals to community resources and support groups for caregivers of patients with memory loss. The ACE team would enact delirium prevention care processes, including attention to mobility and prevention of urinary catheter placement. The ACE team would recognize that his mobility status was limited even prior to admission due to his shortness of breath and he has declined from being ambulatory and independent in his ADLs to now predominantly chair bound and needing assistance with transferring, dressing, bathing, and toileting. A safe mobility care plan would be enacted to help this patient begin to regain his function starting day 1 of hospitalization and would start with placing the patient in a chair daily with the goal to have him leave his hospital room to participate in a group music and occupational therapy session in the unit's congregate room. Based on the daily assessment of his functional status, the ACE team would determine if this patient would benefit from home physical and/or occupational therapy in addition to nursing after discharge, as the goal is to avoid placement in a facility. Through the medical care review, the ACE team would also be more likely to realize that even though the patient's medicine list states he takes a sedative at night for insomnia in reality he stopped taking this medication 2 months prior and should not be receiving

this medication during or after hospitalization. The patient does not become delirious during his hospital stay and is able to return home with a LOS reduced by 2 days. Thus, the ACE model delivers care for the admitting diagnosis in addition to evidence-based geriatric care addressing each patient's individual geriatric syndromes present prior to and during the hospitalization.

ACE Geriatric Interdisciplinary Provider Training

The model of improving geriatric care through nursing practice preceded and now complements ACE Unit care. In 1981, the geriatric resource nurse (GRN) program was launched at Beth Israel Hospital in Boston [33]. This geriatric training for nurses who serve as the geriatric expert and resource for a hospital unit or practice area is now a core component of the national Nurses Improving Care for Healthsystem Elders (NICHE) program (Chap. 5). NICHE provides support for GRN and ACE Unit program development and geriatric training for hospitals and providers. As of 2014 NICHE programs existed in over 530 hospitals and health care facilities in 46 states [33]. Given the emphasis on nurse-initiated care protocols and nursing leadership in patient care on ACE Units, many ACE Units are developed in conjunction with new or existing NICHE programs or other formal geriatric professional development for nurses and other providers.

The ACE Unit is an excellent site for teaching trainees and providers in the non-nursing disciplines as well about geriatric care. Medical students, residents, fellows and attending physicians alike can learn about team work and best practice care of the older adult in the hospital via formal training as well as the hidden curriculum that stems from caring for patients on an ACE Unit. Pharmacy residents can be trained regarding potentially inappropriate medications and the potential pitfalls of prescribing in older adults. Learners in other disciplines, such as physical, occupational, and speech therapist; dietitians; and chaplains should find the ACE Unit an important site in which to learn about the growing aging population. Finally, the ACE Unit can also serve as a site for pilot testing new innovative care processes and models of care for older adults. In this manner, all members of the team, as well as patients and their families, can gain insight into better ways to manage acutely ill hospitalized elders.

Before the ACE Unit opens, all team members should receive general education that usually includes normal aging changes, geriatric syndromes, such as dementia and delirium, and the Beers' Criteria medications that should be avoided in older adults. Team members also need to learn about the ACE model of care with its goal of preserving patient function, and review ACE protocols utilized to prevent potential problems, such as delirium, pressure ulcers or difficulty performing self-care/activities of daily living. Once the unit opens, there should be ongoing education that may occur informally in daily rounds or in formal sessions, such as lunch and learns, workshops, simulation sessions, real-time bedside audits and teaching, journal clubs, nursing grand rounds, or difficult case conferences. Given the change in unit culture required to launch an ACE Unit, in addition to geriatric care training, many successful units provide initial training in the functioning of an interdisciplinary geriatric team. Curricula exist for such training, such as the Geriatric Interdisciplinary Team Training (GITT) curriculum. The GITT Kit includes a training manual, curriculum guide, and training videos that include simulated IDT meetings. This curriculum addresses six key topics for successful IDT development: (1) Teams and Team Work, (2) Team Members Roles and Responsibilities, (3) Team Communication and Conflict Resolution, (4) Care Planning Process, (5) Multiculturalism, and (6) Ethics and Teams [34]. The GITT Kit is available in an online format for a fee through the Hartford Institute for Geriatric Nursing (www.hartfordign.org/education/gitt/). NICHE also provides member hospitals with ACE protocols that can be implemented and a script to guide the daily presentations at IDT rounds. Information on resources NICHE offers and how to become a NICHE designated hospital can be found at the NICHE website (www.nicheprogram.org). A number of other organizations also provide online resources for geriatric education, including the ConsultGeriRN repository of geriatric resources (www.consultgerirn.org), the Portal of Geriatric Online Education (www.pogoe.org), the American Association of Colleges of Nursing (www.aacn.nche.edu), and the American Geriatrics Society (www.americangeriatrics.org).

ACE Unit Setting and Patient Population

Most ACE Units select patients based on age, using a cutoff age of 65 or 70. Other key factors influencing ACE Unit admission criteria are the particular needs of the hospital regarding population management for elders and processes related to patient-placement and flow within each hospital. While there is no published evidence of patients that should be excluded from admission to an ACE Unit, research supports that the ideal patient whom would benefit most from the ACE model is an older community-dwelling adult with a low or moderate case mix index (CMI) with an acute decline in function due to acute illness or acute exacerbation of chronic illness [27]. The CMI is defined as the sum of the relative weights of the Diagnosis-Related Groups (DRGs) of a patient population divided by the number of patients in that population and reflects patient complexity and expected resource consumption [35]. In practice, most ACE Units have found that placing strict criteria for admission to an

ACE Unit leads to logistical complexities without patient benefit and therefore ACE Units will often accept any patient over a selected age as an "ACE patient." The early ACE Units were developed and studied in general medical patient populations and it remains true today that most ACE Units are general medical units staffed by general internists or hospitalists with geriatric consultation or co-management, or alternatively are staffed by geriatricians as the primary attending. However, there has been an emergence more recently of ACE Units for non-general medicine patients such as cancer or stroke patients (see section "Scaling-Up the ACE Model"). Finally, while the ACE Unit can be established in varied sizes of medical centers, smaller rural hospitals may not see as much of a cost-savings benefit if they do not have the patient volume to maintain the ACE Unit at full capacity. Hospitals with at least 100 beds should have capacity to easily maintain and see cost–benefit from an ACE Unit [36].

ACE Unit Outcomes

Process and Clinical Outcomes

Table 1.4 summarizes key ACE Unit studies and outcomes. ACE Units were initially developed with the primary goal to prevent HAD and the first ACE randomized controlled trial (RCT) was designed to test the efficacy of the ACE model in achieving this desired functional outcome. In this study performed at the University Hospitals of Cleveland, general medical patients aged 70 years and older were randomized to the ACE Unit versus a usual care (UC) general medicine ward; the units were staffed similarly regarding nurses and attending physicians with residents. Performance in five basic ADLs (bathing, dressing, toileting, transferring from bed to chair, and eating) was the primary outcome and was assessed via patient or proxy interview for level of independence at 3 time points: 2 weeks prior to hospitalization (baseline), time of hospital admission, and time of hospital discharge. Patients admitted to the ACE Unit had significantly improved performance of basic ADLs from admission to discharge compared to UC. This benefit was also seen when comparing ADL performance improvement from baseline to discharge in ACE vs. UC patients. Fewer ACE Unit patients were discharged to a post-acute facility (included long-term care, subacute care, and acute rehabilitation hospitals) compared to UC patients. Finally, overall health status was rated significantly higher by ACE patients at discharge, even after controlling for health status rating at time of admission [30]. A follow-up RCT from a second ACE Unit developed by the same authors in a community teaching hospital utilized both nonteaching services as well as resident services. Study subjects were 1,531 community-dwelling patients aged 70 years and older randomized to ACE or UC units. The primary outcomes measures were performance of the same five basic ADLs from baseline, time of admission, and time of discharge as well as geriatric processes of care. Process outcome measures included utilization of nine geriatric nurse-driven care protocols; time to consultation of providers such as social work and physical therapy; use of urinary catheters, restraints and potentially inappropriate medications; and orders for bed rest. Additional outcomes measures included patient, caregiver, physician, and nurse satisfaction with geriatric patient care. In the intention-to-treat analysis there was no difference in number of ADLs performed independently from either baseline or time of admission compared to discharge in ACE versus UC patients. In the per-protocol analysis however, the proportion of patients with ADL decline from baseline to discharge was less on ACE compared to UC ($p=.051$). There was a benefit in the composite outcome of either ADL decline from baseline or nursing home placement at time of discharge in ACE compared to UC and this benefit persisted 1 year after discharge. Processes of geriatric care that were statistically significantly improved on the ACE Unit included more use of geriatric nurse-driven care protocols, better physician recognition of patient depression, earlier and more frequent consultation with social workers and physical therapists, reduced bed rest days, reduced restraint use, and reduced use of potentially inappropriate medications within the first 24 h of hospitalization. Patient, caregiver, and provider satisfaction were also higher on ACE than UC [37]. The authors note the attenuated effect on ADL performance at discharge from this community hospital setting provides helpful information regarding the ACE model of care in nonacademic centers in which lack of resident involvement may lead to delays or incomplete adherence to ACE team recommendations due to logistical challenges in ACE team-to-attending communications. This study was conducted prior to the increased use of hospitalists we see today, and the authors note the important role hospitalists can play in achieving the full impact of ACE interventions.

While the primary outcome measure from these two landmark RCTs was the efficacy of the ACE model on HAD, these studies provided a glimpse via secondary outcome measures of additional improvements in elder care that ACE Units provide. This is not surprising, given the inherent improved recognition and management of geriatric syndromes and overall care coordination that stems from the ACE IDT approach. A handful of systematic reviews and meta-analyses of ACE studies have been conducted. In a 2009 meta-analysis, randomized studies of ACE Units demonstrated significantly reduced functional decline at hospital discharge compared to UC as well as significantly higher likelihood of living at home following hospitalization [38]. A key finding of this

meta-analysis is that ACE Units did not have more staff than the usual care units, supporting the notion that the benefits from the ACE model of care come from the standardization of geriatric assessment and management and organization of staff into an interdisciplinary team. The authors recommend as next steps more RCTs of ACE Units studying efficiency by evaluating cost-effectiveness ratios. A 2012 systematic review and meta-analysis included 13 randomized and quasi-experimental trials of ACE Unit care principles of varying doses compared to UC and included 6,839 older adults with a mean age of 81 years. Usual care units were medical, medical-surgical, or orthopedic units. This review also noted geriatric care utilizing one or more components of ACE Units improves outcomes for both patients and hospitals, including significant reductions in delirium, functional decline compared to pre-illness baseline, and LOS, with higher likelihood of being discharged to home rather than a facility [39]. Additional studies of ACE care in varied patient populations have also demonstrated improved processes of care including enhanced nutritional support [40] and medication appropriateness [41].

Health Care Utilization and Cost Outcomes

Hospital LOS has become an ever-important outcome in that shorter LOS reduces exposure to risk from the hospitalization and reduces costs. Multiple ACE Unit studies have demonstrated reduced LOS [39, 42, 43]. Several early ACE Unit studies also included a measurement of hospital charges or costs as a secondary outcome and demonstrated improved clinical outcomes, such as better functional status and less post-acute facility use, without increasing hospital total costs [44]. Over time with the increasing urgency to reduce costs of care without compromising quality, subsequent ACE Unit studies began to investigate resource utilization as a primary outcome measure. In the cost analysis from the first ACE RCT, Landefeld et al. included the start-up costs for environmental redesign, staff training, and development of care protocols, and found this added only $38 per bed day during the duration of their study. However, this cost was off-set with a cost savings experienced from a reduced LOS (7.5 vs. 8.4 days, $p=.449$), with a total cost savings per patient for ACE care compared to UC ($6,608 vs. $7,240, $p=.93$ [44]. In 2012, Barnes et al. conducted a follow-up cost analysis looking at patients over age 70 years cared for on ACE and non-ACE Units between 1993 and 1997 and found a continued pattern of lower LOS (6.7 vs. 7.3 days, $p=.004$) and reduced total costs of care ($9,477 vs. $10,451, $p<.001$) [36].

In a 2006 retrospective case–control study, health care utilization was analyzed as the primary outcome in patients

Table 1.4 Selected ACE Unit studies and outcomes

	Type of study	Study population	Primary service	Primary outcome (ACE vs. UC)	Secondary outcome(s) (ACE vs. UC)	Study limitations	Study strengths
Landefeld et al. [30]	RCT	651 patients aged ≥70 years	Internists with residents for ACE and UC	Significantly improved ADL performance from 2 weeks prior to admission ($p=.05$) and admission compared to discharge ($p=.009$)	Significantly reduced post-acute facility placement (14 % vs. 22 %, $p=.01$) Significantly improved overall health status at discharge, ($p<.001$)	RAs unable to be blinded to patient study group Need for proxy reports of functional and health status	Randomized design Improved outcomes seen in subgroup and multivariate analyses
Covinsky et al. [44]	RCT; Cost analysis from Landefeld et al. study	650 patients aged ≥70 years	Internists with residents for ACE and UC	Nonsignificant reduction in total hospital costs per case ($6,608 vs. $7,240, $p=.93$)	Nonsignificant reduction in LOS (7.5 vs. 8.4 days, $p=.449$) Significantly reduced 90-day facility use (24.1 % vs. 32.3 %, $p=.034$)	Use of total costs included indirect costs Sample size lacked power to determine significance in cost difference	Randomized design Included ACE start-up costs, likely underestimating long-term cost savings
Counsell et al. [37]	RCT	1,531 patients aged ≥70 years, community-dwelling, with LOS ≥2 days	Internist or family practice attending, 62 % without a resident	No significant change in number of independent ADLs from 2 weeks prior to admission to discharge in ACE vs. UC Significant reduction in composite outcome of ADL decline or NH placement in ACE vs. UC (34 % vs. 40 %, $p=.027$)	Significant improvement in processes of care Significant improvement in patient, caregiver, and provider satisfaction In per-protocol analysis, proportion of patients with ADL decline from baseline to discharge was less on ACE (30 % vs. 35 %, $p=.051$).	RAs unable to be blinded to patient study group Need for proxy reports of functional and health status ADL outcome may have been influenced by healthier patient population and shorter LOS than prior studies	Randomized design Large sample size
Asplund et al. [42]	RCT	413 patients aged ≥70 years	ACE—Geriatrician with Internist UC—Internist	No difference in the poor global outcome measure (defined as death and/or severe ADL dependence and/ or poor psychological well-being) at 3 months post-discharge	Significantly reduced LOS (5.9 vs. 7.3 days, $p=.002$) No difference in readmissions or health care resource utilization at 3 months post-discharge Trend toward lower hospital costs on ACE ($p=.08$)	RAs unable to be blinded to patient study group Did not assess 30-day outcomes or readmissions	Randomized design

(continued)

Table 1.4 (continued)

Study	Design	Population	Provider		Limitations	Strengths/Comments
Salvedt et al. [46]	RCT	254 patients aged ≥75 years and meeting frailty criteria	ACE—Geriatrician with residents UC—Internist or Medical Subspecialists with residents	Significantly reduced mortality at 3 (12 % vs. 27 %, $p=.004$) and 6 (16 % vs. 29 %, $p=.02$) months post-discharge	LOS on ACE was significantly longer than UC (15 vs. 7 days, $p<.001$) Significantly more ACE patients with dementia, depression, and delirium diagnoses documented (38 % vs. 7 %, $p<.001$)	Non-USA based study may have influenced LOS Some ACE patients were transferred from other units	Randomized design Targeted frail patients Included medical subspecialty patients Evaluated mortality as a primary outcome
Allen et al. [47]	Descriptive, pre–post comparison of Stroke-ACE model	1,166 acute stroke patients, mean age 72 years	Neurologist	Significantly reduced LOS (3.8 vs. 4.6 days, $p<.0001$)	Significantly increased likelihood of discharge home (62 % vs. 50 %, $p<.001$) Significantly higher proportion of patients without a readmission at 1 year (41 % vs. 18 %, $p<.0001$) Significantly reduced inpatient mortality (11 % vs. 8 %, $p=.02$)	Non-randomized Data from administrative database	Demonstrate scalability of ACE to new patient population
Jayadevappa et al. [43]	Retrospective case–control	1,360 patients aged ≥65 years admitted for CHF, UTI, or pneumonia	ACE—Internist or Geriatrician UC—Internist	Significantly reduced LOS (4.9 vs. 5.9, $p=.01$) and unadjusted mean costs ($13,586 vs. $15,039, $p=.012$)	Readmissions lower on ACE by 11% after adjusting for age, race, comorbidity, and number of prior admissions	Non-randomized Data from administrative database Costs estimated from a cost-to-charge ratio Different attendings on ACE and UC	Adjusted for prior admissions in analyzing readmission rate
Flood et al. [45]	Retrospective cohort	818 patients aged ≥70 years spent entire hospitalization on ACE or UC	Hospitalists	Significantly reduced variable direct costs ($2,109 vs. $2,480, $p=.009$)	Significantly reduced 30-day readmissions (7.9 % vs. 12.8 %, $p=.02$)	Non-randomized Data from administrative database	Study units utilized same staffing ratios and attendings Use of variable direct costs as primary measure Reduced costs despite short and equal LOS

RCT randomized controlled trial, *ACE* Acute Care for Elders, *UC* usual care, *ADL* activities of daily living, *RA* research assistant, *LOS* length of stay, *CHF* congestive heart failure, *UTI* urinary tract infection

aged 65 years and older admitted to either ACE or UC with one of three DRGs: congestive heart failure, pneumonia, or urinary tract infection. This study demonstrated significant reductions in hospital LOS by 1 day and unadjusted mean cost savings of $1,453 per patient on ACE versus UC ($p = .012$). In an analysis adjusting for age, race, comorbidities and number of admissions prior to the index admission, ACE Unit patients had a reduced readmission rate by 11 % [43]. However, this study was limited in that costs were estimated from a cost-to-charge ratio. A subsequent ACE Unit study analyzing costs and readmissions was published in 2013. This retrospective cohort study evaluated variable direct costs in patients age 70 and over who spent their entire hospitalization on either ACE or UC units. Variable direct cost represents the cost stemming directly from daily patient care and therefore provides the best measurement for the impact of the ACE model on costs. This study reduced some of the confounding variables present in prior studies of patient care costs in that patients in both study units had the same attending physicians and the units had the same staffing with the exception of slightly increased availably of rehabilitation therapists on the ACE Unit. In addition, both the ACE and UC units had a daily team meeting. The ACE Unit daily IDT meeting focused on patient function, cognition, and geriatric care coordination and included the bedside nurses, physical and occupational therapists, pharmacists, dieticians, social worker, ACE Unit coordinator, and geriatrician. The UC unit had the traditional "discharge planning" meeting that focused on day of discharge and destination and included only the charge nurse, hospitalists and nurse practitioners, as well as care coordinators and social workers; the UC team meeting did not incorporate formal assessment of patient functional or cognitive status. The ACE Unit model demonstrated significant mean variable direct cost savings of $371 per patient compared to UC. Cost ratios adjusted for age, gender, comorbidity score, and CMI revealed the ACE model reduced costs in patients with low (0.82, 95 % CI 0.72–0.94) and moderate (0.74, 95 % CI 0.62–0.89) CMI scores; care was cost-neutral for patients with high CMI scores (1.13, 95 % CI 0.93–1.37). In addition, significantly fewer ACE patients were readmitted within 30 days of discharge compared to UC [45]. Both the 2009 and 2012 meta-analyses of ACE Unit studies also found overall patient-care related costs savings from the ACE model. Thus, these more recent ACE studies confirm findings from early studies that ACE results in "higher-valued care": more geriatric care delivered without increases in hospital costs. In fact most often ACE leads to cost savings via reduced LOS, reduced readmissions, and decreased adverse events and HAD. See Table 1.4 for a summary of ACE outcomes [46, 47].

Future for ACE

Scaling-Up the ACE Model

While it is not known definitively how many ACE Units exist, as of 2014, it is estimated that there may be approximately 200 units in the USA that have been established in both community and academic hospitals [48]. In addition, ACE Units are found not only in the USA but are also present in hospitals in other countries and will likely become increasingly prevalent as the global population ages. Despite the increasing number of ACE Units, one disadvantage to applying the model to a small subset of patients in a geographically distinct location is that the proven improved health outcomes only reach a minority of hospitalized older adults. Wide-spread incorporation of the ACE Unit principles focusing on maintaining and improving function, avoidance of adverse events, and care coordination requires an approach that is not limited by physical walls and which integrates seamlessly into provider work-flow.

The mandate for hospitals to implement an EHR provides an opportunity to leverage this technology to more widely disseminate ACE care principles throughout a hospital and, therefore, offer a means for scaling-up ACE. Dr. Malone and colleagues at Aurora Health Care in Wisconsin created an EHR tool called "ACE Tracker." ACE Tracker is a software program that queries for specified geriatric care data from the EHR to create a unit-based spreadsheet report for patients age 65 and over that summarizes this geriatric clinical information (i.e., results of cognitive screens, functional status, albumin level, total number of prescribed and high-risk medications, use of urinary catheters, use of restraints, orders for physical and occupational therapy and social service assessments). ACE Tracker has been validated; the data collected electronically correlate with in-person observation of care of hospitalized older adults [49]. In essence, these unit-based ACE Tracker reports serve as an electronic spreadsheet summary of each patient's functional and cognitive status and risks for HAD which can be addressed by unit providers functioning as an IDT. At Aurora Health Care, non-ACE Units use the ACE Tracker reports to discuss each patient's geriatric-specific needs and implement an interdisciplinary plan to meet those needs to prevent HAD and guide care transition planning. For those units who have access to a geriatrician, the geriatrician attends the IDT meeting twice weekly. For those units without a geriatrician, the teams use an "e-Geriatrician." The e-Geriatrician is an off-site geriatrician who participates in multiple unit IDT meetings through teleconferencing. In the Aurora Health Care model, the e-Geriatrician spends 30–45 min on the conference call and is reimbursed at an hourly rate for the service. An initial evaluation of the e-Geriatrician and ACE Tracker model showed a decrease in the use of urinary catheters and an increase in the referrals for physical therapy after implementation. ACE Tracker was developed with the goal to improve quality of older adult hospital care. In the Aurora Health Care System, many different hospitals share the same medical record system, providing the opportunity to use ACE Tracker to create quality bench mark reports for each hospital. The same could be done among hospital units within one hospital. Limitations of the ACE Tracker and e-Geriatrician models to disseminate ACE principles include dependence on assessment and documentation for data accuracy, inability to track implementation of recommendations, and lack of data on patient outcomes [49]. See Chap. 4 for details regarding ACE Tracker and e-Geriatrician.

Since the launch of geographically distinct ACE Units, there is an emergence of models which utilize a roving ACE team that performs consults for frail elders throughout the hospital on non-ACE Units, sometimes called "ACE without walls" or "mobile ACE" (Chap. 3). In one such model, a geriatrician and GNP identified hospitizalized medical patients with advanced age (≥85 years), or older age (≥70 years) with cognitive and/or functional difficulties, and provided proactive consultation. This model demonstrated potential for cost savings for the hospital. Thus, the ACE Tracker/e-Geriatrician and mobile ACE initiatives are promising means of scaling-up the ACE Unit model and require future research on patient and health-system outcomes.

Another means of increasing the scale of ACE is the dissemination of key components of the ACE Unit model to surgical and other specialty and medical subspecialty patient populations. At the Summa Health System Akron City Hospital, ACE processes including screening assessments, protocol implementation, and daily IDT rounds were implemented on a stroke unit, thus creating a Stroke-ACE Unit. Analysis of hospital and Medicare administrative databases before and after launch of the Stroke-ACE Unit demonstrated significantly reduced LOS and 1-year post-discharge readmissions with increased likelihood of discharge to home. Medicare data also noted significantly reduced stroke-specific and risk-adjusted inpatient mortality rates despite an increase in patient age and illness acuity during the post-stroke unit time period compared to care prior to the ACE intervention [47]. As another example, Barnes-Jewish Hospital in St. Louis implemented an Oncology-ACE (OACE) Unit that was geographically distinct from cancer wards [50]. The OACE Unit employed the five core components of the ACE model of care for all cancer patients age 65 and over and demonstrated improved nutritional support [40] and medication appropriateness [41]. Implementing the ACE model in a surgical patient population remains an opportunity yet to be fully implemented and studied. Thus, an over-

arching goal of this approach is that the core ACE Unit components become the standard of hospital care for all vulnerable patients on every hospital unit, regardless of admitting diagnosis. A 2013 systemic descriptive review of the primary components of the ACE model of care suggests the multi-component approach including patient-centered care, medical review, and early mobilization contribute most to improved outcomes seen in ACE studies published to date and signal a starting point for care delivery redesign throughout a hospital [32]. However, the effect size of these components individually was low, further supporting the notion that geriatric care requires not just one intervention, but the multi-component approach that ACE Units employ.

Another example of imbedding these ACE Unit principles into non-ACE Unit care is programs targeting specific clinical domains or syndromes. In Australia, the "Eat Walk Engage" program involved IDT development of protocols to increase patient's oral intake, increase mobility, and increase cognitive stimulation on a general medical unit [51]. Evaluation of the first 18 months of this program showed improved nursing documentation on these domains, improved patient-reported mobility and access to cognitive activities, and shorter LOS (6 vs. 9 days; statistical analysis not performed). Another program which utilizes this syndrome-focused strategy is the Hospital Elder Life Program (HELP). HELP (Chap. 2) provides multicomponent interventions targeting patients' risk factors for delirium and can be delivered on any hospital unit [17]. HELP has demonstrated reduced incident delirium, functional decline, and hospital cost [17, 52, 53].

Potential barriers for all of these models include sustainability, accountability, and ownership of the implementation process. Successful scaling-up of the ACE Unit model requires a business approach: instilling beliefs and behaviors, connecting with the right people, linking solutions to hospital problems, and cascading excellence and successes [54] (see section "ACE Unit Development: Leveraging ACE in the Current Health Care Environment").

Future Direction of ACE Outcomes Research

Given that the ACE model of care remains relatively new and underutilized, opportunity exists for additional patient-centered and health systems outcomes research from ACE care principles. There remains only a handful of RCTs studying the efficacy, effectiveness, and efficiency of ACE Units and none since 2000. However, there are practical challenges in achieving randomization in complex health care environments with periods of limited inpatient capacity precluding "holding" hospital beds for a RCT. While it is encouraging that the model can be scaled to benefit a diverse group of patients, the diversity makes it difficult to combine patient populations to study larger population outcomes related to ACE Units. The authors of a 2010 literature review of ACE Unit studies noted only 20 published studies at that time met inclusion criteria for an ACE Unit review and conclusions were limited by lack of clearly defined ACE Unit operations and outcome variables [27].

Specific geriatric syndromes and hazards of hospitalization that are likely improved from the ACE model remain understudied. For example, few studies have specifically examined the impact of the ACE model on polypharmacy and use of potentially inappropriate medications during and after hospitalization. The effect of the ACE model on delirium and fall prevention, caregiver stress, and provider satisfaction and professional development are opportunities for further research. Additional studies also need to be done to determine the impact and opportunities for ACE Units to improve care transitions and patient status in the weeks to months following a hospitalization. In an early attempt to evaluate the impact of ACE Units on outcomes after hospital discharge, a RCT from Sweden evaluated global patient status in general medicine patients age 70 years and over 3 months after discharge from an ACE or usual care unit. While there was no significant difference in the primary outcome of poor global status (defined as the composite of death and/or severe ADL dependence and/or poor psychological well-being) 3 months after discharge, ACE Unit patients did have a significantly reduced hospital LOS by over one day (Table 1.4) [42]. With more robust care transitions models and studies now available (Chap. 9), opportunity exists for adding care transition specific interventions to the ACE model to study outcomes post-hospital discharge. Finally, the ACE model needs to be implemented and studied in patient populations other than general medical patients.

ACE and Health Care Reform

As early as the 1980s forward thinking champions were advocating for hospital care delivery redesign to address the quality and cost containment imperatives that come with what was then termed the "geriatric imperative" [26]. The challenges portended then are now pressing and urgent realities. Delivering high-quality elder care while containing cost is absolutely essential for the economic stability of our health care system and nation. The financial solvency of the Centers for Medicare and Medicaid Services (CMS) is a primary driver for health care reform in the USA. The Patient Protection and Affordable Care Act (PPACA), commonly called the Affordable Care Act (ACA), was signed into law in 2010 and institutes new quality based CMS rules encouraging hospitals and providers to improve quality of hospital care as well as care transitions [55]. Under the ACA, hospitals will receive reduced CMS reimbursement for excessive 30-day readmissions, hospital-acquired conditions, and other clinical and patient experience outcomes, thus transitioning from a volume-based to a value-based health care system. These quality and patient experience mandates are known as "Value-Based Purchasing" (VBP). The ACE model of care compliments and enhances other disease or unit specific process or quality improvement efforts that achieve VBP mandates and thus provide leverage for hospitals to develop and support an ACE Unit. The ACA also increases educational advancement opportunities for nurses, reinforcing the importance of advanced geriatric training [56] and why hospitals should consider expanding or establishing NICHE programs, which include ACE Units, if not already in existence.

In addition to quality mandates in the acute care setting, the ACA also includes new programs and mandates that span the care continuum. One such program is the Bundled Payments for Care Improvement Initiative with the goal to reduce fragmentation of care by aligning acute care and post-acute care settings and providers through "bundling" payments that require financial and performance accountability [57]. The original ACE RCT demonstrated that for every 15 patients receiving the ACE model of care, one more patient was discharged to home rather than a facility compared to usual care [30]. As ACE studies have continued to demonstrate reduced post-acute facility utilization, the ACE benefits extend across the care continuum and can positively impact bundled payments. Another provision of the ACA designed to reduce costs related to unplanned readmissions is the Hospital Readmission Reduction Program (HRRP) [58]. Under this program, hospitals with above average 30-day readmission rates for three diagnoses (acute myocardial infarction, heart failure, and community acquired pneumonia) began incurring financial penalties in the form of reduced reimbursements in 2013. The number of conditions and the amount of the financial penalties is anticipated to increase annually in the coming years. The readmission rates for specific conditions are publically reported on the Medicare Hospital Compare website. More recent ACE Unit studies indicate reductions in 30-day readmissions, and thus evidence of another benefit of the ACE model under health care reform.

ACE Unit Development: Getting Buy-In from Stakeholders

Barriers to ACE Unit Development

The benefits of the ACE model of care for patients, families, and hospitals are numerous and well documented. However, despite these numerous benefits, challenges remain in developing, sustaining, and disseminating ACE models of care. Commonly cited barriers to development of an ACE Unit include limitations in physical space, change in provider work-flow by adjustment of schedules to incorporate daily IDT rounds, and availability of a geriatrician to lead the initiative [49]. Cost is often the primary barrier for ACE development cited by hospital leaders. In this time of declining reimbursement for health care and constricted hospital capital budgets, the notion of renovating an old unit or creating a new unit may appear prohibitive. In addition to unit renovations, another start-up cost includes time and effort for staff training. Finally, logistical barriers such as finding the ideal time for IDT rounds, revamping provider work-flow, and the challenges inherent with culture change are other possible barriers. However, each of these barriers can and have been overcome by existing ACE Units. The key lies in leveraging the benefits of ACE to clearly demonstrate return on investment (ROI).

Leveraging ACE in the Current Health Care Environment

The foundational principle when engaging stakeholders for ACE Unit development and/or expansion is the fact that the ACE model of care benefits both patients and hospitals in the delivery of higher-valued care. Thus, ACE is an area of focus that hospitals should prioritize given the increasing numbers of elders over the next several decades and the evidence that the benefits outweigh the barriers. Securing support (philosophical and financial) for developing either a geographically distinct ACE Unit or another initiative that embodies ACE principles amongst hospital leadership requires presenting a clear and concise business case that demonstrates ROI. This is more easily accomplished today than it was for the founders of ACE in that mounting evidence continues to support the positive clinical and cost saving outcomes associated with the ACE model of care. The quality mandates that are inherent in the ACA now provide a timely incentive that can be leveraged to garner hospital leadership and stakeholder support for the adoption of ACE. Thus, ROI will not only be in financial savings, but also in the improved processes and outcomes that support VBP and patient safety mandates that hospital leaders are grappling with daily. Linking all of the known improved outcomes from ACE Units, not just the cost-avoidance outcomes, to the hospital leadership's current problems is vitally important for demonstrating ROI. There are multiple domains in which ACE may align with institutional priorities and demonstrate beneficial impact and ROI, including: (1) new staff expertise as demonstrated by pre/post-training tests or performance of new skills, (2) new geriatric care processes such as standardized assessment of cognitive or functional status, (3) clinical outcomes such as reduced rates of hospital-acquired conditions,

and (4) financial goals such as reduced resource utilization, LOS, and readmissions.

Due to these new changes in the health care landscape, health systems are turning more and more to geriatricians for guidance on how to bring the health benefits and cost savings demonstrated by the ACE Unit to their institution. In regard to renovation costs as a barrier to ACE development, the other components of the ACE model are the most vital and a unit can become an ACE Unit with delayed and/or incremental renovations. Covinsky et al. demonstrated that additional start-up costs for a new ACE Unit were recuperated via reduced LOS stemming from the ACE model of care coordination [59]. Additionally, after seeing the patient-centered hospital environment of an ACE Unit, hospitals have been known to extend these features beyond the ACE walls to all units. "Geriatric sensitive" environments are helpful for frail patients with mobility or cognitive limitations regardless of age. Therefore, renovating all units in the ACE model will benefit a variety of patient populations with physical challenges. The well-documented cost savings from the ACE approach easily compensate for any upfront costs in launching ACE. This fact needs to be clearly outlined for stakeholders. The ongoing costs saved by ACE provide one means for sustaining ACE Units and programs. One important financial impact to measure is the role of the ACE model on patient populations who are cost "outliers." This group of complex cases may essentially have even more extensive cost avoidance on ACE Units. Therefore, costs analysis should include these cases in a separate review and not be compared only in aggregate forms. Stakeholders should be shown that the initial costs associated with implementation of an ACE program must be viewed within the context of a cost/benefit ratio over several years.

Steps in ACE Unit Development

Each hospital will have its own unique culture, leadership structure, and processes for new program development. One implementation strategy described by ACE Unit founders as the "ABC's of ACE Unit Implementation" outlines the following stepwise approach for program development: (1) Agreement on the need by key stakeholders, (2) Build the program through interdisciplinary leadership support, (3) Commence the new program with ongoing monitoring, (4) Document every phase of program implementation, (5) Evaluate all processes and outcomes, and (6) Feedback to key stakeholders for ongoing support and direction [60]. Each step has prescribed elements for planning, implementation, and measurement. In addition, an ACE Unit is a laboratory for continuous quality improvement initiatives that align ACE with the quality and safety mission of the hospital.

One specific component of these steps that has proven beneficial to successful ACE Units is the formation of an ACE Unit Development Team. Because an ACE Unit requires interdisciplinary collaboration, successful development of this new model requires support from the leaders of every key discipline as well as hospital administrators. This development team may include department directors for nursing, rehabilitation services, pharmacy, nutrition, volunteer services, and care management; physicians from geriatrics as well as the service line for the targeted patient population (i.e., hospitalists, teaching attendings); key hospital administrative leaders (vice president, chief nursing officer, quality officer, finance officer); development officer; and hospital health information technology and data management personnel. The NICHE program also provides resources for assessing a hospital's readiness for change and current status regarding geriatric care; tools for program development including how to gain support from hospital administration and considerations for renovating/building space; leadership training; and media kits and marketing resources.

Sustaining an ACE Unit

Once an ACE Unit is launched, key members of the Development Team need to continue to serve as an Advisory Council or Steering Committee for sustaining and even expanding ACE programming. As with all clinical programs and the ever-changing health care environment, an ACE Unit will always require adaptation to meet the needs of a growing number of complex patients and hospital goals. Thus, this group serves to ensure ACE programs remain aligned with hospital strategic priories and also serve as informed advocates for ACE throughout the organization. The ACE Unit Advisory Council and clinical teams must work collaboratively to continually identify mutual goals, strategic priorities, and resources to accomplish the shared mission. Health care systems will continue to provide care to an increasing proportion of older adults. Demands from insurers, consumers, and providers for accessible geriatric sensitive care that includes patient experience and quality outcomes in the acute and post-acute care settings will continue to drive market share. Just as every cardiac or oncology patient cannot be cared for on a specialty unit, every older adult cannot be cared for on an ACE Unit. However, ideally the ACE Unit team working collaboratively with the ACE Advisory Council will find ways to care for vulnerable and frail patients that allows the most positive ROI both clinically and financially, while not restricting access or creating admission criteria that adversely affect patient throughput.

Recruiting and maintaining a team of ACE providers is no small feat. Clearly, providers will come with a variety of experiences, perceptions and expectations. Transformative learning recognizes that emotional changes are often involved in effecting change in providers' practices and decision making. For providers from all disciplines to alter their practice style from a disease-focused multidisciplinary approach to a patient-center interdisciplinary model requires providers to *want* to change. The primary reason providers want to change how they deliver care is to understand *why* it is important. Taking time to tell the new ACE Unit frontline providers the *why* behind starting an ACE Unit prior to ACE Unit launch is a good first step in successful culture change. One possible venue for this is a pre-launch workshop or team building event.

Ongoing ACE IDT education is essential to sustaining culture change and team building. ACE training also often fulfills requirements for age specific training mandated by accreditation bodies. The ACE team may be uniquely positioned to provide leadership to help address issues that challenge care hospital-wide such as falls, restraint use, polypharmacy, delirium and care transition planning. Training of the ACE staff can be opened to the entire health care system, thereby expanding reach. This provides an ideal marketing tool as well as demonstrates support for the entire health system. In hospitals today often acute care is provided by hospitalists. Opportunities to provide education to non-geriatric providers such as hospitalists abound on an ACE Unit and should be integrated within the ACE mission. By increasing geriatric expertise throughout the health system, more patients will benefit and ROI is increased. While it is difficult to put a dollar amount on hospital accreditation and evidence-based care, it is nonetheless a very necessary part of doing business and one at which ACE teams often excel.

Conclusion

HAD and other hospital-acquired conditions are unfortunately common in older adults, negatively impacts an older adult's health, and leads to increased health care costs. The increasing size of the older adult population coupled with pressure to reduce hospital costs and improve quality of care provides the impetus to redesign acute care delivery for elders. ACE Units are one model which has been proven to decrease HAD and improve quality of care while reducing health care costs. While a physically distinct ACE Unit provides multiple benefits to patients on the unit, the future of improved acute care for elders involves extension of the ACE model beyond the ACE Unit walls. Because this model of care is "low tech, high touch," development is also relatively low cost given the opportunities for cost-avoidance, but does require thoughtful planning and interdisciplinary leadership support.

References

1. Covinsky KE, Pierluissi E, Johnston CB. Hospitalization-associated disability: "She was probably able to ambulate, but I'm not sure". JAMA. 2011;306(16):1782–93.

2. Boyd CM, Landefeld CS, Counsell SR, Palmer RM, Fortinsky RH, Kresevic D, Burant C, Covinsky KE. Recovery of activities of daily living in older adults after hospitalization for acute medical illness. J Am Geriatr Soc. 2008;56(12):2171–9.

3. Russo CA, Elixhauser A. Hospitalizations in the elderly population, 2003. Statistical Brief #6. Healthcare Cost and Utilization Project (HCUP) Statistical Briefs [Internet]. Rockville (MD): Agency for Health Care Policy and Research (US); 2006 May.

4. Katz S, Ford AB, Moskowitz RW, Jackson BA, Jaffe MW. Studies of illness in the aged. The Index of ADL: A standardized measure of biological and psychological function. JAMA. 1963;185:914–9.

5. Hirsch CH, Sommers L, Olsen A, Mullen L, Winograd CH. The natural history of functional morbidity in hospitalized older adults. J Am Geriatr Soc. 1990;38(12):1296–303.

6. Covinsky KE, Palmer RM, Fortinsky RH, Counsell SR, Stewart AL, Kresevic D, Burant CJ, Landefeld CS. Loss of independence in activities of daily living in older adults hospitalized with medical illnesses: increased vulnerability with age. J Am Geriatr Soc. 2003;51(4):451–8.

7. Palleschi L, De Alfieri W, Salani B, Fimognari FL, Marsilii A, Pierantozzi A, Di Cioccio L, Zuccaro SM. Functional recovery of elderly patients hospitalized in geriatric and general medicine units. The PROgetto DImissioni in GEriatria Study. J Am Geriatr Soc. 2011;59(2):193–9.

8. Goldman LE, Sarkar U, Kessell E, Guzman D, Schneidermann M, Pierluissi E, Walter B, Vittinghoff E, Critchfield J, Kushel M. Support from Hospital to Home for Elders: A Randomized Controlled Trial 2014. Ann Intern Med. 2014;161(7):472–81. doi:10.7326/M14-0094.

9. Gill TM, Allore HG, Holford TR, Guo Z. Hospitalization, restricted activity, and the development of disability among older persons. JAMA. 2004;292(17):2115–24.

10. Brown CJ, Roth DL, Allman RM, Sawyer P, Ritchie CS, Roseman JM. Trajectories of life-space mobility after hospitalization. Ann Intern Med. 2009;150(6):372–8.

11. Goodwin JS, Howrey B, Zhang DD, Kuo YF. Risk of continued institutionalization in older adults. J Gerontol A Biol Sci Med Sci. 2011;66A(12):1321–7.

12. Reuben DB, Seeman TE, Keeler E, Hayes RP, Bowman L, Sewall A, Hirsch SH, Wallace RB, Buralnik JM. The effect of self-reported and performance-based functional impairment on future hospital costs of community-dwelling older persons. Gerontologist. 2004;44(3):401–7.

13. Fried TR, Bradley EH, Williams CS, Tinetti ME. Functional disability and health care expenditures for older persons. Arch Intern Med. 2001;161(21):2602–7.

14. Brown CJ, Friedkin RJ, Inouye SK. Prevalence and outcomes of low mobility in hospitalized older patients. J Am Geriatr Soc. 2004;52(8):1263–70.

15. Inouye SK, Westendorp RGJ, Saczynski JS. Delirium in elderly people. Lancet. 2014;383(9920):911–22.

16. Inouye SK, Charpentier PA. Precipitating factors for delirium in hospitalized elderly persons. Predictive model and interrelationship with baseline vulnerability. JAMA. 1996;275(11):852–7.

17. Inouye SK, Bogardus Jr ST, Charpentier PA, Leo-Summers L, Acampora D, Holford TR. A multicomponent intervention to prevent delirium in hospitalized older patients. N Engl J Med. 1999;340(9):669–76.

18. Zisberg A, Sinoff G, Gur-Yaish N, Admi H, Shadmi E. In-hospital use of continence aids and new-onset urinary incontinence in adults aged 70 and older. J Am Geriatr Soc. 2011;59(6):1099–104.

19. Holroyd-Leduc JM, Sen S, Bertenthal D, Sands LP, Palmer RM, Kresevic DM. The relationship of indwelling urinary catheters to death, length of hospital stay, functional decline, and nursing home admission in hospitalized older medical patients. J Am Geriatr Soc. 2007;55(2):227–33.

20. Bouldin EL, Andresen EM, Dunton NE, Simon M, Waters TM. Liu M Falls among adult patients hospitalized in the United States: prevalence and trends. J Patient Saf. 2013;9(1):13–7.

21. Cameron ID, Gillespie LD, Robertson MC, Murray GR, Hill KD, Cumming RG, Kerse N. Interventions for preventing falls in older people in care facilities and hospitals. Cochrane Database Syst Rev. 2012;12, CD005465.

22. Dykes PC, Carroll DL, Hurley A, Lipsitz S, Benoit A, Chang F, Meltzer S, Tsurikova R, Zuyov L, Middleton B. Fall prevention in acute care hospitals: a randomized trial. JAMA. 2010;304(17):1912–8.

23. Lyder CH, Wang Y, Metersky M, Curry M, Kliman R, Verzier NR, Hunt DR. Hospital-acquired pressure ulcers: results from the national Medicare Patient Safety Monitoring System study. J Am Geriatr Soc. 2012;60(9):1603–8.

24. Covinsky KE, Martin GE, Beyth RJ, Justice AC, Sehgal AR, Landefeld CS. The relationship between clinical assessments of nutritional status and adverse outcomes in older hospitalized medical patients. J Am Geriatr Soc. 1999;47:532–8.

25. Sullivan DH, Sun S, Walls RC. Protein-energy undernutrition among elderly hospitalized patients: a prospective study. JAMA. 1999;281(21):2013–9.

26. Bachman SS, Collard AF, Greenberg JN, Fountain E, Huebner TW, Kimball B, Melendy K. An innovative approach to geriatric acute care delivery: The Choate-Symmes Experience. Hosp Health Serv Adm. 1987;32(4):509–20.

27. Ahmed NN, Pearce SE. Acute care for the elderly: a literature review. Popul Health Manag. 2010;13(4):219–25.

28. Geriatric Evaluation and Management (GEM) Procedures. VHA Handbook 1140.04. Department of Veterans Affairs, Veterans Health Administration. May 2010. Available at: http://www.va.gov/vhapublications/ViewPublication.asp?pub_ID=2237. Accessed 8/14/14.

29. Latour J, Lebel P, Leclerc BS, Leduc N, Berg K, Bolduc A, Kergoat MJ. Short-term geriatric assessment units: 30 years later. BMC Geriatr. 2010;10:41.

30. Landefeld CS, Palmer RM, Kresevic DM, Fortinsky RH, Kowal J. A randomized trial of care in a hospital medical unit especially designed to improve the functional outcomes of acutely ill older patients. N Engl J Med. 1995;332:1338–44.

31. Palmer RM, Landefeld CS, Kresevic D, Kowal J. A medical unit for the acute care of the elderly. J Am Geriatr Soc. 1994;42(5):545–52.

32. Fox MT, Sidani S, Persaud M, Tregunno D, Maimets I, Brooks D, O'Brien K. Acute care for elders components of acute geriatric unit care: systematic descriptive review. J Am Geriatr Soc. 2013;61:939–46.

33. Welcome to NICHE. Available at: http://www.nicheprogram.org. Accessed 7/1/14.

34. Hartford Institute For Geriatric Nursing. GITT Kit Resources. http://hartfordign.org/education/gitt/. Accessed August 25, 2014.

35. Fiscal Year 2011 Final Rule Data Files, Case Mix Index File. Centers for Medicare & Medicaid Services. http://www.cms.gov/Medicare/Medicare-Fee-for-Service-Payment/AcuteInpatientPPS/FY-2011-IPPS-Final-Rule-Home-Page-Items/CMS1237932.html. Accessed September 7, 2014.

36. Barnes DE, Palmer RM, Kresevic DM, Fortinsky RH, Kowal J, Chren MM, Landefeld CS. Acute care for elders units produce

shorter hospital stays at lower costs while maintaining patient's functional status. Health Aff. 2012;31(6):1227–36.

37. Counsell SR, Holder CM, Liebenauer LL, Palmer RM, Fortinsky RH, Kresevic DM, Quinn LM, Allen KR, Covnisky KE, Landefeld CS. Effects of a multicomponent intervention on functional outcomes and process of care in hospitalized older patients: A randomized controlled trial of ACE in a community hospital. J Am Geriatr Soc. 2000;48:1572–81.

38. Baztan JJ, Suarez-Garcia FM, Lopez-Arrieta J, Rodriguez-Manas L, Rodriquez-Artalego F. Effectiveness of acute geriatric units on functional decline, living at home, and case fatality among older patients admitted to hospital for acute medical disorders: meta-analysis. BMJ. 2009;228:b50. doi:10.1136/bmj.b50.

39. Fox MT, Persaud M, Maimets I, O'Brien K, Brooks D, Tregunno D, Schraa E. Effectiveness of acute geriatric unit care using acute care for elders components: a systematic review and meta-analysis. J Am Geriatr Soc. 2012;60:2237–45.

40. Flood KL, Brown CJ, Carroll MB, Locher JL. Nutritional processes of care for older adults admitted to an oncology-acute care for elders unit. Crit Rev Oncol Hematol. 2011;78:73–8.

41. Flood KL, Carroll MB, Le CV, Brown CJ. Polypharmacy in hospitalized older adult cancer patients: experience from an Oncology-Acute Care for Elders Unit. Am J Geriatr Pharmacother. 2009; 7:151–8.

42. Asplund K, Gustafson Y, Jacobsson C, Bucht G, Wahlin A, Peterson J, Blom JO, Angquist KA. Geriatric-based versus general wards for older acute medical patients: a randomized comparison of outcomes and use of resources. J Am Geriatr Soc. 2000;48:1381–8.

43. Jayadevappa R, Chhatre S, Weiner M, Raziano DB. Health resource utilization and medical care cost of acute care elderly unit patients. Value Health. 2006;9(3):186–92.

44. Covinsky KE, King JT, Quinn LM, Siddique R, Palmer R, Kresevic DM, Fortinsky RH, Kowal J, Landefeld CS. Do acute care for elders units increase hospital costs? A cost analysis using the hospital perspective. J Am Geriatr Soc. 1997;45:729–34.

45. Flood KL, MacLennan PA, McGrew D, Green D, Dodd C, Brown CJ. An acute care for elders unit reduces costs and 30-day readmissions. JAMA Intern Med. 2013;173(11):981–7.

46. Salvedt I, Opdahl ES, Fayers P, Kaasa S, Sletvold O. Reduced mortality in treating acutely sick, frail older patients in a geriatric evaluation and management unit. A prospective randomized trial. J Am Geriatr Soc. 2002;50:792–8.

47. Allen KR, Hazelett SE, Palmer RM, Jarjoura DB, Wickstrom GC, Weinhardt JA, Lada R, Holder CM, Counsell SR. Developing a stroke unit using the acute care for elders intervention and model of care. J Am Geriatr Soc. 2003;51:1660–7.

48. Clark C. If ACE Units are so great, why aren't they everywhere? HealthLeaders Media. April 25, 2013. http://www.healthleaders-media.com/page-1/QUA-291513/If-ACE-Units-Are-So-Great-Why-Arent-They-Everywhere. Accessed July 7, 2014.

49. Malone ML, Vollbrecht M, Stephenson J, Burke L, Pagel P, Goodwin JS. Acute care for elders (ACE) tracker and e-geriatrician: methods to disseminate ACE concepts to hospitals with no geriatricians on staff. J Am Geriatr Soc. 2010;58(1):161–7.

50. Flood KL, Carroll MB, Le CV, Ball L, Esker DA, Carr DB. Geriatric syndromes in elderly patients admitted to an oncology-acute care for elders unit. J Clin Oncol. 2006;24(15):2298–303.

51. Mudge AM, McRae P, Cruickshank M. Eat Walk Engage: An interdisciplinary collaborative model to improve care of hospitalized elders. Am J Med Qual. 2015;30(1):5–13. doi:10.1177/10628606 13510965. 2013 Nov 22 Epub ahead of print.

52. Inouye SK, Bogardus ST, Baker DI, Leo-Summers L, Cooney LM. The Hospital Elder Life Program: a model of care to prevent cognitive and functional decline in older hospitalized patients. Hospital Elder Life Program. J Am Geriatr Soc. 2000;48(12): 1697–706.

53. Rizzo JA, Bogardus Jr ST, Leo-Summers L, Williams CS, Acampora D, Inouye SK. Multicomponent targeted intervention to prevent delirium in hospitalized older patients: what is the economic value? Med Care. 2001;39(7):740–52.

54. Sutton RI, Rao H, Shapiro R. Scaling up excellence: Getting to more without settling for less. New York: Crown Business; 2014.

55. U.S. Department of Health and Human Services. About the law. http://www.hhs.gov/healthcare/rights/index.html. Accessed July 12, 2013.

56. Brody A, Sullivan-Marx EM. The patient protection and affordable care act: implications for geriatric nurses and patients. J Gerontol Nurs. 2012;38(11):3–5.

57. Centers for Medicare & Medicaid Services. Bundled Payments for Care Improvement (BPCI) Initiative: general information. http://innovation.cms.gov/initiatives/bundled-payments. Accessed August 18, 2013.

58. Centers for Medicare & Medicaid Services. Readmissions Reduction Program. http://www.cms.gov/Medicare/Medicare-Fee-for-Service-Payment/AcuteInpatientPPS/Readmissions-Reduction-Program.html. Accessed July 18, 2013.

59. Covinsky KE, Palmer RM, Kresevic DM, Kahana E, Counsell SR, Fortinsky RH, Landefeld CS. Improving functional outcomes in older persons: lessons from an acute care for elders unit. Jt Comm J Qual Improv. 1998;24(2):63–76.

60. Palmer RM, Counsell S, Landefeld CS. Clinical intervention trials: the ACE Unit. Clin Geriatr Med. 1998;14(4):831–49.

Hospital Elder Life Program (HELP)

2

Jirong Yue, Tammy T. Hshieh, and Sharon K. Inouye

Hospitalization has long been recognized as a time of high risk, often a pivotal event in the life of a vulnerable older person [1], with exposure to a myriad of hazards and potential "trauma" [2] from immobilization, lack of orienting influences, inadequate sleep, poor nutrition, dehydration, adverse effects of medications and procedures, and emotional stress. The leading complication of hospitalization is delirium, an acute confusional state, which is common, serious, and often fatal. Delirium occurs in up to 50 % of hospitalized elders, and costs more than $164 billion per year in the USA (2011 estimates) [3]. Delirium leads to high rates of functional decline, prolonged hospital stays, high rates of institutionalization and readmission, increased need for rehabilitation services, long-term cognitive decline, and increased mortality [3–5]. Importantly, delirium is preventable in 30–40 % of cases [3], highlighting its significance as a target for intervention.

The Hospital Elder Life Program (HELP, www. hospitalelderlifeprogram.org) is an innovative model of care proven to prevent complications of hospitalization for older persons, specifically delirium and functional decline. Given its well-documented efficacy and cost-effectiveness along with its widespread adoption, it is considered the gold standard program for delirium prevention, as well as a means to improve acute care for older persons more generally. This chapter will provide a description of the model of care, its staffing and procedures, evidence of its efficacy and cost-effectiveness, and steps to guide successful implementation.

J. Yue, M.D.
The Center of Gerontology and Geriatrics, West China Hospital, Sichuan University, Chengdu, Sichuan, China

T.T. Hshieh, M.D.
Division of Aging, Brigham and Women's Hospital and Institute for Aging Research, Hebrew SeniorLife, Boston, MA, USA

S.K. Inouye, M.D., M.P.H. (✉)
Department of Medicine, Beth Israel Deaconess Medical Center and Institute for Aging Research, Hebrew SeniorLife, Harvard Medical School, Boston, MA, USA
e-mail: agingbraincenter@hsl.harvard.edu

With our rapidly aging population, HELP provides a real-world approach to enable our health-care system to provide safe and high quality care to older persons.

Overview

HELP is an innovative, hospital-based, patient-centered, multidisciplinary integrated model of care. It utilizes evidence-based multicomponent strategies for preventing delirium and functional decline in hospitalized older persons [4, 6]. The goals of the HELP program, as originally outlined in 1993 [4] are to: (1) maintain physical and cognitive functioning throughout hospitalization, (2) maximize independence at discharge, (3) assist with the transition from hospital to home, and (4) prevent unplanned readmission.

The program was originally developed in 1993 and since then, has been updated regularly. Recently in 2013, HELP protocols were adapted to allow fulfillment of the NICE guidelines [7]. In the past 15 years, this program has been implemented in over 200 hospitals in at least eight countries. HELP has been implemented in every type of hospital unit (medical, medical subspecialty, surgical, surgical specialty, mixed medical-surgical, orthopedic, palliative care, intensive care, step-down, rehabilitation, emergency department), post-acute and long-term care settings. At least ten studies have documented effectiveness of HELP for prevention of adverse hospital outcomes, including incident delirium, cognitive and functional decline, and hospital falls [4, 6, 8–16]. In addition, HELP has been documented to be effective in decreasing length of hospital stay [6, 8–12], institutionalization [10], and sitter usage [10]. The HELP program has proven cost-effectiveness, saving hospital costs of about $1,200–2,700 per person per hospitalization [8, 17] and about $13,000 per person in the year following discharge [16] (updated to 2014 USD). Extrapolating nationally, if HELP were implemented in one-half of US hospitals, the savings to the health-care system would amount to over $18 billion per year [18].

The HELP model presents many advantages over other geriatric models of care. HELP is intended to integrate the principles of geriatrics into standard nursing and medical care on any hospital unit, and to bring geriatric expertise to impact management of patients throughout an institution. Thus, HELP does not require a dedicated geriatric unit, serving a broader proportion of patients across a hospital, yet integrating well with existing geriatric services. Since HELP provides the expertise and trained staff to conduct interventions, a separate geriatric consult team is not required. Establishing HELP facilitates integration and coordination of interdisciplinary geriatric experts across the hospital setting. Quality assurance procedures are built in across all levels of HELP, thus maximizing quality of care and patient safety.

Key Points

- The Hospital Elder Life Program utilizes multicomponent strategies to provide optimal care for older adults during hospitalization.
- The primary goals of the program are to: maintain cognitive and physical functioning throughout hospitalization, maximize independence at discharge, assist with the transition from hospital to home, and prevent unplanned readmissions.
- The HELP program was created in 1993 and has been continuously updated. In 2013, updated protocols enhanced the scope of the program and allowed fulfillment of NICE guidelines for delirium prevention.

Program Structure and Interventions

All patients are screened for eligibility as detailed below and assigned to intervention protocols according to delirium risk factors present (Table 2.1). Once enrolled, a skilled interdisciplinary team assisted by trained volunteers implements standardized non-pharmacologic intervention protocols

Table 2.1 Risk factors and corresponding HELP intervention protocol

Risk factors	HELP protocol
Cognitive impairment	Orientation protocol/therapeutic activities
Sleep deprivation	Sleep enhancement protocol
Immobility	Early mobilization protocol
Hearing/vision impairment	Hearing/vision protocol
Dehydration/constipation	Fluid repletion/constipation protocol
Poor nutrition	Feeding assistance
Pain	Pain management protocol
Hypoxia	Hypoxia protocol
Infection	Infection prevention protocols
Multiple medications	Psychoactive medications protocol

(Table 2.2). Adherence to interventions is tracked daily. Geriatric nursing interventions and interdisciplinary team rounds occur regularly. These processes are described in further detail below (Fig. 2.1).

Eligible Patients and Enrollment Process

Once admitted, every patient aged 70 years and older is screened for eligibility using a standardized assessment including a brief cognitive screen (such as the Short Portable Mental Status Questionnaire), basic and instrumental activities of daily living, screening of vision and hearing, and chart review for Blood Urea Nitrogen/Creatinine (BUN/Cr) ratio. The inclusion criteria (see below) are presence of at least one risk factor for cognitive or functional decline and ability to communicate either verbally or in writing. The reasons for exclusion are primarily inability or refusal to participate in the intervention protocols.

Enrollment Criteria for Hospital Elder Life Program

Inclusion Criteria
- Age 70 years and older
- Admitted to a HELP unit
- At least one risk factor for cognitive or functional decline. Risk factors include:
  - Cognitive impairment by any cognitive screening test, e.g., Short Portable Mental Status Questionnaire (SPMSQ) with 2+ errors
  - Any mobility problems or impairment on activities of daily living
  - Vision impairment: <20/70 best corrected vision
  - Hearing impairment: <3 of 6 whispers in each ear on Whisper Test
  - Dehydration: BUN/Cr ratio >18
- Able to communicate verbally or in writing. Nonverbal patients who can communicate in writing are included.

Exclusion Criteria
- Coma
- Mechanical ventilation
- Aphasia (expressive and/or receptive) if communication ability severely impaired
- Terminal condition with death imminent, comfort care only
- Combative or dangerous behavior
- Severe psychotic disorder that prevents participation in interventions
- Severe end-stage dementia with inability to communicate
- Neutropenia precautions

Table 2.2 Hospital Elder Life Program (HELP) interventions

Interventions	Staff	Description
Core interventions		
Orientation/Therapeutic activities	ELS, volunteers	Orientation board with names of care team members and daily schedule; orienting communication
		Cognitive stimulation activities three times daily
Sleep enhancement	ELNS, ELS, volunteers	At bedtime, warm milk or herbal tea, relaxation tapes or music, and back massage. Unit-wide noise reduction strategies and schedule adjustments to allow uninterrupted sleep
Early mobilization	ELNS, ELS, volunteers	Ambulation or active range-of-motion exercises three times daily; minimizing use of immobilizing equipment
Vision protocol	ELS, volunteers	Visual aids (e.g., glasses or magnifying lenses) and adaptive equipment (e.g., large illuminated telephone keypads, large print books, and fluorescent tape on call bell), with daily reinforcement of their use
Hearing protocol	ELNS, ELS, volunteers	Portable amplifying devices and special communication techniques, with daily reinforcement. Ear wax clearing by ELNS as needed
Fluid repletion/constipation	ELNS, ELS, volunteers	Encourage fluids; promote mobility and regular toileting; increase fiber in the diet; laxative treatment as needed
Feeding assistance	ELS, volunteers	Feeding assistance and encouragement during meals
NICE-to-HELP interventions		
Pain management	ELNS, ELS, Volunteers	Begin pain management plan and modify as needed, with non-pharmacological and pharmacological management
Hypoxia protocol	ELNS	Seek advice regarding oxygen administration; check oxygen flow; elevate head of bed to 45°
Infection prevention		
Hand Hygiene Protocol	All staff	Hand washing protocol; generalized infection control measures
Aspiration prevention	ELNS	Oral care every 4 h or per hospital protocol; head of bed to 60° during meals; monitor for signs of pneumonia
Preventing catheter-associated urinary tract infections	ELNS	Sterile insertion technique, early catheter removal
Other program interventions		
Geriatric nursing assessment and interventions		
Delirium protocol	ELNS	Creating a calm, orienting environment; communicate with the patient in a pleasant manner; encourage family involvement, referral to physicians if needed
Dementia protocol	ELNS	Collaborate with medical staff and family; avoiding psychoactive medications
Psychoactive medications	ELNS, interdisciplinary group	Screen medication list for medications associated with delirium daily; collaborate with interdisciplinary group about potential and actual adverse medication outcomes, and make recommendations
Discharge planning	ELNS	Assessing home environment and social supports for possible discharge needs
Optimizing length of stay	ELNS	Identifies risk factors that indicate a need for intensive discharge planning and anticipates discharge needs
Additional areas	ELNS	Nursing assessment and interventions for emotional health, nutrition, functional status, incontinence and elimination issues, skin, social issues
Interdisciplinary interventions		
Interdisciplinary rounds	ELNS, ELS, geriatrician, primary nurses, interdisciplinary team	Regular (2–3× weekly) rounds to discuss each Elder Life patient, set goals and review all Elder Life issues with interdisciplinary input (e.g., physical therapist, dietitian, pharmacist, chaplain, social work, care coordination, psychiatric liaison nursing, and consultants). Interventions are recommended and tracked
Interdisciplinary consultation	Interdisciplinary team	Provide as-needed consultation and input about Elder Life patients upon referral by staff
Geriatrician consultation	HELP Geriatrician	Targeted consultation on Elder Life issues, as requested by program staff or primary team. Formal geriatric consultation on a limited basis as requested
Community linkages and Telephone follow-up	ELNS, ELS,	Referrals and communication with community agencies to optimize transition to home. Telephone follow-up phone call within 7 days after discharge for all patients
Provider education program	ELNS, geriatrician	Formal didactic sessions, one-on-one interactions, and resource materials to educate nursing and physician staff about Elder Life issues

ELNS Elder Life Nurse Specialist, *ELS* Elder Life Specialist

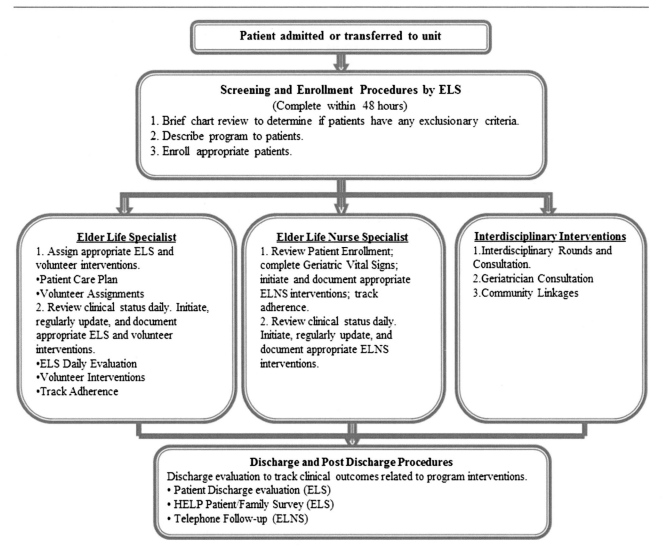

Fig. 2.1 The clinical process

Intervention Process

The program consists of core interventions and other program interventions (Table 2.2). Core interventions include protocols for daily visiting and orienting communication, therapeutic activities, sleep enhancement, early mobilization, vision and hearing adaptation, fluid repletion, and feeding assistance. These core interventions are conducted by the HELP staff assisted by trained volunteers. NICE-to-HELP interventions include prevention of infection, management of constipation, pain, and hypoxia. Other program interventions include geriatric nursing assessment and intervention, interdisciplinary rounds, ongoing staff educational programs, post-discharge community linkages and telephone follow-up. Table 2.2 describes the HELP program interventions and staff intended to carry them out. While the intervention protocols are standardized, the assigned interventions are individualized and tailored for each patient according to their abilities and preferences.

The HELP Interdisciplinary Team

Critical to the effectiveness of HELP is a skilled interdisciplinary team (Fig. 2.2), which interfaces with the primary medical team and nurses, and coordinates the HELP program and interventions. The team includes an advanced practice or geriatric-trained nurse (the Elder Life Nurse Specialist), geriatrician, and program coordinator (Elder Life Specialist), along with interdisciplinary team members across many fields, such as rehabilitation therapy (physical, occupational, and speech therapy), clinical pharmacy, nutrition, chaplaincy, social work, and care coordination. The team is assisted by trained volunteers. These roles are further described below.

Fig. 2.2 The Hospital Elder Life
Program: staffing model

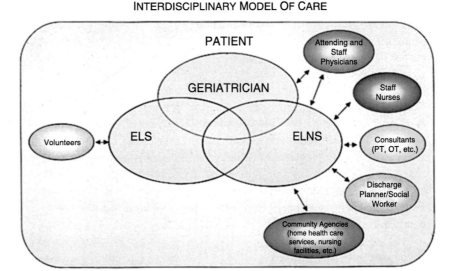

THE HOSPITAL ELDER LIFE PROGRAM
INTERDISCIPLINARY MODEL OF CARE

Elder Life Nurse Specialist

The Elder Life Nurse Specialist (ELNS) is a masters-level
nurse with experience and knowledge in geriatrics. The
ELNS performs patient assessments and interventions, provides ongoing educational in-services regarding the HELP
principles and protocols for nurses, aides, and other hospital staff, and acts as a liaison between the primary nurses
and physicians and other interdisciplinary professionals,
communicating HELP recommendations and ensuring
follow-up.

Key Responsibilities of the ELNS

1. Geriatric nursing assessment of all included patients, and
   implementing HELP nursing protocols. Daily communication with unit nursing staff.
2. Coordinating interdisciplinary geriatric team rounds on
   each HELP unit and assuring implementation of recommendations. Serving as a liaison between the HELP
   geriatrician, primary physicians and other health-care
   specialties in the hospital.
3. Monitoring adherence to nursing interventions and outcomes. Serving as liaison between HELP team and nursing staff, and assuring coordination with regular nursing
   care.
4. Identifying and addressing reasons for non-adherence
   and implementing changes to improve services.
5. Continually reevaluating program interventions and outcomes to respond to patient's care needs and outcomes.
6. Serve as a clinical resource and role model for providing
   optimal geriatric nursing care.
7. Providing regular didactic educational sessions, case
   conferences and one-on-one bedside teaching for all
   nursing staff.

8. Providing clinical and administrative support for the
   ELS and volunteers.
9. Developing in-depth knowledge of community resources
   and facilities. Working with the primary team and care
   coordination, the ELNS helps to facilitate referrals to
   appropriate community agencies and to build effective
   support systems for patients and their families in post-
   discharge care planning.
10. To assist with transitions, developing knowledge of and
    a mechanism for regular communication with key staff
    of community agencies to which older patients are com-
    monly discharged, including visiting nursing agencies,
    congregate housing, and skilled nursing facilities.

Elder Life Specialist

The Elder Life Specialist (ELS) is a unique role created for
HELP. Preferred background includes a bachelor or master's
degree in human services or a health-care related field, 1–3
years working in clinical program development with super-
visory and training skills, and experience working with older
patients. The ELS screens and enrolls patients into the program, orients patients and families to the program and
assigns appropriate intervention protocols. The ELS also
trains and oversees volunteers, and develops individualized
care plans for volunteer interventions. The ELS oversees
daily operations of the HELP program.

Key Responsibilities of the ELS

1. Screening and enrolling patients into HELP.
2. Evaluating the risk factors and tailoring HELP intervention protocols. Providing equipment and updating care
   plans daily according to the patients' evolving needs.

3. Implementing intervention protocols and making volunteer assignments. Ensuring staff/volunteer coverage of all interventions, including weekends and holidays.
4. Monitoring and recording adherence to all protocols, and addressing reasons for non-adherence.
5. Coordinating volunteer schedules. Providing daily volunteer supervision and support, with continuous feedback.
6. Collaborating with the Volunteer Services in volunteer recruitment. Coordinating quarterly HELP Volunteer Trainings. Ongoing educational programs and retention activities for existing volunteers. Quarterly competency-based checklists with volunteers to assure interventions are correctly implemented.
7. Educating patients and families prior to discharge about community resources and needs.

Geriatrician

The background requirements of the geriatrician include board certification in geriatric medicine and two years clinical experience in geriatric medicine preferred. The geriatrician serves as the medical liaison with the hospital medical staff, providing ongoing educational programs in geriatric medical care and collaborating with an interdisciplinary group of health care professionals. In addition, the geriatrician provides consultation to the ELNS and other HELP staff upon request. Likewise, the geriatrician performs formal geriatric medicine consultations upon request from the primary medical team. The geriatrician often serves as program champion and clinician leader, providing a crucial role for HELP program maintenance and sustainability. Some of these last mentioned roles can also be played by the ELNS or ELS.

Key Responsibilities of the HELP Geriatrician

1. Provide comprehensive geriatric medicine evaluation with emphasis on prevention of delirium risk factors. Monitor clinical progress and outcomes.
2. Provide bedside consultation to HELP patients.
3. Participate in HELP interdisciplinary team rounds. Participate in house-staff rounds for complex patients.
4. Serve as a liaison with medical staff and assure coordination of HELP services.
5. Provide formal geriatric consultation upon request of primary medical team.
6. Provide education to physicians and other health-care staff via formal lectures, case conferences, rounds, and regular one-on-one interactions.

Volunteers

The volunteer component is a unique aspect of the HELP program, providing program interventions directly at the bedside three times a day, 7 days a week. Volunteers help to provide sympathetic support, encouragement and companionship to older patients and their families. The volunteer interventions include daily visits with orienting communication, therapeutic activities, early mobilization, vision and hearing enhancement, oral volume repletion, feeding assistance, and sleep enhancement protocols. Volunteers are recruited and screened for characteristics including responsibility, empathy, maturity, communication skills, respect for older patients, confidentiality, and enthusiasm. Volunteer training is extensive, to provide the necessary skills to safely provide the HELP interventions, and includes: (1) at least 16 h of classroom learning using the volunteer training manuals, training videos, and cases for small group discussion; (2) at least 16 h of one-on-one training paired with an experienced volunteer or HELP staff member on the hospital unit; (3) competency-based checklists to assess each volunteer's performance on all interventions, completed and validated by HELP staff before working independently with patients. Volunteers are carefully instructed that they must not interfere with a patient's medical treatment or give medical advice, and all dietary and activity interventions must be cleared with the patient's nurse. Subsequently, volunteers undergo quarterly competency checks. After completion of training, volunteers are assigned regular shifts to provide interventions to 4–6 patients per shift. The presence of volunteers introduces a valued humanistic element to the program, provides high-quality hospital care, and maximizes cost-effectiveness.

A study of 13 HELP sites in the USA found that all sites used trained volunteers [19], and these were recruited from local colleges (100 % of sites), hospital volunteer services (92 %), general community organizations (92 %), local churches or religious organizations (62 %), hospital employees (46 %), and other sources (high schools, summer programs, ladies' auxiliary groups, and retired senior volunteer programs) (39 %).

Interdisciplinary Rounds

The HELP program conducts regular interdisciplinary rounds on all HELP patients (at least 2–3 times per week). The goal is to provide a mechanism for interdisciplinary expertise to focus on the geriatric issues for each HELP patient in a timely manner. The HELP interdisciplinary model of care is shown in Fig. 2.2. The rounds, coordinated by the ELNS, bring together HELP staff, primary team nurses and physicians, rehabilitation therapists (physical, occupational, and speech therapy), clinical pharmacist, dietitian, chaplain, social workers, care coordination, and relevant consultants. The primary nurse presents each patient, providing name, age, date and reason for admission, past medical history, and geriatric vital signs (cognition, psychoactive medication use, sleep, functional status, mobility, vision and hearing, nutritional status, hydration, elimination, skin, emotional health, social concerns, and discharge plans). Each team member reports on the patient's progress, new findings, and any problems delivering recommended interventions. The ELNS records recommendations and tracks adherence. Interdisciplinary rounds are critical to assuring the effectiveness and clinical impact of the program.

Staff Overview

- Key HELP staff includes Elder Life Nurse Specialist (ELNS), Elder Life Specialist (ELS), volunteers, geriatrician, and interdisciplinary experts.
- The program provides skilled interdisciplinary staff and trained volunteers to implement intervention protocols targeted towards delirium risk factors.

Quality Assurance Procedures

Standard, consistent quality assurance procedures are integral to HELP. Continuous feedback to improve program quality and intervention adherence is a central paradigm of the program philosophy. Quality assurance procedures cover five major categories: intervention adherence, staff role functioning, volunteer performance, patient-family survey, and ongoing program improvement.

Quality Assurance to Improve Intervention Adherence

On a daily basis, the ELS reviews documentation on completion of volunteer and staff interventions. Any interventions not completed are reviewed, exploring the reasons. Barriers to adherence are addressed immediately. In addition, the HELP team meets as a working group twice monthly. Monthly summaries of intervention adherence are reviewed, and any changes in adherence rates are discussed. Recommendations to improve adherence are implemented and tracked. Examples of successful recommendations include volunteer feedback and retraining, advance scheduling of interventions with patients, adaptation of procedures to improve patient acceptability, providing missing equipment, and enlisting support of nursing and medical staff to reinforce intervention with patients.

Quality Assurance to Improve Staff Role Functioning

The program director meets with each staff member four times per year to review their satisfaction and effectiveness in their role. At these meetings, any barriers to adherence with program procedures are discussed, and the staff member sets short-term and long-term goals. Initially and on a yearly basis, staff members undergo paired standardization and performance checks for all program screening, enrollment, and intervention procedures, as part of the HELP reliability assessment process.

Quality Assurance of Volunteer Performance

Volunteers undergo quarterly competency evaluations by the ELS to assure correct and complete adherence with all intervention protocols. These sessions allow volunteers to ask questions, clarify any program procedures, and enhance their skills.

Patient-Family Survey

At the time of discharge, all patients and/or a family member are asked to complete an anonymous survey regarding their satisfaction with the program, as well as suggestions for program improvement. The HELP team reviews this information regularly, and program modifications based on this feedback are implemented.

Ongoing Program Quality Improvement

The ethos of HELP is ongoing quality improvement based on all the checks and balances above, as well as feedback from patients, families, nurses, physicians, and hospital administration. During an annual reporting process, HELP tracks clinical and cost outcomes. Programmatic improvement efforts also focus on continuous improvement in achieving targeted outcomes (see Table 2.3).

Strategies to Improve Adherence

The HELP program's effectiveness depends on adherence to the intervention protocols. Complete adherence is defined as a patient receiving all parts of the assigned protocol for the number of times it was designated to be given. In a previous study [20], adherence had a significant independent protective effect against delirium (adjusted OR = 0.69, 95 % CI 0.56–0.87). Higher adherence to HELP interventions was associated with lower delirium rates. In fact, for the highest adherence group, the delirium rate was only 2.9 % (89 % risk reduction). The major reasons for non-adherence were lack of availability of staff or volunteers (32 %), patient refusal (26 %), medical contraindication (22 %), and patient unavailability (13 %) [6].

Table 2.3 Effectiveness of HELP for clinical outcomes

Reference	Sample size	Rate in HELP	Rate in controls	Improvement with HELP
Incidence of Delirium				
Caplan and Harper [10]	37	6 %	38 %	32 %
Chen et al. [9]	179	0 %	17 %	17 %
Inouye et al. [6]	852	10 %	15 %	5 %
Rubin et al. [11]	704	26 %	41 %	15 %
Rubin et al. [8]	>7,000	18 %	41 %	23 %
Zaubler et al. [12]	595	12 %	20 %	8 %
Falls				
Babine et al. [13]	158	2.5/1,000 pt-dy	5.2/1,000 pt-dy	52 % reduction
Caplan and Harper [10]	37	6 %	19 %	13 %
Inouye et al. [14]	–	2 %	4 %	2 %
Length of stay				
Caplan and Harper [10]	37	5.3 days	6.0 days	0.7 days
Chen et al. [9]	179	17.4 days	19.4 days	2.0 days
Inouye et al. [6]	852	8.4 days	8.0 days	0.4 days
Rubin et al. [11]	704	–	–	0.3 days
Rubin et al. [8]	>7,000	22.5 days	26.8 days	4.3 days
Zaubler et al. [12]	595	5.2 days	7.4 days	2.2 days
Cognitive decline				
Chen et al. [9]	179	2 %	5 %	3 %
Inouye et al. [4]	1,507	8 %	26 %	18 %
Functional decline				
Chen et al. [15]	189	19 %	65 %	46 %
Inouye et al. [4]	1,507	14 %	33 %	19 %
Institutionalization				
Leslie et al. [16]	801	241 days	280 days	14 % reduction
Caplan and Harper [10]	37	25 %	48 %	23 %
Sitter use				
Caplan and Harper [10]	37	330 h	644 h	49 % reduction

A target goal for each hospital is to provide 7 days per week coverage and to meet a minimum of 80 % adherence with HELP interventions.

Guiding Principle

Coverage by staff for weekends, volunteer absenteeism and vacations needs to be built into the program. The HELP staff is ultimately responsible for completion of all interventions.

General Strategies

1. The HELP staff and experienced volunteers work staggered shifts to provide evening, weekend, and holiday coverage.
2. Increase staff interactions with complex or special needs patients.

3. Patient/family education strategies: Review goals of interventions and clarify importance of interventions with patient/family to gain their engagement.
4. If observed by HELP staff or experienced volunteers, patients can walk or exercise alone or with family or visitors.
5. Train and encourage family participation in interventions, including orientation, therapeutic activities, mobility, feeding, and fluid repletion.
6. Enlist support of physicians and nursing staff to encourage patient participation.

Volunteer-Related Strategies

1. Ongoing recruitment and quarterly training sessions with volunteers to assure all shifts are filled and adequately covered.
2. Ensure volunteer absence coverage:
   - Schedule at least two volunteers per shift to allow for volunteer absences.

- Develop list of available on-call volunteers to fill in.
- Volunteers call each other to arrange coverage.
- Provide volunteer training to deal with refusals or complex patients.
3. Stress the importance of completing all assigned interventions in training and newsletters.
4. Ensure volunteers are well-educated regarding the importance of their interventions.
5. Ongoing volunteer performance reviews and training to handle challenging situations.

HELP Outcomes

Before initiating a HELP program, hospitals are encouraged to obtain baseline rates of outcomes considered to be important at their sites for a three-month period (see below). One year after successful implementation, outcomes should be measured again and then yearly thereafter. The types of outcomes tracked will need to be customized at each hospital, and ideally should be: (1) important to the hospital leadership; (2) routinely tracked as part of HELP procedures; or (3) feasible to collect from other hospital sources. It is recommended that an annual report be presented to the hospital leadership with numbers of patients served, clinical outcomes, patient satisfaction results, and potential cost savings. Such ongoing reporting may be critical to program sustainability. It is important to note that new HELP programs need to allow adequate time, at least 12–18 months, to realize clinical benefits and cost savings.

Tracking outcomes requires careful planning and ongoing data collection. To collect delirium rates, brief cognitive screening (such as with the Short Portable Mental Status Questionnaire [21] or Mini-Cog [22]) followed by the Confusion Assessment Method (CAM) [23] or another validated delirium instrument is required. The five leading outcomes that were tracked across 13 HELP sites in a previous study [19] were use of physical restraints (92 % of sites), falls (92 %), delirium (85 %), use of sitters (85 %), and LOS (85 %). Despite their importance, only 31 % of sites were able to track hospital costs. The major obstacle is that accurate tracking of costs at the patient level requires data from hospital fiscal services or Medicare, expertise in cost analyses, and typically external funding.

Potential Outcomes to be Tracked at HELP Sites

Process Measures
1. Total number of patients enrolled per year
2. Total number of volunteers and volunteer-hours per year
3. Total number of HELP interventions conducted per year
4. Adherence rates with interventions (overall and by type)

5. Intermediary variables: use of Foley catheters, polypharmacy or use of Beers criteria medications, iatrogenic complication rates

Clinical Outcomes
1. Delirium: prevalent and incident
2. Falls
3. Use of physical restraints
4. Use of bed alarms
5. Length of stay
6. Nursing home placement
7. Patient of family satisfaction scores
8. Decline on cognitive testing
9. Decline in basic activities of daily living (admission to discharge)
10. Decline in instrumental activities of daily living (admission to discharge)
11. Hospital and post-hospital cost savings
12. Nurse retention or satisfaction scores
13. Aide retention or satisfaction scores
14. Pressure ulcers
15. Catheter-associated urinary tract infections
16. Malnutrition
17. Immobility
18. Pain management
19. Constipation
20. Use of sitters (constant companions)
21. Incident reports or legal actions
22. 30-day mortality rate
23. 30-day readmissions rate

Evidence for Efficacy and Cost-Effectiveness

Efficacy Studies

Over the past 15 years, at least ten studies (Table 2.3) have documented the efficacy of HELP for prevention of delirium, falls, decreasing length of stay, functional decline, cognitive decline, institutionalization, and use of sitters (constant companions). The efficacy of HELP for prevention of incident delirium is well-established in at least six studies [6, 8–12] with the absolute risk reduction ranging from 5 to 32 %. HELP has also been documented to decrease the rate and duration of prevalent delirium [8, 11, 12]. In three studies, HELP reduced the incidence of falls by a 2–13 % absolute reduction [10, 13, 14]. Six studies demonstrated that length of stay was consistently 0.3–4.3 days shorter with HELP [6, 8–12]. Reduced rates of cognitive and functional decline/frailty have been demonstrated in three previous studies [4, 9, 15]. Institutionalization has been examined in two studies. In one study of 801 patients, HELP did not impact the rate of institutionalization following discharge; however,

Table 2.4 Documented cost savings with HELP

Reference	Sample size	Cost savings[a]
Zaubler et al. [12]	595	>$1.1 million per year in hospital costs, >$2,700 per patient
Rubin et al. [8]	>7,000	>$7.3 million per year in hospital costs, > $1,480 per patient
Rizzo et al. [17]	852	$1,187 per person-year in hospital costs
Leslie et al. [16]	801	$13,489 per person-year in nursing home costs
Caplan and Harper [10]	111	$162,696 per year in hospital sitter costs

[a]Adjusted for 2014 US dollars

receiving the HELP intervention significantly reduced the probability and duration of long-term nursing home stays [16]. In another small study, Caplan and Harper [10] demonstrated a 23 % reduction in the rate of institutionalization after discharge. Only one study specifically examined sitter use, and demonstrated a nearly 50 % reduction in sitter hours required with HELP [10].

Cost-Effectiveness Studies

The HELP program has proven cost-effectiveness (Table 2.4), saving hospital costs of between $1,187 and 2,700 per person per hospitalization [8, 12, 17], decreasing long-term nursing home costs by $13,489 per person-year [16] and saving $162,696 per year in sitter costs per hospital unit [10] (estimates adjusted to 2014 USD). HELP has been estimated to save over $7.3 million per year at one hospital [8]. If HELP were implemented in one-half of US hospitals, the savings to the health-care system would amount to over $18 billion per year [18]. Since HELP reduces total costs across the continuum of care, the program has been adopted in many capitated health-care systems and poses potential advantages for accountable care organizations or models that assume more global risk for health care.

Challenges to Implementation

Challenges in Starting a Program

With its innovative, interdisciplinary approach, establishing HELP can require transformation of organizational culture. One study involving 58 interviews with 32 HELP staff at nine sites identified common challenges in initiating a new HELP program [24]. The common challenges are identified below.
- Gain internal support for HELP from clinical and administrative leaders
- Ensure effective clinician leadership with at least one program champion
- Integrate HELP with existing geriatric programs

- Maintain program fidelity as much as possible to assure effectiveness
- Document and publicize positive outcomes locally
- Realize that the program must shift organizational culture to transform care

Challenges in Sustaining HELP

To identify factors required to sustain a program, a subsequent qualitative study [25] involved 102 interviews with 42 HELP staff across 13 sites. This study identified the success factors for sustaining HELP at least 12 months after its implementation. Three critical elements for sustaining HELP appear below.
- Ensuring effective clinician champions and senior leadership support
- Adapting program to local circumstances while maintaining key HELP principles
- Obtaining long-term resources and funding through the hospital operating budget

Surviving in Difficult Economic Times

HELP is facing an extremely challenging fiscal environment with tremendous scrutiny and cost-cutting across all clinical programs. In 62 interviews across 19 successful HELP sites, qualitative interviews were conducted with HELP staff and hospital administrators to probe successful strategies to justify the program and secure long-term funding for continued operations. These strategies are presented below.

Challenges for Surviving in Difficult Economic Times
- Interact meaningfully with decision-makers in formal meetings and informal settings
- Document success with metrics that resonate with decision-makers
- Garner support from influential hospital staff at all levels (physicians, nurses, administration, support services)

Learning from Closure of Operational Sites

Between 2006 and 2011, six fully operational HELP sites closed. A qualitative study was conducted involving 14 staff and hospital administrators at these six sites [26]. The major problems underpinning site closure involved two interrelated areas: the financial crisis of 2008 and/or restructuring at the hospital or health system level. The major themes were identified below.

- Crisis created new vulnerabilities:
  - Restructuring with loss of champions ⇒ multiple champions required
  - Demand for immediate revenue-generation ⇒ document cost-effectiveness
- Crisis exacerbated underlying vulnerabilities:
  - Insufficient support by hospital staff ⇒ Engage physician and nursing leaders
  - Program not widely known ⇒ Publicize the program
  - Program not believed to be important ⇒ Demonstrate program's effectiveness and report outcomes to hospital leadership at least annually

The HELP Dissemination Process

HELP represents an effective translation of scientific evidence into clinical practice. The process of dissemination is supported by dissemination materials and website (www. hospitalelderlifeprogram.org), a dedicated dissemination team, a virtual community, and national meetings. The HELP dissemination materials include program manuals, business tools, training videotapes or compact discs. The materials facilitate simple and consistent implementation, low start-up costs, and consistent performance. The business tools include an executive summary, power point presentation, data collection questionnaire, and customizable financial spreadsheets. These tools are intended to provide an initial approach to evaluate patient volume, staffing needs, volunteer needs, and potential cost savings at the hospital. Sites can receive support, training, and site visits from HELP Centers of Excellence, nine experienced sites who represent HELP master-trainers. Other sources of support for HELP sites include an on-line discussion forum (Google groups) to enhance exchange of information, annual HELP conferences, twice-yearly HELP Special Interest Groups at the American Geriatrics Society and Gerontological Society of America Annual Meetings, and electronic and telephone support from the central HELP Dissemination Team.

Support for the HELP Dissemination Process

- HELP website (www.hospitalelderlifeprogram.org)
- Program materials (how-to guides), training manuals, video tapes, business tools

- HELP Centers of Excellence, experienced master-trainer sites
- Central HELP dissemination team
- HELP Google Groups, virtual on-line community
- HELP Annual Conference and Special Interest Groups and national meetings (3/year)

Feasibility of Family Participation

Family participation has been an important part of the HELP program since its inception. All of the volunteer protocols have been adapted for use by family members; however, they are intended to be used in conjunction with training and supervision by the HELP staff in the hospital setting. Thus, they are not designed for use by family members outside the context of a HELP program. Family members (who have received training) are encouraged to continue their activities after hospital discharge.

A previous study tested the feasibility of the Family-HELP Program (FAM-HELP), an adaptation that included a subset of the HELP volunteer protocols (orientation, therapeutic activities, early mobilization, vision, and hearing protocols). For this study, 15 family caregivers were trained by the HELP geriatric nurse or geriatrician [27], and engagement of family caregivers in these preventive interventions was demonstrated to be feasible and acceptable. Outcomes were not tracked in this pilot study. It should be noted that FAM-HELP is only recommended for use in the context of a HELP program and careful training of family members is required.

Integration of HELP with Other Geriatric Models of Care

In the current environment of accountable care and horizontal health-care delivery, HELP is a particularly relevant model that effectively integrates multiple disciplines, brings hands-on expertise to the bedside, improves outcomes and reduces costs [28]. Thus, incorporation of HELP into the portfolio of strategies hospitals can use to address the multifaceted needs of older adults should be considered. HELP fills an important niche and is highly complementary to many other geriatric models of care (such as specialized geriatric units or geriatric nursing programs), with which it frequently coexists.

Acute Care for Elders (ACE) [29, 30] and Geriatric Evaluation and Management (GEM) [31–33] units provide prepared environments, specially trained interdisciplinary staff, and geriatric care protocols which can optimize care for older hospitalized adults. However, they can only serve a small proportion of older patients at a given hospital and often do not have the staffing to provide the hands-on bedside care provided by HELP. Thus, over a third of current HELP sites coexist with ACE units. HELP is also strengthened by the existence of strong geriatric nursing expertise, and often coexists with Nurses Improving Care for Healthsystem Elders (NICHE) [34] and Geriatric Recourse Nurse programs. Many HELP hospitals have achieved Magnet status or commendations from the Joint Commission on Accreditation of Healthcare Organizations (JCAHO) based on their HELP models. HELP programs are currently exploring use of the ACE Tracker system, a computer-based system [34] that consolidates information from multiple areas of the electronic medical record to identify geriatric risk factors for functional decline and poor outcomes. The ACE Tracker would greatly facilitate screening of high-risk patients for HELP and tracking outcomes of interest.

Summary

The HELP model fulfills the triple aim of improved healthcare quality and patient satisfaction, improved health outcomes for the older population, and reduced per capita costs. The care of acutely ill hospitalized older persons is inherently complex, and necessitates multicomponent care with several geriatric models of care operating in a coordinated fashion. With its broad nature, extending from bedside care with volunteers and a skilled interdisciplinary team to creating coordinated high-value health care within an organization, HELP often provides the scaffolding on which a comprehensive geriatric health-care model can be built.

HELP is a successful program that provides high quality, high value geriatric acute care overall, with benefits that extend far beyond the goal of delirium prevention. Under the Medicare fee-for-service program, HELP will remain a sustainable geriatric model of care, yet it is particularly well suited for the accountable care and value-based purchasing environment where hospitals and health systems assume greater risks of health care. This is due in part to the well-demonstrated cost-effectiveness of HELP with cost-savings of over $13,000 per patient-year extending well beyond the acute hospital episode, as well as improved health outcomes, including reducing delirium incidence and duration, decreasing falls, length of hospital stay, institutionalization, functional and cognitive decline. HELP has been demonstrated to be sustainable in difficult economic climates. To date, HELP has been implemented in hundreds of hospitals worldwide, improving geriatric care on a wide scale. Thus, the HELP model provides an effective means to improve the quality and effectiveness of hospital care for older persons and prepares our health care system to cope with our rapidly aging society.

Acknowledgments This work is dedicated to the memory of Joshua Bryan Inouye Helfand and Bradley Yoshio Inouye. We gratefully acknowledge the HELP Dissemination Team (Shin-Yi Lao, Asha Albuquerque, Eva Schmitt, Dulce Pina), HELP Advisory Board and Centers of Excellence, dedicated clinicians and staff members at all the HELP sites, and the patients and family members that we serve. Grazie mille!

Grant Funding
This report was supported in part by Grants No. K07AG041835 (SKI) and T32AG000158 (TTH) from the National Institute on Aging, Grant No. 2013-87 from the Retirement Research Foundation (SKI), the Irma and Paul Milstein Program for Senior Health (JY, SKI), and the Hospital Elder Life Program. Dr. Inouye holds the Milton and Shirley F. Levy Family Chair.

References

1. Creditor MC. Hazards of hospitalization of the elderly. Ann Intern Med. 1993;118(3):219–23.
2. Detsky AS, Krumholz HM. Reducing the trauma of hospitalization. JAMA. 2014;311(21):2169–70.
3. Inouye SK, Westendorp RG, Saczynski JS. Delirium in elderly people. Lancet. 2014;383(9920):911–22.
4. Inouye SK, Bogardus Jr ST, Baker DI, Leo-Summers L, Cooney Jr LM. The Hospital Elder Life Program: a model of care to prevent cognitive and functional decline in older hospitalized patients. Hospital Elder Life Program. J Am Geriatr Soc. 2000;48(12):1697–706.
5. Witlox J, Eurelings LS, de Jonghe JF, Kalisvaart KJ, Eikelenboom P, van Gool WA. Delirium in elderly patients and the risk of postdischarge mortality, institutionalization, and dementia: a meta-analysis. JAMA. 2010;304(4):443–51.
6. Inouye SK, Bogardus Jr ST, Charpentier PA, Leo-Summers L, Acampora D, Holford TR, et al. A multicomponent intervention to prevent delirium in hospitalized older patients. N Engl J Med. 1999;340(9):669–76.
7. National Clinical Guideline Centre. Delirium: diagnosis, prevention and management (full guideline). Published July 2010. www.nice.org.uk/nicemedia/live/13060/49908/49908.pdf. Accessed 3 May 2011
8. Rubin FH, Neal K, Fenlon K, Hassan S, Inouye SK. Sustainability and scalability of the hospital elder life program at a community hospital. J Am Geriatr Soc. 2011;59(2):359–65.
9. Chen CC-H, Lin M-T, Tien Y-W, Yen C-J, Huang G-H, Inouye SK. Modified hospital elder life program: effects on abdominal surgery patients. J Am Coll Surg. 2011;213(2):245–52.
10. Caplan G, Harper E. Recruitment of volunteers to improve vitality in the elderly: the REVIVE* study. Intern Med J. 2007;37(2):95–100.
11. Rubin FH, Williams JT, Lescisin DA, Mook WJ, Hassan S, Inouye SK. Replicating the Hospital Elder Life Program in a community hospital and demonstrating effectiveness using quality improvement methodology. J Am Geriatr Soc. 2006;54(6):969–74.
12. Zaubler TS, Murphy K, Rizzuto L, Santos R, Skotzko C, Giordano J, et al. Quality improvement and cost savings with multicomponent delirium interventions: replication of the Hospital Elder Life Program in a community hospital. Psychosomatics. 2013;54(3):219–26.
13. Babine RL, Farrington S, Wierman HR. HELP(c) prevent falls by preventing delirium. Nursing. 2013;43(5):18–21.
14. Inouye SK, Brown CJ, Tinetti ME. Medicare nonpayment, hospital falls, and unintended consequences. N Engl J Med. 2009;360(23):2390–3.
15. Chen CC, Chen CN, Lai IR, Huang GH, Saczynski JS, Inouye SK. Effects of a modified Hospital Elder Life Program on frailty in individuals undergoing major elective abdominal surgery. J Am Geriatr Soc. 2014;62(2):261–8.

16. Leslie DL, Zhang Y, Bogardus ST, Holford TR, Leo-Summers LS, Inouye SK. Inouye SK Consequences of preventing delirium in hospitalized older adults on nursing home costs. J Am Geriatr Soc. 2005;53(3):405–9.

17. Rizzo JA, Bogardus Jr ST, Leo-Summers L, Williams CS, Acampora D, Inouye SK. Multicomponent targeted intervention to prevent delirium in hospitalized older patients: what is the economic value? Med Care. 2001;39(7):740–52.

18. Leslie DL, Marcantonio ER, Zhang Y, Leo-Summers L, Inouye SK. One-year health care costs associated with delirium in the elderly population. Arch Intern Med. 2008;168(1):27–32.

19. Inouye SK, Baker DI, Fugal P, Bradley EH. Dissemination of the hospital elder life program: implementation, adaptation, and successes. J Am Geriatr Soc. 2006;54(10):1492–9.

20. Inouye SK, Bogardus Jr ST, Williams CS, Leo-Summers L, Agostini JV. The role of adherence on the effectiveness of nonpharmacologic interventions: evidence from the delirium prevention trial. Arch Intern Med. 2003;163(8):958–64.

21. Pfeiffer E. A short portable mental status questionnaire for the assessment of organic brain deficit in elderly patients. J Am Geriatr Soc. 1975;23(10):433–41.

22. Borson S, Scanlan J, Brush M, Vitaliano P, Dokmak A. The minicog: a cognitive 'vital signs' measure for dementia screening in multi-lingual elderly. Int J Geriatr Psychiatry. 2000;15(11):1021–7.

23. Inouye SK, van Dyck CH, Alessi CA, Balkin S, Siegal AP, Horwitz RI. Clarifying confusion: the confusion assessment method. A new method for detection of delirium. Ann Intern Med. 1990;113(12):941–8.

24. Bradley EH, Schlesinger M, Webster TR, Baker D, Inouye SK. Translating research into clinical practice: making change happen. J Am Geriatr Soc. 2004;52(11):1875–82.

25. Bradley EH, Webster TR, Baker D, Schlesinger M, Inouye SK. After adoption: sustaining the innovation. A case study of disseminating the hospital elder life program. J Am Geriatr Soc. 2005;53(9):1455–61.

26. SteelFisher GK, Martin LA, Dowal SL, Inouye SK. Learning from the closure of clinical programs: a case series from the Hospital Elder Life Program. J Am Geriatr Soc. 2013;61(6):999–1004.

27. Rosenbloom-Brunton DA, Henneman EA, Inouye SK. Feasibility of family participation in a delirium prevention program for hospitalized older adults. J Gerontol Nurs. 2010;36(9):22–33.

28. Landefeld CS. Improving health care for older persons. Ann Intern Med. 2003;139(5 Pt 2):421–4.

29. Counsell SR, Holder CM, Liebenauer LL, Palmer RM, Fortinsky RH, Kresevic DM, et al. Effects of a multicomponent intervention on functional outcomes and process of care in hospitalized older patients: a randomized controlled trial of Acute Care for Elders (ACE) in a community hospital. J Am Geriatr Soc. 2000;48(12):1572–81.

30. Fox MT, Persaud M, Maimets I, O'Brien K, Brooks D, Tregunno D, et al. Effectiveness of acute geriatric unit care using acute care for elders components: a systematic review and meta-analysis. J Am Geriatr Soc. 2012;60(12):2237–45.

31. Cohen HJ, Feussner JR, Weinberger M, Carnes M, Hamdy RC, Hsieh F, et al. A controlled trial of inpatient and outpatient geriatric evaluation and management. N Engl J Med. 2002;346(12):905–12.

32. Rao AV, Hsieh F, Feussner JR, Cohen HJ. Geriatric evaluation and management units in the care of the frail elderly cancer patient. J Gerontol A Biol Sci Med Sci. 2005;60(6):798–803.

33. Van Craen K, Braes T, Wellens N, Denhaerynck K, Flamaing J, Moons P, et al. The effectiveness of inpatient geriatric evaluation and management units: a systematic review and meta-analysis. J Am Geriatr Soc. 2010;58(1):83–92.

34. Malone ML, Vollbrecht M, Stephenson J, Burke L, Pagel P, Goodwin JS. Acute Care for Elders (ACE) tracker and e-Geriatrician: methods to disseminate ACE concepts to hospitals with no geriatricians on staff. J Am Geriatr Soc. 2010;58(1):161–7.

The Acute Care for Elders Consult Program

3

William W. Hung, Jonny A. Macias Tejada, Soryal Soryal, Saima T. Akbar, and Ella Harvey Bowman

Acute Care for Elders: Background and Introduction

Older adults, the fastest growing segment of the United States (US) population, often suffer from multiple chronic diseases and are more prone to acute illnesses. They also account for a disproportionately high number of acute care admissions and hospital days. While older adults aged 65 and older constitute only about 15 % of the total US population, they currently account for about 43 % of inpatient hospital days and are responsible for more than 50 % of total hospital expenditures. The US Census Bureau predicts that we will continue to witness a tremendous growth in our population of older adults over the next several decades, so that by 2050 the number of Americans aged 65 and older is projected to be 88.5 million, more than double the population of 40.2 million reported in 2010. Hence, this particular population plays a vitally important role in the fiscal outcomes for individual acute care hospitals as well as for our entire national healthcare climate [1].

Older adults are particularly vulnerable to adverse events during and immediately following hospitalization for acute medical problems, including pressure ulcers, falls, hospital-acquired infections, functional decline, institutionalization, and early readmission to the hospital after discharge. Furthermore, for many elderly hospitalized patients who often have multiple chronic comorbid conditions and geriatric syndromes, the period of time following hospitalization can be hallmarked by an overwhelming flurry of often confusing changes for the patient, their caregiver(s), and all of their healthcare providers involved across the care continuum. A widely utilized measure of hospitals' successful care transitions for patients is the 30-day readmission rate. A study of 2004 Medicare claims data revealed that nearly 20 % of discharged beneficiaries were rehospitalized within 30 days; 34 % were rehospitalized within 90 days. Half of patients discharged back to the community and rehospitalized within 30 days lacked a documented follow-up visit with their primary care physician (PCP) prior to rehospitalization. The authors estimated that the cost to Medicare for these unplanned readmissions in 2004 was $17.4 billion [2]. To help address these and many other challenges of caring for older adults in acute care settings, geriatric consultative services have gradually evolved over the past two decades as a resource for busy clinicians spanning the various medical specialties in order to better manage the patients they have admitted.

Such geriatric consult services historically have aimed to assist in the care of elders hospitalized in various inpatient sites throughout the hospital, spanning medical, surgical and other specialty units. As an example, geriatric consultative services might be considered when an elderly patient with known dementia is admitted to the hospital after falling and sustaining a hip fracture. The geriatric consultant in this case would be called by the orthopedic and/or possibly the anesthesia team for evaluation prior to or immediately following surgery to assist with managing pain, potential postoperative delirium, and helping with identifying potential needs at the time of discharge such as rehabilitation plans. Other possible scenarios might include the elderly patient in the Cardiac Intensive Care Unit who has developed confusion after suffering a myocardial event, or assisting in the management of a patient admitted on the medicine service for weight loss,

W.W. Hung, M.D., M.P.H.
Brookdale Department of Geriatrics and Palliative Medicine, James J Peters VA Medical Center, Geriatric Research, Education and Clinical Center, Icahn School of Medicine at Mount Sinai, New York, NY, USA

J.A.M. Tejada, M.D. • S.T. Akbar, M.D.
University of Wisconsin School of Medicine and Public Health, Aurora St. Luke's Medical Center, Milwaukee, WI, USA

S. Soryal, M.D.
Aurora West Allis Medical Center and University of Wisconsin School of Medicine and Public Health, Milwaukee, WI, USA

E.H. Bowman, M.D., Ph.D. (✉)
Department of Medicine, Sidney & Lois Eskenazi Hospital, Indiana University School of Medicine, Indianapolis, IN, USA
e-mail: elbowman@iu.edu

anorexia, and inability to care for self, whereby the geriatrics consult team is called in to assist with assessment, identification of underlying reasons leading to the presenting findings, and helping to address specific goals of care along with an individualized care plan. All three of the above scenarios present significantly different needs of the patients and also of the consulting providers, and yet in all cases the geriatrician can help guide the clinician who may have little education on the management of older adults, ultimately helping to provide care that is both appropriate and sensitive to older adult patients' needs, while making care safer and more effective.

Acute Care for Elders (ACE), also initially described as "the ACE Unit," is a direct outgrowth of the maturation of the prototypical inpatient geriatrics consult service. A patient-centered model of care tailored to promote independent function and ease the return to home while preventing functional decline, ACE is an evidence-based systematic process of patient care, serving to improve the management of acutely ill hospitalized older adults while avoiding unnecessary procedures and medications which might have detrimental outcomes in the older person [3]. ACE was specifically designed at the outset to address the unique needs of acutely ill elders from the moment of admission to the hospital. This concept has been integrated into a physical unit, "the ACE Unit," in many hospitals across the nation, and has been seen as a sentinel step for improving the care of older adults. The archetypal ACE Unit was a specific medical-surgical ward in the hospital specifically selected, where an interdisciplinary team of geriatrics-trained professionals transformed the environment with modifications designed with the unique needs of elderly patients in mind [3]. For instance, the physical environment of the ACE Unit was designed with special flooring, lighting, and noise control to maximize patient independence while avoiding iatrogenic complications such as delirium and falls. The entire atmosphere was designed to allay the often disorienting and depersonalizing hospital environment to promote a more home-like experience, from geometric carpeting to decrease noise, enhance distance perception and encourage ambulation, to the careful placement of calendars and clocks to promote orientation. Everything from the walls and ceilings to the lighting and furniture was carefully selected with the older adult in mind, recognizing the prevalence of sensory impairment in this population. Care on the ACE Unit was designed to be highly patient-centered, with nursing-implemented protocols promoting self-care; recognition of physical, cognitive, and psychosocial functional needs early on; and implementation of comprehensive discharge planning utilizing vigilant daily medical care review that begins right from the day of admission. Over the last two decades the concept of the ACE Unit has taken on many shapes and sizes, morphing and accommodating to fit the unique needs and environment of every type of inpatient acute hospital setting. As such, the concept

of "ACE" has expanded beyond that of a dedicated, physical unit, to now involve the use of "virtual" and/or "mobile" consult teams that still address those very same core nursing-based principles of the original ACE Unit, but often in a very different environment that no longer is limited by the walls of a unit, and as described below, may not even exist within the confines of a single structure at all, as in the case of "ACE Tracker" and other completely electronic database-designed ACE teams that are improving the care of hospitalized older adults often with many miles separating the patient and the actual team. From here on out, the term "ACE" will be used in reference to *all formats* of the ACE Model, not just the prototypical ACE Unit, unless otherwise specified.

The Dysfunctional Syndrome, the ACE Prehabilitation Model, and the ACE Interdisciplinary Team

Despite appropriate treatment for the acute illness necessitating hospitalization, older adults are vulnerable to developing significant hospital acquired disability which includes delirium, depression, pressure ulcers, falls, and generalized functional decline, all of which can have both immediate but most importantly long-term consequences including nursing home placement, permanent functional impairment, and increased mortality. These untoward outcomes ultimately lead to increased cost to the patient, the family/caregivers, and our society. For instance, about one-third of elderly adults who survive hospital discharge on a medicine service will die in the year following discharge [4], and the same proportion of older adults will experience a decline in baseline function at discharge that will continue indefinitely, leading to one in five developing a new disability in the year following discharge [5]. Hence, although functional outcomes are typically not the focus of care during hospitalization, in the end especially for older adults they are often critical determinants of the quality of life, physical independence, cost of care, and prognosis. This hospital-acquired functional decline was initially conceptualized as "The Dysfunctional Syndrome," from which the multi-component ACE concept developed to address these adverse events by combining the principles of geriatric assessment with quality improvement to achieve better outcomes in older hospitalized adults [6].

The theoretical model of "The Dysfunctional Syndrome" relates to the often hostile environment in which an older patient may find oneself when admitted to the hospital: a functional older person enters the hospital with an acute illness, whereby cluttered hallways and tethers such as intravenous lines and cardiac telemetry wires discourage independent ambulation; poorly timed procedures and team rounds lead to sleep deprivation and even malnutrition from

Fig. 3.1 Conceptual model for how ACE can prevent hospitalization-associated disability (From Pierluissi E, Francis DC, Covinsky KE. Patient and hospital factors that lead to adverse outcomes in hospitalized elders. In: Malone M, Capezuti E, Palmer RM, editors. Acute care for elders—a model for interdisciplinary care. New York, NY: Springer Science and Business Media; 2014:21-47 with permission.)

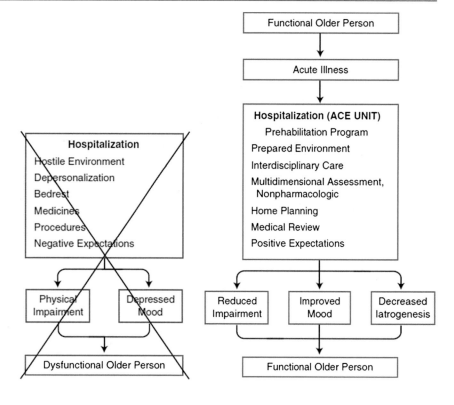

missing meals and prolonged NPO status; medications that are prescribed in inappropriate doses lead to serious adverse events such as delirium, falls, and further debility, all of which combine and lead to a dysfunctional adult at discharge who is unable to directly return to independent living. This further leads to depressed mood, negative expectations, and poor functional as well as deleterious medical outcomes. The ACE concept strives to prevent this detrimental cascade through the presence of a physical climate offering a "prehabilitation" program of patient-centered care fostering multidimensional assessment and careful medication reconciliation utilizing an interdisciplinary team linked with early discharge planning, whereby iatrogenic dysfunction is diminished, hope is maintained, and a functional older person emerges at the time of discharge to resume a normal productive life (Fig. 3.1) [6, 7].

The ACE Model was thus developed as a multi-component intervention specifically designed to address this hospital-acquired dysfunction, focusing on improving the management of acutely ill hospitalized older adults. ACE Consult Programs have been around since the 1990s, and implement specific practices targeting the comprehensive biopsychosocial and functional needs of the hospitalized older adult, starting at the moment of hospital admission. The four core principles of ACE include: (1) a prepared environment promoting mobility and orientation; (2) patient-centered care using nursing-initiated protocols for the promotion of inde-

pendence spanning self-care to assessment of mood and cognition; (3) multidimensional assessment linking nonpharmacologic recommendations with promotion of optimal medication prescribing; and (4) interdisciplinary team rounds linked with comprehensive discharge planning that begins the day of the initial consultation in order to optimize the eventual care transition from the hospital.

ACE Consult Team

Comprised of a geriatrician as well as nursing leaders working together to lead an interdisciplinary team that might include any combination of physical and/or occupational therapy, social services, geriatric pharmacy, and dietary services, ACE programs aim to preserve the function of hospitalized elders, minimize iatrogenic events, minimize the use of potentially inappropriate medications, and decrease the rate of discharges to nursing homes [8]. As already briefly described above, the original concept of ACE was embodied in a discreet physical location of the hospital known as "the ACE Unit," where the interdisciplinary team led by a geriatrician serving in a consultative role would review the plan of care and round daily on older adults hospitalized on the unit [3]. The typical process that evolved consists of the admitting physician contacting a point person on the ACE team to help evaluate and guide care for his/her most vulnerable seniors with complex medical and/or psychosocial needs. These needs might include the more commonly recognized geriatric functional syndromes as well as perhaps some less often appreciated conditions: delirium; depression and cognitive impairment; dizziness, syncope, falls and difficulty walking; generalized functional decline; incontinence and toileting needs; constipation; insomnia; malnutrition and weight loss; pressure ulcers; sensory impairment; and even helping to identify specific goals of care to assist with the eventual transition from hospital, which might require identifying a rehabilitation site aside from the patient's home. In some programs, these syndromes and conditions are made available to consulting teams as a list of "triggers" that might help them target patients who would benefit from ACE consultation. ACE consults in other settings might be directly facilitated by the ACE team themselves, through a process of case finding performed during daily interdisciplinary team rounds which might involve reviewing the hospital census to identify elderly patients in a certain age category, such as those over age 85 years.

Regardless of the method by which the ACE team receives consults, the standard consultation process has distinctive components performed by core team members that are fairly consistent across sites, often including any combination of the following disciplines: geriatrician, advanced practice nurse (APN), registered nurse (RN), medical social worker (MSW), case manager (either RN or SW as this role varies by facility), physical therapist (PT), occupational therapist (OT), pharmacy (PharmD), dietician, and pastoral care. Most core interdisciplinary ACE teams typically consist of at least a board-certified geriatrician along with any number of nursing leaders, such as an APN or Nurse Practitioner (NP) with specialized gerontological training who works together with the MD to lead the team. The Geriatrician's role is to coordinate the comprehensive evaluation of the patient's medical and geriatric functional issues as well as to conduct daily rounds which might have a heavy teaching component depending upon the setting (i.e., university or medical school-based vs. community-based hospital), whereas the role of the APN is typically to organize and help lead interdisciplinary rounds, assist in the assessment of complex cases, and to help educate all nursing and interdisciplinary staff about geriatric matters. The ACE team's RN, sometimes given the title of "ACE Resource Nurse," has the vital role of conducting prompt bedside assessment of the patient's physical, cognitive, and emotional status, communicating this information to the attending physician, and monitoring the patient for ongoing safety issues such as recognizing the use (and recommending the discontinuation) of unnecessary tethers such as Foley catheters. After comprehensive bedside assessment, the RN further assists the team's efforts by implementing nursing based protocols designed to address specific geriatric functional syndromes. When the role of the

RN includes that of Case Manager, the ACE nurse also performs utilization management and coordinates discharge planning for each patient seen by the interdisciplinary team, all the while making sure the primary (admitting) team is apprised of the most updated recommendations to assure a smooth care transition. Some programs also have a Medical Social Worker (MSW) who further assists in collecting a comprehensive psychosocial history, helps with completion of Advance Directives, and might assist nursing in coordinating referrals to post-discharge sites of care such as skilled rehabilitation. The specific tasks will likely vary according to the composition of the ACE team and the needs of the hospital.

In addition to nursing and social services, the therapists and pharmacist are also essential members of the core ACE team. Physical, occupational, and sometimes even speech therapy are core team members who assist in the comprehensive geriatric functional evaluation and help guide the team regarding disposition, safety recommendations, and other highly practical information such as recommending specific durable medical equipment from which the patient will benefit. In addition to providing their opinions on the best discharge level of care and educating family members on safe transfers, devices, and overall home safety, physical therapy assists in evaluating patients for mobility problems and addresses the need for any devices to ultimately prevent functional decline, while occupational therapy focuses on the assessment of patient self-care skills and any necessary treatment needed to address specific debilities encountered. The pharmacist will typically have specific geriatric training and plays a critical role in completing comprehensive medication reconciliation on all new consults as well as performs a daily medication review on patients who have already received consultation, assisting the team in making appropriate recommendations which take into account the Beers List as well as trying to minimize polypharmacy. The Pharmacist might even serve the important role of assisting the geriatrician as a team teacher, especially if there are medical trainees and other learners on the team. Some ACE teams also include a nutritionist or dietician who will monitor the patient for weight changes as well as identify any unique dietary needs. A special geriatric focus of a dietician includes educating patients and caregivers about nutritional requirements for specific conditions or need for special diets (such as low fat or sodium restriction), and helping provide all medical personnel with recommendations for improving the patient's oral intake. Dieticians therefore also play a very important role in the hospital setting by advocating for patients by helping to recognize and hopefully avoid prolonged lengths of time when the patient might not be allowed to eat: for planned necessary testing, for suspected oropharyngeal dysphagia, and other conditions where an older adult might be admitted with *nil* per os status ("NPO") and rendered unable to eat for sometimes days until planned testing or evaluation is

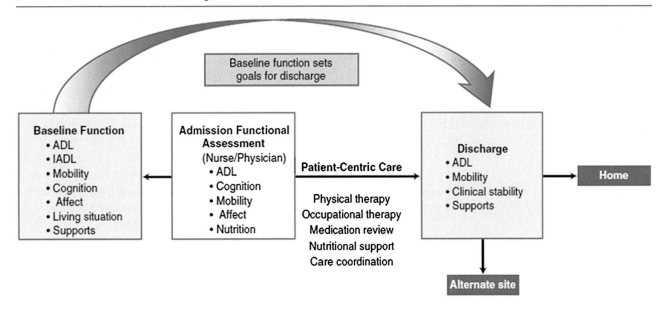

Fig. 3.2 Clinical pathway: the functional trajectory. *ADL* activities of daily living, *IADL* instrumental activities of daily living (From Palmer RM. Acute hospital care: future directions. In: Yoshikawa TT, Norman DC, editors. Acute emergencies and critical care of the geriatric patient. New York, NY: Marcel Dekker Inc; 2000:461-86 with permission.)

completed. The presence of pastoral care on a team assists through ministering to the spiritual needs of patients and families to help provide comprehensive, "total" care. Hence, the core ACE team might ultimately consist of over a half dozen individuals, all working together to develop a personalized and comprehensive plan of care for each patient seen. If a specific member is not included on the team in a particular healthcare system, it is critically important that such professionals are identified within the hospital and that they work closely with the ACE team to create a successful and comprehensive consult service whose ultimate focus is on helping transition of the patient from hospital to the safest site possible that maximizes the functional, medical, and personal care needs—ideally, back to the patient's home (Fig. 3.2) [6].

Given the sheer number of experts comprising the core ACE team, it is not surprising that ACE consultations are by nature comprehensive, detailed, and patient-centric. Collaboration between the interdisciplinary team members, and furthermore excellent communication of the team's recommendations to the consulting primary team, is critically important for a successful outcome. This interdisciplinary team collaboration is a hallmark that makes ACE consultation stand out from most other specialties and services, and even more unique in that it allows all team members to weigh in evenly in regard to the care of the patient, much unlike most modern medical teams that are organized in a physician-lead hierarchy. While the geriatrician is typically the leader of the ACE team, helping to energize and lead by example in providing excellent and passionate care for seniors, the

successful geriatrician, and in turn the successful team, will have recognized that the most comprehensive consultative recommendations are comprised with the collective input of the whole team, taking into account each member's unique skill sets, and also recognizing the specific needs and goals of the patient and the family/caregiver(s). Once the initial ACE consultation is completed, it is rather customary that the ACE team will continue to follow the patient daily throughout hospitalization in a consultancy role, while the primary (admitting) team remains the one driving the overall care and management of the patient. This is a broad generalization, and as such there are exceptions to this standard. For instance, for ACE teams who have their own nurse-case manager, the ACE team might take over the actual discharge disposition of the patient, such as coordinating post-discharge community-based services including home health and other assistance to help assure a safe and sound patient care transition. This disposition is typically activated only after the primary team initiates an order to start the actual discharge process.

Given the detailed and informative set of recommendations that typically develop from the interdisciplinary team approach during an ACE consult, documentation of the team's findings and suggestions for optimizing care is critical. It is as important that these recommendations be documented thoroughly as it is they be entered timely into the patient's chart to efficiently direct care and safety needs. As electronic medical records (EMRs) have developed and disseminated over the nation, like many other hospital-based services, ACE teams have also taken advantage of technology to develop tools varying from geriatric order sets to electronic triggers to even entire templates for documentation of the typically lengthy geriatric cognitive and functional assessments that result from interdisciplinary team member input. These electronic order sets, triggers, and templates vary greatly from setting to setting, for they can be easily adapted to meet the highly specialized and unique needs of every individual healthcare system where ACE has made its mark.

Challenges Faced by ACE Consult Programs

Given that the concept of the ACE team-facilitated comprehensive geriatrics assessment seems like a win-win for patient, family, nursing and other hospital staff, and medical teams themselves, it might be surprising that there are still inherent challenges to this model of care. Such challenges include at least three general themes which must be candidly addressed when developing an ACE Program in any setting: implementation rate of team recommendations, gaining hospital support to fund large (and sometimes even small) interdisciplinary teams, and the ongoing difficulties of maintaining and leading a team comprised of individuals with their own unique personalities, strengths, and weaknesses. For instance, for any consultation to be effective, the recommendations suggested by the consultant should be effectively communicated and ultimately implemented. The institution must therefore have the resources necessary to carry out the team's suggested recommendations in a timely fashion, whether this be various teams holding rounds that occur in physical proximity to each other, collaboration areas where inter-team communication can conveniently occur, an electronic medical record that supports expeditious sharing of recommendations in a format that is readily accessible to all involved in the care of the patient, or any combination thereof. In addition, the likelihood of consultant recommendations being readily implemented is also increased if the expectations of the consulting team are met through a limited number of concisely documented suggestions that are prioritized according to the most urgent needs at hand, versus a "laundry list" of recommendations spanning the alphabet. Other factors contributing to low adoption of the ACE team's recommendations include faulty communication, inappropriate timing, inadequate detail in the recommendations, difference in opinions, lost paperwork, and administrative or systems-based barriers [9].

The various barriers to implement a successful ACE Consult Model will naturally vary by institution, and might include availability of geriatrics-trained providers and personnel, accessibility of financial subsidy, and institutional backing from organizational leadership. Gaining hospital support and overall institutional buy-in is often the most significantly cited challenge to building and sustaining an inter-disciplinary ACE team. Some consulting physicians might be under the misconception that the ACE service is in effect the "discharge planning service." To address such misjudgments, geriatric consultation programs can assist in both formal and informal ongoing staff education about common geriatric syndromes as well as the many other direct measurables by which ACE can help consultants, and ultimately the entire hospital, meet its "bottom line," whether the driving impetus is decreasing early readmissions, cutting length of stay, or some other determinant. The ACE consultation service may even develop a role in educating specialty physicians who care for older patients, thus sustaining an important function in "geriatricizing" the whole hospital.

Maintaining any team comprised of individuals with their unique personalities, strengths, and weaknesses takes exceptional leadership, dedication, support, and a passionate vision for the team's mission. The ACE team is no different; a mature team that practices effective interdisciplinary communication can improve patient outcomes, prevent iatrogenic complications, and promote efficient transitions in care. That said, as disciplinary boundaries broaden and sometimes overlap, which is often necessary in providing comprehensive management of complex patients, there is the risk of "stepping on toes" and having team members who might have conflicting opinions about best approaches. The geriatrician who has sought additional skills in team management and conflict resolution will be especially adept at bringing out the very best of the team, valuing everyone's individual input, while assisting the team to arrive at its common goal of improved patient care.

ACE Consult Program: Evaluation Measures

Tracking basic outcomes to demonstrate the impact of the ACE consult model is of paramount importance to ensure that the model is well implemented, has a positive impact on patient outcomes, and assure future team sustainability. Researchers may track additional findings to demonstrate model impact, but this effort often necessitates additional resources that may not be available to the average clinician, clinical department, or hospital planning to adopt the model. Recent advances in information technology, electronic ordering and medical record systems may help mitigate some challenges in data collection, but there are still limitations. The primary challenge for every ACE consult team is to determine what outcomes are most essential to track for the purposes of improving the team's processes and outcomes that enable the delivery of the highest quality care to hospitalized elders. These measurable outcomes should also take into account what is necessary to demonstrate the team's impact to hospital administration so that future support for the interdisciplinary team can be sustained.

A list of measures that can be easily tracked to understand the processes and impact of the ACE consult service includes: volume of the service (daily, weekly or monthly census); data on the type of patients served including demographics; data on providers seeking consultation (what services primarily request ACE consults, what types of consult questions are posed, etc.); and the success/rate of implementation of consult recommendations. Tracking the actual implementation of recommendations suggested by the consultant team, however, is often a more difficult task. One way to analyze the number of recommendations which are ultimately executed by the consulting team is to take a sampling of consults performed, and track the consistency of implementation of recommendations. If the ACE team determines that implementation rate is suboptimal, then perhaps follow up consultation might be performed to investigate this gap, potentially enabling the team to develop strategies to enhance future uptake.

As with processes and team impact, patient outcomes can be similarly tracked, and might include any of the following: 30-day hospital readmission rates; length of stay for patients receiving ACE consultation; avoidance of adverse events during hospitalization; functional status of patients at baseline and at time of hospital discharge; patient satisfaction; and patient disposition/discharge location. Of all these measures, the 30-day readmission rate is currently one of the most heavily scrutinized measures of hospital performance, by which individual services, hospitals, and even entire healthcare systems are being compared. For the ACE consult team attempting to track readmission rates, it will be extremely important to consider how these data should be interpreted given that readmission rates, without an adequate comparison group, might not be very useful in demonstrating the impact of the ACE team. For example, an ACE team that achieves exceptional patient outcomes with decreased mortality might actually have *increased* readmissions, as patients with complex comorbid conditions will invariably have ongoing acute care needs. Attempts to avoid adverse hospital-acquired events might include demonstrating a reduction in the documented number of catheter-associated urinary tract infections, falls, pressure ulcers, restraints, and cases of delirium—many of which are already tracked on the hospital level. Functional status, often included in studies on older adults and geriatric models of care, can be measured using a number of instruments such as the Katz Index of Activities of Daily Living. However, this may be challenging to measure for all patients seen in ACE consultation, for it may include tracking additional data beyond the availability of team resources. To get around this limitation, a team might decide to track a surrogate marker of functional status such as rate of institutionalization at the time of discharge. Patient satisfaction utilizing standardized instruments is often already tracked at the hospital level using the Hospital

Consumer Assessment of Healthcare Providers and Systems survey (HCAHPS) and may therefore be an easier measure by which to demonstrate success. Regardless of which patient level measures an ACE team chooses to track, one important note is that outcome data might be very unhelpful in attempting to demonstrate the model's impact without a clearly and well defined comparison group. For instance, *with* an adequate comparison group, it will be possible to compare these outcomes and estimate the potential benefits of the ACE consult team. However, *without* a comparison group, these measures can still be tracked, but will likely be useful only in the sense of following trends for future quality improvement.

Studies have demonstrated improved clinical outcomes and cost savings from the ACE Unit model of care. More recent studies have also pointed toward the additional benefit of an ACE Model on care transitions. Flood et al. demonstrated lower costs and fewer all-cause rehospitalizations within 30 days for ACE Unit patients compared to similar patients cared for on a usual care unit [10]. Hung et al. describe a Mobile Acute Care for Elders (MACE) service utilizing a mobile interdisciplinary team that seeks to decrease the hazards of hospitalization, facilitate transitions of care, and provide patient and family education. In this study, the MACE service, a variant of the ACE Model, acts as the primary care team for patients from an outpatient geriatric clinic, and consists of a team including an attending geriatrician hospitalist, geriatric medicine fellow, social worker, and clinical nurse specialist. Although not part of the MACE team, providers of other disciplines, such as physical and occupational therapists and dieticians, are often consulted and work closely with the core MACE team. In the single-center, matched cohort study, MACE service patients were less likely to experience adverse events such as catheter-associated urinary tract infection, pressure ulcers, restraint use and falls, had shorter length of stay (LOS) by 0.8 days on average, and rated the quality of their care transition (as measured by the Care Transitions Measure [11]) higher than patients managed in general medicine as the comparison group; however, the rate of hospital readmission was not substantially different between the groups [12]. Researchers at Johns Hopkins University also sought to develop and pilot-test a model that combined the strengths of inpatient geriatric evaluation, co-management, and transitional care in a cluster-randomized trial of 717 hospitalized older adults on 4 general medicine services. In the two treatment groups, a geriatrician–geriatric nurse practitioner dyad assessed patients, co-managed geriatric syndromes, provided staff education, encouraged patient self-management, communicated with PCPs, and followed up with patients soon after discharge. The intervention was associated with greater patient satisfaction with inpatient care and slightly higher quality care transitions (though not statistically significant) [13].

Other studies have produced mixed results. In a 2012 published systemic review and meta-analysis of over 6,800 hospitalized elderly patients, Fox et al. demonstrate that acute geriatric unit care based on all or part of the ACE Model improves patient- and system-level outcomes, including fewer fall risks, less delirium, less functional decline at discharge from baseline 2-week pre-hospital admission status, shorter LOS, fewer discharges to nursing home, lower costs, and more discharges to home. There were no significant differences found in hospital readmissions, mortality, or post-hospitalization functional status compared with functional baseline before hospital admission [14]. Sennour et al. described a proactive geriatrics consultation service implemented in collaboration with hospitalists that incorporated the basic principles of ACE to prevent functional decline and improve the care of older hospitalized patients admitted with geriatric syndromes. This proactive consultation service demonstrated high level of satisfaction by hospitalists—96 % rated the service as excellent in helping them provide better care—while analysis of hospital administrative data revealed a shorter LOS and reduced hospital costs in patients receiving a geriatrics consultation [15]. This study was not designed to examine post-hospitalization care transitions or rehospitalization outcomes though the reduction in LOS is promising and evaluating the impact of this intervention on care transitions is a next step.

The Business Case for ACE Consult Programs

Under the current reimbursement system structure in the US, hospitals and large healthcare organizations must be able to proactively integrate evidence-based programs into their institutions in order to guarantee their financial survival. The situation is no different for ACE; regardless of how much focus is placed on comprehensive, exceptional care for the geriatric patient that the system knows is "right," if the program lacks vision for future funding, it will fail in the current economic climate. The healthcare system recognizes that patients with multiple medical problems like our elderly population are more likely to have multiple admissions with longer lengths of stay. The ACE consult service with its biopsychosocial approach to care as well as interdisciplinary team focus can minimize the cost and downstream financial repercussions of these hospitalizations. As described above, the ACE Model has aptly demonstrated that it can reduce functional decline, decrease length of hospital stays, diminish likelihood of nursing home placement at discharge, and in some cases lower unnecessary and expensive readmissions for which hospitals are now being fiscally penalized. The very nature of the ACE Model can thus be utilized to equip hospitals with the skills and strategies that have shown a positive result on the quality of care of hospitalized seniors, while at the same time lowering costs. A sound business model will thus ideally match the needs of the organization with the specific design of ACE team that research has demonstrated will best meet these demands.

The key components of the business case for any geriatrics model of care program include: (1) defining the actual challenge or scope of problem to be addressed; (2) describing the program clearly and concisely, while highlighting the high quality evidence demonstrating how the ACE Model of Care has been shown to improve outcomes; (3) outlining an executive summary of the program including all services involved with associated costs; (4) describing specifically the key components the proposed service is planning to address; (5) defining how the service will be evaluated including specific measures and outcomes to be tracked; (6) delineating all roles and responsibilities of the proposed team and how members will integrate into the current system; (7) developing a strategy for communicating outcomes to administration; (8) outlining an implementation schedule; and perhaps most importantly, (9) developing a sound financial plan that will demonstrate improvement in cost savings in the era of today's value-based healthcare market. Each of these components are vitally important, and can take much time and planning to develop. Without them, however, no matter how passionately dedicated, hard-working, and successful the team is, the chance for future failure is high whether program termination is due to economic downturn, changes in organizational structure or leadership, or someone else devises a "better" model that supplants interest in the original model of care. The successful ACE Models supported in the literature and described above all developed from an initial concept that began with a thorough and rigorous business model.

The Future of Acute Care for Elders

In May 2013, the Centers for Medicare and Medicaid Services (CMS) issued immediately actionable guidelines regarding discharge planning for condition of participation (CoP) for hospitals. These new requirements, extensive in expanding the scope of "discharge planning" to "transition planning," require that "a registered nurse, social worker, or other appropriately qualified personnel must develop, or supervise the development of, the evaluation" of care transition needs. The guidelines furthermore cite the benefits of an interdisciplinary team approach to hospital discharge planning, scheduling follow-up appointments and filling prescriptions prior to discharge, and follow-up phone calls within 24–72 h of discharge to ensure adherence to the care transition plan and identify any barriers. These are functions that may be performed by non-physician team members, should be coordinated with patients and families, and are

Table 1. Example of Printout from ACE Tracker Summarizing Risk Factor for Patients Aged of 65 or Older on a Hospital Unit

Patient Room/Bed	Age	Length of Stay	History of Dementia	CAM	Number of Meds	Beers	Morse	HX of Falls	Bed Rest	P/T	O/T	RES	ADL	Cath	Press Ulcer	Wound Care	Braden Scale	Albumin	Social Services	Advance Directives
Patient A	76	2	N	N	13	N	60	Y	N	Y	Y	N	8	Y	Y	Y	17	ND	Y	N
Patient B	74	1	Y	N	7	N	50	Y	Y	N	N	N	6	Y	Y	Y	9	2.9	N	Y
Patient C	78	12	Y	Y	10	Y	50	Y	N	Y	Y	N	7	N	N	Y	14	3.9	Y	Y
Patient D	72	1	N	N	5	N	50	N	N	N	N	N	12	N	N	N	15	ND	N	N
Patient E	91	6	Y	N	8	N	60*	N	N	Y	Y	N	6*	N	N	N	14	ND	Y	N
Patient F	78	1	N	N	7	N	70	Y	Y	N	N	N	6	Y	N	N	16	ND	N	N
Patient G	75	1	N	N	0	N	45	N	N	Y	Y	N	12	N	N	N	14	4.3	N	N
Patient H	93	1	Y	N	12	N	65	Y	N	Y	Y	N	6	N	N	N	15	ND	Y	Y
Patient I	91	1	Y	N	1	N	95	Y	N	Y	Y	N	7	N	N	N	12	3.5	N	Y
Patient J	74	5	N	N	20	N	45	Y	N	Y	Y	N	7	Y	Y	Y	12*	ND	Y	Y
Patient K	72	6	N	Y	14	N	20	N	N	Y	Y	N	8	N	N	N	17	3.2	Y	Y
Patient L	83	3	N	Y	12	N	80*	Y	Y	Y	Y	N	8	Y	N	N	12	2.3	N	Y
Patient Totals			5	3	11	1		8	3	9	9	0		5	3	4			6	7

Report Date: 02/27/08.

Report Time: 17:17.

History of Dementia – Cognition as defined by nursing admission assessment of history of dementia or Alzheimer's disease.

CAM – Confusion Assessment Method[10] as performed by nursing staff on admission and repeated daily on high-risk patients.

Meds – Number of total prescribed medications given to the patient on a scheduled basis.

Beers – Administration of potentially inappropriate medications for use in older adults within the prior 48-hours.[9]

Morse – Morse falls risk from calculated on admission and daily by nursing staff. A score >45 indicates an increased risk of in hospital falls.[11]

Hx of Falls – Any history of falls prior to hospitalization as recorded on nursing admission assessment.

Bed Rest – Bed rest as determined by daily nursing database describing the patient's activity level.

PT – Physical therapy consultation ordered.

OT – Occupational therapy consultation ordered.

Res – Current use of a physical restraint device as recorded on nursing daily assessment.

ADL – Activity of daily living score for bathing, dressing, transferring, walking, using the toilet and eating. 0 score for requiring total assistance; 1 score for requiring some assistance; 2 score of independent. These data from nursing admission assessment are repeated every other day.

Cath – Urinary catheter in place as noted on nursing daily assessment.

Press Ulcer – Pressure ulcer noted on nursing daily assessment.

Wound Care – Wound care consultation ordered.

Braden Scale – Calculated Braden Scale: 15–18 at risk, 13–14 at moderate risk, 10–12 at high risk, and 9 or below at very high risk.[12] These data are from nursing daily assessment.

Albumin – The most recent serum albumin value with an asterisk noting a value of 3.5 mg/dL or lower.

Social Services – Any documentation of a social service assessment.

Advance Directives – Any documentation of the presence of the patient's advance directives.

Y – Yes.

N – No.

ND – Not drawn.

* This score is less favorable than the admission score.

Fig 3.3 ACE tracker printout identifying geriatric risk factors for patients aged 65 or older on a hospital unit (From Malone ML, Vollbrecht M, et al. Acute Care for Elders (ACE) Tracker and e-Geriatrician: methods to disseminate ACE concepts to hospitals with no geriatricians on staff. J Am Geriatr Soc 2010;58:161–67 with permission.)

crucial components of a successful care transition. Most importantly, *they are the very tasks that are inherent to what an ACE team already does exceptionally well.* In addition to the new financial rules, CMS is also addressing the quality of transitions through new process mandates, holding hospitals accountable for successful care transitions, and expecting them to achieve these mandates by assessing the patients' functional and cognitive abilities, types of post-hospital care that will be needed, and patient caregiver/support systems in order to determine capacity for self-care and needs for appropriate post-hospitalization care settings. Encouraged is the development of collaborative relationships between hospitals, facilities, and providers who care for discharged patients [16]. Again, these tasks are inherent to the interdisciplinary comprehensive geriatrics functional evaluation performed by an ACE team, and thus can serve as a means by which the ACE Model can continue to emphasize its very essential role in achieving hospital outcomes as well as excellent all-inclusive patient care.

As the healthcare climate continues to evolve, the ACE Model of Care will need to acclimate to these constant changes to ensure its success and survival. One means by which the ACE Model can adapt is through harnessing the advances in information technology through the use of the electronic medical record (EMR) and computerized physician order entry (CPOE). The ability to identify vulnerable hospitalized older adults using an EMR is an innovative method whose design has already come to fruition with the "ACE Tracker." To address the barriers in dissemination of the ACE Model of Care, Malone and colleagues from the Aurora Health Care System have developed the software program ACE Tracker for use in several EMR systems in northern Wisconsin (Fig. 3.3). The ACE Tracker program collects existing data from a patient's EMR in real time to generate an individual patient level summary of geriatric clinical data and a unit-based summary spreadsheet of key geriatric risk factors in all hospitalized patients age 65 and older. These items include information such as LOS to date, total number and potentially inappropriate medications prescribed, risk of falls and skin breakdown based on nursing assessment screens, use of urinary catheters, and formal consultation to disciplines such as physical and occupational therapy and social services. In 2010, Malone and colleagues published a descriptive pilot study using ACE Tracker as a means of disseminating the ACE Model of Care to hospitals and units that do not have consistent access to a geriatrician. Units using ACE Tracker experienced significant reductions in use of urinary catheters and significant increase in consultations for physical therapy. While changes in LOS or 30-day readmissions were not the primary objective of this study, the use of this novel health information technology in improving care transitions serves as an impetus for further research [17]. For example, such research might focus on aligning hospital-based ACE principles with telehealth and other home-based interventions to improve outcomes in disease-specific populations, including those living with certain chronic diseases such as congestive heart failure and chronic obstructive lung disease.

Medicare Rule Changes for Care Transitions, and How ACE Principles Can Minimize the Impact on Hospitals

Two certainties in health care are inevitable: costs will continue to rise, and the aging of baby boomers will exert further pressure on our country's healthcare system. Current systems of healthcare delivery are not designed to care for the aging population, and often older adults cared for in the hospital may experience inefficient, fragmented care that is costly but does not yield better health outcomes.

In a fee-for-service payment model, interventions that decrease rehospitalizations have not been financially rewarded historically due to the time required by providers to improve care coordination particularly during transitions of care. However, the Patient Protection and Affordable Care Act (PPACA), signed into law in 2010 institutes new quality-based Medicare rules encouraging hospitals and providers to improve care transitions and other quality of care processes [18]. The alignment of patient outcomes on the hospital level with reimbursement may further accelerate the adoption of models and practices that have demonstrated their potential in improving patient outcomes. Geriatric-focused models of hospital care offer effective ways to transform inpatient treatment for older adults, making care more efficient and safer for hospitalized elders. The support for the adoption of these evidence-based care models that improve outcomes and lower costs is an area of focus as hospitals anticipate increasing numbers of elders and become more driven by improvements in patient outcomes and quality. The ACE Consult Model has not only demonstrated evidence to support its efficacy, but it serves as a very accessible model of care for hospitals to adopt. Furthermore, ACE teams that are more mobile, focused on seeing patients anywhere in the hospital and not just on a dedicated "ACE Unit," will evoke even fewer barriers in terms

of financing and logistics and thus will remain a very tangible and affordable means by which quality-focused outcomes can be achieved. In summary, as hospitals develop strategies to deliver better care to older adults and adopt models and practices that have the potential to improve patient care quality and safety, the ACE Consult Team is a demonstrable solution that is suitable for adoption.

Conclusions

Regardless of structure and form, the core of ACE remains the same: to improve outcomes in hospitalized elders by emphasizing patient-centered care, frequent interdisciplinary team rounds designed to manage geriatric syndromes, and early transition planning designed to achieve the best outcomes. Research demonstrates improved care, better prescribing practices, improved physical functioning, less restraint use, increased patient and provider satisfaction, and reduced length of stay and institutionalization rates. The Triple Aim of health care (improving care of the individual, improving the health of the population, and to do so while reducing per capita costs) [19] is a formidable challenge, but with care delivery and payment reforms encouraging a shift from episodic, segmented care toward integrated patient-centered care, it is achievable even for our most complex older patients. The ACE Model of Care stands at the very nexus of this continuously evolving climate, whether implemented on a dedicated ACE Unit or as an ACE Consult Program.

References

1. Vincent, GK, Velkoff VA. (2010, May). The next four decades the older population in the United States: 2010 to 2050. In U.S Census Bureau. Retrieved from http://www.census.gov/prod/2010pubs/p25-1138.pdf
2. Jencks SF, Williams MV, Coleman EA. Rehospitalizations among patients in the Medicare fee-for-service program. N Engl J Med. 2009;360:1418–28.
3. Landefeld CS, Palmer RM, Kresevic DM, Fortinsky RH, Kowal J. A randomized trial of care in a hospital medical unit especially designed to improve the functional outcomes of acutely ill older patients. N Engl J Med. 1995;332(20):1338–44.
4. Walter LC, Brand RJ, Counsell SR, et al. Development and validation of a prognostic index for 1-year mortality in older adults after hospitalization. JAMA. 2001;285(23):2987–94.
5. Boyd CM, Landefeld CS, Counsell SR, et al. Recovery of activities of daily living in older adults after hospitalization for acute medical illness. J Am Geriatr Soc. 2008;56(12):2171–9.
6. Palmer RM, Counsell SR, Landefeld SC. Acute care for elders units: practical considerations for optimizing health outcomes. Dis Manage Health Outcomes. 2003;11(8):507–17.
7. Pierluissi E, Francis DC, Covinsky KE. Patient and hospital factors that lead to adverse outcomes in hospitalized elders. In: Malone M, Capezuti E, Palmer RM, editors. Acute care for elders—a model for interdisciplinary care. New York: Springer Science and Business Media; 2014. p. 21–47.

8. Counsell SR, Holder CM, Liebenauer LL, et al. The acute care for elders (ACE) manual: Meeting the challenge of providing quality and cost-effective hospital care to older adults. Summa Health System: Akron, OH; 1998.

9. Were MC, Abernathy G, Hui SL, Kempf C, Weiner M. Using computerized provider order entry and clinical decision support to improve primary-care physicians' implementation of consultants' medical recommendations. J Am Med Inform Assoc. 2009; 16:196–202.

10. Flood KL, MacLennan PA, McGrew D, Green D, Dodd C, Brown CJ. An Acute Care for Elders Unit reduces costs and 30-day readmissions. JAMA Intern Med. 2013;173(11):981–7.

11. Coleman EA, Smith JD, Frank JC, Eilertsen TB, Thiare JN, Kramer AM. Development and testing of a measure designed to assess the quality of care transitions. Int J Integr Care. 2002;2:e02.

12. Hung WW, Ross JS, Farber J, Siu AL. Evaluation of a Mobile Acute Care for the Elderly (MACE) service. JAMA Intern Med. 2013;173(11):990–6.

13. Arbaje AI, Maron DD, Yu Q, Wendel VI, Tanner E, Boult C, et al. The geriatric floating interdisciplinary transition team. J Am Geriatr Soc. 2010;58(2):364–70.

14. Fox MT, Persaud M, Maimets I, O'Brien K, Brooks D, Trequnno D, et al. Effectiveness of acute geriatric unit care using acute care for elders components: a systematic review and meta-analysis. J Am Geriatr Soc. 2012;60:2237–45.

15. Sennour Y, Counsell SR, Jones J, Weiner M. Development and implementation of a proactive geriatrics consultation model in collaboration with hospitalists. J Am Geriatr Soc. 2009;57:2139–45.

16. Department of Health and Human Services, Centers for Medicare & Medicaid Services. Center for Clinical Standards and Quality/ Survey & Certification Group. Ref: S&C:13-32-HOSPITAL [Internet].   http://www.cms.gov/Medicare/Provider-Enrollment-and-Certification/SurveyCertificationGenInfo/Downloads/Survey-and-Cert-Letter-13-32.pdf. Accessed August 10, 2014.

17. Malone ML, Vollbrecht M, et al. Acute Care for Elders (ACE) Tracker and e-Geriatrician: methods to disseminate ACE concepts to hospitals with no geriatricians on staff. J Am Geriatr Soc. 2010;58:161–67.

18. U.S. Department of Health and Human Services. About the Law [Internet]. http://www.hhs.gov/healthcare/rights/index.html. Accessed August 10, 2014.

19. Berwick DM, Nolan TW, Whittington J. The triple aim: care, health, and cost. Health Aff. 2008;27(3):759–69.

Acute Care for Elders (ACE) Tracker and e-Geriatrician Telemedicine Programs

Marsha Vollbrecht, Aaron Malsch, Mary L. Hook, Michelle R. Simpson, Ariba Khan, and Michael L. Malone

Introduction to ACE

The Acute Care for Elders (ACE) Program was developed, implemented, and results published by Dr. Seth Landefeld, Dr. Robert Palmer, and colleagues [1] 20 years ago. The basic elements of ACE focus on preventing functional decline, medical care review with a geriatrician, early discharge planning, interdisciplinary team rounds, and patient-centered plan of care. The ACE model of care is designed to standardize and improve the care for hospitalized seniors age 65 and older. Multiple comorbidities and complex medical needs are common among this population. The ACE Program serves seniors at risk for developing geriatric syndromes and functional decline. This model of care has been described more fully in this book by other authors.

M. Vollbrecht, M.S., C.S.W., N.H.A. (✉)
Department of Senior Services, Aurora Health Care,
Plymouth, WI, USA
e-mail: marsha.vollbrecht@aurora.org

A. Malsch, M.S.N., R.N.
Department of Senior Services, Aurora Health Care,
Milwaukee, WI, USA

M.L. Hook, Ph.D., R.N.-B.C.
Department of Knowledge-Based Nursing (KBN),
Aurora Health Care, Milwaukee, WI, USA

M.R. Simpson, Ph.D., R.N.
Center for Nursing Research and Practice, Aurora Health Care,
Milwaukee, WI, USA

A. Khan, M.D., M.P.H.
Department of Geriatrics, Aurora Sinai Medical Center,
Milwaukee, WI, USA

M.L. Malone, M.D.
Aurora Senior Services and Aurora at Home, Aurora Health Care,
Milwaukee, WI, USA

University of Wisconsin School of Medicine and Public Health,
Milwaukee, WI, USA

ACE at Aurora Health Care

Aurora Health Care in Wisconsin is a large, not-for-profit health system that has widely disseminated the ACE model of care through multiple strategies. Aurora provides hospital care to approximately 30,000 seniors per year within their 14 hospitals in Eastern Wisconsin. Due to this large senior population and the unique vulnerabilities of older individuals during their acute illness, Aurora adopted the ACE model of care. The first ACE unit in Wisconsin was started in 2001 at Aurora Sinai Medical Center, led by Dr. Ellen Danto-Nocton and Dr. Michael Malone. This first ACE unit demonstrated improved patient quality, interdisciplinary collaboration, and improved processes of care. Continuous improvement led to enhancement to the Aurora's ACE model. ACE Tracker was developed in response to our goal of measuring outcomes and processes of care on a real-time basis. The e-Geriatrician service was implemented as a strategy to spread the limited resource of geriatricians. The addition of the ACE Tracker tool and the e-Geriatrician service differentiate the ACE model of care at AHC. The implementation of these elements facilitated wide dissemination of ACE within a large health system.

Geriatricians are the foundation of ACE at Aurora Health Care. Geriatricians attend daily team rounds at the large urban area hospitals where they are typically based. Aurora employs about ten geriatricians, all within the metropolitan Milwaukee area. To accommodate the needs of the smaller, non-urban and rural sites where there are no geriatricians on staff, the e-Geriatrician service was developed. This model requires the geriatricians to join rounds remotely twice per week through teleconferencing technology described below. Currently at Aurora Health Care there are more than 40 inpatient units that implement the ACE principles of care through use of evidence-based practices, electronic health record content and functionality, and the use of multiple quality improvement strategies [2].

The Structure of Aurora Health Care's Senior Service Line

Aurora Health Care leaders chose a matrix organizational structure for their senior service line (SSL) to serve the entire system. The service line leaders work at the health system level, reporting to Chief Medical and Nursing Officers. The service line leaders also work with each hospital site leaders and staff. This matrix structure allows authority, accountability, and resource control for the program to be balanced between system level leaders and local facility managers [3]. The SSL is comprised of an interdisciplinary team to address the complex and diverse needs of the senior population. This SSL leadership team is comprised of a geriatrician, a geriatric social worker with administrative credentials, and an advanced practice nurse with gerontological board certification. These SSL leaders are charged with improving care for seniors throughout the Aurora system by developing, disseminating, and sustaining geriatric models of care. The SSL has a department budget, which supports the dissemination of geriatric models and geriatric professional education throughout the system.

The SSL is responsible for achieving optimal geriatric program outcomes by working with clinicians and site level leaders. The SSL leaders work with each site to: (1) teach the principles of ACE care, (2) increase the number of clinicians utilizing ACE principles, (3) support ACE interdisciplinary team members, and (4) measure quality outcomes and processes of care. The SSL leaders also assist in developing and guiding site-based ACE advisory teams, described below.

Leadership Support for Acute Care for Elders

The SSL leaders at Aurora Health Care started by building a business case for the ACE based on needs and return on investment assessment. They established direct linkages to system and site-based leaders who work to ensure that ACE is aligned with the organization's strategic plan and goals. The plan defined the required resources, identified a budget, leadership responsibilities, outcome measures, and a timeline. Small pilot projects were used to facilitate the identification and refinement of key metrics and test processes. Outcome data demonstrated the success and value of the program. Leaders planned early for program dissemination by inviting future unit/site representatives to serve on the planning/advisory team. This facilitated a more rapid implementation to those additional units and created frontline staff buy-in.

Education, Direction, and Communication

The SSL leaders work with the site leaders to identify opportunities to improve care for seniors by implementing the ACE model of care. The decision is typically based on the volume of seniors served on the unit, staff maturity and experience level, culture of the unit, and quality measures. Unit implementation starts by identifying a site leader who provides guidance to the team for model implementation, barrier identification and mitigation, and tracking outcome data. The site leader then identifies members for their site-based team that includes frontline staff representing all the disciplines, nursing leaders, and physician champions. The SSL and site-based leader provide educational sessions for the interdisciplinary staff team members on key topics including the ACE Program, ACE concepts, and geriatric syndromes. The team learns about using the assessment tools and interventions and how and when to use them. Education alone is not enough to change practice. The geriatrician leader who works with the interdisciplinary team can help guide the clinician practice through feedback and recommendations at the daily interdisciplinary team rounds. This "just in time" teaching method applies feedback to clinicians when the impact is most poignant.

The site-based ACE advisory teams meet monthly when the program is new to provide additional education and support. As teams mature, the meetings may be scheduled less frequently. Some of the ACE advisory teams include a patient representative, and representatives from local long-term care facilities. This facilitates a community approach to the ACE Program. The SSL leaders share outcomes from the local hospital and from other Aurora Health Care hospitals. This allows the team to develop quality improvement plans and to celebrate successes. It also demonstrates value of ACE to hospital leaders. Multilevel communication needs to occur on a regular basis in order to keep the momentum going and sustain the program. Further, we have found value in sharing patient stories which describe the care provided to older persons by the team. This brings the ACE concept into real practice.

A Description of ACE Tracker

Acute Care for the Elderly (ACE) Tracker (Fig. 4.1) is an innovative near-real-time electronic clinical decision-support tool that extracts key demographic, assessment, and care parameters documented in the EHR and displays the information for all hospitalized patients who are 65 years and older at each facility, on a daily report used by interdisciplinary team members to facilitate care [2]. ACE Tracker was developed at AHC by a team of software programmers, geriatricians, nurses, a social worker, and pharmacists in 2003. Geriatricians identified the need to efficiently review an entire unit's senior population during daily interdisciplinary rounds. The original ACE Tracker utilized query tools available in a platform provided by the Cerner Corporation.

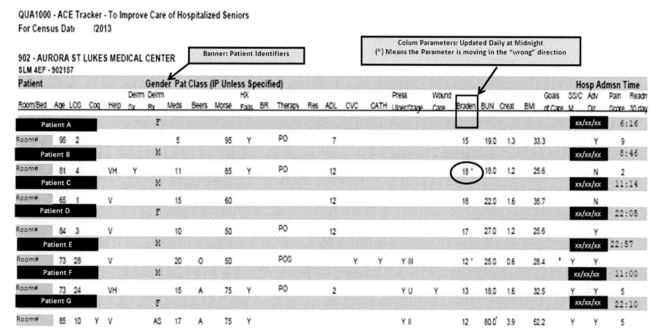

Fig. 4.1 ACE Tracker printout

Table 4.1 Daily ACE Tracker patient variables

		Blood urea
Room/Bed	History of falls	Nitrogen/Creatinine ratio
Patient age	Bed rest order	Body mass index
Length of stay	Therapy orders	Goals of care discussion trigger
Cognitive impairment	Restraints	Social work/Case manager consult
Elder Life Program Trigger (sensory impairment)	Activity of Daily Living Score	Advance directives (in place)
Delirium symptoms	Central venous catheter (in place)	Numeric Pain Score
Antipsychotic drugs (ordered or administrated)	Urethral catheter (in place)	30-Day Readmission
Number of scheduled medications	Pressure ulcer stage	Beers Criteria Drugs (ordered or administrated)
Morse Fall Scale Score	Wound Consult	Braden Pressure Ulcer
		Risk score

The tool was refined in Cerner over the course of 8 years. When the organization transitioned to an Epic-based EHR platform in 2011, the ACE Tracker report layout and parameters were maintained with the inclusion of additional parameters.

The current ACE Tracker utilized by Aurora Health Care is formatted with SAP Business Objects (BO) Crystal Reports using Structured Query Language (SQL) to communicate to the Epic Clarity 2010 relational database. The report is set to refresh daily against a copy of the production environment that occurs at midnight with data entered into the EHR from multiple sources over the previous 24–48 h depending on the parameter. The tool provides a unit-based patient list of every hospitalized older adult who is currently admitted to each facility as an inpatient or observation case. The data for 30 parameters (Table 4.1) are displayed using abbreviations with a legend provided at the bottom of each page that contains details about the source for each parameter to aid in interpreting and troubleshooting the report as needed. A clinical "red flag" signified by an asterisk (*) is used to depict findings that indicate when the patient status appears to be changing in an undesirable direction. Clinicians use the report tool to monitor patient progress and consider adding supportive care interventions during the stay and post-discharge.

ACE Tracker Validation

The caregivers who use the tool must understand what each of the clinical decision support parameters mean and develop confidence that the data reported on the tool are accurate. Inaccurate or misleading results can occur for several reasons—including inaccurate or late data entry or incorrect programming. It could also mean that the results are accurate and that the data appear the way it does because of the known limitations in the functionality (e.g., data will be missing if entered after the established cut off time for the report). Clinicians are encouraged to monitor the accuracy of the report and to contact the ACE Tracker team if discrepancies are identified.

The accuracy of the ACE Tracker report was clinically evaluated for accuracy by an interdisciplinary team using a convenience sample of patients receiving care on eight medical/surgical inpatient care units in one urban tertiary medical center. The validation was carried out with a sample ($n = 94$) of older adults (mean age = 78 years; SD = 8; range = 65–95) with more than half (55 %) male. Most patients were evaluated several days into their hospital stay (average day of stay was 7.6 days; range 1–53). Many older adults were at risk for falls (59 % had a Morse Fall Scale of $\geq$45) and pressure ulcers (46 % had a Braden Score of <18). Three-fourths of the patients had an order for therapy. The average patient was on 12.5 scheduled medications (SD = 13.8; range 0–25). Many (54 %) had orders for drugs that are on the Beers list of potentially inappropriate medications for older adults. Most Beers list drug orders originated from the standard "as needed" (PRN) medication computerized physician order set. Only 28 % of patients actually received medications on the Beers list. The Beers list drugs that were used included lorazepam and zolpidem for sleep. No patient required the use of restraints during the clinical evaluation.

The ACE Tracker values matched the clinical values for all parameters except restraints and urethral catheters. The ACE Tracker identified six patients with restraint documentation that was not appropriately discontinued in the EHR at the time when the patients were receiving care in an intensive care unit. The clinical reviewers identified two patients with urinary collection bags that were later found to be associated with condom (not indwelling) catheters, indicating a documentation error, rather than a problem with the ACE Tracker functionality. This validation study demonstrated that the ACE Tracker provided a unit- and patient-level summary of accurate and reliable data from EHR for review by the interdisciplinary team during rounds. The tool also provides unit leaders with an opportunity to view correct documentation, before it becomes a permanent part of the patient record. Just as one would standardize a new instrument (e.g., a blood pressure cuff or a glucometer) in a clinical setting, the authors of ACE Tracker require validation of the tool, prior to the implementation of this report in clinical sites beyond Aurora Health Care.

How the ACE Tracker Is Used

Daily interdisciplinary rounds are held in every nursing unit in Aurora Health Care to discuss and plan each patient's care. The rounds are the primary locus of developing and implementing the patient's plan of care from admission to discharge. The rounds are attended by the staff RN, unit RN manager, unit clinical nurse specialist (CNS), social worker, case manager (CM), therapy representative, pharmacist, and the scheduled e-Geriatrician. The staff nurse presents each patient per a standardized list of topics and then each discipline will contribute to the overall discussion and develop a plan for discharge. Each patient's discussion is limited to 2–3 min to efficiently review all patients on the unit.

The ACE Tracker was originally envisioned as tool for the geriatrician to efficiently assess an entire unit's census during their attendance at the daily unit level interdisciplinary rounds. Being efficient was necessary because the interdisciplinary team has 2–3 min to discuss each patient. Previously, the geriatrician would review the patient chart, record relevant details, and develop questions prior to the daily interdisciplinary rounds. This behavior was inefficient and did not require the expertise of a geriatrician. The development of the ACE Tracker provides a checklist of patient's key risk indicators. This report allows the geriatrician to provide recommendations to the assembled interdisciplinary team.

Although the ACE Tracker was originally developed as a tool for geriatricians, it also facilitates the non-geriatrician by providing a broad overview of geriatric risk factors and nursing practice indicators. The ACE Tracker is easily downloaded from within the EHR. The unit nursing leaders can access the ACE Tracker as a daily tool to assess nursing practice on a unit, provide a "geriatric" perspective and "just-in-time" teaching to staff when the e-Geriatrician is not at daily rounds. The power of the tool stems from the fact that the clinical staff can efficiently assess an entire unit's census from the tool, as well as risk factors for each senior. For example, the CNS can quickly see that a 91-year-old patient with a body mass index (BMI) of 17 and Braden score of 10 is at high risk for skin breakdown. The CNS can then verbally follow up with the nurse during daily rounds to employ proper interventions. Additionally, the CNS can assess if skin precautions are employed in the patient room and that proper documentation in the nursing teaching record and the interdisciplinary care plan are present. In short, the ACE Tracker provides a real-time checklist which can increase the number of health care professionals who use geriatric principles as they care for older patients.

Additionally, the power of the ACE Tracker as a tool for practice improvement can be illustrated by its use at differing levels within the organization. The patient level information is used on a daily basis during interdisciplinary rounds. Data from the ACE Tracker are also aggregated by unit and month, and then reported to each hospital in the system to provide a broader overview of practice. Outcomes from these reports are monitored by ACE advisory teams and compared with other system hospitals. The following outcomes are commonly monitored at all Aurora Health Care hospitals: indwelling urinary catheter use, rate of early therapy assessment, and rate of documentation of patients' advance directives. These variables illustrate longitudinal site level analysis of care reports, which provides feedback directly to the frontline clinical staff. Furthermore, these reports are also shared with site and system leaders to demonstrate the value of this model of care.

Role of the "e-Geriatrician"

An integral component of the Aurora Health Care ACE model is the "e-Geriatrician." Geriatricians who live and work in Milwaukee are assigned to a hospital at a non-urban, remote site. To access patient information, the e-Geriatrician is provided basic privileges at these distant hospitals. Daily interdisciplinary team rounds are held on each hospital unit and the e-Geriatrician participate twice per week. At the appointed time for the interdisciplinary team meeting, the e-Geriatrician simply calls to the remote team meeting. The e-Geriatrician does not bill for services, as they are consulting with the team, and not providing direct patient care. Each hospital pays for the e-Geriatrician's time through their budgets. The e-Geriatrician has access to the EHR and to ACE Tracker. The role of the e-Geriatrician at rounds is to provide academic detailing and practice recommendations in an educational environment. Using the patient variables on ACE Tracker, the e-Geriatrician is able to speak to the needs of vulnerable older patients.

To have an optimal experience the team follows basic rules of communication. The team clearly reports the name and room number of the patient. The phone is placed close to the person who is talking. The e-Geriatrician picks a quiet area to minimize background noise, while the team discusses each patient. The e-Geriatrician is given adequate time to give input that helps guide the development of the plan of care.

Although the e-Geriatrician is joining the team remotely, via teleconferencing technology, it is also important to develop a relationship with the team in person. If the e-Geriatrician is simply a "voice on the phone," recommendations are not likely to be implemented and the program will not be sustainable. As the program is being established the e-Geriatrician needs to be with the team in person to build relationships and credibility. When the program is up and running, the geriatrician needs to visit the team periodically to maintain the relationship by participating in rounds, attending ACE advisory team meetings, providing educational sessions and meeting with leaders and/or hospitalists. Due to the challenges of on-going staff turnover, and competing priorities, it is important to maintain a good working relationship. Without an on-going relationship, the e-Geriatrician may be reduced to a voice on the phone, and may be dismissed by the team and site leaders.

Measuring Outcomes

The Acute Care for Elders model has been shown to improve quality of care for older hospitalized patients. When implemented in varying degrees, ACE significantly impacts patient and system-level outcomes [4]. A systematic review and meta-analysis has demonstrated the following outcomes associated with one or more components of the ACE model: less falls, a lower rate of delirium, less functional decline, shorter length of stay, fewer discharges to the nursing home, more discharges to home, and lower costs. In addition, Flood [5] reported a reduction in cost and 30-day readmissions for patients receiving care on units with the ACE model in place.

The ACE Tracker [2] can be used as a near real-time outcomes information report. Traditionally, data collection specific to outcomes of interest require targeted collection efforts. The ACE Tracker reporting approach moves beyond collecting data on key indicators and reporting them at a later date, but rather extracts data from the electronic health record in near real-time. The tracking of key geriatric inpatient care indicators provides pertinent information for gauging how well the ACE model is being implemented on any given unit. These data measure processes of care and provide a basis for where to intervene—at the individual patient and/or unit level. In addition to the daily review of individual patient data at the unit level, the ACE Tracker development team has created a mechanism to summarize key outcome indicators reported on the ACE Tracker on a monthly basis. These Monthly Production Reports are intended to provide objective data and identification of variation of care performance over time at each hospital.

The top five most common complications experienced by hospitalized older adults include delirium, serious adverse drug events, functional decline, urinary dysfunction, and falls with possible fracture [6]. Consistent with the ACE model and the known complications experienced by older adults in the acute care setting, the individual patient data elements (reported per unit) displayed on the ACE Tracker report include: patients' age, length of stay, history of cognitive impairment, HELP (vision or hearing risk factors; see

Chap. 2), delirium symptom assessment result, total number of medications, ordered or administered beers medications, Morse fall score, history of falls, presence of bed rest order, therapy involvement (physical, occupational, speech), use of restraints, presence of sitter, activities of daily living score, use of central venous catheter, use of urinary catheter, presence of pressure ulcer and stage, wound care orders, Braden score, serum albumin level, BUN and creatinine, presence of goals of care, pain score, and readmission within last 30 days (Table 4.1).

Findings from a quality improvement project completed in 2010 [7] provide support for the use of the ACE Tracker for improvement of geriatric inpatient outcomes. Between October 2007 and September 2008, 28.0 % of hospitalized older adults who received inpatient care throughout Aurora Health Care had an indwelling urinary catheter in place as of Day 2 of hospitalization. Over a comparison time period of January through December of 2010 (when ACE Tracker was fully implemented), 22.1 % had a catheter in place as of Day 2 of their hospital stay. Thus, the use of indwelling urinary catheters among older adults in Aurora Health Care hospitals decreased after full implementation of ACE Tracker. This analysis demonstrates that the use of the near-real-time ACE Tracker, when used during in interdisciplinary rounds and daily evaluation of vulnerable hospitalized seniors, may improve care for this patient population. Future efforts are needed to examine the impact of interdisciplinary use of the ACE Tracker on health outcomes.

Lessons Learned and Future Implications

Aurora Health Care has had over a decade of experience with the ACE model. Clinicians at Aurora have enhanced ACE with ACE Tracker and the e-Geriatrician service. This experience provides lessons learned and highlights future implications. The e-Geriatrician is not able to bill for the services under the current Medicare fee for service program. The service is sustained by providing time and salary support by the hospital administration. This model may be a good fit under the Affordable Care Act with its focus on value-based purchasing and accountable care organization reimbursement. Identifying vulnerable patients within a population allows clinicians to target care plans to those who are in greatest need. The ACE Tracker and e-Geriatrician may be early steps in managing patients toward improved outcomes and reduced costs.

The variables noted on the ACE Tracker are populated by the clinical staff documentation of patient care. The accuracy of the variables is dependent on the knowledge and documentation of the clinical staff. If the information on the ACE Tracker is not accurate, it may be due to inadequate or missing documentation. In the process of improving the use of electronic health record tools, Aurora Health Care leaders have found opportunities to improve clinician documentation.

Communication is a vital component of the e-Geriatrician program. To enhance the communication and pilot new technologies, video conferencing was piloted at one site. It was not successful due to the complexity, video quality issues, logistics, and clinical staff not being comfortable with the medium.

The variables noted on the ACE Tracker are chosen based on previous literature showing an association with adverse outcomes. Further work is needed to address the predictive ability of the ACE Tracker for improved outcomes.

While the e-Geriatrician program is effective for the majority of patients, there are a few complex patients who may benefit from a formal (or video telemedicine geriatrics [8]) consult.

References

1. Landefeld CS, Palmer RM, Kresevic DM, Fortinsky RH, Kowal J. A randomized trial of care in a hospital medical unit especially designed to improve the functional outcomes of acutely ill older patients. N Engl J Med. 1995;332(20):1338–44.
2. Malone ML, Vollbrecht M, Stephenson J, Burke L, Pagel P, Goodwin JS. Acute Care for Elders (ACE) tracker and e-Geriatrician: methods to disseminate ACE concepts to hospitals with no geriatricians on staff. J Am Geriatr Soc. 2010;58(1):161–7.
3. American Geriatrics Society 2012 Beers Criteria Update Expert Panel. American Geriatrics Society updated Beers Criteria for potentially inappropriate medication use in older adults. J Am Geriatr Soc. 2012;60(4):616–31.
4. Fox MT, Persaud M, Maimets I, Brooks D, O'Brien K, Tregunno D. Effectiveness of early discharge planning in acutely ill or injured hospitalized older adults: a systematic review and meta-analysis. BMC Geriatr. 2013;13:70.
5. Flood KL, Maclennan PA, McGrew D, Green D, Dodd C, Brown CJ. Effects of an Acute Care For Elders unit on costs and 30-day readmissions. JAMA Intern Med. 2013;173(11):981–7.
6. Pierluissi E, Francis DC, Covinsky KE. Patient and hospital factors that lead to adverse outcomes in hospitalized elders. In: Malone ML, Capezuti EA, Palmer RM, editors. Acute Care for Elders: a model for interdisciplinary care. 1st ed. New York: Springer Science+ Business Media; 2014. p. 21–48.
7. Meyer H. Using teams, real-time information, and teleconferencing to improve elders' hospital care. Health Aff. 2011;30(3):408–11.
8. Martin-Khan M, Flicker L, Wootton R, et al. The diagnostic accuracy of telegeriatrics for the diagnosis of dementia via video conferencing. J Am Med Dir Assoc. 2012;13(5):487.e19–e24.

The NICHE Program to Prepare the Workforce to Address the Needs of Older Patients

Linda Bub, Marie Boltz, Aaron Malsch, and Kathleen Fletcher

NICHE Program History

The idea of a nurse-driven program to improve the care of older adults began in 1981 with Dr. Terry Fulmer, former Dean of the New York University College of Nursing. She implemented a program that centered on a Geriatric Resource Nurse (GRN) model at Boston's Beth Israel Hospital. These unit-based GRNs provided consultation to fellow nurses on the care of older adults to address medical problems also referred to as geriatric syndromes. These GRNs created standard protocols to address these common geriatric problems and ultimately felt that this improved the care provided as well as advanced their expertise [1, 2].

Following on the success of the original program, Dr. Fulmer and a team at Yale New Haven Hospital adapted the GRN model to a geriatrician led model of care as part of a multisite initiative. The Hartford Foundation's Hospital

L. Bub, M.S.N., R.N. (✉)
NICHE Nurses Improving Care of Healthsystem Elders,
NYU College of Nursing, 726 Broadway, New York,
NY 10003, USA
e-mail: linda.bub@nyu.edu

M. Boltz, Ph.D., C.R.N.P., F.A.A.N.
Connell School of Nursing, Boston College,
140 Commonwealth Avenue, Chestnut Hill, MA 02467, USA
e-mail: marieboltz@yahoo.com

A. Malsch, M.S.N., R.N.
Department of Senior Services, Aurora Health Care,
945 North 12th Street, OHC-4037, Milwaukee, WI 53233, USA
e-mail: aaron.malsch@aurora.org

K. Fletcher, R.N., D.N.P.-B.C.
Riverside Health System, Newport News, VA 23601, USA
e-mail: kathleen.fletcher@rivhs.com

Outcomes Program for the Elderly (HOPE) focused on increasing nurse expertise through a nurse-driven program [3]. The HOPE program addressed clinical issues such as nursing-sensitive indicators as well as clarification of goals and addressing medication concerns.

In 1992, the success of these two programs prompted the development of a new program funded by the John A. Harford Foundation in New York and the Education Development Center, Inc. called Nurses Improving Care for Hospitalized Elders (NICHE). In 1996, it became part of the Hartford Institute of Geriatric Nursing in New York University Division of Nursing. Over that time, NICHE grew to approximately 150 hospitals in the United States and Canada. In 2006, NICHE received funding from the Atlantic Philanthropies (U.S. Aging Programme) Foundation to develop a sustainable business plan to bring the program to hospitals across the country, serve member sites through support and evidenced-based practice and position NICHE as a leader in nurse-driven, innovative program aimed at improving the care of older adults. The 5-year program expansion from 2007 to 2012 resulted in the following resources and programmatic development for NICHE:

- Development of an internal business infrastructure
- Expanded NICHE-specific resources
- Creation of a web platform
- Increased the number of participating NICHE facilities (hospitals as well as nursing homes, home care agencies, rehabilitation centers, etc.)
- Enhance the NICHE benchmarking service
- Supported research that generates evidence-based practices
- Fostered inter-organizational collaboration
- Developed sufficient diversified revenue sources
- Increased the penetration and level of activity of current NICHE sites [4]

Current NICHE Program

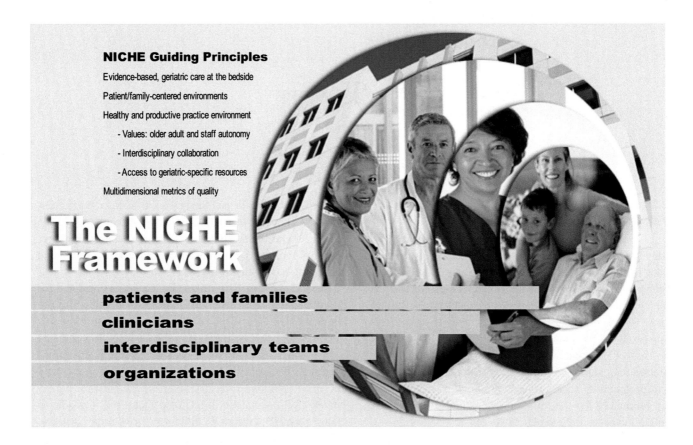

NICHE Guiding Principles

Evidence-based, geriatric care at the bedside

Patient/family-centered environments

Healthy and productive practice environment

   - Values: older adult and staff autonomy

   - Interdisciplinary collaboration

   - Access to geriatric-specific resources

Multidimensional metrics of quality

The NICHE Framework

patients and families

clinicians

interdisciplinary teams

organizations

Currently, NICHE has over 540 hospitals and healthcare facilities in the United States, Canada, Bermuda, and Singapore as well as current collaboration with the Mexican government to expand services in a pilot program focused on public hospitals in four states in Mexico. The Knowledge Center or member-only online learning management system hosts the resources for the NICHE program and currently has over 35,000 participants using the resources.

Originally developed to address the needs of the older adult in the hospital setting, the NICHE program along with the healthcare environment has evolved over the last 30 years to an environment that has reimbursement and regulatory changes that promote and in some cases require the care of a patient across the care continuum. NICHE has recognized this change and with the Atlantic Philanthropies assistance was able to develop a plan that addresses the care and practice deficits in the long-term care and home health settings. Currently, NICHE is updating and expanding content in courses as well as other resources with subject matter and content experts to address the unique needs of patients in all healthcare environments while fostering resources that support nurse and allied health professional education needs across the spectrum of care environments.

Addressing the needs of the older adult in the acute setting has a financial incentive for hospitals. Despite the fact that older adults (those over the age of 65) comprise only 13–14 % of the general population of North America, older adults in the hospital setting comprise approximately 37 % of hospital discharges and 43 % of hospital days [5]. Length of stay for older adults is approximately 5.5 days compared to 5.0 days for patients aged 45–64 and 4.8 days for all ages [5]. The CDC reports that older adults also have higher rates of 30-day hospital re-admissions as well as higher rates of functional decline and medical errors during hospital stays (U.S. Dept. of Health and Human Services, Centers for Disease Control).

Other areas of care are expected to see an increase in the number of older adults along with the hospital setting. Care for the older adult in the community setting is expected to grow at an exponential rate with, again, staff that are ill prepared to care for this population. Currently, long-term care for the older adult includes care in the Skilled Nursing, LTC, Home Health and residential care settings and costs range from $210.9 billion to $306 billion annually.

Approximately 59,000 residential providers care for roughly eight million older adults in the community setting

and long-term care service recipients will increase from approximately 15 million in 2000 to 27 million in 2050. Approximately two-thirds of older adults will need long-term care services at some point in their life [6].

With these growth trends of the older adult as well as use of services across the care spectrum, the need to ensure quality care of this population is imperative. NICHE is the only nurse-driven program designed to improve the care of older adults in the three identified venues of care. Seamless adoption of geriatric care principles and evidenced-based, practice-focused, protocols are available to all NICHE sites. Other venues of care that are in the pilot phase of implementation include programs such as PACE (Program for All inclusive Care of the Elderly), ACOs (Accountable Care Organizations), and large health system work that includes dozens of hospitals and other care sites across the continuum. The primary care setting is currently not in pilot stage of program development but has been identified as a need in the future. In the acute care setting, there are approximately 500 hospitals across the country with NICHE, which is the most successful, nurse-driven program designed to meet the needs of patients and their families as well as to grow nursing practice. The expansion to the LTC and HH setting as well as others in the future is intended to create a seamless, collaborative care environment for geriatric nursing practice in all venues of care.

Population

The older adult population is growing at exponential levels across the globe. The older adult population will continue to grow with projections in the US reaching 20 % of the population by 2030 with an additional 80 million adults reaching 65 or older. This is expected to put an extraordinary amount of stress on the healthcare system that is ill equipped to manage the care of this population. Because of this rapid growth of older adults, healthcare expenditures by Medicare will increase from $555 billion yearly to $903 billion by 2020. Older adults are increasingly complex and the current healthcare system is not designed to care for this population. NICHE is designed to bridge the gap in knowledge and practice for nurses as well as allied health professionals.

Older adults have been shown to be particularly vulnerable to complications during hospital stays [7]. The following are potential complications of hospital stays
- Functional decline—reduction in ability to perform activities of daily living including walking
- Fall-related injury
- Under/malnutrition
- Pressure ulcer
- Urinary infection (usually secondary to catheter) and urinary incontinence

- Delirium
- Adverse drug effects
- Sleep deprivation
- Inadequate pain management
- Dehydration

The NICHE program focuses on reducing these complications by providing resources and tools to improve their care as well as create an infrastructure in the facility to identify high-risk older adults, prevent these complications or quickly intervene to minimize impact on the older adult. Because older adults are cared for in all specialty areas in the hospital including the emergency department, intensive care, surgical and other specialty areas such as orthopedics, cardiac, pulmonary and psychiatry, all these settings in the hospital are appropriate for the NICHE program. With the growing expansion of resources for LTC and HH, older adults in all these settings are also appropriate for the NICHE program.

The NICHE program strongly encourages the inclusion of the family in the care of the older adult. Often, the older adult is cared for in varying levels by the family. For those older adults that are not able to care for themselves or speak for themselves due to chronic or acute cognitive impairment, the family is often the primary source of information and teaching. NICHE sites vary in the level of family involvement protocols and practice but all are encouraged to include the family in discharge teaching, management or prevention of complications and transitions in care. Some NICHE sites have patient and families participate in their steering committee or have a patient/family advisory panel or council. This is imperative for successful and comprehensive care of the older adult as well as give feedback on the care that is provided to the older adult.

Program Setting

The NICHE program has been implemented in many types of hospitals from rural and critical access to academic medical centers with bed size as large as 900+ beds. The program is adaptable to any size hospital with varying percentages or amounts of older adults in the setting. NICHE sites range from GRNs on one unit (either a medical surgical unit) to a program that has GRNs on all appropriate units (those with greater than 40 % older adults). As sites develop programming and resources, all are encouraged to have as many units participate in the program as is manageable by staffing financial resources in order to improve the care of all older adults. NICHE units are not limited to medical/surgical units; specialty units are encouraged for implementation as well. Increasingly, specialty units are the initial site and in some case the main unit of the NICHE program as they are not immune to the growing number and percentage of older adults. NICHE sites are looking to improve the care of the older adults starting with the initial experience in the facility starting with the Emergency room or will focus on critical care or with specialty units such as orthopedics or cardiac care.

Many NICHE sites have Acute Care of the Elderly (ACE) units along with the GRN program. Of the 500+ sites, 99 or approximately 25 % have ACE units. For the other 400 sites, this is not a possibility due to the cost of setting up an ACE unit and staffing when many of the units in the hospital have older adult populations that are greater than 40–50 %. One site, UC San Diego built their program around their ACE unit which happens to be a geropsychiatric unit. This works particularly well for their population and the staff on the unit provide consultation on behavioral issues particularly delirium on other units in the hospital.

Conceptual Basis for NICHE

The GRN

The NICHE program and resources are designed to meet the multidimensional needs in designing, implementing, evaluating, and sustaining change in practice in the care of the older adult. The theoretical basis of the NICHE program is twofold, in order to create lasting change with measurable impact on the care of older adults in any setting the nursing staff need to be empowered with education and resources as well as practice in an environment that supports staff development and empowerment. This has been studied since introduced by [36] but not often referred to in a geriatric practice environment. Educational resources for nurses develop a basic understanding of the unique needs of the geriatric patient and geriatric syndromes that impact the overall outcomes of the older adult; resources that empower nurses to consider geriatric specialization and advocate for patient care and nursing practice, and be a role model as an agent for change in practice in collaboration with all disciplines caring for the older adult. This nursing practice needs organizational support for a positive nursing practice environment that improves outcomes for older adults, their families and caregivers as well as nurses and the hospital setting [8–10]. Within this positive practice environment, the NICHE Guiding Principles impart these essential concepts:
• Evidence-based geriatric knowledge
• Patient–family-centered care
• Healthy-productive practice environment
• Multidimensional metrics of quality

Central to the care of the older adults is a solid clinical understanding of the complexity and unique nature of the aging patient. The NICHE program imparts this knowledge of the aging process, the complications and vulnerability of the older adult in the hospital setting and now across the venues of care. In order to meet the needs of this population, the nurse must care for the entire person, not just a body system, in collaboration with the multidisciplinary team. This idea has been the core of the GRN since conception [11]. This type of care depends on geriatric practice developed through evidenced-based education, protocols, and collaboration.

Nurses are central to quality care of the older adult in the hospital or any setting. When hospitals, health systems, LTC sites, and HH agencies are looking to improve clinical outcomes, it is the nurse that is central to the monitoring of current practice, implementation of change, and subsequent evaluation of outcomes. With the proper geriatric education, the nurse at the bedside (whether in the hospital, LTC setting, or in the home) is able to identify potentially harmful geriatric syndromes and act quickly with the proper tools and resources. In order for the nurse to be able to practice in this manner, there must be good support from leadership as well as an environment of continuous learning and striving for change.

For many NICHE sites, the nurse that becomes a GRN is open and ready for knowledge and understanding that geriatrics is a specialty and has the support from leadership to have the time to participate in education that is not interrupted by other staffing needs, patient care and other distractions that can take time and concentration from learning. After the education, there must be time for the nurse to have mentoring to put this knowledge into practice. If there is not mentoring and modeling of behavior, there is minimal change in practice. Typically, nurses are based on a unit where there is an educator and an advanced practice nurse that ensures the implementation of the site-specific NICHE program. If there is not either of these in place the implementation may not be as effective and can cause program fatigue.

The NICHE GRN Curriculum is available online in the NICHE Knowledge Center learning management system or LMS, and includes a series of interactive e-learning presentations organized into individual content modules based on topics of the NICHE Evidenced-Based Protocol Book [8]. The modules contain the following content and supplemental materials:
• Interactive e-learning slide presentations with voice over
• Post test
• Handout(s)—applicable tables and case examples developed based on the chapter and module content
• Pertinent issue(s) of the Try This Series

The GRN Core Curriculum includes the following topics:
• Why Geriatric Nursing?
• Age Related Changes in Health
• Cognition: Depression, Delirium, and Dementia
• Falls
• Family Caregiving
• Function

- Healthcare Decisions
- Medications
- Nutrition, Hydration, and Oral Health
- Pain
- Pressure Ulcers and Skin Tears
- Restraints
- Sleep
- Urinary Incontinence

Also important to the growth of the nurse is the idea of recognizing practice [12, 13]. For many NICHE sites, the role of the GRN is recognized on the clinical ladder and/or certification in geriatrics. This has an impact on the type of nursing care provided as well as the caliber of nurses that are employed in any setting. The NICHE program is a prominent aspect of many sites that have gone for initial Magnet designation and re-designation due to the consistent theme of empowering the nurse at the bedside, nurse-driven protocol development, positive patient impact as well as nurse and patient satisfaction. Many sites have shown reduction in nurse turnover and at one site in particular, all of the GRNs at some point have applied for clinical leadership positions with only one nurse leaving for another institution.

The second aspect of the NICHE model is growing the institutional capability to have a geriatric program. Prior to 2010, hospitals would become a NICHE site after attending an in-person 2-day training session led by instructors that were from NICHE sites called the Leadership Training Program or LTP. These instructors were coordinators, nurse leaders, nurse researchers, and the NICHE faculty staff. In 2010, the LTP transitioned to a blended learning format with online education led by faculty mentors with recorded webinars, interactive phone call sessions, assignments, and discussion board postings. The faculty mentors are NICHE coordinators from sites that have strong levels of implementation. The LTP covers multiple topics all aimed at introducing the hospital sites to implementing a best practice program aimed at improving the care of older adults in the hospital setting. The 13 modules cover the following topics:

- Introduction to NICHE
- Review of the need for Geriatric Specialty Program
- The Geriatric Resource Nurse Model
- The Acute Care for Elders Unit
- SWOT Analysis and developing priorities based on this assessment
- Developing and embedding geriatric best practice
- Funding sources including grant writing
- The Geriatric Institutional Assessment Profile
- Magnet and NICHE initiatives
- And finally developing an action plan (including budget and determining a pilot unit) to implement their own NICHE program tailored to meet the needs of their facility.

After completing the LTP and the action plan being approved by the NICHE staff, the site is considered designated. The sites are encouraged to begin the implementation of their site-specific program with the feedback from the NICHE faculty mentors and staff.

In 2013, the program was revised and updated of all previous recorded webinars and included webinars with instructions for the assignments. Live webinars were included to introduce the participants to the course as well as a call 2 months after the LTP to provide additional support and guidance in the implementation of their program. Currently, calls are transitioning to live webinars to allow for the participants to review at a later date if not available to participate in the designated time or for additional review. All changes have also been the result of user feedback to ensure quality courses and instruction for implementation.

After initial designation, sites begin the process of implementation that builds on the work done in the LTP including the SWOT analysis, priority development based on clinical outcomes, and staffing needs as well as the action plan. Most begin with an assessment of the baseline knowledge and attitude of the staff in the care of geriatrics with the GIAP (this will be covered in more detail in a later section of this chapter) to determine baseline needs as well as benchmark growth with the introduction of best practice education. Sites are encouraged to assess all units as well as all disciplines to ensure broad understanding of baseline data. Within the first 6–12 months sites begin the education program development to consist of multiple formats including online or didactic learning. All sites are encouraged to develop a program that mentor nurses in developing expertise and promote change in their work environment. Some sites have developed programs that include GRNs picking an area of practice development or improvement to create program development and sustain change. The Meridian and Christiana Care Healthsystems have developed this role for the GRN with positive impact on clinical outcomes as well as satisfaction with the GRN role. All sites are encouraged to have GRN engagement and empowerment central to their program. Sites are able to develop the GRN role to best fit their facility needs as well as the capabilities of the NICHE coordinator.

Along with the initial education that the GRNs are given, continuing education is imperative to retain and grow skills of the GRN. Many sites have learning opportunities in group sessions led by the GRNs or NICHE coordinator that include site-developed education, NICHE resources such as live or archived webinars that are available two times monthly or case study review. This allows for program growth and skill development for non-GRN staff including other disciplines. Other aspects of the model include development of the interdisciplinary team and inclusion of the patient and family in care as well as hospital and program development.

Role of the Interdisciplinary Team

The GRN role and the NICHE program center on the idea of meeting the needs of the older adult and family in a team model. This interdisciplinary team includes the geriatrician and all of those trained in geriatrics. Many of the NICHE sites do not have a medical director or geriatrician due to lack of available geriatricians. When this is not available, sites rely on Nurse Practitioners or Clinical Nurse Specialists trained in geriatrics to develop and sustain their program. The NICHE program success and positive patient outcomes are also dependent on an interdisciplinary team trained in geriatrics focused on implementing best practice across disciplines.

Barriers to the Program

Information gained from the program evaluations has shown common themes in barriers to implementation and sustaining the NICHE program. The most common themes focus on leadership support, staff participation and buy-in to the program, recognition of accomplishments as well as having a coordinator or leader that will maintain the fidelity of the program and sustain the level of implementation [12]. Without leadership support and buy-in, sites are not able to have the ability to reimburse or even recognize the time and effort needed to finish the education. Recognition of geriatric expertise and specialty is also important in sustaining interest in a NICHE program [12]. Staff participation is imperative to program success. If staff do not understand the importance of evidenced-based practice that is grounded in clinical expertise and empowerment, the program will have sustained difficulties. And finally, the NICHE coordinator is key to the strength of any program. A strong coordinator is enthusiastic and competent and brings recognition of geriatric excellence in a hospital.

NICHE Measurement

The NICHE benchmarking service provides ongoing evaluation of the following quality metrics: assessment of the "institutional milieu" surrounding care of older adults using the Geriatric Institutional Assessment Profile (GIAP) [14–16] and relevant unit level measures including clinical outcomes, and measures of staffing volume and certification [17]. These measures are ideally evaluated at baseline, i.e., prior to program implementation, and tracked on an ongoing basis to monitor progress in quality improvement activity. The NICHE Benchmarking Service provides web-based data entry and automated benchmarking reports to NICHE member sites [17].

The GIAP is a 133-item self-report survey instrument that includes participant demographic information, three major scales (staff knowledge, perceptions of the care environment, and views on professional issues) and several subscales [14, 17–20]. Most questions are posed as statements, which respondents rate on a 5-point scale similar to the Likert scale ranging from 0 (strongly disagree) to 4 (strongly agree). At the end of the survey, respondents are asked to write in comments:

- *What are the most pressing issues you currently face in caring for older adults?*
- *Do you have any reactions to a particular issue raised by this questionnaire?*
- *What would help you improve care for older adults?*

The NICHE Benchmarking Service analyzes the GIAP data and produces a report for the individual hospital. There are three categories of reports: (1) individual hospital data; (2) comparison (benchmarked) data from "peer" hospitals (matched by teaching status and bed size); and (3) data benchmarked by type of unit (within the hospital and against similar hospitals nationally). Individual hospital results provide information about staff perceptions of, attitudes toward, and knowledge about common geriatric disorders, and thus are useful in prioritizing staff education and protocol development. Additionally, the GIAP provides information about institutional strengths to build upon while exposing barriers staff confront in providing effective care to older adults [17]. Benchmarked data are used for strategic planning, design of new or redesign of existing services, and staff/professional development programming.

How Have Organizations Used GIAP Data?

GIAP data are used to evaluate organizational readiness to change. Results are then used to garner support and help overcome resistance to change by providing objective evidence of knowledge deficiencies and operational areas of weakness. Data then provide a baseline against which to measure effectiveness of quality improvement efforts [4]. Additionally, the GIAP can assist administrators and researchers to document improvement in knowledge and care delivery through pre- and post-test analysis, with results tracked annually. Hospitals have used the GIAP as evidence of improvements necessary for Joint Commission accreditation and Magnet initiatives and to support efforts to negotiate contracts with insurers [13].

What Have GIAP Results Demonstrated in NICHE Hospitals?

Research with the GIAP has demonstrated that nurses perceive institutional support for geriatrics (valuing the unique needs of older adults, access to geriatric-specific resources, and interdisciplinary collaboration) significantly impacts the quality of care to older adults and families [14, 19]. Furthermore, those perceptions improve after NICHE implementation [14, 21] as does gero-specific nurse competence and knowledge [22]. Thus NICHE recommends that knowledge tests and competency evaluations found on the website be utilized to track proficiency in care of the older adult.

GIAP data report staff knowledge and perceptions in clinical areas related to care of the older adult, but do not measure actual clinical care. GIAP data are best utilized when triangulated with clinical data, including outcome and process measures, and staffing reports from individual units. The GIAP responses around the care environment, considered in tandem with these unit-level measures, help explain additional factors, besides staff knowledge that influence patient outcomes [17].

Unit Level Data: Clinical and Staff-Related

Hospital units vary considerably in many ways, including patient acuity, clinical foci, staff areas of expertise, physical design, deployment of medical staff and other human resources, and leadership priorities. Thus quality performance is evaluated at the unit level, and NICHE collects clinical performance and staffing measures at the time of GIAP submission.

Clinical performance measures include total falls and injury falls per 1,000 days; community-acquired, hospital-acquired, and unit-acquired pressure ulcer prevalence; and the prevalence of physical restraint use, ventilator-acquired pneumonia, central line-associated blood stream infections, and catheter-associated urinary tract infections. These data may be extrapolated from reports submitted to the National Database of Nursing Quality Indicators (NDNQI®), if the hospital submits to the database [21]. Additionally, the number of geriatric resource nurses and certified nurses are tracked; these data can be aligned with clinical data to determine the "dose" of geriatric expertise required to support positive outcomes.

Additional Unit-Level Measures

NICHE sites augment the GIAP and Unit Performance Measures with measures of patient satisfaction, staff satisfaction, the rate of 30-day readmissions, and length of stay. Process measures (e.g., compliance with a clinical protocol such as delirium screening, prevention, and management) are important, especially when implementing a quality initiative.

How Have Organizations Used Unit-Level Data?

Unit-level data are benchmarked against units of the same type in similar hospitals (considering bed size and teaching status) [17]. Data have been used to:

- Compare performance to same-type units in other NICHE facilities
- Compare performance of units within the hospital
- Track performance over time
Data are reviewed along with GIAP results to evaluate:
- Does staff knowledge contribute to outcomes?
- Also, do factors in the Geriatric Care Environment contribute to outcomes?
- Additionally, do pressing issues explain results? Do staff offer recommendations for improvement?

What Have Unit-Level Results Demonstrated in NICHE Hospitals?

NICHE units have demonstrated improved clinical and organizational outcomes. Here are some examples.
- A NICHE Gerontology unit of Christ Hospital used a series of environmental and social interventions to improve patient satisfaction scores and reduced the incidence of falls by 25 % [23]
- The University of Alabama at Birmingham ACE unit implemented a drug alert system that resulted in significantly fewer older adult patients receiving diphenhydramine (11.4 % vs. 15.3 %, $p < 0.0001$) and promethazine (6.8 % vs. 10.3 %, $p < 0.0001$), demonstrating compliance with evidence-based protocols [24]
- Mount Sinai Hospital and Long Island Jewish Medical Center provided an educational program to prepare nursing staff to deliver culturally competent care to older adults. The program significantly increased nurses' cultural awareness levels ($t = 3.95$, $p < 0.001$, $n = 133$) and cultural competence levels ($t = 8.13$, $p < 0.001$, $n = 134$) [25]
- A multi-component delirium protocol (staff education, access to hearing amplifiers and activity cart, pharmacist review of medications, and early mobility program) was associated with: (1) a decrease in the average length of stay for delirium patients from 9 to 2.8 days; (2) an increase in delirium patients discharged to home as opposed to a skilled nursing facility (4 % over a 3-year period), and (3) a reduction in the average total costs for delirium patients (dropped nearly $3,000 over a 2-year period) [26].

More examples are available at the NICHE website (see www.nicheprogram.org).

NICHE Program Evaluation

The NICHE web-based program evaluation provides a mechanism to set goals, track progress, and sustain and grow individual programs [27]. This self-evaluation is a 49-item

Table 5.1 NICHE program evaluation dimensions and summary of items

Dimensions	Summary of items
Guiding principles $a=0.96$	Mission statement endorsement by the governing body and dissemination
Organizational structures $a=0.76$	NICHE steering committee composition and activity
	Model implementation and dissemination: Geriatric
	Resource Model (GRN) and ACE (Acute Care of Elders) Model
Leadership $a=0.70$	Role and qualifications of the NICHE Coordinator and Educator
	GRN leadership functions
	Dissemination and mentoring roles: regional and national
Geriatric staff competence $a=0.97$	Geriatric education across disciplines
	Staff development programs integrated into clinical ladder or advancement program.
	Evaluation of staff capacity to meet the needs of older adults
Interdisciplinary resources and processes $a=0.98$	Use of interdisciplinary evidence-based guidelines
	Transitional care processes
Patient and family-centered approaches $a=0.98$	Patient and family engagement in education decision-making, and program development and evaluation
	Partnerships and consumer outreach
Environment of care $a=0.99$	Systematic evaluation and modification of the physical environment
Quality metrics $a=0.74$	Breadth of quality measures
	Sharing results
	Utilization of metrics to guide program development

tool that measures the depth (degree of application of evidence-based resources) and penetration (dissemination throughout the hospital) of programs. The program evaluation is submitted by the NICHE Coordinator via a web-based portal; it is conducted yearly as part of NICHE recommitment, required for continued designation as a NICHE site. In addition, NICHE at NYU utilizes results to develop resources and cooperative initiatives to support care of the older adult at a national level [17, 27].

The dimensions of the NICHE program evaluation were identified through research conducted with older adult consumers, clinicians, educators, researchers, managers, and administrators. The research yielded components and characteristics of quality care for older adults in the acute care setting, and identified the dimensions of an acute care geriatric model. Each dimension is associated with a set of items that demonstrate the level of NICHE penetration (units engaged in NICHE) and depth and scope of program development. Table 5.1 shows the dimensions and associated Cronbach's alpha (measure of internal consistency) of the self-evaluation, and summarizes the items associated with each dimension [28].

The 49 items are weighted 1–4 for level of complexity (with four as highest) and yield a scoring system to calculate four levels of implementation. For example, one of the items for the dimension, quality metrics, is "a minimum of two measures are evaluated (the GIAP and at least one clinical outcome)." This item is scored a "one" indicating a beginning approach to program evaluation. A more involved NICHE site evaluates a comprehensive set of measures,

including patient, organizational and clinician outcomes and processes, which would be associated with a score of four for that item. The sum of items results in the following implementation levels:

- *Early implementation level*—developing infrastructure: oversight, leadership, staff development, and evaluation (score 0–13)
- *Progressive level*—comprehensive geriatric acute care model, including the GRN model, implemented on at least one unit (score 14–27)
- *Senior friendly level*—geriatric initiatives on multiple units; has assumed a regional leadership role (score 28–41)
- *Exemplar level*—geriatric initiative throughout and beyond the organization and national leadership role (score 42–49)

A recent analysis of program evaluation data showed that hospital size and teaching status were not factors influencing level of NICHE implementation. However, hospitals that have ACE programs and comprehensive geriatric assessment (CGA) programs tend to have higher levels of NICHE implementation, reflective of the interdisciplinary collaboration and clinical leadership of geriatric specialists associated with these programs [27].

In 2013, the NICHE team developed additional measures to ensure the validity of the program assessment which includes NICHE staff review of every submitted evaluation to ensure that answers are complete and appropriate. If a coordinator submits an answer that does not fully answer the question appropriately, the coordinator is not given credit for the answer or if there is subsequent documentation but the coordinator did not take credit for the answer the score is adjusted to reflect this. Along with this initial review, there is also an auditing process developed by the NICHE staff for less developed programs in the Early Adopter phases, sites that have shown significant improvement or decline from the previous year and those that have reached the Exemplar status or highest level of implementation. This gives sites the opportunity to share their unique program implementation and or learn about additional program interventions to adapt to their setting. Finally, the yearly evaluation includes submission of site data such as bed size, nurse data, and specialty certification for NICHE to monitor trends in sites participating in the program.

NICHE Business Plan Development

Most healthcare administrators agree that it is important to provide the highest quality of care to all patients as well as the older adult. Nevertheless, what they will require in order to make the investment in NICHE is a business or action plan that provides the roadmap for NICHE program implementation and includes a demonstration of the return on investment that is unique to that specific system. The business case effectively communicates the importance of action and builds confidence that the investment of time, attention, and resources will yield tangible and measurable results [29]. The business plan needs to project expected NICHE success over a time frame of about 2–5 years. Suggested components of the plan are described below.

Prior to 2009, initial interest in NICHE was typically shown by a nurse on a unit and was brought to the hospital leadership as a program to implement. The LTP was developed to empower the staff nurse or advanced practice nurse (APN) to bring the idea of a comprehensive, geriatric program to the hospital setting and have measureable impact on nursing practice and clinical outcomes. Over time with the changing landscape of healthcare, leaders such as CNOs and CEOs of healthcare systems have approached NICHE for implementation. Healthcare leaders have identified that improving the care of older adults will ensure that penalties from Value-Based Purchasing or other CMS penalties will be minimized. This means developing a business plan that identifies both the cost of the program and the benefit in order to gain acceptance and sustain the program.

During the LTP, the NICHE Coordinator participates in a full assessment of the current status of the facility and or health system that is central to the development of a business plan for a NICHE program. The NICHE Coordinator has the tools to create an executive summary (a snapshot of NICHE plan) that reflects how NICHE supports the mission, vision, and goals of the organization, and provides leverage with site and system leaders to implement a nurse-driven program to improve outcomes for older adults. The target market needs to be fully described, including the aging population currently being cared for in proportion of care, bed days, costs, readmissions, avoidable events, and outlier cases, with the data framed in a way that captures the opportunity for improvement or gaps from benchmark [29, 30]. The target market should also detail current aging and future projections in the service area along with any community needs assessment identifying gaps in aging services and reflecting aging as a priority. Identify briefly what the local competitors are doing or not doing to address this need and the potential for NICHE to capture market share for the health system.

After presenting the executive summary, the coordinator should provide a detailed action plan of what was developed in the LTP that is to be accomplished and by when, including the milestone events which will be measured on an annual basis with the NICHE program evaluation. This action plan includes details about the measurement of need with the nursing staff obtained through the NICHE GIAP. This serves as the needs assessment for geriatric staff competence. Since it is well-known that nurses have minimal education in geriatrics in nursing school, the GIAP is an assessment of baseline knowledge for staff and will guide the program development. Having the executive summary along with the assessment of staff need is an integral part of the business plan. All participants of the LTP detail this in an action plan that is approved by the NICHE team before designation. To ensure success, participating LTP sites also have to establish a budget that includes the costs associated with the NICHE program including staffing needs. This includes the following areas:

- What percentage of time will the NICHE coordinator devote to implementation of NICHE activities?
- What percentage of their time will additional members of the NICHE team devote to project activities
  - Nurse Managers, Geriatrician, Nurse Researcher, Nurse Educator
- How much staff time will administration allow for participation in continuing education
- Estimated number of hours for continuing education
- Estimated number of staff participating in continuing education activities
- NICHE Coordinator salary or partial time from another position

As well as other budget items that the NICHE coordinator should allow for

- Supplies needed for interactive learning sessions
- Travel for conferences
- FTE's dedicated to NICHE
- NICHE Conference fees (Include air and hotel)
- In-house training (FTE Time for in-person trainings)
- Materials
- Refreshments

- Replacement FTE's (Coverage for GRN training, etc.)
- Publicity
- Gifts
- Other

NICHE sites are also encouraged to improve the care environment to be more geriatric friendly or implement an ACE (Acute Care for the Elderly) unit. The costs associated with design or re-modeling the unit should be included in the budget with the business plan.

- Adaptive devices (e.g. meal aids, mobility devices such as canes, walkers)
- Sensory support equipment (e.g. magnifiers, amplifiers, hearing aid batteries)
- NICHE unit(s) aging-sensitive principles
  - Non-glare flooring
  - Adequate lighting
  - Grab bars
  - Access to adjustable height beds
  - Easy to use call lights and controls
  - Sensor alarms or exit alarms
  - Adequate family seating
  - Patient orientation items and whiteboard

After developing the budget along and action plan, the NICHE coordinator is mentored to develop a plan to evaluate the improvement in patient outcomes and staff competence to determine the return on investment of the program. Because the NICHE program is non-prescriptive and can take various forms of program dissemination, the site takes the responsibility of measuring the impact. The program evaluation has been used by many sites as part of this evaluation. A portion of the 49 questions in the program evaluation request measurement of NICHE sites use of the NDNQI data that they are already submitting but focus on data from the units that have GRNs and separate out older adult outcomes. This allows for measurement of impact on the units involved and compare to non-GRN or ACE units. Patient satisfaction is also encouraged as a measurement of impact of NICHE programs and should be included in the business or action plan.

The entire business plan should be concise with clear language, with measureable outcomes. It is natural to develop a plan that describes unprecedented success but it is advisable to acknowledge weaknesses or potential vulnerable areas in the plan. Focusing on measureable impact will ensure success of your NICHE Plan, do not use language such as "the quality of care will improve," or the "the length of stay will go down," focus on baseline data to give estimates that are specific and credible [31]. The NICHE business plan should be a working and guiding document helping to communicate NICHE vision, goals, and objectives to stakeholders in the organization and the community. NICHE sites are encouraged to update their business or action plan every 2 years at a minimum.

In order to assure sustainability of a NICHE program, some sites are able to secure additional support from outside of the organization through requests to local, state, and national foundations and individual donors. Gifts from donors might be restricted or unrestricted to a specific activity related to NICHE and such gifts may be one time or an ongoing contribution with limited expectations and reports, while grants typically require a more rigorous and competitive application process and detailed outcomes reporting [32]. Grants and gifts have supported individual initiatives such as funding nursing leaders to participate in the NICHE Leadership Training Program (LTP), providing equipment or supplies for patient care such as pocket talkers, funding the music/art therapy program, or supporting continuing education for geriatric resource nurses.

Patients and families have been involved in business plans or action plans. Holy Cross hospital in Maryland developed the first Geriatric Emergency Room and the driving force behind the physical and care environment changes was the feedback from the older adult patients that had been invited to be on an advisory council. Their feedback was instrumental to including additional seating and room for family, white boards to share test timing and discharge as well as warming blankets for patients. This feedback was not expected by the staff and was an important aspect to the improved satisfaction after implementation.

Some NICHE action or business plans have stalled or even failed because of unanticipated problems such as the loss of an administrative or clinical champion, changing priorities within the system, or a competitor's advantage. If or when this occurs, it is advisable to review the NICHE business plan with the NICHE steering committee to refocus or gain clarity of the program to reflect the strategic plan of the facility or health system.

Scaling the Niche Model: The Aurora Health Care Experience

With the change in the healthcare environment, the utilization of NICHE in a health system with multiple hospitals and practice settings is increasing. As noted earlier, the original adopters of NICHE were staff nurses that had identified the need for geriatric best practice at the unit or hospital level. Currently, the interest for NICHE has also started coming from clinical and administrative leaders who have requested implementation on a system scale that includes multiple hospitals that are newly acquired, smaller-scale health systems, that include all hospitals, to very large integrated health systems that cover dozens of hospitals and other settings over multiple states. Examples of NICHE being scaled to meet the needs of a large integrated health system included Wisconsin's Aurora Health Care. Aurora Health Care was an early adopter of the ACE model [33] and a pioneer in an EHR electronic clinical decision-support (CDS) tool called the ACE tracker [34]. (This is covered in more detail in another chapter in this book.) The ACE model has been disseminated to 14 of Aurora's acute care hospitals starting in 2000. The ACE model at Aurora Health Care focuses on preventing functional decline, Geriatrician review of medical care, early discharge planning, patient-centered plan of care, and interdisciplinary team rounds. These elements were the foundation to the health system and NICHE was identified to assist in expanding the knowledge base of staff in 2009.

The Aurora Senior Services department looked to expand their program with the development, dissemination, and assessment of the ACE model principles in more than 40 in-patients units. Although ACE principles were used by the geriatricians and nursing leaders at daily interdisciplinary rounds to provide patient care recommendations to staff and "just-in-time" teaching, the need for consistent foundational nursing education concerning geriatric concepts was identified as a system need. An assessment of in-house developed resources by the Senior Services department determined that the NICHE program's array of courses, resources, webinars, etc., was a cost effective means to educate Aurora's approximately 6,000 registered nurses. Additionally, Senior Services department partnered with Extendicare, a national long-term skilled nursing and rehabilitation company, to increase the scope of learning and collaboration between facilities.

In 2008, Aurora Senior Services and Extendicare began a collaboration to commit to NICHE and formed a steering committee to develop a needs assessment and action plan. The steering committee reviewed the process and cost to start NICHE and created a proposal for piloting the project at interested acute care sites. The needs assessment identified ongoing foundational geriatric education, ease of access, and alignment with nursing professional development as focus points. The NICHE curriculum and services fulfilled these points, but the steering committee sought to augment the GRN training to create a path to ANCC Gerontological Nurse certification as part of the pilot project. The creation of a path to certification was beneficial in that it provides nursing education, strategies to improve patient care, as well as aligned NICHE membership with the Aurora System nursing career development ladder. Additionally, the Gerontological nursing certification pathway aligned with the Aurora's goal of pursuing Magnet designation by providing simplified "pre-packaged" service to support nursing professional development that is scalable for the needs of a large health system. The alignment with the nursing development ladder was a key point in securing site nursing executive buy-in. Eventually, four community hospitals ranging in size from 100 to 250 beds and three long-term care and rehabilitation sites expressed interest to pilot NICHE. The site leadership teams were identified and jointly enrolled in the 2010 NICHE LTP.

The NICHE steering committee and site leadership teams within Aurora and Extendicare created the infrastructure to reach the large and diverse caregiver workforce that jointly care for senior patients along the continuum of care. Joint collaboration and regular communication provided the opportu-nity to tailor the approach for caregivers of different disciplines (GPCA) and multiple locations and care environments. The steering committee meets monthly to assess progress, support sites-specific initiatives, and learn from shared experiences. An example of the benefit of partnership has been establishing contacts between the acute care and long-term facilities to problem solve in difficult discharge situations and readmissions. This collaboration has resulted in a greater understanding of the needs between the transition points for the patient.

As Aurora expanded with NICHE, additional sites were added including a large tertiary hospital, a small community hospital, and an urban hospital serving an underserved population. While the needs for foundational geriatric education was common among all sites, each site had unique needs secondary to the community they served. The steering committee supported the development and coordination of a NICHE GRN team between two of Aurora's small community hospitals that was tasked to create RN competencies for use at their combined sites. The utilization of GRNs to expand the knowledge base for all staff at the sites maximizes limited resources and supported nursing professional development. The Senior Services department has also collaborated with the Aurora certified nursing assistant training program to standardize geriatric education and supply the system with nursing assistants prepared for the challenge of at-risk seniors. Furthering the scale and scope of NICHE to meet the needs of the workforce, the Aurora-Extendicare team collaborated with NICHE to develop a long-term care GIAP and curriculum tailored to their specifics needs and regulations. The utilization of NICHE within a large healthcare system, when combined with coordinated system oversight, is an excellent means to prepare the workforce for the changing demographics.

Other systems have reported the success of implementing NICHE on a larger scale. This includes the adaptation of the NICHE model best suited for each site to ensure success while having a system team to support each of the sites. The Advocate system in Illinois, the Medstar and BonSecours systems in Virginia both have varying levels of designation and implementation at their sites but all of these systems have a system steering team or clinical team that allows for sharing of resources and best practice in their facilities to create a cohesive support system. Other systems have implemented the NICHE program in varying ways with differing steering committees unique to each facility with a nurse leader such as a CNO or CNE that follows their progress and level of designation on a more informal scale.

Integration into the Electronic Health Record (EHR)

For many of the NICHE programs, integrating evidenced-based protocols is essential for success. The use of tools for assessing vulnerable elders and implementing interdisciplinary plans of care is the difference between a site that is beginning to implement geriatric best practice and a site that has established geriatric care. Having the ability to monitor patient outcomes, identify transitional needs and documenting patient and family teaching is necessary to communicate seamless care in a fragmented system. All sites during the LTP are instructed on the importance of the EHR and improving care of the older adult. Many sites develop their own version of established tools or implement established tools such as the SPICES tool [11] into the EHR for rounds to assess vulnerable elders daily, the Confusion Assessment Method or CAM [35] to identify delirium or other assessments that are specific to the needs of the older adult. Aurora Health Care's ACE Tracker [34] is an example of a comprehensive geriatric clinical decision support (CDS) tool that extracts key demographic, assessment, and care parameters documented in the electronic health record (EHR). The ACE Tracker displays the information for all hospitalized patients at each facility who are 65 years and older on a daily report used by interdisciplinary team members to facilitate care (*see* Chap. 4 *for more details*). This allows for monitoring of quality indicators, has specific plans of care or evidenced-based practice at the fingertips of the caregivers to promote consistent use. Because NICHE is not prescriptive but allows for sharing of best practice at the bedside developed by experts in the field, the sites are able to identify a practice area of need and implement a site-specific version of work other sites have done to ensure adoption at the user level.

Healthcare Reform and Cost of the Program

With the changing landscape of healthcare, preventing loss of revenue and improving the quality of care for the older adult is imperative. Based on the identified needs of each institution, the NICHE coordinator is able to determine programmatic and clinical care needs and develop their own geriatric best practices to improve care. This includes never events such as CAUTIs, falls with injury, readmissions, and beginning now patient satisfaction. Having resources that are available to improve care of older adults including medication problems, preventing pressure ulcers and reduction of restraints are clearly defined in starting a program to address, monitor, and sustain change. All are needed in the current regulatory and reimbursement environment.

Coming in 2015, there will be a strong push to improve the care across the continuum at NICHE with the addition of LTC and HH education and programming. With the change to a bundled payment environment and the need to collaborate across care sites, improving nursing and staff education as well as evidenced-based care across the continuum is imperative.

The NICHE program began as a free resource for hospitals across the country. Sites that were interested in becoming a NICHE hospital would attend the annual conference held in New York City and receive materials to take back to their site and adapt to their setting and begin instructor led courses or in some cases create courses on line for staff. Starting in 2010, NICHE became a member organization and began charging fees. These fees include the LTP fees based on the amount of attendees as well as the type and size of hospital participating. Then every year, the sites have a membership fee that is based on status of hospital (lead or flagship) and those in the system that are add-ons. These fees create a sustainable, independent organization for NICHE and provide hospitals and now LTC and HH sites access to tools, resources and education for a workforce that is in dire need of specialization in geriatrics. This access allows sites to have the opportunity to current, evidenced-based resources that they are able to replicate in their specific setting all based on the individual needs of their organization. Many sites do not have a geriatric expert as the lead but rather a nurse or other leader that has a passion for geriatrics has identified this as a specialty or need in their facility and needs the exposure to staff. The LTP provides the opportunity to develop a plan of implementation and the Knowledge Center provides the tools and resources for staff to improve their geriatric skills and knowledge. Many sites do not have content experts in geriatrics; the NICHE Knowledge Center provides resources and education that would not be possible without significant time and effort by educators or nurse leaders. This is a cost-effective means of providing evidenced-based, current education as well as outstanding, tested protocols and programming that NICHE sites across the country have developed and are able to share with the NICHE community.

When looking at Value-Based Purchasing (VBP) and the impact on hospitals across the country, NICHE is poised to create geriatric-sensitive care environments that improve clinical outcomes by developing the knowledge base and clinical practice of staff; potentially to minimize penalties and maximize the reimbursement points. NICHE sites across the country share their efforts to improve the quality of care of older adults through poster and podium presentations at the NICHE Conference yearly. This creates a wealth of information for participating sites to replicate best practice in their settings. The measures of the Clinical Process and Patient Experience of Care Measures monitored by CMS through VBP have been presented at the conference and developed further into live webinars, Solution Series or other resources such as Clinical Improvement Models that address the three domains:

– Clinical Process of Care (13 measures)
– Patient Experience of Care (eight HCAHPS dimensions)
– Outcome (three mortality measures)

NICHE coordinators and GRNs are also able to query fellow NICHE participants on the discussion board about best practice solutions to specific areas of care of the older adult. The education and resources offered by the NICHE program provide real solutions to many of the performance measures that impact the bottom line for health systems. The resources also provide means for systems and facilities to have better patient engagement and satisfaction. For many sites, cost avoidance is the best way of managing costs and limiting penalties as described. Sites are able to improve care over time thus gaining achievement or improvement points in the VBP system by systematically improving the care of older adults in areas such as

- Clinical Process measures
  - HF-1 Discharge Instructions
  - SCIP–Inf–9 Postoperative Urinary Catheter Removal on Postoperative Day 1 or 2
- Patient Experience measures
  - Nurse Communication
  - Hospital Staff
  - Responsiveness
  - Pain Management
  - Medicine Communication
  - Hospital Cleanliness and Quietness
  - Discharge Information
  - Overall Hospital Rating

Sites have access to resources on developing, measuring, and sustaining nurse-driven protocols as well as interdisciplinary protocols in both the LTP and the supplemental reading in the Planning and Implementation guide. This gives step-by-step instructions that assist the site in developing their own resources to improve the care of older adults. The site is able to have a vast amount of clinical resources as well as the tools to adapt and implement geriatric protocols makes the NICHE program an essential tool in the current healthcare environment.

References

1. Fulmer T. The geriatric resource nurse: a model of caring for older patients. Am J Nurs. 2001;102:62.
2. Francis D, Fletcher K, Simon LF. The GRN model of care: a vision for the future. Nursing Clinics of North America. 1998;33(3):481–96.
3. Inouye SK, Acampora D, Miller RL, Fulmer T, Hurst LD, Cooney LM. The Yale geriatric care program: a model of care to prevent functional decline in hospitalized elderly patients. J Am Geriatr Soc. 1993;41(12):1345–52.
4. Capezuti EA, Briccoli B, Boltz MP. Nurses Improving the Care of Healthsystem Elders: creating a sustainable business model to improve care of hospitalized older adults. J Am Geriatr Soc. 2013;61(8):1387–93.
5. Hall MJ, DeFrances CJ, Williams SN, Golosinskiy A, Schwartzman A. National hospital discharge survey: 2007 summary. National health statistics reports; no 29. Hyattsville, MD: National Center for Health Statistics; 2010.
6. http://www.cdc.gov/nchs/data/nsltcp/long_term_care_services_2013

7. Permpongkosol S. Iatrogenic disease in the elderly: risk factors, consequences, and prevention. Clin Interv Aging. 2011;6:77–85.
8. Boltz M, Capezuti E, Zwicker D, Fulmer T, editors. Evidence-based geriatric nursing protocols for best practice. 4th ed. New York, NY: Springer; 2012.
9. Capezuti E, Boltz M, Cline D, Dickson V, Rosenberg M, Wagner L, Shuluk J, Nigolian C. NICHE – a model for optimizing the geriatric nursing practice environment. J Clin Nurs. 2012;21:3117–25.
10. Leff B, Burton L, Mader SL, Naughton B, Burl J, Inouye SK, et al. Hospital at home: feasibility and outcomes of a program to provide hospital-level care at home for acutely ill older patients. Ann Intern Med. 2005;143(11):798–808.
11. Fulmer T, Abraham IL. Rethinking geriatric nursing. Geriatr Nurs. 1998;33(3):387–94.
12. Pfaff J. The geriatric resource nurse model: a culture change. Geriatr Nurs. 2002;23(3):140–4.
13. Conley DM, Burket TL, Schumacher S, Lyons D, DeRosa SE, Schirm V. Implementing geriatric models of care: a role of the gerontological clinical nurse specialist – Part II. Geriatr Nurs. 2012;33(4):314–8.
14. Capezuti E, Boltz M, Shuluk J, et al. Utilization of a benchmarking database to inform NICHE implementation. Res Gerontol Nurs. 2013;6(3):198–208.
15. Fletcher K, Hawkes P, Williams-Rosenthal S, Mariscal CS, Cox BA. Using nurse practitioners to implement best practice care for the elderly during hospitalization: the NICHE journey at the University of Virginia Medical Center. Crit Care Nurs Clin North Am. 2007;19:321–37.
16. Kim H, Capezuti E, Boltz M, Fairchild S, Fulmer T, Mezey M. Factor structure of the geriatric care environment scale. Nurs Res. 2007;56:339–47.
17. Boltz M, Capezuti E, Shuluk J, Nickoley S. NICHE measurement and program evaluation. In: Boltz M, Capezuti E, editors. NICHE planning and implementation guide. New York, NY: Nurses Improving Care for Healthsystem Elders; 2013.
18. Abraham IL, Bottrell MM, Dash KR, et al. Profiling care and benchmarking best practice in care of hospitalized elderly: The Geriatric Institutional Assessment Profile. Nurs Clin North Am. 1999;34:237–55.
19. Boltz M, Capezuti E, Bowar-Ferres S, et al. Hospital nurses' perceptions of the geriatric care environment. J Nurs Scholarsh. 2008;40(3):282–9.
20. Tavares JP, da Silva, AL, Sá-Couto P, Boltz M, Portuguese nurses knowledge of and attitudes toward hospitalized older adults. Scand J Caring Sci. 2015;29(1):51–61.
21. American Nurses Association. The National Database of Nursing Quality Indicators (NDNQI®) website. Available at: http://www.nursingworld.org/Research-Toolkit/NDNQI. Accessed July 16, 2014.
22. St. Pierre J, Twibell R. Developing nurses' geriatric expertise through the geriatric resource nurse model. Geriatr Nurs. 2012;33(2):140–9.
23. Wright, S. Environmental and social approaches to improve outcomes for the hospitalized older adult. Solutions series. 2010. Available at: http://nicheprogram.org/uploads/File/solutions/NICHE_Solutions_9.pdf. Accessed July 16, 2014.
24. Flood K. Improving medication safety in older adults at the University of Alabama at Birmingham Hospital. Solutions series. 2010. Available at: http://nicheprogram.org/uploads/File/solutions/Solution%201_Final_Screen.pdf. Accessed July 16, 2014.
25. Salman A, McCabe D, Easter T, et al. Cultural competence among staff nurses who participated in a family-centered geriatric care program. J Nurses Staff Dev. 2007;23(3):103–11.
26. 2012 NICHE conference poster: a rural hospital's approach to prevention and treatment of delirium in the elderly hospitalized patient improves outcomes. Arun Nagpaul, MD, Pam Elsberee, RN, BSN,

CCM and Karole Shafer, DNP, ACNP, Newark Wayne Community Hospital, Wayne County, New York.

27. Boltz M, Capezuti E, Shuluk J, et al. Implementation of geriatric acute care best practices: initial results of NICHE sites self-evaluation. Nurs Health Sci. 2013;15:518–24.

28. Nickoley S. Aligning NICHE and magnet initiatives. In: Bub L, Boltz M, Capezuti E, editors. NICHE planning and implementation guide. New York, NY: NYU; 2013.

29. Flood KL, MacLennan PA, McGrew D, Green D, Dodd C, Brown CJ. Effects of an acute care for elders unit on costs and 30-day readmissions. JAMA Intern Med. 2013;173:981. doi:10.1001/jamainternmed.2013.524.

30. Boltz M, Capezuti E, Bower-Ferres S, Norman R, Secic M, Kim H, et al. Changes in the geriatric care environment associated with NICHE. Geriatr Nurs. 2008;29(3):176–85.

31. Bond C, Rodenhausen N, Spragens L, Yellig R. Developing a NICHE action plan. In: Bub L, Boltz M, Capezuti E, editors. NICHE planning and implementation guide. New York, NY: NYU; 2013.

32. Wurmser TA. Obtaining financial support through grants and gifts. In: Bub L, Boltz M, Capezuti E, editors. NICHE planning and implementation guide. New York, NY: New York University; 2013.

33. Landefeld CS, Palmer RM, Kresevic DM, Fortinsky RH, Kowal J. A randomized trial of care in a hospital medical unit especially designed to improve the functional outcomes of acutely ill older patients. N Engl J Med. 1995;332(20):1338–44.

34. Malone ML, Vollbrecht M, Stephenson J, Burke L, Pagel P, Goodwin JS. Acute Care for Elders (ACE) tracker and e-Geriatrician: methods to disseminate ACE concepts to hospitals with no geriatricians on staff. J Am Geriatr Soc. 2010;58(1):1.

35. Inouye S, van Dyck C, Alessi C, Balkin S, Siegal A, Horwitz R. Clarifying confusion: the confusion assessment method. Ann Intern Med. 1990;113(12):941–8.

36. Aiken LH, Clarke SP, Sloane DM, Sochalski J, Silber JH. Hospital nurse staffing and patient mortality, nurse burnout, and job dissatisfaction. JAMA. 2002;288:1987–1993.

Palliative Care as a Consultation Model

Bethann Scarborough and Diane E. Meier

Background

Which Healthcare Problems Are Addressed by Palliative Care?

Palliative care addresses fundamental problems in the healthcare system (such as sub-specialization, fragmentation, lack of training in care of the chronically and seriously ill, absent communication and coordination among providers and settings) by aligning the care delivered to patients with the care they desire, treating physical and psychosocial distress, focusing on skilled communication with patients, families, providers, and settings, and thereby improving the quality of care to the most frail, vulnerable patients in the society [1]. Numerous studies have shown that seriously ill patients often do not receive the kind of care they want [2, 3]. Specifically, in the last 6 months of life Medicare beneficiaries spend between 1.3 and 5.7 days in the Intensive Care Unit (ICU) [4] while 10.5–22.5 % of Medicare deaths were associated with an ICU admission [5] and approximately 20 % of Americans who died during a hospitalization spent time in an ICU during their final admission [6]. Intense healthcare utilization is not specific to the ICU—a retrospective review of Medicare data showed that 75 % of decedents visited an Emergency Department (ED) in the last 6 months of life; half visited the ED in the last month of life and 68 % of those patients who were admitted subsequently died in the hospital [7].

B. Scarborough, M.D. (✉)
Brookdale Department of Geriatrics and Palliative Medicine, Mount Sinai Hospital, One Gustave L. Levy Place, New York, NY 10029, USA
e-mail: bethann.scarborough@mssm.edu

D.E. Meier, M.D.
Department of Geriatrics and Palliative Medicine, Icahn School of Medicine at Mount Sinai, 55 West 125th Street, Suite 1302, New York, NY 10027, USA
e-mail: diane.meier@mssm.edu

Figure 6.1 shows national geographic variances in acute care admissions in the last 6 months of life for Medicare beneficiaries. Dying in the hospital is associated with poor quality of life for patients and portends an increased risk of psychiatric disorders in their bereaved caregivers [8]. Frail, elderly patients are also at risk of frequent and burdensome transfers between care sites, with an average of 3.2 transitions in the last 6 months of life. Such repeated transfers put patients at risk for adverse outcomes and lower family members' trust in healthcare professionals [9].

Which Patients Will Be Best Served by Palliative Care?

Seriously ill patients should be screened for common palliative care needs including pain, non-pain symptoms, practical needs such as transportation, food, housing, and financial support, family caregiver burden, and lack of understanding of the likely disease course and its associated treatment options. Palliative care services can be delivered by the patient's primary team if they have been appropriately trained and supported in the necessary knowledge and skills. A primary team may be unable to meet a patient's palliative care needs if they have received inadequate training on conducting successful goals of care discussions or managing physical symptoms or if they perceive they do not have the time to address the needs of seriously ill patients. Patients with more complex or challenging needs may require specialist-level palliative care teams working alongside and in support of the primary team [10]. Screening for palliative care may occur on a patient level where patients are identified based on their physical symptoms, psychological symptoms, spiritual distress, practical needs, or family distress. Alternatively, screening may occur via a systems-based approach using the presence of any potentially life-limiting or life-threatening condition in combination with past utilization (frequent readmissions for example) as a trigger for either primary palliative care (the basic skills required of all physicians and other

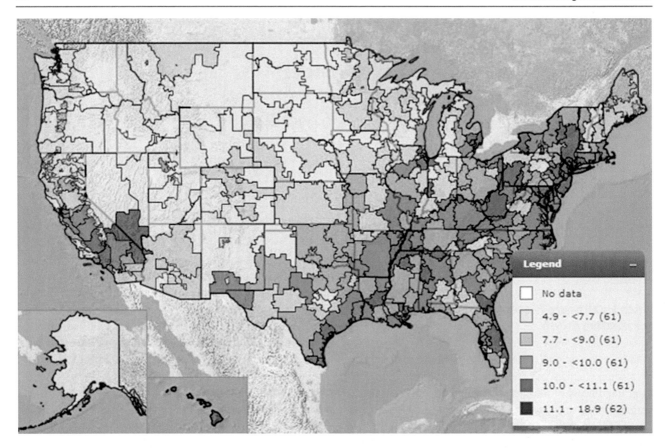

Fig. 6.1 Inpatient days per decedent during the last 6 months of life (Year: 2007) (from The Dartmouth Atlas Project, The Dartmouth Institute, http://www.dartmouthatlas.org/data/topic/topic.aspx?cat=18 with permission)

healthcare professionals) or for a specialty level palliative care consultation. The provision of a palliative care consultation service that provides secondary (specialty level) or tertiary palliative care (provided at a tertiary medical center where specialist knowledge for complex symptom management and goals of care is taught, researched, and practiced) is critically important in caring for patients whose needs exceed those that can be met through primary palliative care [10]. For example, preliminary observations from a pilot program providing inpatient palliative care consultations to patients who met trigger criteria based on disease stage, readmission risk, or uncontrolled symptoms improved the frequency of palliative care consults while reducing readmission rates, increasing hospice use, and improving the mortality index for the patient population studied [11].

What Are the Barriers to the Provision of Palliative Care?

Access to palliative care may be decreased both by critical shortages in the workforce and misconceptions about palliative care.

Workforce Challenges

Despite a 150 % increase in the prevalence of palliative care programs in the US over the past decade [12], a shortage of trained palliative medicine physicians and nurses is still a major barrier to accessing palliative care. Approximately 2 % of hospitalizations in the United States end in the patient's death, and an additional 4–8 % of patients are discharged with serious illnesses—extrapolating from this, one could estimate that approximately 10 % of hospitalized patients require either primary or specialty level palliative care. Palliative care programs currently see a median of 2.6 % of all hospital admissions [13]; quadrupling the number of patients evaluated from this current rate to meet the estimated need of seeing 10 % of all hospitalized patients requires a major expansion in the available workforce [1]. A recent workforce shortage study estimated that between 2,787 and 7,510 full-time physicians are needed just to meet the immediate palliative care needs of the hospital and hospice population in the United States [14], and this does not include estimates of workforce demands for community-based palliative care now or in the future. In 20 of the 50 United States, no postgraduate medical education in specialty level palliative care is available, and in states that do provide such training slots are limited to about 150 trainees per year, far short of current and projected demand [1].

Perception of Palliative Care

Lack of public and professional understanding about what palliative care entails or incorrectly equating palliative care with hospice are significant barriers to access to palliative care. National public opinion research revealed differences between how healthcare providers and the lay public view palliative care and the importance of using very specific language to define the type of care provided by a palliative medicine team. The language with the most positive impact for patients included that which described it as "specialized medical care and an added layer of support for people with serious illness focused on improving quality of life for both the patient and the family" [15]. Recent research also specifically compared the term "palliative care" with "supportive care" for oncology patients and found that the term "supportive care" was associated with better oncologist understanding and more favorable impression of the type of care provided by a palliative medicine team [16]. The misconceptions regarding the benefits of palliative care and the population of patients best served by this specialized care may lead to a mismatch between needs and access that is dependent upon an individual physician's training, bias, and practice patterns [1] or upon patient and family misunderstanding of the benefits of palliative care alongside their regular medical care. Educating healthcare providers on the scope and benefits of palliative care while modeling behavior can effectively increase an individual's understanding of palliative care. Oftentimes, physicians only fully appreciate the benefit of palliative care after receiving assistance with a particularly challenging case. This may be accomplished by having palliative care conduct a family meeting with the physician who requested the palliative care consult present, so he can witness first-hand how effectively specialty-level palliative care can meet the needs of the patient and family.

What Are the Benefits of Palliative Care?

There is an increasing literature on the benefits of palliative care on quality of life for patients and caregivers, survival, and cost savings [2, 17, 18].

Quality Outcomes

Palliative care has been shown to improve symptom management, caregiver burden, satisfaction with communication, and emotional and spiritual support during serious illness. Patients receiving palliative care have also been shown to have higher satisfaction with their hospital care and are more likely to have advance directives when compared to patients who receive usual care [2, 17, 18]. One randomized controlled trial showed that patients who received an inpatient palliative care consultation had higher patient satisfaction scores, fewer ICU admissions if readmitted to the hospital, and longer hospice stays compared with patients who received usual hospital care [17]. One randomized controlled trial of patients with newly diagnosed metastatic non-small cell lung cancer enrolled patients within 8 weeks of diagnosis; those who were randomized to the palliative care group met with a palliative medicine specialist (either a physician or advanced-practice nurse) within 3 weeks of enrollment, in addition to usual oncology care. The patients who received early palliative care concurrently with standard oncologic care had improved quality of life, less depression, and were more likely to have resuscitation preferences documented compared with patients who received standard oncologic care alone. In addition, the patients randomized to receive early palliative care had significantly longer survival than those who received standard oncologic care only despite (or perhaps because of) receiving less hospital-based care near end of life [19].

Cost Outcomes

Healthcare value is defined as the ratio of the quality of care to the cost of care. Palliative care increases the value of care by improving responsiveness to patient and family needs, resulting in reduced emergencies, 911 calls, and hospitalizations [1]. In the current US healthcare system's method of reimbursing higher fees for procedural interventions, palliative care and other so-called "cognitive services" remain relatively poorly compensated, requiring supplementation from both health system operating dollars and philanthropy.

A review of data from eight hospitals with established palliative care programs showed the clear benefits in cost savings due to palliative care consultations. The cost savings for a patient discharged alive who had an inpatient palliative consult averaged $1,696 in direct costs per admission. Of patients who died during the admission, those who had been seen by a palliative care team had an adjusted net savings of $4,908 in direct costs per admission. Based on these statistics, an average 400-bed hospital with a palliative care consultation team that sees 500 patients a year could reap a net savings (costs avoided) of 1.3 million dollars per year. Part of the cost savings comes from a natural reduction in unwanted tests, procedures, and intensive care unit use as palliative care aligns treatments with informed patient goals and preferences [20].

How Does Palliative Care Help Align the Care Delivered to Patients with the Care They Desire?

Conducting successful goals of care discussions involves open communication and information-sharing to facilitate delivery of care the patient wants. Each team member (physician/advanced practice nurse (APN), social worker, chaplain) has a different skill set, making the most productive family meetings those in which all members of the interdisciplinary team are present. When team members have a seamless working relationship, they can each respond to the concerns the patient may have (a social worker may address home situation, coping with illness, or realistic discharge planning; a chaplain may help to explore how religion or spirituality affects the patient or caregiver's coping style or may identify the presence of existential suffering). There are several key steps for conducting a successful goals of care discussion. One method often used is "SPIKES" with six standard steps outlined below [21]:

1. *Setting*: Before meeting with a patient, discuss the case with the other providers involved in the patient's care so that the most current clinical information (i.e., diagnosis or potential treatment plans) is known. Although it may seem like common sense, the importance of creating the appropriate setting for a serious conversation cannot be underestimated. Hospitals and outpatient practices are under increasing time and space constraints, so one must ensure that there is enough time and space for the patient, his loved ones, and the entire healthcare team to sit down together to discuss the case. Part of this initial process often involves asking non-medical questions about the patient to assess what is most important to the patient and family while building rapport. The information garnered during this time can become critical to helping the physician keep the meeting on track later on by focusing on the patient's goals and personal values.

2. *Perception*: Assess the patient's view and understanding of the medical situation—this allows the physician to develop a picture of what the patient understands, the level of healthcare literacy, and any elements of denial that may be present. All of these components can alter the manner in which information is shared during the meeting.

3. *Invitation*: Obtain permission to share information before doing so. While many patients may want detailed information, others may only want the "big picture" of their illness, and some may want information-sharing deferred to their surrogate or healthcare proxy.

4. *Knowledge and information-sharing*: Warn the patient that you are about to share bad news. When information is shared, avoid medical jargon. Give information in small pieces, allowing time for the patient to process it and respond before continuing.

5. *Emotions and Empathy*: Prepare for patients and family members to become emotional as news is shared. Respond to the emotion by empathically naming the emotion and using silence to allow the patient to express whatever emotions are most prominent. Addressing the emotion is often a critical way of moving the conversation forward efficiently.

6. *Strategy and Summary*: After hearing new information, some patients become immediately focused on the next steps, while others may be too overwhelmed to even think of what will happen next. Assess if the patient is ready to discuss a treatment plan or whether he needs more time to process the information shared. If the patient is not ready to discuss next steps, set a time to regroup and do so. For a hospitalized patient this may happen the following day, while for an outpatient this may happen days to weeks later depending on the urgency of the situation.

Notably, these steps may not always occur in the exact order outlined above or even in one meeting. A physician with a longstanding relationship with a patient may already know how the patient perceives his illness, making the "assessment of perception" a smaller part of the process. An emotional response may occur at any time during a conversation and a physician should not wait to try and address all the emotions after delivering information; the emotion must be addressed in real-time [21].

The length of time for a family meeting depends on both the physician's skill in eliciting values first to frame the conversation and stay on target with medical recommendations and on "where the family is"—whether patient and family members are aligned in what they hope for and if they have already discussed the issue at hand. Focusing the family on the acute problem and addressing the underlying emotion helps move the conversation forward, and responding to emotion has been shown to lengthen a typical physician–patient encounter by less than 30 s [22]. In addition, taking a few minutes to first let the patient verbalize his hopes actually saves time later on, because it allows the healthcare team to make a recommendation for care based on the patient's individual values and preferences. A sample conversation is outlined below:

Mr. Benning is an 89-year-old man with dementia who requires assistance with ADLs and is declining oral intake. He is living at home and has a home health aide 5 h per day 5 days per week. His daughter, Lisa, lives with him and cares for him when the home health aide is not working. This is his third admission in the last 5 months for pneumonia, he has lost 15 lb and now has a BMI of 20. The primary team requests a palliative care consultation for assistance with decision-making as the daughter is requesting PEG placement.

MD: Lisa, I am just meeting you and your father. I'd like to take a step back and hear a little bit about what your father was like before he developed dementia. Can you paint me a picture of what was most meaningful and enjoyable to him before he got sick?

Lisa: He was always outdoors…he used to take my son fishing every weekend in the spring, and he loved reading the paper and doing the daily crossword puzzle. He never gave up on that puzzle until it was completed! [tearful].

Chaplain: It sounds like there were a lot of things he loved to do, and I can see that this is really hard for you.

Lisa: Yes, it is.

MD: The doctors caring for your father asked us to talk with you about a feeding tube. Can you tell me what you've heard from them about the risks and benefits?

Lisa: Well, I don't want him to starve to death. And now that he can't eat on his own, he needs the tube so he won't starve. I don't see any risks to that. I think a tube will also help keep him out of the hospital. I don't want him to have to keep coming back here every time he isn't eating normally.

MD: I hear that you are worried about him "starving" and that you want to keep him at home if possible. Can I share some other information with you about a stomach tube for someone who has dementia, so we can decide if a tube will help you achieve your goals for him?

Lisa: Sure.

MD: Actually, there's a lot we know about what happens with people who have dementia and get pneumonia [shares medical information] [23]. One of the things I hear you saying is that you want to keep him out of the hospital if possible—I'm worried a stomach tube will not help you achieve this goal because of the risk of pneumonia associated with it [*MD first elicited Lisa's goals for her father and then used this information to show how a PEG is not aligned with this goal*].

Lisa: I hadn't really thought about it like that before. If he doesn't get the tube, how is he going to stay at home?

SW: I see that your father has Medicare insurance but not Medicaid. After we finish talking with the doctor, why don't you and I speak about some of the options for home care, and if home care isn't possible we can talk about nursing facilities.

MD: I think we covered a lot of information today. You don't need to make a decision now; why don't we give you some time and check in with you tomorrow to see what other questions you may have.

In this example, the physician was able to quickly elicit the patient's previously demonstrated values and the daughter's understanding of a PEG and then provides specific information on how a PEG would not help her achieve her goals. By eliciting the daughter's hopes and understanding first, the conversation is efficiently tailored to these specific issues.

With So Many Choices, How Do Hospitals and Health Systems Know Which Model to Pick?

Every hospital and health system will need to choose a model of care that is best suited to meet the needs of their patient population while helping the hospital system achieve its own goals and overall mission. Some of the choice may be based on operational issues (for example, not having the available staff or hospital beds for a dedicated inpatient unit) while the culture of the institution may also play a role. A system assessment can identify strengths and areas for improvement within an institution and help guide planners to the palliative care model that best fits their existing framework. Some of the basic components of a system assessment include:

- Overall vision—does the hospital system's strategic plan include palliative care?
- Practice standards—Do standardized policies support advance care planning, expert pain and symptom management, interdisciplinary palliative care, bereavement support, psychosocial and emotional support, communication between patients and providers and amongst providers?
- Education—Do continuing education programs include palliative care content for interdisciplinary staff members, patients, and families?[24]

Funding and Building a Program

How Do You Get Buy-in From Health System Leaders?

Buy-in from leadership starts with an assessment of what the health system needs to meet its goals, whether these goals are to lower cost by improving quality of care for highest risk, highest cost patients, increase patient satisfaction, decrease unnecessary healthcare utilization, or any combination of these outcomes. First, gather hospital-level data on clinical outcomes and financial impact to understand the global needs of the system. Next, speak with colleagues within the institution to identify their needs and how they view the needs of their most complex patients. It is helpful to speak with people in various leadership roles (chief medical and nursing officers, case management, local hospice agencies; directors of oncology, geriatrics, critical care, and social work). The most successful proposal will be one that can demonstrate how a palliative medicine team serves as a solution to system problems and fills a gap in the care provided by the current system. Finally, a persuasive proposal should show how the program can be piloted to fit local realities, scaled to meet need, leverage existing staff resources in the hospital system, be viable over time, and have a low risk of failure [24].

How Do You Develop a Business Plan to Determine the Costs and Benefits of the Model?

A good business plan is one that is tailored to the hospital's needs and contains the language used by the institution with the level of detail desired by hospital leadership. The required components are:

1. Executive summary, including a statement of program goals, milestone, and strategy
2. A financial/budget summary
3. An operational plan for implementation
4. Institutional and market analysis (a summary of the system and needs assessment)
5. Marketing plan
6. Appendix

Highlighting the value of care is important, as is including other locations of care throughout the health system (hospice, long term care, home care) that may experience higher future demand and utilization as a result of palliative care consultations for hospitalized patients [24].

Figure 6.2 shows an example of a palliative care business plan [24]; guidelines can also be found online at: https://www.capc.org/payers/palliative-care-payer-provider-toolkit/ [25].

"What Can We Implement and How Can We Get It for the Least Cost?"

When developing a new palliative care consultation service, it is vital to accurately estimate costs based on current needs and projected future growth while being creative in accessing various funding sources. This process ensures that a program implements everything feasible in the most cost-effective manner. An operational plan must describe the resources needed for the program to succeed and estimate the revenues it will generate over time. Each program needs to assume and prepare for rapid growth in order to meet the expectations of the physicians and patients who will continue to request palliative care consultations over time. For example, cost considerations may influence a decision on whether to open an inpatient unit or outpatient practice, as both require extensive staffing and infrastructure needs in comparison with an inpatient consultation service.

Two other ways to be cost-efficient are to leverage current hospital resources by collaborating with volunteer organizations and starting philanthropic efforts to support a new or growing program. Philanthropy can be particularly important as clinical income from physician and APN billing may not be sufficient to cover staff salaries and hospital funding may be unreliable. Philanthropic support—whether from an individual donor, corporation, or foundation—provides an additional source of funding that can help ensure the palliative care program is supported and sustained over time. To garner donations, palliative care leadership staff must prepare to commit the time necessary to forge personal relationships with potential donors and granting entities, while marketing the need for, and benefits of, palliative care [24].

The basic steps that lead to major gifts are:

1. Prospect identification: Identify sources of potential gifts. Sources may include patients, family members, volunteers, or community businesses or organizations.
2. Prospect research: Conduct background research on prospective sources to understand the source and what is important to the individual person or organization.
3. Cultivation and education: Build relationships and provide education on palliative care.
4. Preparing the case: Be prepared, at any time, to be able to explain the needs of the patients and families who benefit from palliative care, the competency and training of the interdisciplinary team members, and how vital philanthropic gifts are to ensuring the long-term success and feasibility of the program.
5. Solicitation: When a potential donor offers to help, set a time to follow-up and ask for a financial gift. When making a request, have data to show how gifts in varying amounts will benefit the program and the population it serves. Do not hesitate or avoid eye contact before asking for money—direct, confident requests are the most successful ones.
6. Stewardship: After someone has supported the program, maintain regular contact. Tailor the method of contact—by phone, email, or in person—to the donor's wishes. Engage willing donors in future activities to ensure they see the tremendous value of, and need for, ongoing philanthropy [24].

Will the Care Be Paid for Under the Medicare Fee-for-Service Program and Who Will Bear the Costs as Health Systems Transition to Value-Based Purchasing?

Palliative care consults and follow-up visits from physicians and advance practice nurses are reimbursed under Medicare Part B fee-for-service payment. The actual reimbursement rate varies depending on the payer's fee schedule and the copayment (determined in advance by a negotiation between the hospital system and insurance companies). The Current Procedural Terminology (CPT) codes used most often by palliative medicine providers are evaluation and management (E&M) codes. CPT E&M codes establish the history, physical examination, decision-making, and counseling conducted during a physician's visit. Palliative care physicians may bill based on visit complexity or on time spent counseling patients. The extent of the history and physical examination and the complexity level of medical decision-making determine the overall intensity of the visit. Palliative medicine visits often have a high level of complex medical decision making; components include the number and stability of medical problems, the complexity of data reviewed (including

Category	Year 1				
	Start-Up Expense	Outreach Activities	Patient Care	Systems Support	Total Year 1
Revenue:					
Professional fees					
Inpatient Hospice Revenue					
Donors & grants					
Contracted services (nursing homes, etc)					
Institutional support (hospital)					
Department support					
Total					
Expenses (should be organized to reflect direct and indirect classifications of institution):					
Program Director					
Physician time					
Staff/team time					
Supplies/software/computers					
Patient materials/education outreach					
Physician & caregiver education					
Billing & reporting service					
Space costs for beds, offices, etc					
Overhead charges (rent, utilities, insurance)					
Travel & conferences					
Total					
Contribution/deficit (before cost avoidance)					
Cost Avoidance Impact Targets:					
Cost avoidance (LOS)					
Cost avoidance (cost per day)					
Capacity management (ICU usage)					
Total Estimated Impact (Indirect $)					

Fig. 6.2 Financial summary for a palliative care program (from Center to Advance Palliative Care with permission)

chart review, discussing the case with another provider, or discussion of test results with the performing physician, such as a radiologist) and the level of risk for the patient. Palliative care patients are high risk if they are critically ill, have multiple chronic conditions and organ failure(s), have a severe exacerbation of an underlying illness, are on parenteral-controlled substances, have a code status changed to do-not-resuscitate, or are receiving any drug therapy that requires intensive monitoring for toxicity—all of which may apply to patients hospitalized with a serious illness while requiring intravenous administration of opioids or benzodiazepines for intensive symptom management [26].

Alternatively, a lengthy palliative care consultation including counseling and exploring goals of care for a patient who is neither critically ill nor actively dying may be billed based on face-to-face *time* spent counseling the patient. Regardless of whether the visit is billed based on complexity or time spent counseling, the medical record must contain enough documentation to support the level of billing being submitted. APN billing varies by state, but APNs can bill for inpatient palliative care services only if they are paid by a non-hospital budget source. They cannot bill if they are paid from the hospital budget because hospital budgets are required to pay for all nursing care under Medicare's DRG payment to the hospital [27].

In contrast to the fee-for-service model that renders payment for the quantity of services delivered, value-based purchasing (VBP) pays based on outcomes. A change from fee-for-service to VBP is anticipated to reduce Medicare spending by approximately $214 billion over the next 10 years. There are several key features of VBP:[28]

- *Standardized measurements*: Crucial to measuring outcomes in VBP—if payment depends on outcomes, the manner of measuring outcomes must be standardized across various systems
- *Data collection*: Allows system-wide data sharing
- *Publicly reported results*: Measurement and reporting facilitate quality improvement and foster collaboration and shared accountability
- *Reforming the payment system to reward quality, value, and ongoing improvement*: A change from rewarding the high-volume service delivery under the current fee-for-service model, VBP rewards and motivates systems for engaging in practices that improve the quality outcomes and value of care over time
- *Engaging purchasers/consumers*: Physicians and patients may define quality in different ways; both patients and physicians must be engaged in health care in the VBP system
- *Managing expenses (providers)*: Cost containment is critical; the focus shifts from providing more care and tests of low quality to truly focusing on high quality care and good outcomes.

The concept behind VBP—providing high quality care and rewarding good outcomes rather than incentivizing increased volume of healthcare utilization—is aligned with the type of care already provided by palliative medicine.

Developing a Program to Meet the Hospital's Needs

What Are the Key Components and How Does the Model Work?

An effective consultation team must meet the needs of the patients, families, and staff as well as align with the mission and strategic plan of the hospital. Consider asking these questions when determining how the model will work [24]:

- *Who are the team members?* A 100-bed hospital may start a program with a part-time physician or APN, while a 1,000-bed hospital may need to start with a full interdisciplinary team. Regardless of the scale on which it starts each system needs to be prepared for growth over time. When starting a new service, including individuals who are respected by their colleagues and known and liked throughout the institution may help cultivate trust in and respect for the program. Collaboration with colleagues from many backgrounds (internal medicine, hospitalists, oncologists, cardiologists, surgeons, social work, nursing leadership) may increase the likelihood that physicians from multiple disciplines throughout the institution will refer patients to a new program [24].
- *How will the program be marketed?* Building a palliative care program is not enough to generate referrals. Hospital staff members must know that the program exists, how to contact the program to generate a new consult/referral, and which issues the palliative care team will address. Education and outreach, *prior* to the program's launch, is a vital part of success. Attending physicians, physicians-in-training, nurses, social workers, and patients and families all must know how to reach the palliative care team so that consults can be generated immediately [24].
- *How will patients be referred for consultation?* Depending on the hospital's individual culture, referrals may be generated based on current needs of the patient (symptom management, advance care planning) or via predetermined triggers for unmet needs (patients at high risk of readmission, high symptom burden, or with a DRG diagnosis that has a high inpatient mortality risk). Decide in advance if referrals will be accepted only from the primary attending physician (thereby ensuring that physician's buy-in for palliative care to see the patient) or if consults may be requested by any member of the patient's primary team and whether patients and family members may request a consult directly [24, 29].
- *How does the team interact with referring providers?* Determining the method by which the palliative care team will interact with referring providers is key to maintaining

open communication regarding patient care. It ensures that referring physicians have a consistently positive experience regardless of which member of the palliative care team evaluates a particular patient. Depending on hospital culture and acuity of the patient, palliative care team members should (in addition to leaving clear, concise, and timely consult notes in the medical record) call the referring provider, speak with the referring provider in person, or send an email or other secure communication with a brief update, thanking him or her for the consultation and ensuring that the reason for consultation was indeed addressed [24].

- *Where will the consultation service see patients?* Many consultation programs are housed within a hospital and see patients throughout the hospital. Some programs may include a dedicated inpatient palliative care unit or see patients in an outpatient palliative care practice (which may be housed within another department, such as oncology or geriatrics, or function as a stand-alone practice). Other programs may exist primarily as an inpatient consultation service in the hospital while partnering with a local hospice agency to seamlessly transfer patients across care sites. Each model has its own strengths and weaknesses and must be developed in the context of the local realities [24].

- *Which patients will "qualify" for palliative care consultation?* Any seriously ill patient may benefit from palliative care. A palliative care consultation is a request for help and signals that the primary team caring for a seriously ill patient recognizes unmet needs and wants assistance, whether with expert symptom management, goals of care discussions, or addressing another unmet need of the patient. Even if the individual calling the consult cannot eloquently describe the issue at hand, the success of the palliative care team depends on providing timely, respectful assistance when it is requested. Simply acknowledging the complexity and challenges of care for a colleague's patient can reduce professional distress and burnout (the so-called "blessing of the second opinion"). A palliative care team member should be available 24 h/day, 7 days/week (even if only by phone at night depending on staffing availability) to provide assistance to colleagues in need. To turn down a request for palliative care involvement is to close the door on someone who needs help. Once this door is closed, it is unlikely the requesting physician will reach out to palliative care in the future. The longevity and reputation of the palliative care consultation service depends on a willingness to help and reliable availability [24].

Who Are the Interdisciplinary Team Members?

The team structure varies depending on the available resources. In addition to a prescribing physician or APN, potential team members may include a social worker, chaplain, psychiatrist or psychologist, massage therapist, art and music therapist, and/or child life specialist. If funding is not available for all complementary services, volunteers may be leveraged until funding can be secured.

Social Work

Palliative care social workers fill a critical and unique role on the team. Social determinants (such as housing, transportation, literacy, history of trauma, access to food) account for nearly 50 % of all healthcare spending. While a hospitalized patient may have an assigned social worker as part of his care, this general social worker's role may be to primarily focus on discharge planning or logistical aspects of care rather than on providing practical and psychosocial support to seriously ill patients and caregivers in need. In addition, although other palliative care team members may uncover psychosocial issues, they may not have the specialized training in clinical counseling that is provided by a palliative care social worker. The palliative care social worker has a discrete role in patient care that is not provided by either the regular hospital social worker or the rest of the palliative care team [30].

Spiritual Care

Questions of meaning and purpose are of highest priority for people living with serious illness, and skilled chaplains are trained to help patients and families articulate and explore these issues. Spiritual support provided as part of a palliative care team can have benefits even for patients who already have a personal relationship with a community religious leader. Spiritual care provided by a member of the medical team has been shown to be associated with better quality of life before death and higher hospice use for patients who are terminally ill [31], in contrast to the outcomes of patients reporting high spiritual support from a member of their religious community [32].

Complementary Therapists

Many patients may be interested in complementary therapies as an adjunct to pharmacologic management of symptoms, to manage non-physical aspects of suffering, or due to a desire to avoid medications for personal, religious or cultural beliefs. Patients who suffer from "total pain" (existential, spiritual, family, physical, practical, and emotional distress) seek "inner stillness or peace" which may be fostered by complementary therapy. Massage, art, and music therapy may be used to treat both physical symptoms and meet emotional and existential needs. Even small studies have shown statistically significant improvement in symptom burden as reported by patients, suggesting that the results may be clinically significant since the outcome is subjective in nature [33].

A massage therapist also serves a role in educating family members about the benefits of massage and safe ways to touch very ill patients. Oftentimes, caregivers are at a loss for what they can offer a loved one in times of need; a recent study showed that education via a massage DVD or reading materials resulted in a decrease in symptoms. Caregivers also showed increased confidence, comfort, and self-efficacy in using massage as a form of care [34].

Art therapy and child-life specialists also help patients and families cope with serious illnesses. Art therapy provides an opportunity for both patients and their family members to explore existential suffering and have a creative outlet for feelings that may be difficult to articulate in words [35]. Child-life specialists fill a crucial role in providing support and exploring fears of children who either have a seriously ill family member or are seriously ill themselves [36, 37].

How Do Interdisciplinary Team Members Work Together?

For an interdisciplinary palliative care consult team to truly succeed each individual must have a clear and well delineated role on the team and regular structured inter-team communication should occur. Patients often share important details of their lives with social workers and complementary therapists, and these details may be vital to facilitating goals of care discussions and understanding the factors that influence the patient's decisions about care. Ideally all team members can view and document in the same medical record system. Each department should also ensure interdisciplinary team rounds are held and decide how often team members should meet together to discuss their active patients.

Ensuring that each team member understands his or her value in providing patient care is vital to the long-term success of the team. The literature on interdisciplinary team dynamics has revealed several common themes, including the importance of clear role boundaries and how to maintain them amongst team members. One example of this is in the challenge of physicians, nurses, social workers, and chaplains all attempting to provide psychosocial and spiritual support to a patient. O'Connor et al. raised the idea of a "contested role" with each team member struggling to find their niche in providing psychosocial support [38]. Outlining clear role boundaries while seamlessly working together as a team requires a delicate balance and an intentional, proactive plan for fostering interdisciplinary teamwork.

Leveraging the Electronic Medical Record

Electronic Medical Records (EMRs) are increasingly used in hospitals and outpatient practices. EMRs may improve the quality of care [39] and can be a powerful tool for collecting data to improve patient outcomes and enact change throughout a healthcare system. Electronic note templates can improve workflow efficacy and ensure consistency and reliability between palliative care providers of the same team. They can track symptom burden, record discussions regarding advance care planning, and monitor changes in patient outcomes including intensity of care, hospice use, and mortality. Figure 6.3 shows an example of an electronic note template:

Can Adult Patients/Family Caregivers Be Involved in the Planning and Advising of the Model of Care?

Both patients and caregivers may be involved in planning a new palliative care consultation service. Once the target patient population for palliative care consultations is identified, it may be helpful to form a focus group or advisory board of similar patients in the community. The group may be surveyed to determine their baseline beliefs about and expectations of palliative care. The input from older adults and family caregivers provides critical insight into the planning process and what will be most effective for the community's patient population [24].

What Training Is Required for Providers?

Each team member should have training and/or work experience in palliative care or hospice. Physicians should be board certified/board eligible in hospice and palliative medicine. If they have not already been grandfathered into board eligibility they will have to complete an ACGME-accredited fellowship program in palliative medicine. Other care providers including nurses, APNs, chaplains, and social workers should also seek training and specialty certification in palliative care. Basic competencies include expert communication skills, strong symptom management capabilities, skill in handling complicated family dynamics, mediating distress between (and among) primary teams and patients/families, providing support (emotional, spiritual, and psychosocial), discussing and honoring patient wishes to assist with discharge planning and treatment decisions, and an ability to think broadly and see the big picture in complicated situations [24].

How Can the Fidelity of the Implementation be Maintained?

To scale up to meet the needs of seriously ill patients and their families, a palliative care consult service must conduct frequent needs re-assessments and track outcomes to ensure that the service is fulfilling its mission statement. These actions will secure the role of palliative care in the broader healthcare system. Questions to ask include:[24]
- *Have there been changes in patient population?* Evaluate whether referral volume is decreasing, increasing or

Mount Sinai Palliative Medicine Initial Consult Note

Referred by:
Reason for referral:
Referring physician will be alerted to this visit and have access to this note.

History

Chief Complaint:

History obtained from (patient, family, chart, discussion with referring provider):

HPI:

Review of Symptoms:
ESAS:
Source: ESAS SOURCE: (patient, team, family):
Depression: (0-none, 1-mild, 2-moderate, 3-severe):
Anorexia: (0-none, 1-mild, 2-moderate, 3-severe):
Inactivity: (0-none, 1-mild, 2-moderate, 3-severe):
Dyspnea: (0-none, 1-mild, 2-moderate, 3-severe):
Anxiety: (0-none, 1-mild, 2-moderate, 3-severe):
Nausea: (0-none, 1-mild, 2-moderate, 3-severe):
Drowsiness: (0-none, 1-mild, 2-moderate, 3-severe):
Constipation: (0-none, 1-mild, 2-moderate, 3-severe):
Agitation: (0-none, 1-mild, 2-moderate, 3-severe):
Physical Discomfort: (0-none, 1-mild, 2-moderate, 3-severe):

Dementia: Yes/No:
Delirium: Yes/No:
Coma: Yes/No:

Review of Systems:
Constitutional:
Ears, Nose, Mouth, Throat:
Cardiovascular:
Respiratory:
GI:
GU:
Musculoskeletal:
Skin:
Neurological:
Endocrine:
Hematological/Lymphatic:
All other ROS have been reviewed and are negative.

Past Medical History:
Family History:
Social History:
Medications:
Allergies:

Complementary Therapies:

Fig. 6.3 Electronic note template

Spiritual History
Religious/spiritual orientation:
Involvement in Spiritual Community:
Need for further Chaplaincy support:
Are you religious or spiritual? Yes/No:
Where do you draw your strength from in difficult times like these?

Advance Care Planning

Awareness and Information Sharing
Patient's awareness/understanding of illness:
Information-sharing preferences:
Family's awareness of illness:

Information shared:

Advanced directives
Health Care Proxy:
Location of Proxy document:
Primary decision maker other than HCP:
Durable Power of Attorney:
Attitude towards place of death:
Funeral arrangements:

Limitations on Life Sustaining Treatments:

Data

I have personally reviewed and interpreted the following studies:
Radiology:

Labs:

PHYSICAL EXAM
Vitals:
Constitutional:
Ears, Nose, Mouth, Throat:
Eyes:
Neck:
Cardiovascular:
Pulmonary/Chest:
Breast:
Gastrointestinal:
Genitourinary:
Musculoskeletal:
Neurological:
Skin:
Psychiatric:

Fig. 6.3 (continued)

ASSESSMENT & PLAN

@name@ is a @age@ @sex@ with a history of *** who is seen by palliative care today for:

Physical Symptoms:

Advance Care Planning:
Extensive discussion, including both disease-directed treatment plans and plans for care if disease advances without being controlled by current treatment
- Will follow up with referring physician
- Encourage completion to end-of-life care tasks, including legal issues, legacy and leave-taking
- DPOA and code status discussed***

Counseling:

TIME SPENT
Visit consisted primarily of counseling and education dealing with the complex and emotionally intense issues of symptom management and palliative care in the setting of serious and potentially life-threatening illness.
Total MD face-to-face time: ***
Total MD counseling/education time: ***
Start time: ***
End time: ***
More than 50% time spent on counseling on education as noted above.

Fig. 6.3 (continued)

remaining stable and if there are particular specialties that refer frequently or do not refer at all [24]. If there are physicians who do not refer patients for palliative care, it may be necessary to conduct another needs assessment to identify barriers to collaboration and find ways to provide primary and specialist-level palliative care to patients in need.

- *Have there been changes in the hospital system*? A major change in the health system, such as a change in leadership, the addition of a new intensive care unit, nursing home, or hospice agency, will also change the demographics of the population. In addition, a new practice within the hospital (including pain management, volunteer services, or major staffing changes) may also begin to change the culture and resources available to patients. Ensure that there is ongoing education about palliative care and how it interacts with other disciplines in the hospital [24].

- *How is palliative care accountable for its outcomes within its own department and throughout the greater hospital system*? Accountability for outcomes requires constant reevaluation of how well the palliative care team is serving the needs of patients, families and colleagues. Monitoring data on clinical and financial impact of the service is important to hospital leadership and is prerequisite to securing ongoing support for the program. Outcome data may also be used to prompt changes in the program, whether from clinical staffing or fiscal support [24].

What Is the Role of the Geriatrician in Developing and Leading the Model?

A palliative care team that serves patients who are frail, elderly, and have multiple chronic co-morbidities will need to work closely with geriatricians in the health system. Collaboration is particularly important as patients transfer between care sites. Some palliative care programs may include physicians who are board certified in both geriatrics and palliative medicine. Geriatricians often lead programs designed to provide inclusive care to the elderly or work at local nursing homes, which would allow palliative care to be provided seamlessly across care sites [24].

How Can Health Systems Integrate the Geriatrics and Palliative Medicine Practice Models to Provide a Portfolio of Strategies to Address the Needs of Patients?

Interdisciplinary geriatric practice models are ideally suited to integrate palliative care principles and practices because they focus on quality of care, quality of life, patient values, and psychosocial needs of patients and families. Geriatric practice models in different care settings (i.e., an acute care hospital, subacute rehabilitation facility, long-term nursing facility, home or inpatient hospice) may leverage the expertise of both geriatricians and palliative medicine physicians to provide seamless transitions of care across care sites. This allows patients and caregivers to feel comfortable knowing that pertinent information related to chronic co-morbid conditions, symptom management, or advance care planning is communicated across care sites [40]. Hospital-based palliative care programs can facilitate communication with external agencies (nursing homes or office-based practices) that may assume care for a patient after discharge. However, even finely tuned discharge plans can fall apart for unpredictable reasons, which may lead to unnecessary readmission or unintentional lack of compliance with discharge regimens due to patient, family, and/or provider confusion. Some healthcare systems have piloted post-discharge interventions to facilitate the transition of care in the weeks or months after hospital discharge. These programs may be led by nurses who met the patient during the hospitalization, providing patients with an extra layer of support from a healthcare provider who is inherently familiar with their recent hospitalization, medical co-morbidities, and any critical medication changes made during the admission [41].

Monitoring Outcomes and Planning for Future Directions

Is the Model Scalable?

Most palliative care consult programs are started on a small or pilot scale, affording the opportunity to refine operational flow and document positive impacts of the program before expanding to a larger scale. A program may start with only one physician and as consult volume grows it becomes more feasible to support both additional physicians and full-time non-physician team members. All aspects of a palliative care program are scalable and can be tailored to meet the specific needs of each community's patient population [42].

How Do We Know the Model Is Improving Care?

Monitoring outcomes is necessary to sustain a program over time and ensure that the program is meeting the needs of the patients it serves, the physicians requesting consultations, and the hospital or health system. Different data need to be collected depending on the concerns and priorities of the audience to whom it is being presented. Palliative care providers and patients may be most interested in clinical data such as symptom control, while healthcare leadership may want financial data on cost savings, 30-day readmissions, hospital mortality rates, or decreases in unnecessary health-

care utilization. Both patients and healthcare system leadership may be interested in qualitative data such as patient satisfaction surveys [43].

What Are the Future Directions of Palliative Care Consultation Services?

Once a palliative care consultation program demonstrates its benefits to the health system by providing high quality care to frail hospitalized patients, there are opportunities to move palliative care consultations upstream and see patients before they are sick enough to be admitted to the hospital. There is growing evidence that outpatient palliative care programs improve the symptom control, satisfaction, and quality of life for patients while reducing healthcare utilization by preventing need for crisis hospitalizations [44] and in certain populations may prolong survival [19].

Outpatient palliative medicine may be particularly important for patients at high risk of frequent hospitalizations. Small outpatient palliative care programs have begun to document the role of outpatient palliative care in addressing symptom burden and exploring advance care planning including resuscitation status and hospice [45]. Benefits of outpatient palliative care are also noted by patients and families, who have reported improved quality of life for patients and lower caregiver burden [46]. In the context of healthcare reform, value-based purchasing and new delivery and payment models focused on improving value by increasing quality and in so doing, reducing costs, the opportunity for bringing palliative medicine to scale is unprecedented. Both providers and payers accepting financial risk (Accountable Care Organizations, patient centered medical homes, bundled payments, Medicare Advantage, managed Medicaid, and commercial insurers) have aligned interests in improving quality for the sickest most complex patients driving more than half of all health spending [1]. Examples of payer–provider relationships driving improved access to palliative care may be found (see http://www.capc.org/payertoolkit/). The key issue is making sure that costs are reduced as a consequence of better quality as opposed to stinting on needed care for vulnerable populations. Close monitoring of valid and standardized quality measures is critical to achieving this goal [1].

References

1. Meier DE. Increased access to palliative care and hospice services: opportunities to improve value in health care. Milbank Q. 2011; 89(3):343–80.
2. Teno JM, Clarridge BR, Casey V, Welch LC, Wetle T, Shield R, et al. Family perspectives on end-of-life care at the last place of care. JAMA. 2004;291(1):88–93.

3. Steinhauser KE, Christakis NA, Clipp EC, McNeilly M, McIntyre L, Tulsky JA. Factors considered important at the end of life by patients, family, physicians, and other care providers. JAMA. 2000;284(19):2476–82.

4. National Center for Health Statistics (US). Hyattsville, MD. 2011. Accessed on 2014 April 14. Available from: http://www.ncbi.nlm. nih.gov/books/NBK54374

5. The Dartmouth Atlas of Health Care. Accessed on 2014 April 14. Available from: http://www.dartmouthatlas.org/data/distribution. aspx?ind=14&loct=5&tf=23&fmt=27

6. Angus DC, Barnato AE, Linde-Zwirble WT, Weissfeld LA, Watson RS, Rickert T, et al. Use of intensive care at the end of life in the United States: an epidemiologic study. Crit Care Med. 2004;32(3): 638–43.

7. Smith AK, McCarthy E, Weber E, Cenzer IS, Boscardin J, Fisher J, et al. Half of older Americans seen in emergency department in last month of life; most admitted to hospital, and many die there. Health Aff (Millwood). 2012;31(6):1277–85.

8. Wright AA, Keating NL, Balboni TA, Matulonis UA, Block SD, Prigerson HG. Place of death: correlations with quality of life of patients with cancer and predictors of bereaved caregivers' mental health. J Clin Oncol. 2010;28(29):4457–64.

9. Teno JM, Mitchell SL, Skinner J, Kuo S, Fisher E, Intrator O, et al. Churning: the association between health care transitions and feeding tube insertion for nursing home residents with advanced cognitive impairment. J Palliat Med. 2009;12(4):359–62.

10. Weissman DE, Meier DE. Identifying patients in need of a palliative care assessment in the hospital setting: a consensus report from the Center to Advance Palliative Care. J Palliat Med. 2011; 14(1):17–23.

11. Adelson Kea. Standardized criteria for required palliative care consultation on the solid tumor oncology service. 2013 Quality Care Symposium. Abstract 37. Presented November 1, 2013.

12. Center to Advance Palliative Care (CAPC). Accessed on 2014 May 22. Available from: http://www.capc.org/capc-growth-analysis-snapshot-2013.pdf

13. Center to Advance Palliative Care (CAPC). Accessed on 2014 July 1. Available from: https://registry.capc.org/cms/

14. Lupu D. Force AAoHaPMWT. Estimate of current hospice and palliative medicine physician workforce shortage. J Pain Symptom Manage. 2010;40(6):899–911.

15. Center to Advance Palliative Care. 2011 Accessed on 2014 April 16. Available from: http://www.capc.org/tools-for-palliative-care-programs/marketing/public-opinion-research/2011-public-opinion-research-on-palliative-care.pdf

16. Maciasz RM, Arnold RM, Chu E, Park SY, White DB, Vater LB, et al. Does it matter what you call it? A randomized trial of language used to describe palliative care services. Support Care Cancer. 2013;21(12):3411–9.

17. Gade G, Venohr I, Conner D, McGrady K, Beane J, Richardson RH, et al. Impact of an inpatient palliative care team: a randomized control trial. J Palliat Med. 2008;11(2):180–90.

18. Casarett D, Pickard A, Bailey FA, Ritchie C, Furman C, Rosenfeld K, et al. Do palliative consultations improve patient outcomes? J Am Geriatr Soc. 2008;56(4):593–9.

19. Temel JS, Greer JA, Muzikansky A, Gallagher ER, Admane S, Jackson VA, et al. Early palliative care for patients with metastatic non-small-cell lung cancer. N Engl J Med. 2010;363(8): 733–42.

20. Morrison RS, Penrod JD, Cassel JB, Caust-Ellenbogen M, Litke A, Spragens L, et al. Cost savings associated with US hospital palliative care consultation programs. Arch Intern Med. 2008;168(16): 1783–90.

21. Baile WF, Buckman R, Lenzi R, Glober G, Beale EA, Kudelka AP. SPIKES - a six-step protocol for delivering bad news: application to the patient with cancer. Oncologist. 2000;5(4):302–11.

22. Kennifer SL, Alexander SC, Pollak KI, Jeffreys AS, Olsen MK, Rodriguez KL, et al. Negative emotions in cancer care: do oncologists' responses depend on severity and type of emotion? Patient Educ Couns. 2009;76(1):51–6.

23. Mitchell SL, Teno JM, Kiely DK, Shaffer ML, Jones RN, Prigerson HG, et al. The clinical course of advanced dementia. N Engl J Med. 2009;361(16):1529–38.

24. CAPC. Center to Advance Palliative Care. A Guide to Building a Hospital-Based Palliative Care Program 2004.

25. Center to Advance Palliative Care (CAPC). Improving care for people with serious illness through innovative payer-provider partnerships. https://www.capc.org/payers/palliative-care-payer-provider-toolkit/ Accessed 5 March 2015.

26. Centers for Medicaid and Medicare Services. 2014. Accessed on 2014 May 29. Available from: http://www.cms.gov/Outreach-and-Education/Medicare-Learning-Network-MLN/MLNEdWebGuide/EMDOC.html

27. Meier DE, Beresford L. Billing for palliative care: an essential cost of doing business. J Palliat Med. 2006;9(2):250–7.

28. James MG, O'Kane ME, Salgo P, Weissberg J. Module 2: policy and value-based purchasing. Am J Manag Care. 2013;19(9 Suppl):s168–73.

29. Center to Advance Palliative Care. A Guide to Building a Hospital-Based Palliative Care Program 2004.

30. Meier DE, Beresford L. Social workers advocate for a seat at palliative care table. J Palliat Med. 2008;11(1):10–4.

31. Balboni TA, Paulk ME, Balboni MJ, Phelps AC, Loggers ET, Wright AA, et al. Provision of spiritual care to patients with advanced cancer: associations with medical care and quality of life near death. J Clin Oncol. 2010;28(3):445–52.

32. Balboni TA, Balboni M, Enzinger AC, Gallivan K, Paulk ME, Wright A, et al. Provision of spiritual support to patients with advanced cancer by religious communities and associations with medical care at the end of life. JAMA Intern Med. 2013;173(12): 1109–17.

33. Berger L, Tavares M, Berger B. A Canadian experience of integrating complementary therapy in a hospital palliative care unit. J Palliat Med. 2013;16(10):1294–8.

34. Collinge W, Kahn J, Walton T, Kozak L, Bauer-Wu S, Fletcher K, et al. Touch, caring, and cancer: randomized controlled trial of a multimedia caregiver education program. Support Care Cancer. 2013;21(5):1405–14.

35. Safrai M. Art therapy in hospice: a catalyst for insight and healing. J Am Art Ther Assoc. 2013;30(3):122–9.

36. Sutter C, Reid T. How do we talk to the children? Child life consultation to support the children of seriously ill adult inpatients. J Palliat Med. 2012;15(12):1362–8.

37. Kühne F, Krattenmacher T, Beierlein V, Grimm JC, Bergelt C, Romer G, et al. Minor children of palliative patients: a systematic review of psychosocial family interventions. J Palliat Med. 2012;15(8):931–45.

38. O'Connor M, Fisher C. Exploring the dynamics of interdisciplinary palliative care teams in providing psychosocial care: "Everybody thinks that everybody can do it and they can't". J Palliat Med. 2011;14(2):191–6.

39. Aspesi AV, Kauffmann GE, Davis AM, Schulwolf EM, Press VG, Stupay KL, et al. IBCD: development and testing of a checklist to improve quality of care for hospitalized general medical patients. Jt Comm J Qual Patient Saf. 2013;39(4):147–56.

40. Unroe KT, Meier DE. Research priorities in geriatric palliative care: policy initiatives. J Palliat Med. 2013;16(12):1503–8.

41. Meier DE, Beresford L. Palliative care's challenge: facilitating transitions of care. J Palliat Med. 2008;11(3):416–21.

42. Center to Advance Palliative Care. Accessed on 2014 April 12. Available from: http://www.capc.org/palliative-care-leadership-initiative/curriculum/pclc_core#module-2

43. Center to Advance Palliative Care. 2014. Accessed on 2014 April 12. Available from: http://www.capc.org/building-a-hospital-based-palliative-care-program/measuring-quality-and-impact

44. Rabow M, Kvale E, Barbour L, Cassel JB, Cohen S, Jackson V, et al. Moving upstream: a review of the evidence of the impact of outpatient palliative care. J Palliat Med. 2013;16(12):1540–9.

45. Bekelman DB, Nowels CT, Allen LA, Shakar S, Kutner JS, Matlock DD. Outpatient palliative care for chronic heart failure: a case series. J Palliat Med. 2011;14(7):815–21.

46. Groh G, Vyhnalek B, Feddersen B, Führer M, Borasio GD. Effectiveness of a specialized outpatient palliative care service as experienced by patients and caregivers. J Palliat Med. 2013;16(8):848–56.

The Wisconsin Star Method: Understanding and Addressing Complexity in Geriatrics

Timothy Howell

The Wisconsin Star Method (WSM) is a simple concrete way to map and visually process the numerous interacting factors in the complex situations so typically common in geriatrics. How to effectively address multiple co-occurring problems is one of the greatest challenges facing those who develop models of geriatric care, as well as those who provide such care directly. The number of comorbid medical conditions and psychosocial issues, often inextricably intertwined, seem to multiply with age. Some problems are acute, many are chronic, and most change over time. In addition, what each problem means can vary according to the unique perspectives and feelings of those involved at every level of the care system.

The effort required not only to assess but also to address such a sizable number of simultaneously interacting factors taxes both cognitive and emotional resources. Further compounding these challenges is the high degree of variability from one older adult or population to the next, generated by multiple factors ranging from age-related physiological heterogeneity to different sets of psychosocial experiences over the course of lifetimes. Under such circumstances, evidence-based guidelines, developed from studies of single problems in homogeneous populations, are of limited utility at best. And not only do providers and planners of care for older adults encounter higher levels of complexity with higher degrees of frequency, but they also face higher levels of ambiguity in terms of diagnosis, prognosis, and plausible interventions stemming from those complexities.

This dilemma has long called for the development of a user-friendly method to facilitate addressing such challenging situations more efficiently and more effectively with greater clinical integrity [1–4]. The WSM is not a rigid or static model, but rather a continuously emerging and flexible method, and has been undergoing development with input from care providers, medical educators, students and clinical trainees, administrators, patients, and family members for more than 10 years. Using the WSM can potentially enhance the implementation of the models of geriatric care described elsewhere in this book, especially in how it seamlessly integrates behavioral health into comprehensive geriatric care.

Evidence-Bases for the Wisconsin Star Method

The structure and function of the Wisconsin Star Method (WSM) are supported by the principles of heuristics [5–7], cognitive science [6–9], information visualization [10, 11], visual analytics [12], ecological interface design [13], team functioning [6, 11], and network theory [14, 15]. The method begins with fashioning a low-tech graphic user interface—drawing a small five-pointed star (Fig. 7.1) on a surface, such as paper or whiteboard—then mapping out natural clusters of clinical data in list form [16] in the appropriate field or domain. Each datum becomes an element in a network of potentially interacting variables, with the links between them varying in strength, from very weak (i.e., negligible) to very strong (i.e., directly causal or interdependent). The primary identifiable clinical challenge (e.g., failure to thrive) is written in the center of the star. In some cases, the primary challenge may not be entirely clear at the outset, but emerges gradually as the situation is reviewed.

Each arm of the star represents a single domain: medications, medical, behavioral, personal, and social. The medication arm includes all of an individual's current medications (e.g., prescribed, over-the-counter, and "borrowed") and other relevant substances (e.g., dietary, recreational). The medical and behavioral arms list known diagnoses and/or symptoms, as well as functional status (e.g., abilities to perform activities of daily living [ADLs] and instrumental ADLs).

T. Howell, M.D., M.A. (✉)
Geriatrics Research, Education, and Clinical Center,
Madison VA Hospital, Madison, WI, USA

Geriatrics Division, Department of Medicine,
University of Wisconsin School of Medicine and Public Health,
Madison, WI, USA
e-mail: thowell@wisc.edu

M.L. Malone et al. (eds.), *Geriatrics Models of Care: Bringing 'Best Practice' to an Aging America*,
DOI 10.1007/978-3-319-16068-9_7, © Springer International Publishing Switzerland 2015

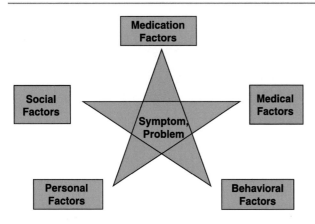

Fig. 7.1 Understanding and Addressing Complex Clinical Problems: The Wisconsin Star Method

Table 7.1 Executive functions of the human brain

- Attention
- Response inhibition: blocking distractions
- Working memory
- Abstract thinking
- Planning: sense of the future, generating options
- Implementing plans: deciding/initiating/sustaining/stopping
- Set-shifting: flexibility
- Organizing: categorizing, sequencing
- Multi-tasking: divided attention
- Problem-solving: new (vs. familiar/learned)
- Monitoring: awareness of self (internal) and others (external)
- Evaluating: assessing
- Modulating: perceptions; feelings/emotions; thoughts; actions; ego

The personal arm highlights a person's situation awareness, individual personality traits, values, loyalties, and usual ways of coping. These include the conscious and unconscious rules of thumb used to guide responses to situations, learning and communication styles, and general approaches in dealing with stressful experiences. The social arm covers interpersonal and environmental problems, assets and access to needed resources (e.g., family support, finances, housing, transportation, legal issues, etc.).

Each arm of the star also represents a different network at a different ecological level within the nested hierarchy of the network of networks that constitute each person. The medication arm corresponds to the biochemical or molecular interface; the medical arm, the level of organ systems; the behavioral, the interface mediating between the brain, the body, and the environment; the personal arm, the interface of the "mind and heart"; and the social arm, the interactions of interpersonal and environmental factors. The WSM's visual approach, by mapping multiple interacting factors onto a single field, affords a bird's eye view, taps into the most powerful information processing system of the human brain. It can facilitate insight into the ways in which the elements in these networks are influencing each other, switching easily between focusing on the linear–causal links and viewing the holistic, overall "big picture" [10, 13, 17].

Note that it is essential for the data be written down—effective implementation is simply not possible in complex cases by attempting to keep all the data in one's head, because the carrying capacity of the conscious human brain is limited to about four simultaneously interacting variables [14]. The WSM flattens the nested hierarchy of networks into a user-friendly [10] two-dimensional map. This map becomes an extension of the users' working memory [8] and, whether used by individuals or a team, enhances executive functioning (Table 7.1) for situation awareness and problem-solving.

Writing the elements down also creates a small but significant distance between the user(s) and the problems, thus providing both cognitive and affective perspectives.

Using the Wisconsin Star Method

With its visual approach, the WSM facilitates attending simultaneously to multiple interacting variables and identifying those data that are most relevant. One simply travels around the star, assessing and highlighting those elements in each arm that appear to connect significantly with the challenge at hand. Recursive iterations of this process additionally allow the user(s) to identify potentially relevant data that are missing (e.g., can the person manage all the steps required to refill a prescription?), thereby reducing the risks stemming proverbially from "not knowing what you don't know." Such processing also enables reconsiderations of whether data initially considered noncontributory may be relevant after all.

Some factors by themselves may not be sufficient to contribute to the central problem, but become so by interacting synergistically with other factors. One can identify these by using a process of triangulation (analogous to surveying and navigation procedures) to "connect the dots." Having discovered a possible connection between such two factors, one can look for additional factors that may also be contributing causes or emergent consequences. These additional factors may be already known—e.g., relocation to a long-term care facility (LTCF) and high personal value on autonomy → refusing cares (Fig. 7.2)—or has not yet occurred but could be predictable—e.g., high loyalty to family and conscientiousness plus pending snowstorm → shoveling snow to help family → angina (Fig. 7.3)—and potentially preventable by an astute intervention.

There may also be factors not yet perceived, but about which hypotheses can be generated and checked out—e.g.,

Fig. 7.2 Star map for an elderly patient refusing cares

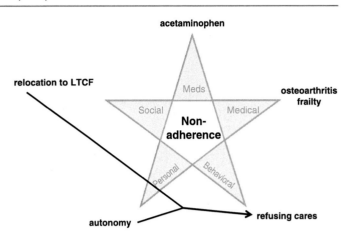

Fig. 7.3 Star map for very old patient with angina planning to help family with shoveling snow

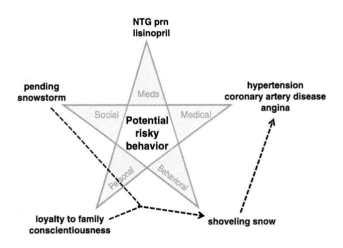

dementia + relocation to a LTCF + ? → wandering, where the unknown factor(s) might be a medication side effect, pain, a delusion (e.g., of having to go to work), and/or an effort to return home (Fig. 7.4).

Using the WSM helps to ascertain which problems have multifactorial origins (e.g., where the triangulated factors turn out to be a cluster of causal factors) and thus avoid a common error in complex situations, that of coming to premature closure [8, 18]. It can ease shifting sets when considering pairs of problems at different levels that might have linear–causal relationships (e.g., poor blood pressure control despite three antihypertensive medications + an inability to afford medication and/or an unrecognized problem with alcohol abuse). It can also be applied holistically to identify how multiple problems may be interconnected, such as parkinsonian gait instability, falls, loss of usual means for coping, depression (low mood and motivation), and social isolation. The resulting map provides a big picture of the case, with strong and weak ties highlighted, and can be viewed as the person's unique ecosystem.

By integrating holistic and linear–causal perspectives into an ecological approach, the Wisconsin Star Method can enhance the recognition of diagnostic patterns both within and between domains, including the identification of vicious cycles, e.g., recurrent falls + concern about appearance → embarrassment about using a walker → declining to use walker → decreased activity → physical deconditioning → recurrent falls (Fig. 7.5).

The WSM also facilitates novel problem-solving: generating hypotheses, prioritizing and sequencing interventions, integrating clinical pearls [19] with evidence-based guidelines [20]. Using the WSM to more readily recognize vicious cycles as well as to identify and address their most critical link(s), care providers can work together on transforming them into virtuous cycles—e.g., arranging for a friendly visitor (someone who also needs a walker) to visit and walk with the person regularly.

Fig. 7.4 Star map for a patient
with dementia who is wandering

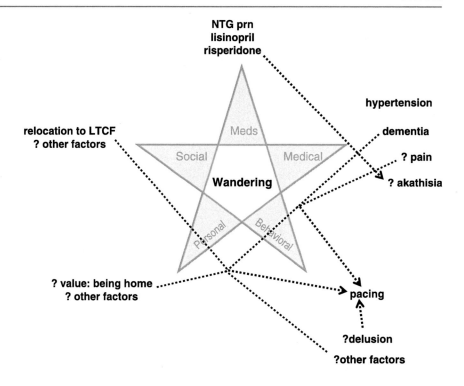

Fig. 7.5 Star map for patient
with frequent falls who declines
using a walker

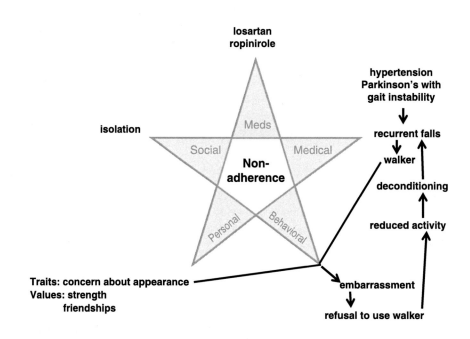

Meaning-Centered Care with the Wisconsin Star Method

The factors clustered in the personal arm of the star can be thought of as those which contribute to what any given situation means to an individual or a team. Attending to their personal knowledge (e.g., health literacy) and experiences, traits, values [21], loyalties, and rules of thumb which inform their usual ways of coping can promote better appreciation of the meaning of otherwise puzzling behaviors and the underlying anxieties that drive them, such as a patient's refusal to use a walker despite recurrent falls stemming from feelings of embarrassment at being seen in public as dependent on a walker.

An important adjunct to the WSM is listening to how one feels when confronted with a challenging situation. Doing so can enhance one's emotional effectiveness and reduce the likelihood of affective errors [22]. The stress responses of patients, teams, and systems are driven by underlying anxieties generated by the gaps between perceived challenges and perceived resources, with these perceptions strongly colored by how they construe the meaning of the situation. Listening to how one feels can provide valuable additional clues to more readily and effectively understand the how and why of the responses to stressors, by means of measured reflecting (vs. just immediately reacting) on the emergent feelings and then generating testable hypotheses. If one feels sad with an elderly male patient, one may be indirectly picking up on his sadness. For care providers and planners of models of care who experience some anxiety or confusion emerging from interactions with others, these feelings may reflect the latter's underlying anxiety or confusion about some issue that they are having trouble identifying or directly communicating.

The way to effective clinical outcomes is often through the personal arm of the star. Exploring the factors operative in this arm of the star can guide clinicians, teams, and planners to sounder appreciation for what problems mean to someone else, in contrast to what they mean to themselves. By monitoring and reflecting on the differences, they can reformulate their explanations and recommendations with greater sensitivity and specificity, to be "on the same page," thereby enhancing mutual communication via shared meaning.

Remembering in dialogs to take time to paraphrase what someone has said, before proceeding with articulating answers, explanations, or plans, demonstrates not only that one has been listening well and truly heard what has been said, but also communicates what one has understood. This either provides confirmation of shared meaning or the opportunity to correct any misunderstandings through further dialog. Thus use of the WSM to provide "meaning-centered" care or planning can help to cultivate collaborative relationships, and avoid relationships characterized by misunderstandings or confrontations (e.g., blaming them for refusing to use a walker or adopt a guideline). Sharing star maps with others, and developing such maps even further with their help, may further enhance the likelihood of those involved becoming literally, as well as figuratively, "on the same page," through shared ownership as well as shared meaning.

Applying the Wisconsin Star Method to Teams and Systems

There are additional levels to the WSM. One is the ad hoc team star (Fig. 7.6) and the others are the system level stars (Fig. 7.7). The figures include potential members, and are not exhaustive lists. Most teams consist of only a few members, but a key to their effectiveness can be the extent to which their membership is diverse. There is evidence that teams (especially those with diverse membership, as opposed to a panel of experts) generally address complex issues more effectively than individuals [6]. Systems stars are analogous to team stars, and can be thought of as "team of teams" or "community of practice star" maps. These can be deployed on an ad hoc basis to delineate factors at higher or lower levels which frequently have a bearing on any particular star

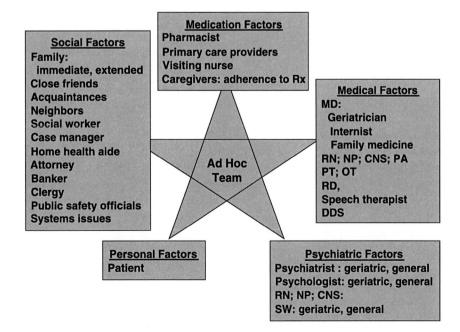

Fig. 7.6 Ad hoc team star map

Fig. 7.7 Systems star mapping: "team of teams" or community of practice star map

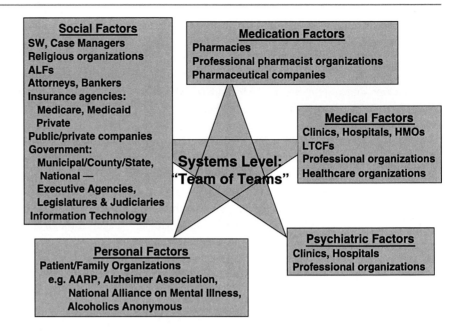

map. Problems at the patient and team levels may be affected by factors at higher levels, such as organizational constraints locally, and/or state, regional, or national policies, and vice versa. Team and systems star mapping can also help to identify missing resources.

Even in situations where there is no formal team, one can create an ad hoc team star map to identify other individuals, teams, or organizations who may be of assistance. Those who spend the most time with the patient (e.g., primary caregivers such as family or care staff) or working on the frontlines of the care organization may be the richest sources of some kinds of important information. In clinical or organizational situations which seem intractable, one can seek out a "weak tie," such as a colleague or an acquaintance, through whom to connect with someone beyond one's local network, who can provide knowledge or resources not locally available (e.g., a chaplain for pastoral counseling), and/or the perspective of someone at a greater distance from the situation (e.g., a colleague working in another system). This is often helpful in complex sets of problems, and not infrequently essential. Where problems are multi-factorial, one can organize and mobilize a team, officially or unofficially ("ad hoc") to take on the interacting issues—different people are helpful for different issues—to assist with monitoring, implementing plans, and advocacy. One can use analogous methods with organizations to address systems level issues.

Using the WSM has the potential not only to enhance proficiency at providing comprehensive care, but also to reduce cognitive and emotional burdens and errors [8, 23]. It can assist individuals and teams, as well as patients and their families, to become more confident, mindful, and resilient in addressing the complex interacting physical, emotional, and social issues of older adults with greater sensitivity and speci-

ficity to each one's uniqueness. The WSM also has the potential to be integrated into electronic health record systems, which are currently quite limited in their abilities to facilitate situation awareness in complex clinical situations [24].

Since 2002 the Wisconsin Geriatric Psychiatry Initiative (WGPI) has been developing and refining the application of the Wisconsin Star Method to challenging problems at a number of systems levels [25]. The WGPI is a small but growing group of geropsychiatry and geriatrics professionals (including state and local government staff) attempting to develop systems to enhance mental health services for older adults in Wisconsin and beyond. Given the widespread and growing shortage of expertise in the mental health and substance abuse problems of older adults, the WGPI is dedicated to widely disseminating basic principles of geriatric psychiatry to care providers in different settings, including health care, long-term care and aging network.

The WGPI approach consists of a collaborative effort to develop, from existing resources, a sustainable geriatric mental health infrastructure by means of an indirect care model with three basic components: (1) evidence-based teaching, via on-site, case-based consultations, of evidence-based principles of geriatrics and geriatric psychiatry, utilizing the Wisconsin Star Method; (2) providing external validation and moral support to frontline care teams struggling to cope with scarce resources; and (3) employing a social entrepreneurial approach to enhance the effectiveness of limited existing resources through network weaving.

WGPI educational activities utilizing the Wisconsin Star Method have included: (1) biweekly geriatric psychiatry colloquia at the Geriatric Medicine and Geriatric Psychiatry Fellowship Programs at the Geriatric Research, Education, & Clinical Center (GRECC) of the Madison VA Hospital

(MVAH) and the University of Wisconsin-Madison (UW-Madison), and the Geriatric Medicine Fellowship Program at Aurora Health Care in Milwaukee; (2) difficult cases conferences (averaging nearly 100/year) with community health care teams, such as Community Care, Inc. (PACE, Partnership, and Family Care teams) in the southeastern Wisconsin region; (3) three monthly Geriatrics Fellows' Most Difficult Case Conferences coordinated by the Aurora Health Care in Milwaukee, each telephonically linked to teams at up to ten other geriatric medicine fellowship sites in the Eastern, Central, or Pacific Time zones [26]; (4) quarterly telephonic Most Difficult Case Conferences at memory clinics throughout Wisconsin affiliated with the Wisconsin Alzheimer's Institute; (5) a continuing education program at UW-Madison's Department of Professional Development, the Mental Health and Older Adult Certificate Series; (6) periodic presentations at regional and national meetings (including the American Geriatrics Society, the American Association for Geriatric Psychiatry, and the International Psychogeriatric Association); (7) a pilot project to reduce the need to hospitalize patients with dementia-related behavioral problems, by creating behavioral health collaboration teams composed of behavioral health teams from participating nursing homes and hospitals in Ladysmith, WI; and (7) a geriatric behavioral health resource website (currently wgpi.org, with plans for wgpi.wisc.edu later in 2015).

Over the past decade, the Wisconsin Star Method has been implemented in geriatric clinics and geriatric services at the MVAH (in Madison, Wisconsin); the Aurora Health Care System (in the eastern Wisconsin region); and Ladysmith Nursing Home and Rusk County Memorial Nursing Home in Ladysmith, Wisconsin. Since 2006, Abundant Life Manor, a community-based residential facility in Milwaukee for older adults with chronic mental illnesses and/or dementia-related behavioral problems, as well as multiple medical comorbidities, has based its system of care on the Wisconsin Star Method. This has been associated with significantly lower staff turnover compared with similar local facilities, and with marked enhancement of outside reviews by staff of the state's Division of Quality Assurance [27]. Most recently, the Wisconsin Star Method has been incorporated into the MVAH's GRECC-Connect program, which is designed to enhance geriatric health care for aging veterans in rural areas by means of interdisciplinary team-based support for primary care providers in community-based outpatient clinics.

Summary

In contrast with the usual piecemeal approaches to problems involving multiple interacting comorbidities, the Wisconsin Star Method represents a user-friendly way for clinicians and planners of care models to obtain a grasp on complex situations, not only more rapidly but also more effectively, in terms of providing initial and ongoing care and planning with greater sensitivity and specificity. Using the Wisconsin Star Method requires mindfully mapping and iteratively processing the numerous interacting factors that comprise the increasingly common challenge of clinical complexity. As such, adopting and using it has the potential to achieve clinical and systems outcomes that are more meaningful to all involved. It could do so by helping to reintegrate the otherwise disparate, fragmented efforts and communication barriers that tend to characterize current healthcare systems.

The WSM also has the potential to help care providers and planners to acquire clinical wisdom. Among the components of wisdom identified in a recent cross-cultural review were a "prosocial attitude" (altruism), a rich body of factual knowledge and procedural skills, "emotional homeostasis," a capacity for reflection, an openness to different perspectives, and the ability to acknowledge and deal effectively with uncertainty and ambiguities [28]. Using the WSM cannot guarantee a prosocial attitude. Nor does it does add much to the clinical knowledge and skills base of its users. But it can facilitate the implementation of those skills and knowledge in the face of complex situations, by more effectively engaging their capacities for reflection and consideration from multiple perspectives.

Higher levels of complexity increase the cognitive and affective loads on the human brain. By providing a useful tool to address complex situations, the WSM can lower the level of complexity-induced stress, thereby enhancing cognitive and emotional effectiveness. This, in turn, can reduce the likelihood of errors. Finally, by not being a static model employing too-rigid guidelines, but rather becoming a flexible, continuously emerging "open" method, capable of undergoing modifications to more effectively fit varying circumstances, the Wisconsin Star Method retains the potential for further development. This can continue to come through input from a diverse virtual "team" comprised of those involved in providing and receiving care—be they clinicians, educators, patients, families, administrators, advocates, developers of geriatric care models, teams, organizations, or systems—well into the future.

Acknowledgements Over the past 14 years of the development of the Wisconsin Star Method, many individuals have made much appreciated contributions. I would like to thank Dean Krahn at the Mental Health Service Line of the Madison VA Hospital (MVAH) for pointing out the star pattern in what was originally an ecological diagram of clusters, and Catherine Swanson-Hays for naming the method after the state of Wisconsin. I have benefited extensively from discussions with colleagues in the MVAH's GRECC and the Geriatrics Division of the UW-Madison's Department of Medicine, most particularly Steve Barczi. I have also learned from colleagues in Milwaukee, including especially Michael Malone at the Aurora Geriatrics Program, Holly Onsager at the Community Care Organization, Meg Gleeson at

Abundant Life Manor, Suzanna Waters-Castillo of the UW-M's Department of Professional Development, and members of the older adult teams at the Milwaukee County Department on Aging and in Ladysmith. Ongoing feedback from fellows, residents, and students (both medical and social work) in the Geriatrics Evaluation and Management Clinic at the MVAH has been very helpful with successive iterations of the WSM, as has that from the staff of numerous medical and social organizations devoted to the care of older adults around the state of Wisconsin. I am grateful to Ron Burnette at the School of Pharmacy of the University of Wisconsin for his years of patiently mentoring me about network theory and complexity science.

Conflicts of Interest: None

Sponsors' Role: None. The opinions expressed in this publication are those of the author and do not necessarily reflect the views of the Veterans Administration or the UW-Madison's School of Medicine and Public Health.

Disclaimer: The Wisconsin Star Method is published in the public domain, and as such may not be copyrighted, trademarked or patented. Permission is granted to use, reproduce and or adapt the Wisconsin Star Method provided this Disclaimer is included in any and all such materials, including the following acknowledgement:

The Madison Veterans Administration Hospital, the University of Wisconsin-Madison School of Medicine and Public Health, the Division of Mental Health and Substance Abuse Services of the Wisconsin Department of Health Services, NAMI Wisconsin, and members of the Wisconsin Geriatric Psychiatry Initiative have provided in kind support for the development of the Wisconsin Star Method.

References

1. Tinetti ME, Bogardus Jr ST, Agostini JV. Potential pitfalls of disease-specific guidelines for patients with multiple conditions. N Engl J Med. 2004;351(27):2870–4.
2. Boyd CM, Darer J, Boult C, Fried LP, Boult L, Wu AW. Clinical practice guidelines and quality of care for older patients with multiple comorbid diseases: implications for pay for performance. JAMA. 2005;294(6):716–24.
3. Tinetti ME, Fried TR, Boyd CM. Designing health care for the most common chronic condition–multimorbidity. JAMA. 2012;307(23): 2493–4. Erratum in: JAMA. 2012 Jul 18;308(3):238.
4. American Geriatrics Society Expert Panel on the Care of Older Adults with Multimorbidity. Patient-centered care for older adults with multiple chronic conditions: a stepwise approach from the American Geriatrics Society: American Geriatrics Society Expert Panel on the Care of Older Adults with Multimorbidity. J Am Geriatr Soc. 2012;60(10):1957–68.
5. Michalewicz Z, Fogel DB. How to solve It: modern heuristics. 2nd ed. Berlin: Springer; 2004.
6. Page SE. The difference. Princeton, NJ: Princeton University Press; 2007.
7. Gigerenzer G. Gut feelings. New York, NY: Penguin; 2007.
8. Redelmeier DA. Improving patient care: the cognitive psychology of missed diagnoses. Ann Intern Med. 2005;142(2):115–20.
9. Heath C, Heath D. Made to stick. New York, NY: Random House; 2007.
10. Ware C. Information visualization. 3rd ed. Waltham, MA: Morgan Kaufmann; 2013.
11. Sibbet D. Visual meetings. Hoboken, NJ: John Wiley & Sons; 2010.
12. Heer J, Agrawala M. Design considerations for collaborative visual analytics. Inf Vis. 2008;7:49–62.
13. Endsley MR, Jones DG. Designing for situation awareness: an approach to user-centered design. 2nd ed. Boca Raton, FL: Taylor & Francis; 2012.
14. Csermely P. Weak links. Berlin: Springer; 2006.
15. Villoslada P, Steinman L, Baranzini SE. Systems biology and its application to the understanding of neurological diseases. Ann Neurol. 2009;65(2):124–39.
16. Hales B, Terblanche M, Fowler R, Sibbald W. Development of medical checklists for improved quality of patient care. Int J Qual Health Care. 2008;20(1):22–30.
17. Quill E. When networks network: once studied solo, systems display surprising behavior when they interact. Sci News. 2012;182(6): 18–25.
18. Groopman J. How doctors think. Boston, MA: Houghton Mifflin; 2007.
19. Mangrulkar RS, Saint S, Chu S, Tierney LM. What is the role of the clinical "pearl"? Am J Med. 2002;113(7):617–24.
20. Hunink MGM, Glasziou PP, Siegel JE, et al. Decision making in health and medicine: integrating values and evidence. Cambridge, UK: Cambridge University Press; 2005.
21. Epstein RM, Peters E. Beyond information: exploring patients' preferences. JAMA. 2009;302(2):195–7.
22. Epstein RM, Siegel DJ, Silberman J. Self-monitoring in clinical practice: a challenge for medical educators. J Contin Educ Health Prof. 2008;28(1):5–13.
23. Graber ML, Franklin N, Gordon R. Diagnostic error in internal medicine. Arch Intern Med. 2005;165(13):1493–9.
24. Karsh BT, Weinger MB, Abbott PA, Wears RL. Health information technology: fallacies and sober realities. J Am Med Inform Assoc. 2010;17(6):617–23.
25. Howell T, Buel L, Gleeson M, Khan A, Swanson-Hayes C, Waters-Castillo S, APS Team. Addressing complexity in the face of scarcity: the Wisconsin Geriatric Psychiatry Initiative after 6 years. Int Psychogeriatrics. 2009;21 Suppl 2:S176.
26. Khan A, Howell T, Malone M, Colon-Nieves P, Singh K. "Geriatrics Fellows' most difficult case conference": knowledge sharing and teaching through program networking: a one year experience. J Am Geriatrics Soc. 2012;60:S156.
27. Gleeson M. Personal communication.
28. Meeks TW, Jeste DV. Neurobiology of wisdom: a literature overview. Arch Gen Psychiatry. 2009;66(4):355–65.

Part II

Models to Address the Needs of Seniors in Transition from Hospital-to-Home

Care Transitions Intervention and Other Non-nursing Home Transitions Models

8

Ella Harvey Bowman and Kellie L. Flood

Background

A transition from one care site to another is a vulnerable time for all patients and especially for frail older adults. While the care transition from hospital to home or post-acute care facility has garnered most attention, the American Geriatrics Society (AGS) defines transitional care as "a set of actions designed to ensure the coordination and continuity of health care as patients transfer between different locations or different levels of care within the same location" [1]. Thus, a comprehensive view of care transitions includes any site of care spanning hospital, outpatient clinic, home, skilled nursing facility, or any other type of domiciliary setting in which a patient receives care (Fig. 8.1).

This chapter broadly summarizes these core features of care transitions, including a description of various sites of care involved, discussion of patient and system-based factors contributing to adverse events, suggestion of minimum standards necessary for optimizing care transitions, delineation of the importance of medication management and accurate reconciliation, highlights of several evidence-based models shown to improve care transitions, demonstration of the role of health information technology in care transitions, and a summary of potential next steps in care transitions in light of Medicare rule changes regarding transitions.

Optimal transitional care, comprised of both the sending and the receiving features of the transfer, is essential for patients with complex care needs and is dependent upon a number of factors that are complimentary to the traditional roles of primary care, care coordination, discharge planning, and case management [2]. A national study of Medicare beneficiaries found that 22 % experience at least one care transition over the course of a year. Half of these transitions involved a single hospitalization followed by return to the original place of residence, but the remaining involved a complex sequence of transitions to varied sites of care. Few predominant transition patterns were present; most patterns were unique, which makes predicting (and accommodating) patients' care transitions difficult. The heterogeneity of transition patterns of older adults challenges approaches to improving transitions outcomes, as it becomes inefficient to plan for all possible care patterns [3].

Discharge from a hospital is just one example of a healthcare transition, but these transitions have gained heightened attention recently because of the focus on quality and financial imperatives for the U.S. healthcare system. Approximately 30 % of hospitalized older adults will experience more than one transfer across care settings within 30 days of a hospital discharge, with almost 13 % experiencing three or more transitions. In a 1997 sample of Medicare beneficiaries, 46 distinct care transition patterns were observed during the 30-day period following hospital discharge [4]. Hence, for many patients with multiple chronic comorbid conditions and geriatric syndromes, multiple healthcare transitions can be an overwhelming flurry of changes for the patients, their caregivers, and all of their healthcare providers involved across the continuum.

A widely utilized measure of hospitals' successful care transitions for patients is the 30-day readmission rate. A study of 2004 Medicare claims data revealed that nearly 20 % of discharged beneficiaries were rehospitalized within 30 days; 34 % were rehospitalized within 90 days. Half of patients discharged back to the community and rehospitalized within 30 days lacked a documented follow-up visit with their primary care physician (PCP) prior to rehospitalization. The authors estimated that the cost to Medicare for

E.H. Bowman, M.D., Ph.D. (✉)
Department of Medicine, Sidney & Lois Eskenazi Hospital,
Indiana University School of Medicine,
720 Eskenazi Avenue, Fifth Third Faculty Office Building,
2nd Floor, Indianapolis, IN 46202, USA
e-mail: elbowman@iu.edu

K.L. Flood, M.D.
Division of Gerontology, Geriatrics, and Palliative Care,
University of Alabama at Birmingham Hospital,
Birmingham, AL, USA
e-mail: kflood@uabmc.edu

M.L. Malone et al. (eds.), *Geriatrics Models of Care: Bringing 'Best Practice' to an Aging America*,
DOI 10.1007/978-3-319-16068-9_8, © Springer International Publishing Switzerland 2015

Fig. 8.1 Sites of care transitions commonly experienced by older adults in the US healthcare system. *PCP* Primary Care Provider, *ED* Emergency Department, *ICU* Intensive Care Unit, *SAR* Sub-Acute Rehabilitation, *LTACH* Long Term Acute Care Hospital, *LTC* Long Term Care

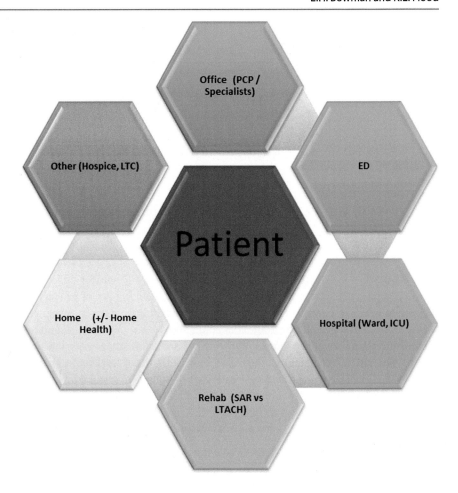

these unplanned readmissions in 2004 was $17.4 billion [5]. Hospitals are now incurring financial penalties for excessive readmissions. The Center for Medicare and Medicaid Services (CMS) announced that in fiscal year (FY) 2014 hospitals had incurred $227 million in readmission penalties, and they anticipate that in FY 2015 the sum of readmission penalties will be much higher, approaching $530 million [6]. Due to this staggering cost to individual hospitals, health systems, and society, an obvious goal is to develop and disseminate clinical decision models to predict those who are at risk for a failed care transition, and then appropriately target this group for interventions to improve outcomes. However, predicting which patients are at risk for 30-day readmission has proven quite difficult. In which patient populations or clinical scenarios and environments is an unplanned readmission avoidable? This question remains a topic of investigation. A 2011 meta-analysis concluded that 23 % of 30-day readmissions were preventable, but that value ranged from 5 to 59 % across studies [7]. Many studies have attempted to identify risk factors for readmission and have largely focused on disease-based factors such as diagnoses and number of comorbidities. Kansagara et al. studied 26 unique models for predicting 30-day hospital readmission and found most per-

formed poorly. The authors noted that most of the models included medical diagnoses as risk predictors, but few contained variables associated with overall health and function, illness severity, or the social determinants of health [8].

One key aspect in determining factors contributing to avoidable readmission is better understanding of the reason for and timing of 30-day readmissions. Currently, the CMS metric for measuring care transitions is the 30-day readmission rate; this metric is not based on a clinical trial demonstrating that 30 days has a clinically meaningful outcome compared to any other time period. In a 2013 study, 30-day readmissions from Medicare beneficiaries from 2007 to 2009 were analyzed for three Diagnosis-Related Groups (DRGs) which represent approximately 15 % of all 30-day readmissions for older adults: heart failure (HF), acute myocardial infarction (AMI), and pneumonia. The proportion of patients readmitted within 30 days was 24.8 % for HF, 19.9 % for AMI, and 18.3 % for pneumonia. Only a minority of the reasons for readmission was for the same diagnosis as the index admission (HF 35 %, AMI 10 %, and pneumonia 22 %). The vast majority of these Medicare patients were readmitted for a problem different than the reason for the first hospitalization. Regarding timing of the readmission, for each DRG over 60 % of the readmissions occurred within the first 15 days post-discharge (HF 61 %, AMI 68 %, pneumonia 63 %). Neither the reason for, nor timing of readmissions varied by patient age, gender, or race [9]. Thus, one opportunity for reducing unplanned 30-day readmissions may be through efforts that target the first 15 days post-hospital discharge. Additionally, care transitions interventions targeting only the admitting diagnoses may not be an effective means of reducing readmissions. Rather, the authors comment on the concept of "posthospitalization syndrome"; that is "a generalized vulnerability to illness among recently discharged patients, many of whom have developed new impairments both during and after hospitalization" [10]. These new impairments often include geriatric syndromes such as loss of function and mobility; hospital acquired delirium, malnutrition, and sleep deprivation; and alterations in medication regimens leading to polypharmacy and adverse drug events. The authors further note that "this heightened vulnerability to a diversity of illnesses may explain why interventions that are broadly applicable to many conditions with multiple components or are delivered by a multidisciplinary team are more likely to reduce readmissions" [9].

In a similar vein, a 2014 study of patients age 65 and over from 126 Veterans Affairs facilities evaluated two geriatric syndromes as predictors of readmissions: (1) frailty and (2) use of high-risk medications. These potential risk factors were chosen because they were known predictors of hospital admission for older adults, they were under-studied, and data regarding presence could be gathered from existing hospital records without requiring additional personnel for data collection. As a proxy marker for frailty, the authors utilized frailty-related diagnoses shown in the literature to be a frailty characteristic or associated with such in studies using the Fried model of frailty. These diagnoses were involuntary weight loss, coagulopathy, fluid and electrolyte imbalance, anemia, and fall or fracture. Amongst these older veterans, the 30-day readmission rate was 18.5 % for FY 2006. In a generalized linear model testing for patient, provider, and facility level variables, having one or more frailty-related diagnosis significantly increased the odds ratio for a 30-day readmission (1.15; 95 % confidence interval 1.11–1.19, $p < 0.001$). Additional factors associated with significantly increased odds of readmission were exemption from copay (a proxy for poverty), increasing comorbidity burden, and Emergency Department (ED) visits or hospitalizations in the prior fiscal year. With the addition of frailty in the model, age was no longer a predictor for readmission. Protective against readmission was increased primary care visits in the previous fiscal year; the impact of this benefit increased with increasing number of primary care visits. Taking a high-risk medication was associated with a reduced risk of 30-day readmission (0.70, 95 % confidence interval 0.66–0.73, $p < 0.001$). However, patients with chronic use of high-risk medications and a frailty diagnosis were not protected from readmission (1.08; 95 % CI 0.97–1.20) [11]. Given that many of the high-risk medications were for symptom management, such as pain control, it is possible that use of these medications resulted in better control of symptoms from chronic illness and therefore fewer readmissions. These recent studies signal that geriatric syndromes such as frailty may inform future readmission-risk models to improve their accuracy. Additionally, readmissions for frail patients may be amenable to reduction via increased primary care visits in the outpatient setting.

In 2009, the American College of Physicians (ACP), Society of Hospital Medicine (SHM), Society of General Internal Medicine, AGS, American College of Emergency Physicians, and the Society for Academic Emergency Medicine published a collaboratively developed Transitions of Care Consensus Policy Statement in an effort to address the well documented quality gaps in care during a transition between inpatient and outpatient settings. This policy statement summarized principles required for a quality care transition, including accountability, communication, timely information exchange, patient/family involvement, respecting the hub of care coordination, providing a medical home for all patients/caregivers, empowering patients to know who is responsible for their care at every transitional point, following national standards, and standardizing metrics to enable quality improvement and accountability. Based on these guiding principles, this consensus panel developed a set of standards describing necessary components for implementation that included coordinating clinicians, care plans/transition record, communication infrastructure, standard communication formats, transition responsibility, timeliness, community standards, and measurement [12].

Sites of Post-hospitalization Care

Older adults may require varying levels of care before and after hospitalization. These sites of care include: (1) private homes with or without home health or hospice; (2) subacute rehabilitation in a skilled nursing facility (SNF); (3) acute inpatient rehabilitation; (4) long-term acute care hospitals (LTACHs); or (5) long-term care (LTC) in a facility (Table 8.1).

The appropriate site of care following a hospitalization is typically based on patient medical and intensity of caregiving needs. Facility and licensed caregiver services in the home require documentation of need, justification for level of care, a payer source, and in some settings, documentation of a timely face-to-face evaluation by the certifying physician. Thus, obtaining the appropriate intensity of services for every patient can often be cumbersome for a busy clinician to facilitate, hallmarking the benefit of implementing

Table 8.1 Sites of care delivery

Site	Care provided	Eligibility requirements	Financing
Independent Living: • House or apartment • Congregate care facilities (CCFs: senior living complex, independent living facility)	• Patients managing ADLs, IADLs, & medical care with or without home health or hospice • CCFs often offer group activities; may provide higher level of services (meals, medication assist) for added $	• Older age for admission to CCFs • Home-bound status & need for skilled services for home health • MD certified terminal diagnosis & anticipated life-expectancy of <6 months for hospice	• Self-pay or some LTC insurances cover CCFs, paid caregivers • MCR Part A covers home health & hospice
Assisted Living Facility (ALF) • Free standing or housed in LTC facility • Specialty Care-Assisted Living Facility (SCALF) for patients with CI	• Services provided varies; most offer assist with meals, some ADLS, laundry, medications, housekeeping, & provide group activities & socialization	• Need for assistance with IADLs and/or ADLs • Most require residents still be able to ambulate or self-propel wheelchair	• Self-pay or LTC insurances • MCD waiver program available in some states • MCR Part A covers home health
Sub-acute Care/Skilled Nursing Facility (SNF) • Free standing facility or housed within hospital or long term care facility	• Skilled nursing or rehabilitation services such as IV medications, enteral tube feedings, wound care, or physical/occupational therapy	• Documented need for daily skilled care following a qualifying hospital stay of at least three inpatient days within the prior 30 days • Some may provide higher levels of care such as trach/ventilator care	• MCR Part A covers up to 100 days (co-pay for days 21–100)
Inpatient (Acute) Rehabilitation • Free standing facility or housed within hospital	• Licensed as an acute hospital • Comprehensive rehabilitation services (physical, occupational, and speech)	• Need for MD supervision of care • Approved diagnosis and able to tolerate and benefit from 3 h of therapy/day, 5 days/week OR, in certain cases, 15 h of therapy over a 7 day period • Does not require preceding hospitalization	• MCR Part A payment based on CMS prospective payment system for rehabilitation diagnoses
Long-Term Acute Care Hospital (LTACH) • Free standing facility or housed within hospital	• Licensed as an acute hospital • Extended medical care requiring prolonged services (e.g., ventilator weaning, TPN, wound care, etc.)	• Need for daily MD and skilled care for patients who may improve with time • Does not require preceding hospitalization	• MCR Part A
Custodial Care/Long-Term Care (LTC)	• Comprehensive medical, personal, & social services care	• Varies by state; in general for persons no longer able to live in community due to functional dependencies and/or chronic illness	• Self-pay, LTC insurance, or MCD • MCR Part A covers MHB

Modified from Bowman EH, Flood KL, Arbaje AI. Models of care to transition from hospital to home. In: Malone M, Capezuti E, Palmer RM, editors. Acute care for elders—a model for interdisciplinary care. New York, NY: Springer Science and Business Media; 2014:175–202 with permission

interdisciplinary teams comprised of members who can help execute these often difficult arrangements—as well as ensure that appropriate payer sources will be enacted.

Factors Contributing to Adverse Events During Care Transitions

A care transition from a hospital to one of these sites of care represents a vulnerable time and exposes patients to risks for adverse clinical events, increased healthcare utilization, and preventable rehospitalizations [2]. In a 2003 prospective study of 400 patients discharged to home following hospitalization, Forster et al found 19 % of patients experienced an adverse event from care management during the care

transition; 30 % of these events were deemed preventable and 31 % ameliorable. The authors identified key targets for improvement during a care transition, including: (1) recognition and communication of unresolved problems across care settings; (2) enhancing patient education and self-management of treatment plans; (3) post-discharge medication therapy monitoring; and (4) overall clinical condition monitoring during the care transition period [13]. A growing body of literature has also identified several additional patient and system-level risk factors among older adults for suboptimal care transitions (Table 8.2).

In addition to these risk factors, the traditional fee-for-service payment models in a fragmented healthcare environment may discourage providers from spending the time required to collaboratively develop an optimal care

Table 8.2 Patient- and system-level factors associated with suboptimal care transitions or early readmission

Patient-level factors	System-level factors
• Age >80 years • Recent hospitalization (within 30 days) • Longer hospital length of stay • Increased number of comorbidities • Functional disability • Unmet functional needs • Male gender[a] • Member of racial/ethnic minority[a] • Unmarried[a] • Low income • History of depression • Living alone • Lack of self-management ability • Limited education • History of substance abuse • Lower self-reported health status	• Failure in implementation of plan of care (durable medical equipment, home health care, follow-up appointments, medications, tests) • Communities with high hospital admission rates • Patients having a usual place to receive health care • Homelessness • Lack of discharge education • Insufficient communication across care settings

Modified from Bowman EH, Flood KL, Arbaje AI. Models of care to transition from hospital to home. In: Malone M, Capezuti E, Palmer RM, editors. Acute care for elders—a model for interdisciplinary care. New York, NY: Springer Science and Business Media; 2014:175–202 with permission
[a]Mixed results in the literature

transition plan and therefore unintentionally contribute to adverse events experienced by the patients discharged to home [13]. Disease-based models of inpatient care and reimbursement rules increasingly bring about patients who are too frail to return home but who also no longer "qualify" for inpatient or rehabilitation settings. This ever-expanding group of patients is therefore at risk for vulnerable care transitions and unplanned readmissions. The uninsured have even fewer (or no) post-hospital care options.

Common Themes in Optimal Care Transitions

A well-documented and comprehensive plan of care and communication transfer, as well as the availability of healthcare providers trained in caring for patients with complex needs, is the central backbone of the care transition. Furthermore, the healthcare practitioner will ideally have some knowledge about (or take the time to elicit) the patient's goals of care, preferences, and current clinical status as well as baseline level of functioning. Finally, the care transition should also take into account the logistical arrangements, care coordination by all healthcare professionals involved in both sides of the transition, and also address the need to educate both patient and family or other involved caregivers. The ideal transition of care thus offers an interdisciplinary

approach to address the patient's individualized care needs, provides accurate and timely medication reconciliation accounting for changes made during the transitional care event, engages patients and families throughout the transitional process using techniques to verify that instructions are understood, and emphasizes the *timely* and *accurate* provision of information to the providers at the receiving site of care. This process has been described as "the Discharge Transitions Bundle" [14].

Communication Across Care Settings

A successful transition from hospital to a new care setting requires efficient, accurate, and timely communication of hospital discharge information from the sending to the receiving care providers. Many studies have revealed that delayed or incomplete transfer of clinical information to PCPs following a hospitalization is common and may contribute to medical errors and rehospitalizations. A systematic review of communication regarding a patient's hospitalization found that only 12–34 % of PCPs received a discharge summary by the time of the patient's first post-hospitalization follow up appointment. Additionally, hospital discharge summaries frequently lacked information essential to a safe care transition, including discharge medications, tests pending at discharge, and counseling provided to patients and families [15]. To address information transfer, many of the studied care transitions interventions utilize a brief personal health record with vital medical and hospitalization information that is transported by the patient across care settings. This will be described in more detail below.

Patient/Caregiver Self-Management

Patient activation, or one's ability and willingness to manage his/her own medical problems and health care, is increasingly recognized as a factor impacting healthcare utilization, costs, and outcomes. According to a 2007 survey conducted by the Center for Studying Health System Change, only 41 % of US adults are highly activated in their health care [16]. This lack of self-management ability has been identified as a risk factor associated with early rehospitalization among Medicare beneficiaries [17]. During a care transition, the only person who is present at all points in time across all settings is the patient (and any existing involved caregivers). The concept of patient activation is optimized in many of the studied care transitions interventions through the use of "coaching" patients and caregivers. Various methods of patient coaching have been employed, including the use of personal nursing coaches or checklists that the patient can use to be reassured they are transitioning

Fig. 8.2 Discharge preparation checklist®. (Courtesy of © Eric A. Coleman, MD, MPH—The Care Transitions Program®, Denver, Colorado. http://www.caretransitions.org/documents/checklist.pdf.)

Discharge Preparation Checklist

Before I leave the care facility, the following tasks should be completed:

❑ I have been involved in decisions about what will take place after I leave the facility.

❑ I understand where I am going after I leave this facility and what will happen to me once I arrive.

❑ I have the name and phone number of a person I should contact if a problem arise during my transfer.

❑ I understand what my medications are, how to obtain them and how to take them.

❑ I understand the potential side effects of my medications and whom I should call if I experience them.

❑ I understand what symptoms I need to watch out for and whom to call should I notice them.

❑ I understand how to keep my health problems from becoming worse.

❑ My doctor or nurse has answered my most important questions prior to leaving the facility.

❑ My family or someone close to me knows that I am coming home and what I will need once I leave the facility.

❑ If I am going directly home, I have scheduled a follow-up appointment with my doctor, and I have transportation to this appointment.

This tool was developed by Dr. Eric Coleman, UCHSC, HCPR, with funding from the John A. Hartford Foundation and the Robert Wood Johnson Foundation

with the critical information they need to accurately follow through with the next stage of their health care [18]. One of the most often used tools is Eric Coleman's Discharge Preparation Checklist® (Fig. 8.2) [19].

How information is communicated to patients and families is important. Despite elders often reporting comprehension of discharge plans, many factors combine to hinder patient understanding and adherence, including cognitive impairment, functional illiteracy and low healthcare literacy, socioeconomic status (SES), multimorbidity, cultural barriers, absent caregivers, and physical limitations [20–22]. Research demonstrates many elders and caregivers misunderstand discharge instructions, lack appropriate follow-up care, and do not receive complete, accurate and legible medication lists at the time of hospital discharge. Healthcare professionals also increasingly recognize the crucial role that culture plays in the health care of patients and families, and the need to communicate in a culturally competent manner [23]. Various strategies and resources must therefore be employed when developing any transitional tool designed to engage the patient to assist in self-management during the care transition. Likewise, tools can be employed to help determine patient comprehension of instructions in a manner that is sensitive to all cultures, levels of education and healthcare literacy. One of these methods is the "teach back" concept, also known as the "show me" method or "closing the loop" in which the healthcare provider confirms that information has been explained to the patient in a way that is truly comprehended, regardless of education or literacy level (Fig. 8.3) [24]. Regardless of culture, SES, race, or literacy level, clari-

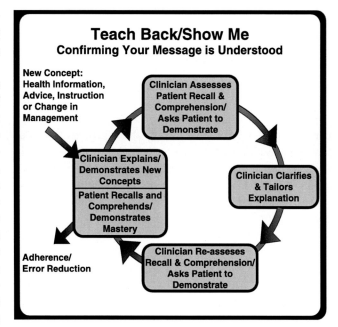

Fig. 8.3 Teach back/show me method®. (Courtesy of Tony DiNuzzo, PhD, Program Director, East Texas Geriatric Education Center-Consortium—Acute Care of the Elderly Clinical Training Program: Improving Communication Skills between Health Professions Students and Older Patients)

fying shared goals is not only important to all patients but critical to patient engagement and activation. Thus, it is vital that the healthcare system work to educate the workforce to master skills of effective communication with patients and caregivers from all economic and cultural backgrounds.

Medication Management and Medication Reconciliation in Care Transitions

Alterations in medication regimens during and after hospitalization are common and lends to another source of vulnerability for patients. Research demonstrates that medication-related care transitions adverse events are common. Forster and colleagues in their prospective study found that 66 % of adverse events from a hospital care transition were adverse drug events [13]. Moore and colleagues found medication continuity errors (discrepancy between hospital discharge medications and medications patient was taking at the time of first follow-up visit) were present in 42 % of patients within 2 months of a hospital discharge [25]. Recurring in the 2013 National Patient Safety Goals is the mandate for hospitals to "maintain and communicate accurate patient medication information." Incorporated in this goal are the following elements of performance: (1) obtain and document a reconciled medication list upon admission to the hospital; (2) provide the patient (or caregiver as needed) with written medication instructions at the time of hospital discharge; and (3) coach the patient (or caregiver) in key elements of medication management, such as the importance of keeping an updated list and taking this list to outpatient appointments [26]. Some key strategies for preparing a patient's discharge medication list include providing: (1) an indication for each medication, stop dates or tapering schedules as appropriate, and clear behavioral triggers for as-needed psychiatric medications; (2) tapering or discontinuation of medications added during the hospital stay (such as analgesics, proton pump inhibitors, or laxatives with as-needed orders); and (3) formal reconciliation of the discharge regimen with the preadmission regimen [27]. Reconciliation results in clear documentation of which medications on the discharge list are new (relative to the preadmission regimen), which of the preadmission medications have been stopped, and which dosages of continued medications have been changed (Fig. 8.4).

Roles of Interdisciplinary Team Members, Patients, and Families in Care Transitions

The 2009 Transitions of Care Consensus Policy Statement comments on the "lack of a single clinician or clinical entity taking responsibility for coordination across the continuum" [12]. The roles of clinicians during care transitions remain poorly defined. A recent study described a conceptual framework summarizing clinicians' roles during care transitions to address this gap in the literature and found incongruence between clinicians' perceptions of their routine versus ideal roles during care transitions (e.g., routine: sending a discharge summary to the receiving clinician; ideal: calling the receiving clinician and discussing the patient's case). The investigators identified factors prompting clinicians to act closer to their ideal roles, such as personally knowing the receiving clinician or major decisions having been made in the hospital regarding goals of care. The conceptual framework highlights the continued ambiguity in accountability during transitions [28]. In addition to the physician role, newly published care transitions interventions emphasize use of all team members. In 2011, Naylor and colleagues published a systematic review of care transition intervention studies focusing on chronically ill adults transitioning from a hospital. Eighteen of the 21 of the RCTs included in the review utilized either a registered or advance practice nurse as the intervention leader or coordinator [2]. Social workers, pharmacists, and other disciplines have also been utilized in interventions. For example, an intervention developed at Rush University, the Enhanced Discharge Planning Program, employs master's-prepared social workers to intervene by phone with patients within 48 h of discharge to support the care plan, address unmet needs, and connect them with needed providers [29]. Several care transitions studies also include family members or caregivers in the intervention [2].

In May 2013, CMS issued new guidelines effective immediately regarding discharge planning for Condition of Participation (CoP) for hospitals. The new requirements are extensive in expanding the scope of "discharge planning" to "transition planning," and emphasize the goal to "consideration of transitions among multiple types of patient care settings that may be involved at various points in the treatment of a given patient." This new CoP requires that "a registered nurse, social worker, or other appropriately qualified personnel must develop, or supervise the development of, the evaluation" of care transition needs. The guidelines cite the benefits of an interdisciplinary team approach to hospital discharge planning, scheduling follow-up appointments and filling prescriptions prior to discharge, and follow-up phone calls within 24–72 h of discharge to ensure adherence to the care transition plan and identify any barriers [30]. These are functions that may be performed by non-physician team members, should be coordinated with patients and families, and are crucial components of a successful care transition.

Interventions to Improve Care Transitions Post-hospitalization

Recently, developed innovative models of transitional care have targeted the previously identified processes in need of improvement during a care transition and have shown promise that specialized programs emphasizing certain key elements including patient and caregiver coaching, early transition planning, and meticulous medication reconciliation can improve outcomes. The majority of published studies regarding care transitions interventions have been in the

Source of Medication Information:

◻Patient self report / medication list
◻Family/caregiver
◻Prescription bottle labels
◻Electronic Medical Record

◻Pharmacy reconciliation
◻Outside facility
◻Prior Discharge medication list
◻Other

Medication Allergies With Noted Reactions:
1. _____
2. _____
3. _____

Please STOP These Preadmission Medications:
(including prescription, over-the-counter, and natural/herbal medications)
1. _____
2. _____
3. _____

Please CONTINUE Only These Preadmission Medications:
(including prescription, over-the-counter, and natural/herbal medications)
1. _____
2. _____
3. _____

Please BEGIN These NEW Medications:
(including prescription, over-the-counter, and natural/herbal medications)
1. _____
2. _____
3. _____

Vaccinations Received During This Hospital Admission:
1. _____
2. _____
3. _____

Additional Information/Recommendations:
1. _____
2. _____
3. _____

Pharmacy / Phone & Fax (If Known): _____
Medication history and reconciliation performed by: _____
Discharge medication counseling provided to patient by: _____
Patient given written and verbal information
and verbalized understanding? _____

Fig. 8.4 Medication reconciliation form template. Thorough medication reconciliation will guide the patient to understand which new medications to start, which old medications to continue or stop taking, assess patient comprehension of instructions, and offer contact information for future questions. (Modified from Bowman EH, Flood KL, Arbaje AI. Models of care to transition from hospital to home. In: Malone M, Capezuti E, Palmer RM, editors. Acute care for elders—a model for interdisciplinary care. New York, NY: Springer Science and Business Media; 2014:175–202 with permission.) *ADL* activities of daily living, *IADL* instrumental activities of daily living, *CI* cognitive impairment, *MCR* Medicare, *MCD* Medicaid, *CMS* Centers for Medicare & Medicaid Services, *TPN* total parenteral nutrition, *MHB* Medicare Hospice Benefit

last 10 years. In Naylor's 2011 systematic review, care transition RCTs were examined in terms of how results (positive or negative) can inform implementation of healthcare reform objectives. All but one study had at least one positive outcome; nine included beneficial outcomes related to hospital readmissions. Each of these nine studies impacting readmissions utilized a nurse as the intervention coordinator and six of the nine utilized home visits [2].

Based on results of prior research, four primary models of care transitions originating in the hospital setting have emerged: (1) Transitional Care Model (TCM); (2) Care Transition Intervention® (CTI); (3) Re-Engineered Discharge (Project RED); and (4) Better Outcomes for Older Adults Through Safe Transitions (BOOST). The first three of these four models will be discussed herein; BOOST will be described in a separate chapter (see Chap. 9). In addition, recent research of Acute Care for Elders (ACE) and Mobile ACE models of care has demonstrated promising impact on care transitions outcomes and will be briefly discussed below and more thoroughly elaborated upon in separate chapters (see Chaps. 1 and 4).

Transitional Care Model

The TCM developed by Naylor and colleagues provides comprehensive, evidence-based transitional care coordination for chronically ill high-risk older adults [31, 32]. The heart of this model is the Transitional Care Nurse (TCN), an advanced practice nurse who follows enrolled patients from in-hospital planning meetings to home, focusing on caregiver and patient needs. The TCN conducts an initial hospital visit and assessment, followed by subsequent home visits focusing on medication management, coaching patients for follow-up visits and even accompanying them to the visits, and conducting follow-up phone calls during weeks without planned home visitation. In this fashion the TCN is available 7 days a week via both home visits as well as telephone access for 1–3 months of post-hospital follow-up. Findings from multi-site RCTs demonstrate reduced readmissions, total hospital days, and costs in addition to increased patient, caregiver, and provider satisfaction [32, 33].

Care Transitions Intervention

The CTI developed by Coleman and colleagues is a 4-week program addressing four primary pillars of a successful care transition: (1) improved communication via a portable record (Personal Health Record) of essential health information the patient carries across care settings; (2) medication reconciliation and self-management training; (3) patient-scheduled follow-up appointments; and (4) improved patient knowledge regarding clinical symptoms signaling worsening status ("red-flags") and how to respond [34, 35]. These components are taught by a nurse Care Transitions Coach®, who provides individualized coaching by conducting an initial hospital visit and assessment, working with the patient to complete the Discharge Preparation Checklist®, coaching the patient how to utilize their own personal health records, and providing oversight of medication management. The Care Transitions Coach® follows the patient for 4 weeks post-discharge via home visits and three follow-up phone calls. A RCT of the CTI demonstrated significantly lower 30- and 90-day rehospitalizations, reduced mean hospital costs at 90 and 180 days, and improved patient disease self-management and increased confidence about their role during care transitions [36].

Re-Engineered Discharge

Project RED developed out of a safety net hospital research group at Boston University Medical Center that develops and tests strategies to improve the hospital discharge processes through promoting patient safety and reducing rehospitalization [37, 38]. Project RED strives to minimize rehospitalizations by seeking to engage patients in disease self-management training, medication reconciliation, matching discharge plans with published clinical guidelines, improving communication through expedited transmission of discharge summaries, and transporting patient health records to all care settings. Patient coaching is again performed by a nurse; post-discharge phone calls by a pharmacist ensure medication reconciliation and reinforcement of the discharge plan. The RED Toolkit is founded on 12 discrete, mutually reinforcing components of a discharge, provides guidance to implement the RED processes for all patients, including those with limited English proficiency and from diverse cultural backgrounds, and helps hospitals reduce readmission rates by replicating the discharge process. In a randomized study, Project RED patients experienced a 30 % decrease in 30-day hospital utilization (combined emergency department visits and readmissions) compared to usual care. Project RED patients reported being more prepared for discharge and had significantly improved knowledge regarding their diagnosis and PCP name. They were also significantly more likely to follow-up with their PCP. The intervention was most effective in patients with a prior hospitalization within the last 6 months [39].

ACE/Mobile ACE

Multiple published studies have demonstrated improved clinical outcomes and cost savings from the ACE Unit model of care. More recent studies have also pointed toward the additional benefit of an ACE model on care transitions. Flood et al demonstrated lower costs and fewer all-cause rehospitalizations within 30 days for ACE Unit patients compared to similar patients cared for on a usual care unit [40]. Hung et al describe a Mobile Acute Care for Elders (MACE) service utilizing a mobile interdisciplinary team that seeks to decrease the hazards of hospitalization, facilitate transitions of care, and provide patient and family education. MACE service patients were less likely to experience adverse events, had shorter length of stay (LOS), and rated the quality of their care transition higher than matched general medicine patients [41]. Other studies have produced mixed results. Researchers at Johns Hopkins University pilot-tested a model that combined the strengths of inpatient geriatric evaluation, co-management, and transitional care in a cluster-randomized trial of 717 hospitalized older adults on four general medicine services. In the two treatment groups, a geriatrician–geriatric nurse practitioner dyad assessed patients co-managed geriatric syndromes, provided staff education, encouraged patient self-management, communicated with PCPs, and followed up with patients soon after discharge. The intervention was associated with greater patient satisfaction with inpatient care and slightly higher quality care transitions (though not statistically significant) [42]. In a 2012 published systemic review and meta-analysis of over 6,800 hospitalized elderly patients, Fox et al demonstrate that acute geriatric unit care based on all or part of the ACE model improves patient- and system-level outcomes, including fewer fall risks, less delirium, less functional decline at discharge from baseline 2-week pre-hospital admission status, shorter LOS, fewer discharges to nursing home, lower costs, and more discharges to home. There were no significant differences found in hospital readmissions, mortality, or post-hospitalization functional status compared with functional baseline before hospital admission [43].

Care Transition Intervention Targeting Patients Experiencing Low Socioeconomic Status

Data regarding care transitions interventions specifically targeting lower socioeconomic status patients are limited. Challenges seen in this patient cohort may include lack of social support, a higher prevalence of mental health and substance abuse disorders, and barriers to accessing healthcare. A 2014 trial developed and tested a Care Transition Innovation (C-Train) specifically designed for socioeconomically disadvantaged adults. In this cluster randomized controlled trial, 382 community-dwelling hospitalized adults without mental illness who were either uninsured or had public insurance and were admitted to a general medicine or cardiology service were randomized to the intervention or usual care tran-

sition planning. The C-Train intervention consisted of: (1) a care transition coach who engaged the patient at the time of admission and conducted post-discharge follow-up phone calls; (2) home visits for highest risk patients; (3) medication reconciliation and oversight by a pharmacist including guidance to the patient's PCP to use low-cost medications and provision of 30 days of medications post-discharge for patient unable to afford medications; (4) arrangement of PCP follow-up; and (5) monthly continuous quality improvement meetings with the goal to continuously improve the intervention. The C-Train intervention did not reduce 30-day readmissions (14.4 % vs. 16.1 %, $p = 0.644$) or ED visits (24.4 % vs. 19.6 %, $p = 0.271$). Based on the 3-item Care Transitions Measure, the intervention did lead to a significant improvement in the quality of the care transition experience compared to usual care (OR 2.17, 95 % CI 1.30–3.64). Intervention patients also had a lower unadjusted mortality rate within 30 days of discharge (0 % vs. 3 %, $p = 0.02$) [44]. One possibility is that improved access to care afforded by the C-Train intervention actually reduces mortality by increasing access to hospitalization. This study cohort consisted of 60 % males, over half of whom were uninsured, over 75 % of whom lacked a usual source for routine primary care, and over 40 % of whom had a history of illicit drug use. Thus, this patient population will likely require a different approach than patient populations without these extenuating circumstances, and the degree to which readmissions are preventable at least in this population remains to be determined.

Outpatient-Based Models Shown to Reduce Unnecessary Hospitalizations/Readmissions

One method of reducing unplanned readmissions in older adults is to prevent an unnecessary initial hospitalization. Several interventions that are outpatient-based follow the principles of Guided Care (also see Chap. 11) and have demonstrated comprehensive geriatric care while preventing unnecessary hospitalization and/or readmissions. These include Palliative Care Programs for patients with life-limiting illness/injury, Geriatric Resources for Assessment and Care of Elders (GRACE), Hospital at Home®, and Program for All-Inclusive Care for Elders (PACE). These are briefly summarized below and thoroughly developed in Chaps. 6, 10, 14, and 24, respectively.

Guided Care (GC) is an outpatient-based interdisciplinary team model of care led by a specially trained registered nurse in partnership with PCPs and caregivers to support a practice's most complex patients by assessing the patient and primary caregiver at home, creating an evidence-based care plan for providers and an action plan for patients and caregivers, promoting patient self-management, monthly monitoring of patients' conditions, coordinating efforts of care providers in all settings, smoothing transitions between sites of care, educating and supporting family caregivers, and facilitating access to community resources. Studies suggest implementing GC is feasible and improves patient, caregiver, and provider satisfaction as well as patient ratings of the quality of chronic care. In a clustered RCT, GC patients tended to utilize fewer home health services but there was no difference in hospital, emergency department (ED), and SNF services or 30-day readmission rates compared to usual care patients [45]. However, this trial targeted patients known to be high risk for healthcare utilization based on predictive models. A lower or moderate risk target population may have benefited more from GC in terms of reducing healthcare utilization.

Other models of care coordination that have been shown to impact care transitions use principles found within GC. Hospital at Home® provides hospital-level care for an acute illness in-home for patients meeting medical eligibility criteria, thereby avoiding admission to an acute care facility. Necessary medical equipment (oxygen, infusions, lab, and radiology testing) is provided. Patients receive nurse and physician visits daily, with additional visits as needed [46]. Hospital at Home® programs demonstrate improved patient and caregiver satisfaction and reduced costs with comparable or improved clinical outcomes compared to traditional hospital admission [47, 48]. The PACE Program is a capitated Medicare and Medicaid community-based managed care program that provides interdisciplinary team care to frail adults. Persons age 55 and over are eligible for PACE if they live in a PACE catchment area and meet state Medicaid criteria for nursing home eligibility. PACE enables frail elders to continue community living via an interdisciplinary team with development of comprehensive, individualized medical, psychosocial, and functional care plans [49]. PACE is associated with improved survival, quality of life, functional status, patient satisfaction, and reduced hospitalizations and nursing home placement [50]. Similar in concept, GRACE helps frail community-dwelling elders age in place by incorporating in-home geriatric assessment of patient and caregiver(s) through a geriatric nurse practitioner and social worker team in conjunction with the PCP. Individualized care plans addressing geriatric syndromes developed by the GRACE team (geriatrician, pharmacist, mental health liaison, nurse practitioner/medical social worker dyad) are approved by the PCP prior to implementation. GRACE has demonstrated improved patient-centered care transitions and reduced hospital readmissions and nursing home placement [51].

Patients with chronic or life-limiting illnesses have many complex post-discharge needs that often do not include the common discharge destination of a rehabilitation facility; therefore this patient population is at risk of readmission due to unmet symptomatic needs. For patients not yet meeting the guidelines for Medicare Hospice Benefit, a palliative care (PC) approach focusing on patient-centered goals of care is often more appropriate. The National Consensus Project (NCP) defines PC as care that is focused on "seriously ill patients and those with advanced disease, who are unlikely to be cured, recover, or stabilize, and their caregivers" [52]. PC focuses on aggressive symptom management as well as providing interdisciplinary support for patients and families with the goal of improving quality of life when cure might not be possible. PC is not exclusively end of life care, should be provided at any stage of illness that symptom burden occurs, and should be offered in conjunction with all other appropriate forms of medical treatment, including curative therapies. The NCP offers a means by which PC can be operationalized through eight different domains to effectively manage pain and other distressing symptoms, while also incorporating psychosocial and spiritual care with consideration of patient/family needs, preferences, values, beliefs, and cultures. These eight domains include: (1) structure and processes of care; (2) physical aspects of care; (3) psychological and psychiatric aspects of care; (4) social aspects of care; (5) spiritual, religious and existential aspects of care; (6) cultural aspects of care; (7) care of the imminently dying patient; and (8) ethical and legal aspects of care. PC is provided by an interdisciplinary team and can be delivered in all care settings. The Medicare Hospice Benefit, just one component of PC, can be activated when the patient's life expectancy is anticipated to be 6 months or less. Research reveals patients receiving PC experience improved symptom control and satisfaction, reduced ED visits and hospitalizations, reduced costs, and greater likelihood of dying at home compared to those receiving conventional care [53, 54].

Other Sites of Care Transitions

The ED is another site for care transitions. Older adults have a higher risk of return ED visit or hospitalization within 30 days of ED discharge compared to younger adults. Preliminary studies have investigated the roles of screening tools and geriatric assessments in the ED to target elders at risk for poor care transitions. The most studied screening tools for identification of high-risk elder ED patients are the Identification of Seniors At Risk Tool (ISAR) tool and the Triage Risk Stratification Tool (TRST) [55, 56]. These brief screens are designed to be completed within a few minutes by ED staff and assess for geriatric syndromes such as cognitive, functional, and visual impairments; difficulties with medication management; and prior history of ED visits or hospitalizations. The TRST also allows for ED staff to include any concerns for patient safety. To date, these tools have demonstrated moderate predictability for identifying elders at risk for return ED visit or hospital admission following ED discharge [56, 57]. Preliminary studies have examined use of screening and targeted geriatric assessment in the ED. In 2001, Mion et al describe the implementation of the Systematic Intervention for a Geriatric Network of Evaluation and Treatment (SIGNET) program, using the TRST to identify elders discharging from ED to home who are at risk of poor outcomes or readmission to receive a geriatric assessment by a geriatric clinical nurse specialist (GCNS). The GCNS coordinates patient and caregiver education and needed referrals to community agencies, PCPs, and/or outpatient geriatric assessment. In a feasibility study, SIGNET significantly reduced the proportion of elders with return ED visits within 30 days and significantly increased the number of referrals to community agencies [58]. The Discharge of Elderly from the Emergency Department (DEED) program does not use a screening tool for targeting patients, but instead utilizes comprehensive geriatric assessment (CGA) performed by a nurse for patients aged 75 and older who are discharged from the ED to home. Based on the CGA findings, an interdisciplinary team develops a care plan, in coordination with the patient, caregivers, PCP, and community resources, and follows the patient for 4 weeks, including home visits. In a RCT, the DEED II study demonstrated a significantly reduced rate of hospitalization within the first 30 days and reduced rate of ED admission for 18 months following index ED visit. Intervention patients also experienced a significantly longer time to the first repeat ED visit [59].

Health Information Technology as a Tool to Assist with Care Transitions

Electronic Health Record and Discharge Summaries

Advances in health information technology and increasing use of electronic medical records (EMRs) provide opportunities to improve timeliness of information transfer following hospitalization. Kripalani and colleagues note in their review that discharge summaries generated electronically (information systems merging administrative and clinical information) tended to result in more complete and timely information transfer from a hospitalization to the PCP compared to dictated summaries. The authors concluded that hospitals should use information technology to populate discharge summaries with required clinical information such as medications, diagnoses, and test results (and pending tests) wherever possible and that discharge summaries should be sent or be available for direct access by the PCP on the day of discharge [15]. In keeping with the crucial theme of timely and accurate information transfer, the SHM's Hospital Quality and Patient Safety Committee assembled an expert

consensus panel to develop the Ideal Discharge of the Elderly Patient Checklist. This checklist focuses on the key transition safety elements of patient status (including function, cognition, and resuscitation status), medication reconciliation, patient education, and follow-up (including pending tests) that should be included in discharge summaries. This checklist has been formally endorsed by the SHM [60]. Additionally, in 2009 a collaborative working group consisting of members from the American Board of Internal Medicine Foundation, ACP, SHM, and the Physician Consortium for Performance Improvement® (PCPI) published the Care Transitions Performance Measurements (CTPM) [61]. The working group defined six process measures that have since been endorsed by the National Quality Forum and should be incorporated into continuous quality improvement efforts to improve care transition outcomes. These process measures are:

- Measure 1: Reconciled medication list received by discharged patients.
- Measure 2: Transition record with specified elements received by discharge patients.
- Measure 3: Timely transition of transition record (to facility or PCP for follow-up care).
- Measure 4: Transition record with specified elements received by discharged patients for ED discharges.
- Measure 5: Discharge planning/post-discharge support for heart failure patients.
- Measure 6: Promote improved patient understanding of and adherence to treatment plans via addition of appropriate questions to patient satisfaction measures.

This set of process measures were chosen because they are linked to the following identified indicators of success in improving care transitions:

1. Reduction in adverse drug events.
2. Reduction in patient harm related to care transition medical errors.
3. Reduction in unnecessary healthcare utilization (e.g., hospital readmissions).
4. Reduction in redundant tests/procedures.
5. Achievement of patient goals, including functional status, comfort care measures, etc.
6. Improved patient understanding of and adherence to the treatment plan.

A list of the SHM endorsed minimal key data elements that should be included in all discharge summaries and the corresponding process measure is summarized in Table 8.3.

ACE Tracker

To address the barriers in dissemination of the ACE Unit model of care, Malone and colleagues from the Aurora Health Care System developed the software program ACE

Table 8.3 Crosswalk summarizing minimal key data elements for: (1) inclusion in all discharge summaries for next site of care/provider; and (2) related care transition process measures

Data element	SHM endorsed key elements to be included in discharge summaries [ref]	Care transition process measure [ref]
Transition record of hospitalization or ED visit		
• Problem that precipitated hospitalization or chief complaint	X	2,4
• Brief hospital/ED course with key events/findings, consultant recommendations, and anticipated problems and suggested interventions	X	2
• Results of key tests/procedures	X	2,4
• Discharge diagnoses	X	2,4
• Condition at discharge, including status of geriatric syndromes such as function and cognition	X	
• Discharge destination	X	
• Transition record transmitted to facility, PCP, or other provider designated for follow-up care within 24 h of discharge		3
Medication reconciliation		
• Discharge medication list reconciled with patients' list of medicines prior to hospitalization (medications to be continued, medications not to be continued, new medications added)	X	1,2,4
• Discharge medication doses, frequencies, instructions, and stop dates (if applicable) included for each continued and new medication	X	1
• Medication cautions (allergies, adverse reactions)	X	1
Follow-up information		
• Follow-up care needed, including appointments made or needed, provider name(s), contact information, and date of appointment	X	2,4
• Tests/studies pending at discharge and contact information for obtaining results	X	2
• 24/7 call back number for questions or new problems related to hospitalization	X	2
Patient/caregiver teaching		
• Patient education/instructions provided	X	2,4
• Documentation of patient/caregiver level of understanding	X	
Advance care planning		
• Summary of goals of care discussions including but not limited to code status, advance directives, surrogate decision maker	X	2

X required element, *SHM* Society of Hospital Medicine, *ED* emergency department, *PCP* primary care physician. (Modified from Bowman EH, Flood KL, Arbaje AI. Models of care to transition from hospital to home. In: Malone M, Capezuti E, Palmer RM, editors. Acute care for elders—a model for interdisciplinary care. New York, NY: Springer Science and Business Media; 2014:175–202 with permission)

Tracker for use in several EMR systems. The ACE Tracker program collects existing data from a patient's EMR in real time to generate an individual patient level summary of geriatric clinical data and a unit-based summary spreadsheet of key geriatric risk factors in all hospitalized patients age 65 and older. These items include information such LOS to date, total number and potentially inappropriate medications prescribed, risk of falls and skin breakdown based on nursing assessment screens, use of urinary catheters, and formal consultation to disciplines such as physical and occupational therapy and social services. In 2010, Malone and colleagues published a descriptive pilot study using ACE Tracker as a means of disseminating the ACE model of care to hospitals and units that did not have consistent access to a geriatrician. Units using ACE Tracker experienced significant reductions in use of urinary catheters and significant increase in early

physical therapy assessments. While this preliminary study did not demonstrate changes in LOS or 30-day readmissions, this was not the primary objective of this study and the use of this novel health information technology in improving care transitions remains an area for further research [62].

Telehealth and Readmissions

The high cost of caring for many patients with certain chronic diseases such as congestive heart failure (CHF) is due largely to frequent rehospitalization for exacerbations. Some studies have looked at disease-specific populations to examine the effect of home-based interventions on readmission rates; results have been mixed. In an attempt to compare the effectiveness of discharging patients hospitalized with CHF exacerbations home with usual outpatient care, nurse telephone calls, and home telecare delivered via a 2-way video-conference device with an integrated electronic stethoscope, a small 1-year randomized trial of 37 patients demonstrated a significant 86 % decrease in CHF-related readmissions in those receiving telecare, as well as an 84 % decreased rehospitalization in those receiving post-discharge phone calls. However, the difference between the groups was not statistically significant, implying that in this small study population, home telecare did not offer incremental benefit beyond telephonic follow-up which can also be done at a significantly lower cost burden [63].

In another study evaluating the efficacy of a telehealth-facilitated post-hospitalization support program in reducing resource use in patients with CHF, patients from the Department of Veterans Affairs were randomized to telephone, videophone, or usual care for follow-up care after hospitalization for CHF exacerbation. The intervention resulted in a significantly longer time to readmission, but had no effect on readmission rates, mortality, hospital days, or urgent care clinic use. Thus, rigorous evaluation is needed to determine whether any target patient population will benefit from specific telehealth applications, as well as identify which technologies are the most cost-effective [64].

Medicare Rule Changes Regarding Care Transitions and Impact on Hospitals

In a fee-for-service payment model, interventions that decrease rehospitalizations have not been financially rewarded in the past due to the time required by providers to coordinate care transitions. However, the Patient Protection and Affordable Care Act (PPACA), commonly called the Affordable Care Act (ACA), was signed into law in 2010 and instituted new quality-based Medicare rules encouraging hospitals and providers to improve care transitions [65]. The support for adoption of evidence-based care transition models that improve outcomes and lower costs is an area of focus as hospitals anticipate increasing numbers of elders.

New Financial Rules

Beginning January 1, 2013, CMS implemented new Transitional Care Management codes for PCPs to receive compensation for time spent in the outpatient setting seeing patients who require moderate or high complexity decision making following discharge from an acute care setting (hospital, psychiatric hospital, inpatient rehabilitation, LTACH), SNF, community mental health center, or observation status in a hospital to a community living setting (home, domiciliary, rest home, ALF living) [66]. The goal of the new codes

is to improve care coordination through incentives for care transition management in the outpatient care setting rather than risk hospital readmission. Along these same lines, in January 2015 providers will begin receiving monthly stipend from Medicare for coordinating the care of complex patients with two or more chronic conditions [67]. This new federal payment policy is aimed at compensating providers for care coordination, thus recognizing the time and effort involved for integrated patient care tasks that have been largely unreimbursed until now. This provision also is intended to help keep patients with multiple chronic conditions out of the hospital, through encouraging providers to assess patients' social and psychological as well as medical needs when devising a comprehensive plan of care. This new policy will operate by paying providers a $42 monthly stipend per Medicare patient, and will be offered regardless of whether the provider is a physician or a mid-level provider such as a physician assistant or nurse practitioner. Approximately 20 % of the monthly $42 stipend (an expense similar to what is already spent on physician services) will ultimately come from the patient. Care management services can be provided only if the patient agrees to it in writing. In turn, the patient will benefit through the requirement that their PCP must offer 24/7 care for any urgent care needs, in addition to the improved comprehensive care coordination that is inherent to the policy. The very act of providing separate payments to providers for chronic care management represents a significant policy change, and the theory behind it is that the improved care coordination intended to result could pay for itself by keeping these complex patients out of the hospital.

Another provision of the ACA designed to reduce costs related to unplanned readmissions is the Hospital Readmission Reduction Program (HRRP) [68]. Under this program, hospitals with above average 30-day readmission rates for three diagnoses (acute myocardial infarction, heart failure, and community acquired pneumonia) began incurring financial penalties in the form of reduced reimbursements in 2013. The number of conditions and the amount of the financial penalties is anticipated to increase annually in the coming years. The readmission rates for specific conditions are publically reported on the Medicare Hospital Compare website. These new financial rules may be contributing to recent slight downward trends in readmissions as hospitals prepared for the penalty phase of the HRRP. From 2006 to 2011, the all-cause 30-day readmission rates declined from 16.0 % to 15.3 % for Medicare patients. Also in 2011, 12.3 % of Medicare beneficiaries experienced a potentially preventable readmission (PPR), a decrease from 13.4 % in 2006. These 2011 PPR rates ranged from 9.9 % in the highest performing hospitals to 15.3 % in lowest performing hospitals [69].

The ACA also includes the Bundled Payments for Care Improvement Initiative with the goal to reduce fragmentation of care by aligning acute care and post-acute care settings and providers through "bundling" payments that require financial and performance accountability. Participants in these new bundled payment models began testing their programs in 2013 [70]. Additionally, the Community-Based Care Transitions Program provides up to $500 million in funding from 2011 to 2015 to community-based organizations partnering with hospitals to improve care transitions services while reducing costs [2, 71]. Finally, the ACA calls for the development of Accountable Care Organizations (ACOs). The new ACOs will be groups of care providers and hospitals that develop a collaborative partnership with the goal to improve coordination of care to ensure patients are receiving the right care at the right time, especially for the chronically ill and complex patient population [72]. Updates on new funding opportunities and the stage of development of ACOs and all of the new ACA care coordination initiatives can be found on the CMS Innovation Center website [73].

New Process Rules

In addition to financial rules, CMS is also addressing the quality of transitions through new process mandates. The 2013 CMS CoP guidelines holds hospitals accountable for four primary phases of care transition planning: (1) developing a formal care transition plan for every inpatient, or screening to identify patients at risk for adverse transitions outcomes; (2) evaluating the post-discharge needs of high-risk patients, or any patient upon patient or physician request; (3) developing an individualized care transition plan; and (4) initiating the care transition plan prior to discharge. To achieve these mandates hospitals are expected to assess the patients' functional and cognitive abilities, types of post-hospital care that will be needed, and the patient's caregiver/support system in order to determine the patient's capacity for self-care (or need for care providers) and needs for appropriate post-hospitalization care setting. Encouraged is the development of collaborative relationships between hospitals and facilities and providers who care for discharged patients [30].

Future/Next Steps in Care Transitions

A consensus document by the National Transitions of Care Coalition outlines 3 perspectives from which information needs to be obtained in order to fully address optimal care coordination and transitions: (1) patient/family; (2) healthcare professional; and (3) healthcare system [74]. Ongoing culture change driven by this diverse group of stakeholders will likely be required to continue to improve care transitions at the patient, caregiver, provider, system, and community levels [75]. Broader thinking represents moving

beyond targeting diagnosis-specific readmission rates (e.g., CHF), because individual patients are diverse and diagnoses alone do not define risk. Focusing excessively on one targeted outcome as opposed to a holistic methodology may have unintended consequences. Reducing readmissions has been a prioritized outcome due to related risk to patients and costs to the healthcare system. However, a hospital readmission may not represent poor quality and may in fact result in improved outcomes for some patients. For example, hospitals with higher readmission rates for CHF have lower CHF mortality rates, highlighting that these patients are living longer and therefore will require hospitalizations. Furthermore, some studies have indicated that as care coordination improves, patients may experience more hospitalizations as their overall access to health care improves [76]. Also, there is a complex relationship between patients' socioeconomic status and risk for readmission. A hospital's share of low-income patients is a strong predictor of 30-day readmissions, and hospitals with large shares of low-income patients tend to have higher readmission rates. Policy makers must guard against deterring hospitals from caring for poor patient populations while also not accepting lower quality standards for hospitals with a larger proportion of low-income patients.

In a 2013 publication, a modified Delphi consensus technique was used to identify five key measurable outcomes of quality of a care transitions: (1) readmission within 30 days of discharge; (2) seeing a primary care physician within 7 days of discharge for high-risk patients; (3) medication reconciliation completed upon hospital admission and repeated prior to discharge; (4) readmission within 72 h of discharge; and (5) time from hospital discharge to first visit by home care nurses [77]. Additional work is also essential in standardized measurement of patient and family needs and experiences during a care transition. One metric used for the purpose of assessing the quality of care transitions is either the 3- or 15-item Care Transitions Measure (CTM) [78]. This questionnaire can be administered over the phone or by mail to patients recently discharged from the hospital. The CTM has been endorsed by the National Quality Forum. Like many survey tools, the CTM may be difficult for patients with cognitive impairment to understand. While the 15-item version can be administered to caregivers in place of the patient, the 3-item version cannot.

While results of care transition studies to date are promising, the number of RCTs is small, and many have an intervention sample size of less than 100 patients or other study limitations [79]. The June 2013 Medicare Payment Advisory Committee Report to Congress recommends a broader research plan that includes the association of readmissions and mortality, health literacy, and patient frailty as well as expansion of research and policy to additional groups such as observation patients and post-acute providers [69]. Additional research is also needed regarding care transitions from EDs and SNFs and the use of information technology. Finally, the healthcare workforce, including informal care providers, will require additional training in care transitions. Currently, this training is not required in healthcare provider licensure and certification processes [2].

Conclusions

To date, published transitional care interventions incorporate common themes, including information transfer strategies, patient/caregiver coaching for self-management, aggressive medication reconciliation, and portable health records. Next-generation interventions may incorporate additional use of health information technology and telemedicine as well as additional sites of care. Ultimately, the "perfect" hospital transitional care program will provide a comprehensive set of key elements that providers and systems are charged with developing and incorporating into their daily practice and will result in improved adherence with discharge instructions, timely outpatient follow-up, and improved patient functioning and satisfaction with reduced adverse medical events, readmissions, costs, and caregiver burden [80]. Given the declining number of geriatricians, exemplary models of care will also provide the means of educating trainees and providers across all disciplines to work as interprofessional teams across the care continuum.

References

1. Coleman EA, Boult C. Improving the quality of transitional care for persons with complex care needs. Position statement of the American Geriatrics Society Health Care Systems Committee. J Am Geriatr Soc. 2003;51:556–7.
2. Naylor MD, Aiken LH, Kurtzman ET, Olds DM, Hirschman KB. The importance of transitional care in achieving health reform. Health Aff. 2011;30(4):746–54.
3. Sato M, Shaffer T, Arbaje AI, Zuckerman IH. Residential and health care transition patterns among older medicare beneficiaries over time. Gerontologist. 2011;51(2):170–8.
4. Coleman EA, Min S, Chomiak A, Kramer AM. Posthospital care transitions: patterns, complications, and risk identification. Health Serv Res. 2004;39(5):1449–65.
5. Jencks SF, Williams MV, Coleman EA. Rehospitalizations among patients in the medicare fee-for-service program. N Engl J Med. 2009;360:1418–28.
6. Department of Health and Human Services, Center for Medicare & Medicaid Services. Hospital inpatient prospective payment systems for acute care hospitals. [Internet] https://s3.amazonaws.com/public-inspection.federalregister.gov/2014-18545.pdf. Accessed 08/28/14.
7. Van Walraven C, Jennings A, Forster AJ. A meta-analysis of hospital 30-day avoidable readmission rates. J Eval Clin Pract. 2011; 18:1211–8.
8. Kansagara D, Englander H, Salanitro A, Kagen D, Theobald C, Freeman M, et al. Risk prediction models for hospital readmission: a systematic review. JAMA. 2011;306(15):1688–98.
9. Dharmarajan K, Hsieh AF, Lin Z, Bueno H, Ross JS, Horwitz LI, Barreto-Filho JA, Kim N, Bernheim SM, Suter LG, Drye EE, Krumholz HM. Diagnoses and timeing of 30-day readmissions after hospitalization for heart failure, acute myocardial infarction, or pneumonia. JAMA. 2013;309(4):355–63.
10. Krumholz H. Posthospitalization syndrome-an acquired, transient condition of generalized risk. N Engl J Med. 2013;382(2):100–2.
11. Pugh JA, Want CP, Espinoza SE, Noel PH, Bolllinger M, Amuan M, Finley E, Pugh MJ. Influence of frailty-related diagnoses, high-risk prescribing in elderly adults, and primary care use on readmission in fewer than 30 days for veterans aged 65 and older. J Am Geriatr Soc. 2014;62:291–8.
12. Snow V, Beck D, Budnitz T, Miller DC, Potter J, Wears RL, et al. Transitions of care consensus policy statement american college of physicians-society of general internal medicine-society of hospital medicine-american geriatrics society-american college of emergency physicians-society of academic emergency medicine. J Gen Intern Med. 2009;24(8):971–6.
13. Forster AJ, Murff HJ, Peterson JF, Gandhi TK, Bates DW. The incidence and severity of adverse events affecting patients after discharge from the hospital. Ann Intern Med. 2003;138:161–7.
14. Kim CS, Flanders SA. Transitions of care. Ann Intern Med. 2013;158(5_Part_1):ITC3–1.
15. Kripalani S, LeFevre F, Phillips CO, Williams MV, Basaviah P, Baker DW. Deficits in communication and information transfer between hospital-based and primary care physicians: implications for patient safety and continuity of care. JAMA. 2007;297(8): 831–41.
16. Hibbard JH, Cunningham PJ. How engaged are consumers in their health and health care, and why does it matter? Res Brief. 2008; 8:1–9.
17. Arbaje AI, Wolff J, Yu Q, Powe NR, Anderson GF, Boult CE. Post-discharge environmental and socioeconomic factors and the likelihood of early hospital readmission among community-dwelling medicare beneficiaries. Gerontologist. 2008;48(4):495–504.
18. National Transitions of Care Coalition. Taking Care of My Health Care [Internet]. http://www.ntocc.org/Portals/0/PDF/Resources/Taking_Care_Of_My_Health_Care.pdf. Accessed August 26, 2014.
19. Discharge Preparation Checklist [Internet]. http://www.caretransitions.org/documents/checklist.pdf. Accessed August 26, 2014.
20. Bodenheimer T. Coordinating care—a perilous journey through the health care system. N Engl J Med. 2008;358(10):1064–71.
21. Lindquist LA, Jain N, Tam K, Martin GJ, Baker DW. Inadequate health literacy among paid caregivers of seniors. J Gen Intern Med. 2011;26(5):474–9.
22. Kangovi S, Barg FK, Carter T, et al. Challenges faced by patients with low socioeconomic status during the post-hospital transition. J Gen Intern Med. 2014;29(2):283–9.
23. National Transitions of Care Coalition. Cultural Competence: Essential Ingredient for Successful Transitions of Care [Internet]. http://www.ntocc.org/Portals/0/PDF/Resources/CulturalCompetence.pdf. Accessed August 26, 2014.
24. Teach Back / Show Me Method [Internet]. http://etgec.utmb.edu/ace.asp. Accessed August 30, 2014.
25. Moore C, Wisnivesky J, Williams S, McGinn T. Medical errors related to discontinuity of care from an inpatient to an outpatient setting. J Gen Intern Med. 2003;18:646–51.
26. The Joint Commission. Hospital: 2013 National Patient Safety Goals [Internet]. http://www.jointcommission.org/hap_2013_npsg. Accessed August 26, 2014.
27. Arbaje AI. Transitional care. In: Durso SC, Sullivan GM, editors. Geriatrics review syllabus: a core curriculum in geriatric medicine. 8th ed. New York, NY: American Geriatrics Society; 2013.
28. Schoenborn N, Arbaje AI, Eubank KJ, Maynor KA, Carrese JA. Clinician roles and responsibilities during care transitions of older adults. J Am Geriatr Soc. 2013;61(2):231–6.

29. Shier G, Rooney M, Golden R. Rush enhanced discharge planning program: a model for social work based transitional care. In: Spitzer W, editor. The evolving practice of social work within integrated care, National Society for Social Work Leadership in Health Care. Petersburg, VA: The Dietz Press; 2011. p. 57–68.

30. Department of Health and Human Services, Centers for Medicare & Medicaid Services. Center for Clinical Standards and Quality/ Survey & Certification Group. Ref: S&C:13-32-HOSPITAL [Internet]. http://www.cms.gov/Medicare/Provider-Enrollment-and-Certification/SurveyCertificationGenInfo/Downloads/Survey-and-Cert-Letter-13-32.pdf. Accessed August 26, 2014.

31. Transitional Care Model [Internet]. http://www.transitionalcare. info. Accessed August 26, 2014.

32. Naylor MD, Brooten D, Campbell R, Jacobsen BS, Mezey MD, Pauly MV, et al. Comprehensive discharge planning and home follow-up of hospitalized elders: a randomized clinical trial. JAMA. 1999;281(7):613–20.

33. Naylor MD, Brooten DA, Campbell RL, Maislin G, McCauley KM, Schwartz JS. Transitional care of older adults hospitalized with heart failure: a randomized, controlled trial. J Am Geriatr Soc. 2004;52:675–84.

34. Coleman EA, Smith JD, Frank JC, Min SJ, Parry C, Kramer AM. Preparing patients and caregivers to participate in care delivered across settings: the care transitions intervention. J Am Geriatr Soc. 2004;52:1817–25.

35. The Care Transitions Program® [Internet]. http://www.caretransitions.org. Accessed August 26, 2014.

36. Coleman EA, Parry C, Chalmers S, Min SJ. The care transitions intervention: results of a randomized controlled trial. Arch Intern Med. 2006;166:1822–8.

37. Agency for Healthcare Research and Quality. Project RED (Re-Engineered Discharge Training Program [Internet]. http://www.ahrq.gov/qual/projectred. Accessed August 26, 2014.

38. Project RED: Re-Engineered Discharge [Internet]. http://www.bu.edu/fammed/projectred/toolkit.html. Accessed August 26, 2014.

39. Jack BW, Chetty VK, Anthony D, Greenwald JL, Sanchez GM, Johnson AE, et al. A reengineered hospital discharge program to decrease rehospitalizations: a randomized trial. Ann Intern Med. 2009;150:178–87.

40. Flood KL, MacLennan PA, McGrew D, Green D, Dodd C, Brown CJ. An acute care for elders unit reduces costs and 30-day readmissions. JAMA Intern Med. 2013;173(11):981–7.

41. Hung WW, Ross JS, Farber J, Siu AL. Evaluation of a mobile acute care for the elderly (MACE) service. JAMA Intern Med. 2013;173(11):990–6.

42. Arbaje AI, Maron DD, Yu Q, Wendel VI, Tanner E, Boult C, et al. The geriatric floating interdisciplinary transition team. J Am Geriatr Soc. 2010;58(2):364–70.

43. Fox MT, Persaud M, Maimets I, O'Brien K, Brooks D, Trequnno D, et al. Effectiveness of acute geriatric unit care using acute care for elders components: a systematic review and meta-analysis. J Am Geriatr Soc. 2012;60:2237–45.

44. Englander H, Michaels L, Chan B, Kansagara D. The care transition innovation (C-Train) for socioeconomically disadvantaged adults: results of a cluster randomized controlled trial. J Gen Intern Med 2014 Nov 10;29(11):1460-7. http://link.springer.com/article/10.1007%2Fs11606-014-2903-0#page-2.

45. Boult C, Reider L, Leff B, Frick K, Boyd CM, Wolff JL, Frey K, Karm L, Wegener ST, Mroz T, Scharfstein DO. The effect of guided care teams on the use of health services: results from a cluster-randomized controlled trial. Arch Intern Med. 2011;171(5):460–6.

46. Hospital at Home [Internet]. http://www.hospitalathome.org. Accessed August 28, 2013.

47. Cryer L, Shannon SB, Van Amsterdam M, Leff B. Costs for hospital at home patients were 19 percent lower, with equal or better outcomes compared to similar inpatients. Health Aff. 2012;31(6): 1237–43.

48. Leff B, Burton L, Mader S, Naughton B, Burl J, Clark R, et al. Satisfaction with hospital at home care. J Am Geriatr Soc. 2006; 54:1355–63.

49. National PACE Association [Internet]. http://www.npaonline.org/. Accessed August 26, 2014.

50. Grabowski DC. The cost-effectiveness of noninstitutional long-term care services: review and synthesis of the most recent evidence. Med Care Res Rev. 2006;63(1):3–28.

51. Counsell SR, Callahan CM, Clark DO, Tu W, Buttar AB, Stump TE, et al. Geriatric care management for low-income seniors: a randomized controlled trial. JAMA. 2007;298(22):2623–33.

52. National Consensus Project for Quality Palliative Care. Clinical Practice Guidelines for Quality Palliative Care, Second Edition, 2009.

53. Morrison RS. Health care system factors affecting end-of-life care. J Palliat Med. 2005;8 Suppl 1:S79–87.

54. Brumley R, Enguidanos S, Jamison P, Seitz R, Morgenstern N, Saito S, et al. Increased satisfaction with care and lower costs: results of a randomized trial of in-home palliative care. J Am Geriatr Soc. 2007;55:993–1000.

55. McCusker J, Bellavance F, Cardin S, Trépanier S, Verdon J, Ardman O. Detection of older people at increased risk of adverse health outcomes after an emergency visit: the ISAR screening tool. J Am Geriatr Soc. 1999;47(10):1229–37.

56. Lee JS, Schwindt G, Langevin M, Moghabghab R, Alibhai SMH, Kiss A, et al. Validation of the triage risk stratification tool to identify older persons at risk for hospital admission and returning to the emergency department. J Am Geriatr Soc. 2008;56:2112–7.

57. Salvi F, Morichi V, Grilli A, Lancioni L, Spazzafumo L, Polonara S, et al. Screening for frailty in elderly emergency department patients by using the identification of seniors at risk (ISAR). J Nutr Health Aging. 2012;16(4):313–8.

58. Mion LC, Palmer RM, Anetzberger GJ, Meldon SW. Establishing a case-finding and referral system for at-risk older individuals in the emergency department setting: the SIGNET model. J Am Geriatr Soc. 2001;49:1379–86.

59. Caplan GA, Williams AJ, Daly B, Abraham K. A randomized, controlled trial of comprehensive geriatric assessment and multidisciplinary intervention after discharge of elderly from the emergency department—the DEED II study. J Am Geriatr Soc. 2004;52: 1417–23.

60. Halasyamani L, Kripalani S, Coleman E, Schnipper J, van Walraven C, Nagamine J, et al. Transition of care for hospitalized elderly patients-development of a discharge checklist for hospitalists. J Hosp Med. 2006;1:354–60.

61. Care Transitions Performance Measurement Set [Internet]. http://www.abimfoundation.org/News/ABIM-Foundation-News/2009/~/media/Files/PCPI%20Care%20Transition%20measures-public-comment-021209.ashx. Accessed August 26, 2014.

62. Malone ML, Vollbrecht M, et al. Acute care for elders (ACE) tracker and e-geriatrician: methods to disseminate ACE concepts to hospitals with no geriatricians on staff. J Am Geriatr Soc. 2010;58:161–7.

63. Jerant AF, Azari R, Nesbitt TS. Reducing the cost of frequent hospital admissions for congestive heart failure: a randomized trial of a home telecare Intervention. Med Care. 2001;39(11):1234–45.

64. Wakefield BJ, Ward MM, Holman JE, Ray A, Scherubel M, Burns TL, et al. Evaluation of home telehealth following hospitalization with heart failure: a randomized, controlled trial. Telemed J E Health. 2008;14(8):753–61.

65. U.S. Department of Health and Human Services. About the Law [Internet]. http://www.hhs.gov/healthcare/rights/index.html. Accessed August 26, 2014.

66. Department of Health and Human Services, Center for Medicare & Medicaid Services. Transitional Care Management Services [Internet]. http://www.cms.gov/Outreach-and-Education/Medicare-Learning-Network-MLN/MLNProducts/Downloads/Transitional-Care-Management-Services-Fact-Sheet-ICN908628.pdf. Accessed August 26, 2014.

67. The New York Times. Medicare to Start Paying Doctors Who Coordinate Needs of Chronically Ill Patients [Internet]. http://www.nytimes.com/2014/08/17/us/medicare-to-start-paying-doctors-who-coordinate-needs-of-chronically-ill-patients.html. Accessed: 8/28/14.

68. Centers for Medicare & Medicaid Services. Readmissions Reduction Program [Internet]. http://www.cms.gov/Medicare/Medicare-Fee-for-Service-Payment/AcuteInpatientPPS/Readmissions-Reduction-Program.html. August 26, 2014.

69. MedPAC. Payment Policy for Inpatient Readmissions. Report to the Congress: Medicare and the Health Care Delivery System. Washington, DC: Medicare Payment Advisory Commission; June 2013.

70. Centers for Medicare & Medicaid Services. Bundled Payments for Care Improvement (BPCI) Initiative: General Information [Internet]. http://innovation.cms.gov/initiatives/bundled-payments/. Accessed on August 26, 2014.

71. Centers for Medicare & Medicaid Services. Community-based Care Transitions Program [Internet]. http://partnershipforpatients.cms.gov/about-the-partnership/community-based-care-transitions-program/community-basedcaretransitionsprogram.html. Accessed August 26, 2014.

72. Centers for Medicare & Medicaid Services. Accountable Care Organizations (ACO) [Internet]. http://www.cms.gov/Medicare/Medicare-Fee-for-Service-Payment/ACO/ Accessed August 26, 2014.

73. Centers for Medicare & Medicaid Services. The CMS Innovation Center [Internet]. www.innovation.cms.gov. Accessed August 26, 2014.

74. [[National Transitions of Care Coalition [Internet]. www.ntocc.org. Accessed August 26, 2014.

75. Rooney M, Arbaje AI. Changing the culture of practice to support care transitions—Why now? Generations. J Am Soc Aging, Special issue: Care Transitions in an Aging America. Winter 2012–2013; 36(4):63–70.

76. Joynt KE, Jha AK. Thirty-day readmissions—truth and consequences. N Engl J Med. 2012;366(15):1366–9.

77. Jeffs L, Law MP, Staus S, Cardoso R, Lyons RF, Bell C. Defining quality outcomes for complex-care patients transitioning across the continuum using a structured panel process. BMJ Qual Saf. 2013;22(12):1014–24.

78. Coleman EA, Smith JD, Frank JC, Eilertsen TB, Thiare JN, Kramer AM. Development and testing of a measure designed to assess the quality of care transitions. Int J Integr Care. 2002;2:e02.

79. Hansen LO, Young RS, Hinami K, Leung A, Williams MV. Interventions to reduce 30-day rehospitalizations: a systematic review. Ann Intern Med. 2011;155:520–8.

80. Kripalani S, Jackson AT, Schnipper JL, Coleman EA. Promoting effective transitions of care at hospital discharge: a review of key issues for hospitalists. J Hosp Med. 2007;2: 314–23.

Project BOOST®: A Comprehensive Program to Improve Discharge Coordination for Geriatric Patients

Jing Li, Mark V. Williams, and Robert S. Young

Hospital discharge is often a stressful and hazardous venture for patients and their caregivers, especially for older adults with complex medical needs. The unfortunately routine discontinuity and fragmentation of care associated with hospitalization generate tangible risks of harm to patients and flummox their caregivers. Project BOOST® (Better Outcomes by Optimizing Safe Transitions) comprehensively aims to enhance transitions of care, improve patient satisfaction, and augment the flow of information between hospitals and primary care and subacute providers. BOOST's ultimate goal is to coordinate patient-centered care during a hospital discharge transition by ensuring patients and/or caregiver comprehension of instructions, improving hospital to post-acute provider communication, and reducing unnecessary emergency department (ED) visits and rehospitalizations. BOOST® focuses on facilitating interdisciplinary care of patients and utilizes a team approach to assess patients' risk for rehospitalization linked to planning and executing risk-specific discharge efforts.

The transition process from hospital to home or other post-acute settings can break down at a number of points, including preparation of the patient and caregiver for self-care, medication reconciliation, communication between providers, or ensuring outpatient follow-up. Traditional health care delivery models typically do not have mecha-

nisms in place for coordinating care across settings; care delivery silos generally keep the focus within individual venues [1]. This gap in coordination of care for older adults is not surprising given the high level of complexity of the US health care system, and the remarkable number of physicians involved in providing care to individual patients. For instance, Medicare patients see an average of two primary care physicians and five specialists during a 2-year period; patients with chronic conditions may see up to 16 physicians in 1 year [2]. The potential breakdowns in attempts to coordinate the continuum of care among so many different care providers (i.e., hospital, home health, skilled nursing facility, and rehabilitation facility) combined with patient-specific factors (e.g., socioeconomic status, caregiver support, health literacy, psychosocial issues) increase the risk of hospitalizations and other adverse outcomes (Fig. 9.1).

Research in the past 20 years clearly documents a number of significant patient safety and quality deficiencies in our current system of care transition. Identified areas behind most failed care transitions include the following:

- *Ineffective patient/family education and lack of patient/ family empowerment*

  Patient activation refers to a patient's knowledge, skills, ability, and willingness to manage his or her own health and care. Higher patient activation is correlated with healthy behavior and better care outcomes [3]. Upon hospital discharge, patients and family caregivers are often expected to assume new self-care responsibilities, to implement new dietary restrictions, to use new medications, and to monitor and respond to new and evolving symptoms. However, patients transitioned from one setting to another often receive little or inadequate information on their medical condition and proposed self-care plan [4]. Sometimes patients and caregivers are even excluded from planning related to the transition process. As a result, the medical conditions of many patients worsen and they may end up being readmitted to the hospital. Even with adequate education, learning in a "passive" way often fails patients to use the new knowledge in

J. Li, M.D., M.S.
Center for Health Services Research, University of Kentucky, 740 South Limestone Street, Kentucky Clinic J523, Lexington, KY 40536-0284, USA
e-mail: jingli.tj@uky.edu

M.V. Williams, M.D. (✉)
Center for Health Services Research, University of Kentucky, 740 South Limestone Street, Kentucky Clinic J527, Lexington, KY 40536-0284, USA
e-mail: mark.will@uky.edu

R.S. Young, M.D., M.S.
Department of Internal Medicine, University of Kentucky, 740 South Limestone Street, Kentucky Clinic J521, Lexington, KY 40536-0284, USA
e-mail: rob.syoung@uky.edu

M.L. Malone et al. (eds.), *Geriatrics Models of Care: Bringing 'Best Practice' to an Aging America*, DOI 10.1007/978-3-319-16068-9_9, © Springer International Publishing Switzerland 2015

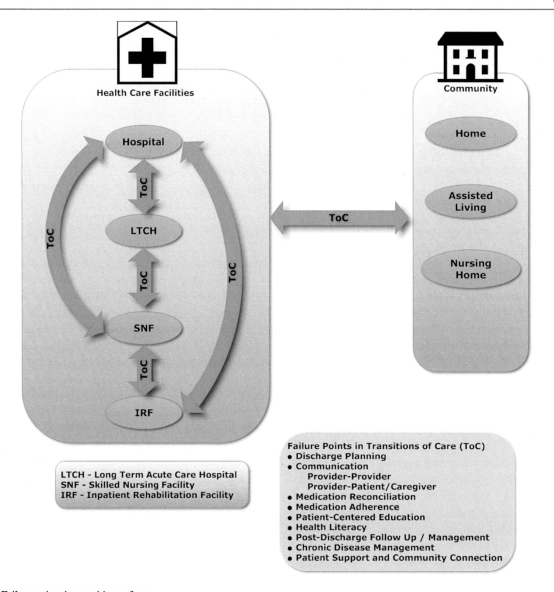

Fig. 9.1 Failure points in transitions of care

their self-care. Health care providers must engage or activate patients and their caregivers to adhere to appropriate care and behaviors.

- *Lack of community connection and health-related supports*

  The lack of coordinated, adequate, and accessible supports for older adults, especially socioeconomically disadvantaged patients, moving between health and social support settings contributes to adverse post-discharge events [5]. Multiple factors serve as barriers to smooth transitions such as insufficient access to outpatient care, unmet transportation needs, lack of community services, limited health literacy, lack of self-management skills, and unmet functional needs; these have all been associated with adverse care transition outcomes including readmission and mortality [5, 6].

- *Lack of provider coordination/communication and information sharing*

  Care providers often do not effectively or completely communicate important information among themselves, to the patient, or to those taking care of the patient at home in a timely fashion. Inconsistencies and miscommunications lead to general inefficiency and ineffectiveness as well as more specific problems such as medical errors, equipment-related problems, and even transitions to inappropriate locations [7]. Often hospital discharge summaries are not available in a timely fashion, and when they are available, they often lack important information such as diagnostic test results, treatment and medication changes during hospital stay, accurate discharge medications, test results pending at discharge, patient or family counseling, and follow-up plans [8].

Fig. 9.2 Comprehensive transition plan

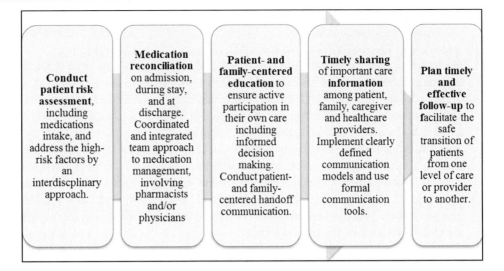

- *Lack of follow-up with primary care providers (PCPs) and other providers*
  Studies demonstrate that increased PCP follow-up is significantly and independently associated with a decreased risk of hospital readmission [9, 10]. Patients often do not consistently receive appropriate follow-up care or ongoing outpatient management of their chronic conditions after leaving the hospital. When patients do not receive timely follow-up care and do not know whom to contact, utilization of inappropriate and costly care in EDs or hospitals is likely to increase. Sadly in the past, for Medicare beneficiaries readmitted to the hospital within 30 days of a discharge, half had no contact with a physician between their first hospitalization and their readmission [11].

  To achieve successful transitions, preparing for the move from hospital to subsequent care should engage an interdisciplinary team including the above stakeholders who interact with the patient and/or caregivers. Project BOOST® takes a multifaceted approach and follows a "comprehensive transition plan" (Fig. 9.2) aiming to help patients smoothly transition from the hospital to the next care setting and achieve successful recovery.

Interventions and Tools in Project BOOST®

The BOOST® interventions and tools were developed from evidence found in peer-reviewed literature established through experimental methods in well-controlled academic settings. Further tool development was informed by recommendations of an advisory board consisting of expert representatives and advocates involved in the hospital discharge process: patients, caregivers, physicians, nurses, case managers, social workers, insurers, and regulatory and research agencies. The key components of BOOST® include the following:

- *Comprehensive suite of interventions and tools*—address multiple aspects of the hospital discharge transition and follow-up with the goal of improving or sustaining health by optimizing the safety of care transitions.
- *8P Risk Assessment*: Numerous risk factors have been identified in the literature as being associated with increased risk of rehospitalization, emergency department visits, or other adverse events post-hospital discharge. The Project BOOST® team (www.hospitalmedicine.org/BOOST) reviewed evidence-based patient-specific risk factors and created a user-friendly tool called the 8P scale.
  - *Problem medications and polypharmacy*
  - *Psychological issues (e.g., depression)*
  - *Principal diagnoses (e.g., heart failure, COPD, cancer, diabetes)*
  - *Poor health literacy*
  - *Patient support*
  - *Physical function (e.g., frailty)*
  - *Prior hospitalizations*
  - *Palliative care*

This risk assessment tool is completed at admission and highlights the need to identify patients at risk and utilize the duration of the hospitalization to mitigate these risks as much as possible.

- *Generalized Assessment of Preparedness (GAP)*: General Assessment of Preparedness (GAP) is a list of potential psychosocial and logistical barriers to patients being able to secure and engage in the intended care plan during and after hospitalization. The checklist reminds users of issues to consider and address with patients and their caregivers. Different GAP elements may be addressed during different phases of the hospitalization. For example, transportation to subsequent follow-up appointments may be a day-of-discharge checklist item, whereas functional status and cognitive status may have to be addressed daily as these may change over time.

- *Teach Back*: Teach back [12] is an essential technique by which a patient's and/or their caregiver's understanding of a concept and a health care provider's ability to educate are assessed. Providers must clearly inform patients and their caregivers of the patient's current health status and care plan. Health providers can fulfill this responsibility by providing education and then confirming comprehension via teach back. This is accomplished by requesting the patient to "teach back" the information to assess their level of comprehension. It is recommended that teach back be performed throughout the hospitalization and at discharge. For example, instructions on new or changed medication should be reinforced throughout the patient's stay at times of dosing.

- *Patient-Centered Discharge Instruction*: It is important that patients leave the hospital with printed reminders of key aspects of their aftercare plan to use as a reference. They do not require many of the elements included in a standard discharge summary and typical discharge instructions, although there may be some overlap. Project BOOST® offers participating hospitals two different tools to assist in creating these instructions containing just the essential educational components: the Discharge Patient Education Tool (DPET), two pages, and the Patient Preparation to Address Situations Successfully (PASS), one page, tool. Key elements of the DPET and PASS include clear statements of why the patient was in the hospital using "living room" language; warning signs of potential complications and whom to contact; date, time, and place of follow-up appointments; and list of medications and directions written in lay terminology. As a whole, these instructions should be easy to read and concise, and highlight the most vital information. Patients and their caregivers only want to know what they actually need to know to care for themselves and continue on a trajectory to improved health or prevent deterioration. They typically are not interested in the physiology of disease that many providers attempt to describe.

- *Timely Follow-Up Appointment*: A timely follow-up visit represents a critical opportunity to address the conditions that precipitated the hospitalization, to prepare the patient and family caregiver for self-care activities, and to prevent deterioration leading to unnecessary rehospitalizations. Evidence among patients with heart failure and COPD indicates that a follow-up visit within 7 days of hospital discharge is ideal, but this should be adapted to the patient's specific situation. The historical "2 to 4 weeks" follow-up appointment is likely not timely enough to identify patient's deteriorating clinical condition post-hospitalization.

- *Standardized Communication with PCPs and Post-Acute Providers*: Upon hospital discharge, patients often are expected to return to their primary care physician or another clinician who may not have direct knowledge about the hospital stay. Hospitals should use information technology to extract information into discharge summaries to ensure accuracy (e.g., medication names and doses) and to facilitate rapid completion of summaries (e.g., within 24 h of discharge, or ideally on the day of discharge). On the day of discharge, a summary document or the actual discharge summary should be sent to the primary care physician or the post-acute facility by e-mail, fax, or with the patient. If a complete discharge summary cannot be sent on the day of discharge, then an interim discharge should be sent or a phone call should be made. At minimum, it should include the diagnoses, discharge medications, results of procedures, follow-up needs, and pending test results.

- *48–72-h Follow-Up Call for High-Risk Patients*: Connecting with patients after they have left the hospital has, in multiple studies, shown the unsurprising fact that many aspects of their care change after patients leave the support of the hospital setting. Telephone follow-up calls made within 72 h of discharge can effectively begin to identify many of the new issues and barriers the patient has faced during the critical initial period after discharge, and also determine who needs to be evaluated urgently to prevent rehospitalization.

NOTE: All the key BOOST® interventions and tools could be integrated into an electric medical record, but this requires collaboration by vendors. Nonetheless, some are actively undertaking this and some health systems are customizing their EMRs to do this.

- *BOOST® Implementation Guide* (www.hospitalmedicine.org/BOOST)—This includes a collection of project management tools to help interdisciplinary teams plan, implement, and evaluate their discharge process. Upon identifying issues, the team can then implement appropriate corrective interventions using essential steps in quality improvement—flow mapping current processes and identifying opportunities for improvement, performance monitoring and evaluation, and maintaining gains.

- *BOOST® Collaborative Community*—Sites who formally participate in Project BOOST® are able to communicate with and learn from each other via the BOOST® listserv, document sharing, newsletters, and webinars.

- *Mentored Implementation*—One unique component of participation in Project BOOST® is individual physician mentoring. The mentoring provides a year of longitudinal technical support to assist BOOST® implementation at a hospital site. The external physician mentors are experts in care transitions and possess quality improvement (QI) skills and experience in process improvement science and change management. Mentors provide continuous support and guidance from the planning through implementation while transferring management skills to the local QI teams and teaching techniques for facilitating effective practice change. The mentor also helps to engage hospital leadership, garner local physician buy-in, motivate the QI team, and address institutional barriers. While ensuring the model fidelity, the mentor guides hospitals to identify opportunities for intervention adaptation and customization. The mentoring is delivered through monthly conference calls, site visit, and ad hoc e-mail or phone communications.

- *Post-Acute Care Transitions Toolbox*—A collaboration of the Society of Hospital Medicine (SHM) with AMDA—The Society of Post-Acute and Long-Term Care Medicine and the American College of Emergency Physicians generated a Web-based Post-Acute Care Transitions Toolkit focused on the transition from acute care hospitals to skilled nursing facilities (SNF). This addition to Project BOOST© supports the efforts of hospitals and SNFs to improve transitions of care between these facilities. The Web-based toolkit guides cross-setting, interprofessional teams through a process improvement framework to work through hospital-SNF-specific transition issues to improve care continuity for the large frail and elderly patient population who use SNF services.

- The website introduces health care providers to the various post-acute care settings and the rehabilitation and medical services they provide. In addition, the website guides interested providers through building their cross-setting teams, acquiring institutional support, and developing data infrastructure to measure and control the outcomes of their process improvement efforts, and provides tools for improving communications between settings, filling in care gaps for transitioning patients, and maintaining governmental regulatory compliance. The website also provides a list of state and national programs addressing the hospital-SNF transition and other relevant care transition resources.

- Already the framework and the material presented in the Post-Acute Care Transitions Toolkits have been successfully used by Project BOOST© mentors to assist their BOOST teams to partner with their SNF providers to improve the care transition to and from SNFs. The contents of the toolkit will be free and available to the public. The website can be accessed at http://www.hospitalmedicine. org/Web/Quality___Innovation/Implementation_Toolkit/ pact/Overview_PACT.aspx.

The key processes and steps in Project BOOST® include the following (Fig. 9.3):

- *Comprehensive planning and risk assessment throughout hospitalization*
Discharge planning begins upon admission with completion of a risk assessment within the first 24–48 h. Patients are assessed by the BOOST® 8P scale for risk factors that may limit their ability to perform necessary aspects of self-care.

- *Enhanced medication reconciliation and management*
Obtaining a "best possible medication history" (http:// www.hospitalmedicine.org/Web/Quality___Innovation/ Implementation_Toolkit/MARQUIS/Med_Rec_ Resources_Medication_Reconciliation.aspx) on admission will increase the accuracy of medication reconciliation. Patients should understand any changes in their medications, how to take each medicine correctly, and important side effects.

- *Interdisciplinary communication and care coordination*
The care team—including the physician, nurse, pharmacist, case manager, social worker, and others as appropriate—conducts daily interdisciplinary rounds to communicate and coordinate each patient's care plan and assure a successful transition. Discharge planning and addressing patient safety issues are key aspects of these rounds.

- *Standardized transition plans, procedures, and forms*
A discharge summary template is used by all discharging physicians and includes pertinent diagnoses, active issues, reconciled medication list with changes highlighted, results from important tests and consultations, pending test results, planned follow-up and required services, warning signs of a worsening condition, and what to do if a problem arises. Project BOOST® encourages hospitals to mandate a process to send completed discharge summaries directly to the patient's primary care physician or next setting of care within 24–48 h of discharge—ideally at the time of discharge.

- *Enhanced patient/family education*
Using the interactive method of "teach back," actively teach patients, families, and/or other caregivers to learn and practice self-care and to follow the care plan, including how to self-manage medications. Create easy-to-understand discharge plans to provide to patients and their caregivers. Encourage patients and their caregivers to ask questions, and then utilize "teach back" to confirm comprehension of responses.

- *Timely follow-up, support, and coordination after the patient leaves a care setting*
Arrange for timely follow-up visits before discharge, and coordinate this with the patient and/or caregiver to ensure ability to make it to the appointment. Telephone or in-person follow-up, support, and coordination by a case

BOOST State of Care Transitions

On Admission:
- Readmission risk factor screen (8Ps)
- Discharge needs analysis
- General assessment of discharge preparedness
- Medication reconciliation
- Readmit root cause analysis (if needed)

During Hospitalization:
- Interdisciplinary team to develop safe transition plan
- Initiate readmission risk reduction interventions
- Develop a patient-centered transitional care plan
- Educate patient & caregiver using Teach Back
- Engage patient/caregiver and aftercare providers

At Discharge:
- Schedule post-discharge appointment
- Patient friendly discharge instructions
- Handoffs (hospital to aftercare)
- Medication reconciliation
- Reinforce education

Post-Discharge:
- Post-discharge follow-up phone call in 72 hours
- Post-discharge follow-up appointment in 7 days
- Transmit discharge summary to PCP or sub-acute setting in 48 hours

project BOOST
Better Outcomes by Optimizing Safe Transitions

Fig. 9.3 Project BOOST® key processes and steps, adapted from Christopher Kim, M.D., M.B.A.

manager, social worker, nurse, or another health care provider 24–72 h after discharge. For patients with complex medication regimens, pharmacists have been found to be effective at this.

Implementation of Project BOOST®

Resources Used and Skills Needed

Staffing
Project BOOST can be implemented with existing discharge planning or nursing staff who can incorporate discharge planning tools into their daily activities.

Costs
The first edition of BOOST® Implementation Guide is available free of charge and the second edition of BOOST® Implementation Guide is available with a small fee ($65)

through the Project BOOST® website. For $4,000, participating hospitals gain access for 2 years to the "BOOST eQUIPS" support package that includes an online learning community and discussion forum, document-sharing capabilities, newsletters, webinars, and a data center. For $24,000, participating hospitals receive 1–2-day kick-off training and a year of implementation support from a physician mentor with expertise in QI and care transitions.

Planning and Development Process

Obtain Senior Administrator Support
To win leadership support, share data on the program's potential to reduce rehospitalizations, improve physician and patient satisfaction, and help the hospital system transform from fee-for-service care to patient-centered value care. A direct line of communication to a senior administrative "champion" is essential.

Estimate Financial Costs and Benefits

Estimates of the program's financial impact (based on factors such as payor mix, occupancy rate, current federal and state delivery and payment reform and demonstrations) and the resources required should be developed. An "ROI calculator" is available on the Project BOOST website to help with this. Unfortunately, traditional fee-for-service payment mechanisms do not create a financial incentive to support activities that reduce ED visits and rehospitalizations. However, as the US health system evolves to payment for value, Project BOOST® is recognized as a promising model in fostering cost-effective continuity of care (http://www. cms.gov/Medicare/Demonstration-Projects/ DemoProjectsEvalRpts/downloads/CCTP_Solicitation.pdf).

Establish an Organizational Framework for QI

Understanding the principles, strategies, and tools for quality improvement is critical for the success of any program to improve the hospital discharge process. In addition to QI recommendations in Project BOOST, hospitals should conduct an organizational readiness assessment and identify system and culture barriers before proposing potential solutions and conducting any needed staff training.

Create an Interdisciplinary Project Team

Achieving successful care transition requires that a number of parties be actively involved. The project team should include representatives from (1) hospital staff including physicians, nurses, case managers, social workers and pharmacists; (2) community physicians (including primary care, especially medical homes, and specialists) and other advance practice providers such as PAs or NPs; (3) post-acute care facilities/services (including skilled nursing facilities, home health, assisted living residences, hospice, and rehabilitation); and (4) patients and their caregivers or families.

Analyze the Existing Processes

The project team should analyze and better understand the existing admission and discharge processes by process flow mapping and identifying key areas for improvement. Important areas for consideration include tools used to assess patient/family preparedness for discharge; the medication reconciliation process, including how polypharmacy issues are addressed; patient handoff, including processes and tools for communicating with physicians and with subsequent care sites; and evaluation methods for assessing the quality of the current admission and discharge processes.

Set Appropriate Project Goals

Goals should be "SMART" (specific, measurable, achievable, realistic, and time defined).

Expect and Prepare for More Patient Questions

Engaging patients in the discharge process will likely encourage them to ask questions or request more information (in fact, clinicians should invite patients to do so). Answering these questions may add some time to the discharge process, but this is time well spent as it will enhance patients' understanding of their condition, treatment, and required follow-up care. This investment during the hospitalization may prevent subsequent inappropriate ED use and potential deterioration of a patient's chronic illnesses.

Implement a New Process

The team should design a new process that incorporates relevant Project BOOST resources, including (but not limited to) a tool to evaluate a patient's risk of readmission (8P Risk Assessment), an assessment of patient preparedness for discharge (GAP), a patient-centered discharge tool (PASS or DPET), medication reconciliation tools, and tools to facilitate and confirm communication with providers at the next level of care.

Evaluation

The team should monitor progress in designing, implementing, and evaluating local QI efforts, and track program characteristics that might influence sustainability.

Structural Measures

These data speak to the adequacy of the support systems needed to implement and sustain a high-quality discharge program. Examples of areas that may be assessed include the following:

- Evidence of engagement with the organization, as shown by existence of an empowered interdisciplinary team that reports to appropriate committees
- Evidence of institutional support, e.g., institution recognizes the issue as a priority, allocates resources to the program
- An active system for collecting data for measuring and reporting project processes and outcomes
- Existence of policies and procedures, educational materials, and decision support tools (e.g., structured discharge documents)

Process Measures

These measures assess the degree to which interventions are being utilized. Examples of processes that may be assessed include:

- Percentage of discharges that received the recommended screening/services

- Percentage of discharges where all crucial information was forwarded to the patient's primary care provider within 48 h of discharge
- Percentage of discharges that required and received post-discharge follow-up phone calls

Outcome Measures

These measures describe the degree to which the program is actually improving care. Examples of outcomes that might be assessed include:

- Patient satisfaction with the discharge process
- Percentage of discharges with ED visits or rehospitalization within 30 days
- Percentage of patients/caregivers who can list their medications and know why they are taking each drug
- Percentage of patients/caregivers voicing understanding of treatments, follow-up care required, and warning signs and response

Ongoing Refinement

Based on findings from the evaluation, the team should continue to improve the discharge process by examining whether the needs of all patients are being addressed, whether hospital staffs have embraced the new process, and/or whether further streamlining of the process is possible.

Effectiveness of Project BOOST®

In a semi-controlled pre-post study involving 11 hospitals that implemented Project BOOST® on one unit (using a physician mentor to assist), readmission rates on BOOST units fell by 13.6 % in the year following implementation (from 14.7 to 12.7 %). Over the same time period, readmission rates on similar units in the same hospitals that did not implement the program remained stable (14.0 % at baseline, 14.1% a year later) [13]. One medium-sized teaching hospital analyzed the 30-day readmission rate for nearly all unplanned rehospitalizations to the hospital retrospectively for the 12 months before and after the implementation of BOOST and the results included a significant reduction in 30-day readmission rates from 4 to 3.7 % and prevented an estimated 119 repeat admissions [14]. The approach of mentored implementation in Project BOOST® was recognized by the Joint Commission and the National Quality Forum with the 2011 John M. Eisenberg Award for Innovation in Patient Safety and Quality at the National Level [15].

Thousands have registered to download the BOOST® Implementation Guide, and Project BOOST® has been implemented in more than 180 hospitals through mentored implementation since October 2008.

References

1. Coleman EA, Fox PD. Managing patient care transitions: a report of the HMO care management workgroup. Healthplan. 2004; 45(2):36–9.
2. Pham HH, Schrag D, O'Malley AS, Wu B, Bach PB. Care patterns in Medicare and their implications for pay for performance. N Engl J Med. 2007;356(11):1130–9.
3. Hibbard JH, Greene J. What the evidence shows about patient activation: better health outcomes and care experiences; fewer data on costs. Health Aff (Millwood). 2013;32(2):207–14.
4. Snow V, Beck D, Budnitz T, Miller DC, Potter J, Wears RL, et al. Transitions of Care Consensus Policy Statement American College of Physicians-Society of General Internal Medicine-Society of Hospital Medicine-American Geriatrics Society-American College of Emergency Physicians-Society of Academic Emergency Medicine. J Gen Intern Med. 2009;24(8):971–6.
5. Arbaje AI, Wolff JL, Yu Q, Powe NR, Anderson GF, Boult C. Postdischarge environmental and socioeconomic factors and the likelihood of early hospital readmission among community-dwelling Medicare beneficiaries. Gerontologist. 2008;48(4): 495–504.
6. Peek CJ, Baird MA, Coleman E. Primary care for patient complexity, not only disease. Fam Syst Health. 2009;27(4):287–302.
7. Solet DJ, Norvell JM, Rutan GH, Frankel RM. Lost in translation: challenges and opportunities in physician-to-physician communication during patient handoffs. Acad Med. 2005;80(12):1094–9.
8. Roy CL, Poon EG, Karson AS, Ladak-Merchant Z, Johnson RE, Maviglia SM, et al. Patient safety concerns arising from test results that return after hospital discharge. Ann Intern Med. 2005; 143(2):121–8.
9. Hernandez AF, Greiner MA, Fonarow GC, Hammill BG, Heidenreich PA, Yancy CW, et al. Relationship between early physician follow-up and 30-day readmission among Medicare beneficiaries hospitalized for heart failure. JAMA. 2010;303(17): 1716–22.
10. Sharma G, Kuo YF, Freeman JL, Zhang DD, Goodwin JS. Outpatient follow-up visit and 30-day emergency department visit and readmission in patients hospitalized for chronic obstructive pulmonary disease. Arch Intern Med. 2010;170(18):1664–70.
11. Jencks SF, Williams MV, Coleman EA. Rehospitalizations among patients in the Medicare fee-for-service program. N Engl J Med. 2009;360(14):1418–28.
12. Schillinger D, Piette J, Grumbach K, Wang F, Wilson C, Daher C, et al. Closing the loop: physician communication with diabetic patients who have low health literacy. Arch Intern Med. 2003; 163(1):83–90.
13. Hansen LO, Greenwald JL, Budnitz T, Howell E, Halasyamani L, Maynard G, et al. Project BOOST: effectiveness of a multihospital effort to reduce rehospitalization. J Hosp Med. 2013;8(8):421–7.
14. Cauwels JM, Jensen BJ, Winterton TL. Giving readmission numbers a BOOST. S D Med. 2013;66(12):505–7. 509.
15. Maynard GA, Budnitz TL, Nickel WK, Greenwald JL, Kerr KM, Miller JA, et al. 2011 John M Eisenberg patient safety and quality awards. mentored implementation: building leaders and achieving results through a collaborative improvement model. Innovation in patient safety and quality at the national level. Jt Comm J Qual Patient Saf. 2012;38(7):301–10.

The GRACE Model

Dawn E. Butler, Kathryn I. Frank, and Steven R. Counsell

Background and Conceptual Model

Studies have confirmed what physicians and healthcare providers caring for older adults have always known, many older adults are living with multiple chronic illnesses and geriatric syndromes. Additionally, this population accounts for a disproportionate share of Medicare expenditures. Unfortunately, older adults receiving their care from primary care settings often fail to receive the recommended standards of care [1, 2].

In response to the need for new delivery models to better address common geriatric conditions and integrate medical and social care, the clinicians and researchers at the Indiana University Center for Aging Research designed and tested a new model of interdisciplinary team care called GRACE, *Geriatric Resources for Assessment and Care of Elders*. The GRACE model was originally developed to improve the quality of care for older adults. The goal of the GRACE model was to optimize health and functional status, decrease excess healthcare use, and prevent long-term nursing home placement. GRACE built on the lessons learned from prior efforts to improve the care of older adults and added several new features including integration of the geriatrics team within the primary care environment, in-home assessment and care management by a nurse practitioner and social

D.E. Butler, M.S.W., J.D. (✉) • K.I. Frank, R.N., Ph.D.
IU Geriatrics and Division of General Internal Medicine,
Department of Medicine, Indiana University School of Medicine,
720 Eskenazi Drive; Fifth Third Bank Building, 2nd Floor,
Indianapolis, IN 46202, USA
e-mail: butlerde@iu.edu; katfrank@iu.edu

S.R. Counsell, M.D.
IU Geriatrics and Division of General Internal Medicine,
Department of Medicine, Indiana University School of
Medicine and Indiana University Center for Aging Research,
720 Eskenazi Avenue; Fifth Third Bank Building, 2nd Floor,
Indianapolis, IN 46202, USA
e-mail: scounsel@iu.edu

worker team, and integration with affiliated pharmacy, mental health, home health, and community-based services [1]. The model was also designed to address barriers found at the system, provider, and patient level that were resulting in older adults having unmet healthcare needs (Fig.10.1). Through a geriatric focused assessment and ongoing proactive care management, GRACE worked through these barriers leading to improved diagnosis and treatment of geriatric syndromes higher quality of care and better outcomes.

GRACE Team Care

Overview

The GRACE model of primary care is a cost-effective, patient-centered team care model that has been proven to improve the health of older adults by working with patients in their homes and in their communities to manage health problems, track changing care needs, and leverage needed social services [3, 4].

There are a number of unique features of GRACE Team Care including multidimensional assessment and interdisciplinary team care. The catalyst for the GRACE intervention is the nurse practitioner and social worker referred to as the GRACE Support Team. The GRACE Support Team meets with each patient in his or her home to conduct an initial geriatric-focused assessment. Following the in-home assessment, the support team meets with the GRACE Interdisciplinary Team composed of a geriatrician medical director, pharmacist, and mental health liaison to develop an individualized care plan using the GRACE protocols [1].

The GRACE Support Team then meets with the patient's primary care physician to review, modify, and prioritize the plan. The support team works in collaboration with the primary care physician and the patient to implement the plan consistent with the patient's goals [1]. The care plan contains strategies to address the medical and psychosocial issues of concern as well as elements related to maintaining quality of life and independence.

Fig. 10.1 GRACE conceptualization (From Counsell SR. The Trustees of Indiana University, Powerpoint Presentation, with permission.)

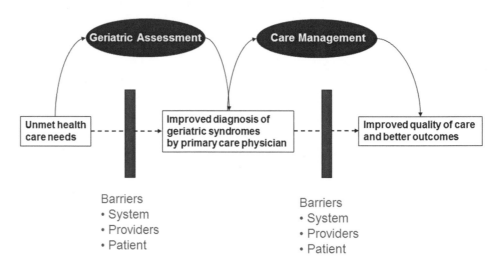

The GRACE Support Team has at least monthly contact with the patient and provides proactive coordination and continuity of care between all healthcare professionals involved in the patient's care. The GRACE team assists with transitions between levels of care by working closely with hospital, emergency department, and nursing facility staff. The GRACE Support Team collaborates with the discharging team to develop an optimal transition plan. Once the patient has returned home, the GRACE Support Team conducts a home visit to ensure the discharge arrangements are in place, complete medication reconciliation, provide support to the patient and caregiver, and connect the patient back to their primary care physician [5].

Key Components

In-Home Geriatric Assessment

There are six key components of GRACE Team Care (Table 10.1) [6]. The first step is an in-home assessment completed by the nurse practitioner and social worker simultaneously allowing for each discipline to hear and learn about issues, problems, concerns, and patient goals related to all aspects of their care. In addition to engaging and establishing the framework for GRACE involvement with the patient, the goal of the in-home assessment is to capture a comprehensive view of the older adult in their environment with the focus on identifying geriatric conditions. The GRACE Support Team's assessment findings and the patient's health goals serve as the basis for developing an individualized care plan.

During the initial home visit, the GRACE nurse practitioner and social worker each complete their respective evaluation that together make up a comprehensive geriatric assessment upon which to develop an individualized care plan

Table 10.1 Key components of GRACE Team Care

1. In-home geriatric assessment by a nurse practitioner and social worker team
2. Individualized care plan using GRACE protocols
3. Weekly interdisciplinary team conference, including a geriatrician, pharmacist, and mental health liaison
4. Review of the care plan with the primary care physician
5. Implementation of the care plan in collaboration with the primary care physician and consistent with patient goals
6. Ongoing care management to ensure coordination of care and smooth care transitions

From IU Geriatrics GRACE Training and Resource Center. GRACE Team Care Training Manual. The Trustees of Indiana University, 2013, with permission

(Table 10.2). The nurse practitioner conducts a medical history, detailed medication review, and brief physical examination. The examination should give special attention to orthostatic vital signs, vision, hearing, and evaluation of gait and balance. The social worker completes a psychosocial history and functional assessment, conducts screens for cognitive impairment and depression, identifies goals of care, discusses advance directives, conducts a caregiver assessment when applicable, and performs a home safety evaluation [1].

To gather a complete assessment, the GRACE Support Team also reviews past medical records and contacts other providers and/or agencies involved in the individual's health care. In addition to collecting pertinent information, agency representatives are invited to participate in the GRACE interdisciplinary team conference to provide input on the care plan development.

Individualized Care Plan and GRACE Protocols

The driver of GRACE is an individualized care plan developed by the GRACE team based on the initial in-home assessment and the patient's goals of care. The care plan is built

Table 10.2 GRACE in-home assessment domains

Nurse practitioner	Social worker
• History of present illness	• Social history
• Past medical history	• Functional status
• Medical review of systems[a]	• Caregiver status
• Geriatric review of systems[b]	• Finances
• Medication reconciliation	• Advance directives
• Orthostatic vital signs	• Depression screen
• Vision/hearing screen	• Cognitive screen
• Gait/balance evaluation	• Home safety evaluation

From IU Geriatrics GRACE Training and Resource Center. GRACE Team Care Training Manual. The Trustees of Indiana University, 2013, with permission
[a]Medical review of systems includes cardiovascular, respiratory, gastrointestinal, genitourinary, musculoskeletal, and neurological
[b]Geriatric review of systems includes nutrition, skin, vision, hearing, dentition, continence, ambulation, feet, and cognition

Table 10.3 GRACE protocols

• Advance care planning[a]	• Caregiver burden
• Health maintenance[a]	• Chronic pain
• Medication management[a]	• Malnutrition/weight loss
• Difficulty walking/falls	• Urinary incontinence
• Depression	• Visual impairment
• Cognitive impairment/dementia	• Hearing impairment

From IU Geriatrics GRACE Training and Resource Center. GRACE Team Care Training Manual. The Trustees of Indiana University, 2013, with permission
[a]Protocol used in initial care plan of all GRACE patients

using the GRACE protocols for common geriatric conditions (Table 10.3). These care protocols and corresponding team suggestions for evaluation and management are based on published practice guidelines and provide a checklist to ensure a standardized and state-of-the-art approach to care [1].

The GRACE Support Team selects the GRACE protocols and corresponding team suggestions as appropriate. The following protocols are selected in all patients: Advance Care Planning, Health Maintenance, and Medication Management. The selection of protocols is up to the clinical judgment of the GRACE Support Team. The GRACE Support Team identifies the contributing factors to the GRACE protocol to provide a rationale for its use. Once selecting the GRACE protocol, the GRACE team selects the corresponding team suggestions. The team suggestions are a combination of medical and psychosocial interventions. All suggestions fall within the scope of practice for an advanced practice nurse and social worker [6].

GRACE Interdisciplinary Team Conference

The GRACE Interdisciplinary Team meets once a week for about 2 h to discuss and finalize care plans for new GRACE patients, follow-up on care plan implementation for established GRACE patients, and discuss those patients identified for an "extra" team review (e.g., unexpected hospital admission).

The GRACE Interdisciplinary Team is composed of the GRACE Support Team, geriatrician medical director, pharmacist, mental health liaison, and program coordinator [6].

New patients are to be presented to the team by the GRACE Support Team. In presenting the patient, the nurse practitioner and social worker provide a brief overview of the patient, the patient's health goals, and findings from the initial in-home assessment. A standard presentation format is used to allow the team members to anticipate information to be shared. The GRACE Support Team identifies the applicable GRACE protocols and shares the draft individualized care plan [6].

The interdisciplinary team members together review the proposed care plan taking one protocol at a time and in order of importance in achieving the patient's health goals. The geriatrician medical director, mental health liaison, and pharmacist each provide input to the care plan by revising and/or adding specific interventions or team suggestions [6].

In addition to new patients, the GRACE Interdisciplinary Team discusses established GRACE patients due for a routine follow-up team review. Scheduled team reviews provide an opportunity to check on progress toward care plan implementation. In addition, the team problem solves barriers to implementing team suggestions and makes adjustments to the care plan as appropriate [6].

Extra team reviews are scheduled if a patient is hospitalized, seen in the emergency department, or otherwise has a change in condition or issue for which the GRACE Support Team would like input from the GRACE Interdisciplinary Team. If following an unplanned hospitalization or emergency department visit, the extra team review should include a discussion of contributing factors and potential interventions that might be applied in the future to prevent recurrence [6].

Primary Care Physician Collaboration

The GRACE model was developed to closely align the GRACE Support Team with the patient's primary care physician (PCP). The GRACE team is meant to compliment and support the PCP in the care of their complex older patients. The GRACE Support Team should be considered an extension of the PCP and office staff, providing regular follow-up and communication with the PCP as needed or requested. Once the GRACE Interdisciplinary Team finalizes a new patient's care plan, the nurse practitioner with or without the social worker meets with the PCP to discuss the care plan, prioritize interventions, and coordinate implementation [1]. Meetings with the PCP occur at a time convenient for the PCP and outside of scheduled clinic time to avoid disrupting patient appointments.

Discussion with the PCP focuses on the high priority items such as medication recommendations, consultations, and labs. The extent of care to be provided by the GRACE team is a key discussion area for the PCP and GRACE nurse practitioner. The comfort level of the PCP with having the GRACE nurse practitioner handle certain issues that are generally done in the office setting (e.g., starting new medications, titrating current medications, and ordering lab tests) should be taken into account and discussed. The focus of the GRACE nurse practitioner should be on implementing the GRACE care plan and providing proactive care management that supports the patient's office-based primary care physician. After reviewing the GRACE care plan and making any necessary revisions as directed by the PCP, the care plan is signed by the PCP and a copy is provided to the PCP for the patient's chart. The GRACE Support Team will bring to the attention of the geriatrician medical director any questions or concerns of the PCP related to the GRACE care plan and team suggestions. A reference file is maintained to include medical literature that can be provided to the PCP in response to questions as needed [6].

Care Plan Implementation and Care Coordination

The nurse practitioner and social worker will collaborate with the PCP to implement the GRACE care plan consistent with the agreed upon goals of care and priorities identified through discussion with the PCP and patient. In the week following the meeting with the PCP, the GRACE Support Team schedules a home visit to review the care plan and begin to implement the highest-priority interventions. During the first follow-up visit to review the care plan, the GRACE Support Team also provides the patient with both verbal and written educational material specific to older adults regarding general health, wellness, and safety. The educational information generally includes medication safety, fitness, nutrition, vaccinations, and community resources and safety tips. The GRACE Support Team keeps the PCP informed of their progress in implementing the care plan, including any difficulties encountered or needed adjustments [6].

As part of the care plan implementation, the GRACE Support Team assists with care coordination across the multiple sites and providers involved in a patient's care. The GRACE team utilizes a collaborative interdisciplinary team approach across the continuum of care to optimize coordination of care and patient function and independence. Patients and their caregivers are encouraged to contact their assigned GRACE Support Team should they feel they need assistance [1].

The GRACE Support Team is often notified if a patient visits the emergency department or is hospitalized to aid in smooth care transitions and care coordination. GRACE teams also monitor upcoming patient appointments to provide patient reminders. Before a GRACE patient's office visit with his/her PCP, the GRACE Support Team will often help prepare both the patient and PCP for the visit. The nurse practitioner and social worker can coach the patient about questions to ask her/his PCP and also inform the PCP or office staff of issues that need to be addressed during the patient's office visit. The GRACE Support Team offers assistance as needed in facilitating the patient's office visit (e.g., help with securing an appointment and/or transportation arrangements) and makes GRACE materials available to optimize the patient's visit (e.g., GRACE care plan, current medication list, completed lab requisitions, etc.) [6].

Proactive Care Management

The GRACE Support Team maintains regular contact with GRACE patients to work toward care plan implementation and to monitor the patient's status and concerns. GRACE patients receive at a minimum a face-to-face visit or telephone call each month. These proactive contacts help build trusting relationships with patients while monitoring and assisting patients in pursuing their health goals. Additionally, these contacts provide an opportunity for the GRACE Support Team to check in on the patient's care plan, identify new issues or problems, discuss medication changes, review physical activity and socialization, and monitor for changes in function, living arrangements, and social supports [1].

The care plan is reviewed with the GRACE Interdisciplinary Team at regular intervals. During these "routine" team reviews, the GRACE Support Team discusses the patient's current status and progress toward implementation of the care plan. Any new problems or issues necessitating team discussion should also be covered during routine team reviews. If the GRACE Support Team has new concerns about a patient or the patient is admitted to the hospital, seen in the ED, or has a change in condition, the patient is brought up for an "extra" team review [1].

GRACE patients who remain with the program receive an annual in-home assessment. The annual assessment process and forms are the same as the initial assessment. A new care plan is drafted by the GRACE Support Team and presented to the interdisciplinary team for input similar to the initial assessment. As with new GRACE patients, the annual assessment and new care plan are reviewed with the PCP and follow the same process of implementation as occurs with new GRACE patients [6].

GRACE Interdisciplinary Team

The strength of GRACE is the team approach. From the initial in-home assessment to implementation of the interdisciplinary team suggestions to ongoing care management, GRACE brings together a support team and expanded interdisciplinary team to work collaboratively with the patient and his/her primary care physician to develop and implement an individualized care plan and provide comprehensive care.

The core GRACE Interdisciplinary Team, in addition to the GRACE Support Teams, includes the geriatrician medical director, mental health liaison, pharmacist, and program coordinator [6]. Additional disciplines have been included as needed for valuable input to care plan development and to serve as a resource to the GRACE Support Team. These disciplines have included a physical therapist, occupational therapist, and community resource liaison [1].

All team members play a vital role in optimizing the health and quality of life of patients enrolled in the GRACE program. Each team member has specific job responsibilities to execute before, during, and after the weekly team conference. By having specific and predetermined responsibilities, each team member knows their role and what information is to be shared and discussed in the interdisciplinary team conference.

The GRACE team geriatrician medical director reviews the nurse practitioner and social worker assessment forms prior to the team meeting. During the team conference, the geriatrician helps clarify the medical problems and geriatric syndromes. While providing input on the care plan, the geriatrician helps the GRACE Support Team draft the care plan in physician language. A key role of the geriatrician is to help the team prioritize implementation of the care plan. Between team meetings, the geriatrician serves as resource to the team members and helps answer questions of the primary care physicians [6].

The pharmacist also plays an important role on the GRACE Interdisciplinary Team. Prior to the weekly team conference, the pharmacist reviews patient pharmacy records looking for medication adherence trends and considers possible medication recommendations. During the team conference, the pharmacist advises the team on potential impact of medications, provides recommendations for alternatives, assists in identifying cost-effective options, and addresses questions from the GRACE Support Team. Between team meetings, the pharmacist is available to the team as an additional resource and as liaison to the pharmacy department [6].

The mental health liaison also plays a valuable role with the GRACE team. As with the pharmacist, the mental health liaison reviews the mental health records of any patients that are due to be discussed in the team meeting. During the team meeting, the mental health liaison provides input to the care plan on symptom management, supportive measures, treatment recommendations, and other potential interventions. The mental health liaison is available to the GRACE team in between team conferences to serve as a liaison between GRACE and mental health providers and as an additional resource for the team [6].

The GRACE program coordinator is responsible for answering all incoming calls on the dedicated GRACE phone line, contacting potential patients to begin the enrollment process and scheduling the initial home visit. The coordinator manages the GRACE databases including the tracking of care plan review schedules and outcome metrics. Before the team meeting, the program coordinator notifies all GRACE team members of the patients that will be reviewed during the upcoming team conference. The program coordinator attends the team meetings to work collaboratively with team members implementing care plans and ensuring follow-up on agreed upon priorities for individual patients. Following the team meeting, the coordinator assists the GRACE Support Team with on-going care management, scheduling appointments, and coordinating transportation [6].

Integration with the Electronic Medical Record

Optimally, all GRACE documentation is made in the health system's Electronic Medical Record (EMR) in a designated area for easy reference by the PCP. If the GRACE initial assessment and care plan documentation are not part of the EMR, a succinct summary is entered or scanned into the EMR including key findings and planned interventions to facilitate coordination of care. A Subjective Objective Assessment Plan (SOAP) note is entered into the EMR after each contact with the patient, including visits and telephone calls. It is important to have this documentation in the medical record to aid in continuity of care and to keep primary care and specialty providers informed regarding the GRACE team's interventions and patient's progress [6].

An Evidence-Based Approach

GRACE Randomized Controlled Trial

The GRACE model was rigorously studied through a large, randomized controlled trial at Eskenazi Health (formerly Wishard Health Services), a public safety-net healthcare system in Indianapolis, Indiana [7]. A total of 951 patients were recruited from six community-based primary care practices affiliated with Eskenazi Health—474 to the GRACE intervention group and 477 to the control group. Patients who were 65 years and older, had one or more visits with their primary care physician in the last 12 months, and had an annual income below 200 % of the Federal Poverty Level were eligible to participate. Patients and primary care physicians were randomized for participation in the study with participants receiving the GRACE intervention for 2 years. Outcome measures were determined based on patient interviews using the Assessing Care of Vulnerable Elders (ACOVE) quality indicators, Medical Outcomes 36-Item Short Form scales, and functional status through metrics from the Assets and Health Dynamics of the Oldest-Old (AHEAD) survey. Acute care utilization including hospital admissions, hospital days, and emergency department visits were obtained from a regional health information exchange.

Patients with a score of 0.4 or higher on the probability of repeated admissions (PRA) screen were considered high risk of hospitalization.

Overall, participants enrolled in the GRACE trial were similar between the GRACE intervention and control groups with mean age of 72 years, 76 % women, 59 % black, and all were socioeconomically disadvantaged. Study participants receiving the GRACE intervention reported improved quality of life and better performance on quality indicators (Table 10.4). Specifically, participants reported improved quality of life in areas of general health, vitality, social function, and mental health. Performance on quality indicators related to general health care (e.g. immunizations, continuity of care) and geriatric conditions (e.g. falls, depression) was also better in the GRACE intervention group compared to control. Patients and their physicians reported high rates of satisfaction with the GRACE model [1, 7].

In patients considered at high risk for hospitalization by their PRA score, those participants receiving the GRACE intervention had fewer hospital admissions compared to the control group (Table 10.4 and Fig. 10.2). Of particular note, the trend in reduced hospitalization rates in the high-risk GRACE intervention group compared to control persisted in the third year, the year following when the GRACE intervention ended. A thorough cost analysis was conducted on the GRACE model. Among high-risk patients, the cost savings from lower acute care utilizations resulted in cost savings in year 2 and 3 while accounting for GRACE program costs [3] (Table 10.4 and Fig. 10.3).

Table 10.4 Results of GRACE randomized controlled trial[a]

Better quality and outcomes in GRACE patients
- Enhanced quality of life by SF-36 scales[b]
  - General health, vitality, social function, and mental health
  - Mental component summary
- Better performance on ACOVE quality indicators[b]
  - General health care (e.g., immunizations, continuity of care)
  - Geriatric conditions (e.g., falls, depression)
- Fewer ED visits
  - 12 % in year 1
  - 24 % in year 2[b]

Decreased hospital admissions and lower costs in high-risk GRACE patients
- Reduction in hospital admissions
  - 12 % in year 1
  - 44 % in year 2[b]
  - 40 % in year 3 (post-intervention year)[b]
- Lower readmission rates
  - 74 % for 7-days[b]
  - 45 % for 30-days
  - 40 % for 90-days[b]
- Lower total costs
  - 2 % in year 1
  - 17 % in year 2
  - 23 % in year 3 (post-intervention year)[b]

Data from Counsell SR, Callahan CM, Clark DO, Tu W, Buttar AB, Stump TE, Ricketts GD. Geriatric Care Management for Low-Income Seniors: A randomized controlled trial. JAMA. 2007;298(22):2623–33
[a]*SF-36* medical outcomes 36-item short-form, *ACOVE* assessing care of vulnerable elders, *ED* emergency department

[b]Statistically significant difference compared to control group ($P<.05$)

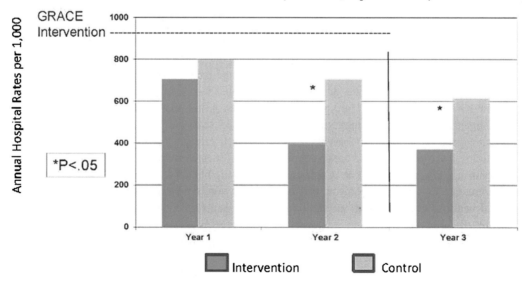

Fig. 10.2 GRACE Randomized controlled trial hospitalization rates of the high-risk group (From Counsell SR. The Trustees of Indiana University, Powerpoint Presentation, with permission.)

Fig. 10.3 GRACE Randomized controlled trial total healthcare costs (From Counsell SR. The Trustees of Indiana University, Powerpoint Presentation, with permission.)

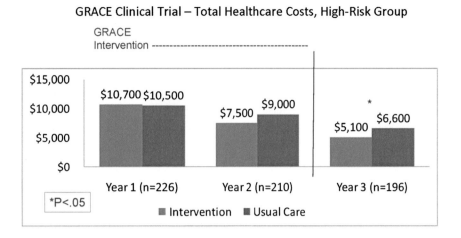

Replication Experience

GRACE Team Care was designed and tested in a public safety net healthcare system and community health centers serving a disadvantaged population including low-income seniors. Since the completion of the randomized control trial, GRACE Team Care has been successfully replicated in a variety of healthcare settings. GRACE has been implemented in health plans, integrated systems, the VA healthcare system, and a large managed care medical group (Table 10.5). In each of these settings, when targeted to high-risk seniors, the GRACE model has demonstrated a positive impact on the quality of care and reduced acute care utilization.

HealthCare Partners in Los Angeles, California implemented the GRACE model in their HomeCare Program serving chronically ill and homebound patients and involving physicians, nurse practitioners, and social workers [8]. HealthCare Partners leadership and staff involved in GRACE implementation rated GRACE as very helpful in providing care to older frail patients and reported that the GRACE model better identified important psychosocial issues and geriatric conditions in their patients, improved medication management and follow-up, and helped coordinate care compared to before GRACE.

The Indianapolis VA Medical Center enrolled older Veterans upon discharge home following a non-elective hospital admission [8]. In this application of the GRACE model, the GRACE nurse practitioner and social worker started with a transition visit in the home soon after hospital discharge and then subsequently, when the patient was more stable, conducted the initial GRACE assessment and developed an individualized care plan using the GRACE protocols. In addition to seeing the gains in recognition and treatment of geriatric syndromes and improved care coordination, older Veterans who enrolled in GRACE had a nearly 50 % reduction in their 30-day readmission rate.

Table 10.5 GRACE Team Care replication partners

Indiana	*Michigan*
• Eskenazi Health (formerly Wishard Health Services)	• University of Michigan Health System
• IU Health Medicare Advantage Plan	• Blue Cross Blue Shield of Michigan
California	*VA Healthcare System*
• HealthCare Partners	• Indianapolis VAMC
• UCSF Medical Center	• San Francisco VAMC
• Health Plan of San Mateo	• Cleveland VAMC
• Whittier Hospital Medical Center & Central Health Plan	• Atlanta VAMC

From Counsell SR. The Trustees of Indiana University, Powerpoint Presentation, with permission

In 2010 the Administration on Aging (now Administration for Community Living) and the Centers for Medicare and Medicaid Services issued funding for "Aging and Disability Resource Centers (ADRC) Evidence-Based Care Transitions Programs." The goal of this funding opportunity was to promote ADRC partnerships with hospitals and physician groups to provide better transitions and care coordination. The GRACE model was one of four evidence-based models that states could implement. Indiana was awarded a grant using the GRACE model, however, with a slightly different staffing model where a social worker from the ADRC served in the GRACE social worker role while the nurse practitioner was from the medical group. Here again, 30-day readmission rates dropped by more than half in patients enrolled in the Indiana ADRC Care Transitions Program [8, 9].

In the replication with Indiana University Health Medicare Advantage plan, health plan members 65 or older were enrolled into the program through various sources including: hospital or skilled nursing facility discharge to home, risk stratification using administrative data, and primary care physician referral [8]. In addition to demonstrated improvements in the quality of care and care coordination, physicians requested expansion of the program from the pilot practice sites to all of the IU Health Physician's primary care practices since they found the program to be especially helpful in providing comprehensive care to their frail older patients.

As seen in the various replications described above, the GRACE model is flexible to meet diverse patient and healthcare system needs, processes and goals. Due to the results outlined above and concomitant demonstration of substantial reductions in hospital admissions in patients served by the programs, the GRACE model has been sustained in each of these healthcare systems.

Who Benefits from GRACE Team Care?

Evidence from the GRACE Trial

The GRACE model was originally tested in low-income seniors obtaining primary healthcare services through one of the community health centers of an urban public safety-net health system. Compared to the control group, the GRACE intervention group was shown at the end of 2 years to have a higher quality of life, received better quality of care, and less frequently visited the emergency department (Table 10.4). High-risk patients enrolled in the GRACE intervention group (25 % of enrollees) were also less frequently hospitalized and had lower total healthcare costs over time compared to high-risk patients in the control group (Table 10.4). In the low-risk patients enrolled in the GRACE intervention group (75 % of enrollees), however, hospitalization rates were similar and total costs were higher (due to the costs of the GRACE intervention) compared to low-risk patients in the control group. Thus, both black and white low-income seniors, and those at low and high risk for hospitalization, appeared to benefit from GRACE related to the quality of healthcare they received and their reported quality of life. Whether or not results of the GRACE trial can be extrapolated to people of higher socioeconomic status and those living in rural communities cannot be determined from the original study [7, 10, 11].

Patient Selection Strategies for Cost Savings

To deploy the GRACE model in a cost neutral or cost savings manner, it is necessary to select patients at high risk of hospitalization or otherwise having high healthcare utilization and costs. It is in these high-risk patients that the GRACE trial demonstrated reduced acute care costs that offset the costs of the GRACE intervention and has the potential for overall cost savings [3]. In the original GRACE trial, "high risk" was determined by the Probability of Repeated

Admission (PRA) Questionnaire which has been used extensively in managed-care settings to identify older adults at high risk for subsequent hospitalization and high healthcare costs [7]. A PRA risk score is calculated based on age, sex, perceived health, availability of an informal caregiver, heart disease, diabetes, physician visits, and hospitalizations. Other surveys and predictive modeling tools exist for identifying high-risk older patients [10, 12]. Selecting an approach that identifies a population of seniors having high baseline rates of hospitalization (e.g., 1,200 admissions per 1,000 per year or greater) helps ensure the opportunity to reduce hospital admissions and costs such that GRACE program expenses are covered and overall cost savings are realized. Enrollment criteria that help identify high-risk and high-cost older patients likely to benefit from GRACE Team Care include: (a) multiple chronic illnesses with functional limitations, (b) one or more non-elective hospitalizations in the prior year, (c) diagnosis of depression or dementia, (d) nine or more prescription medications, (e) lives alone or with a frail spouse, (f) low health literacy, (g) cultural or financial barriers, and (h) dually eligible for Medicare and Medicaid.

The Business Case for GRACE

GRACE Team Care provides a number of clinical and financial incentives to health systems and especially those oriented toward shared risk. Although the specific business case will vary depending on the health system's reimbursement model (fee-for-service, managed care, or accountable care organization), GRACE Team Care has been proven in multiple settings to be a cost-effective program in caring for high-risk older adults. While improving the quality of life for program participants, GRACE has been shown to significantly reduce emergency department visits, hospital admissions, 30-day readmission rates, and stays in skilled nursing facilities. These reductions in acute and post-acute care present savings and value-based opportunities for healthcare systems and managed care organizations [3]. GRACE uses a dashboard to monitor quality indicators to assist organizations in reaching targeted quality goals too; and has consistently received high satisfaction ratings from patients, caregivers, and providers. Thus, GRACE Team Care brings added value to a healthcare system or physician organization by improving quality and lowering costs in high-risk and complex older adults.

As discussed above, cost savings and thus also a "return on investment" for GRACE Team Care can best be achieved by selecting high-risk older patients for enrollment in the program [12]. Examples of enrollment criteria are provided above that help identify patients having a high baseline hospitalization rate and/or that are in the top 20 % of expenditures

Table 10.6 Business case for GRACE[a]

Costs	Return
• 7 FTE (3 nurse practitioners, 3 social workers, 1 coordinator)	• ↓ 30 % Hospital admits
• 0.3 FTE (0.1 medical director, 0.1 mental health liaison, 0.1 pharmacist)	• ↓ 25 % ED visits
• Mileage home visits	• Appropriate risk adjustment
• Increased mental health and rehab utilization	• Better satisfaction and quality scores
• Caseload of 300	• Primary care physician efficiency gains

From Counsell SR. The Trustees of Indiana University, Powerpoint Presentation, with permission
[a]*FTE* full time equivalent employee, *ED* emergency department

in a Medicare managed care plan or accountable care organization. Table 10.6 outlines the basics of a business case for GRACE including program costs and projected return based on results of the original GRACE trial and GRACE replications. A GRACE program having the staffing (Table 10.6) and other costs and operating at steady state with an active census of 300 high risk patients (caseload of 100 per GRACE Support Team) can expect an approximate intervention cost of $175 per patient per month, or $2,100 per patient per year (total annual program staffing and mileage costs of $630,000). Assuming a baseline hospitalization rate of 1,200 per 1,000 per year and $10,000 in cost savings per hospitalization avoided, a 30 % reduction in hospitalization rate will save 108 hospital admissions or $1,080,000. Additional costs are likely to occur associated with the GRACE intervention including an increase in expenses for mental health and physical and occupational therapies, however, additional savings are likely too (e.g., avoided ED visits). Furthermore, there are several less quantifiable benefits of GRACE Team Care that help make the business case and demonstrate added value (Table 10.7).

Implementation of GRACE Team Care

ABC's of Implementation

Successful implementation of GRACE Team Care requires a systematic approach to the implementation process. This process includes obtaining leadership support, documentation of processes, and evaluation of results. To aid in following a structured approach, replication sites are encouraged to follow the "ABC's of Implementation" [13] (Table 10.8). The first step in implementation is to *A*gree on the need for GRACE. Agreement needs to be obtained from key stakeholders and leadership team members. To help obtain agreement, the goals for GRACE

Table 10.7 Less quantifiable benefits of GRACE Team Care

• Improved patient experience and market/patient loyalty
• Reduction in 30-day readmission rates and avoidance of Medicare penalties
• Prevention or delay of institutional long-term care
• Better performance on quality metrics with significant upside potential from incentives in risk contracts
• Greater office efficiency and job satisfaction of primary care providers
• Increased revenue from more appropriate documentation and risk adjustment
• Assistance to patients to optimize health insurance coverage (e.g., Medicaid) and benefits that offset out-of-pocket costs
• More appropriate utilization of home and community-based services
• Keep hospital bed capacity open for higher revenue patients
• Reduced hospitalization rates also reduce pressure for capital dollars and construction of new hospital beds, impacting total cost of care in a community

From Geriatrics GRACE Training and Resource Center. The Business Case for GRACE. The Trustees of Indiana University, 2013, with permission

Table 10.8 ABC's of GRACE Team Care implementation

*A*GREE—Agree on the need for GRACE by key stakeholders

*B*UILD—Build the GRACE model with strong physician leadership and interdisciplinary team approach to planning and development

*C*OMMENCE—Commence GRACE with a focus on patient-centered care and attention to provider issues

*D*OCUMENT—Document implementation of the GRACE model to ensure changes in the process of care take place as planned

*E*VALUATE—Evaluate the program for anticipated benefits to the patients, providers, and healthcare system

*F*EEDBACK—Feedback provided to key stakeholders to update them on the progress of the GRACE program for sustained support

*G*ROW—Grow the GRACE model to serve more older adults

From Counsell SR. The Trustees of Indiana University, Powerpoint Presentation, with permission

should achieve a "win" for patients, providers, and the larger healthcare system. During this first step, a GRACE Steering Committee is formed to develop program goals, identify target populations, and determine outcome measures [14].

The next step is to *B*uild the GRACE model with the aid of key physician leaders. During this phase, a GRACE medical director and physician champion are identified. The GRACE implementation team is also assembled composed of the disciplines involved in the day-to-day operations. Training of staff in the GRACE processes occurs during this stage along with customizing GRACE assessment forms and protocols to meet the needs of the individual health system [14].

*C*ommence is the third stage during which enrollment into the program begins. The GRACE team begins to implement the key components of the model including the in-home assessment and development of individualized care plans. The GRACE interdisciplinary team begins their weekly meetings to review patient care plans [14].

*D*ocumenting GRACE processes are integral to successful implementation. Process metrics should be tracked to ensure changes in the process of care occurred as planned. Documentation related to dates of enrollment, team conferences, and collaboration with primary care physicians is also useful. Monitoring contacts with the patient and continuity of care can provide insight into workloads and complexity of enrolled patients [14].

An important step of implementation is to *E*valuate the model. Evaluation should take into account the anticipated benefits to patient, providers, and the larger health system. During this stage, the Steering Committee should review the evaluation data to determine whether outcome measures were met. Patient and provider satisfaction with the program should be assessed and data regarding care processes, quality metrics, and acute care utilization should be reviewed [14].

After evaluating the data, *F*eedback should be provided to key stakeholders regarding the progress of the program. Through this feedback, support can be gathered for GRACE program sustainability. Feedback should be given routinely to the GRACE Steering Committee and other physician and health system leadership to bolster continued support. Additionally during this stage, focus shifts to the development of a business case for the program [14].

The final stage of implementation is *G*row. As favorable outcomes are achieved and a solid business case developed, the program should warrant expansion to meet the needs of the patient population and healthcare system. Continuous enrollment of new patients is important for long-term sustainability of the GRACE program. During this stage, success of the program should be shared with the larger community through presentations and publications [14].

Barriers and Facilitators to Successful Implementation

Several factors have been identified as being key to successful implementation (Table 10.9). Having a physician champion from the healthcare system who can speak to the program's effectiveness and agree to help with program implementation can be an enormous boost to GRACE implementation. When presenting the program to leadership and key stakeholders, the program should highlight how stakeholders can achieve their goals and priorities. Identifying the "win-win-win" for the health system, providers, and patients is essential to gaining early support. Identifying financial incentives for the health system and

Table 10.9 Facilitators of successful implementations of GRACE Team Care

• "Early adopter" clinical champion
• Key stakeholders support as win-win-win
• Strong primary care and valued clinical geriatrics
• Financial incentives for system and providers
• Shared EMR and care management software
• Dedicated staff for start-up (not "add on" duties)
• GRACE site visit, training, and technical assistance

From Counsell SR. The Trustees of Indiana University, Powerpoint Presentation, with permission

providers can also help gather support. The GRACE model is most effective in a system having a strong primary care service and respected geriatrics or senior health clinicians. Having a shared EMR and care management software can also be an important facilitator in program implementation. The ability for the new program to document and integrate care plans within the same EMR as the primary care providers facilitates communication and relationship building. When beginning a new GRACE program, it is optimal to dedicate staff to the new initiative. This avoids staff with already full workloads getting asked to take on additional duties and becoming overwhelmed. It also allows new GRACE staff time to learn and help implement care processes as they increase their caseload. For successful startup, it can be especially valuable to obtain expert training and technical assistance on the GRACE model. Consultative assistance can help with all phases of GRACE implementation including recommendations on program adaptations for the local health system [14].

GRACE Training and Resource Center

Through experiences in successfully replicating the GRACE model within a variety of health systems across the country, a series of training and technical assistance services have been identified as helpful in aiding organizations (Table 10.10). These services are now offered through the IU Geriatrics GRACE Training and Resource Center at the Indiana University School of Medicine, Indianapolis, IN. Ideally, implementation assistance is offered over the course of several months. With a longer engagement, technical assistance can be provided for all stages of implementation including organization readiness, training on the model, customizing processes and forms, booster training for staff, business case development, and evaluation support. Providing a mix of telephonic, web-based, and in-person training can assist organizations in reaching several audiences such as key stakeholders, physician leaders, and implementation team members.

An optimal engagement for training services is 12 months. During this period, webinars are offered to provide an overview of the GRACE model, discuss implementation, and

Table 10.10 GRACE Training and Resource Center services

- Indianapolis site visit
- Pre-implementation webinars
- Implementation conference calls
- Intensive in-person team training
- GRACE training manual
- GRACE dashboard
- Evaluation and sustainability conference calls
- Evaluation and sustainability session
- GRACE care management tracking system
- On-line tools and resources (Table 10.11)

From GRACE Team Care [homepage on the Internet]. The Trustees of Indiana University; 2013 [updated 2015, January 12th]. Available from: http://graceteamcare.indiana.edu, with permission

identify specific organizational goals. A site visit to Indianapolis to see "GRACE in action" is also offered. Monthly conference calls provide individualized program support and instruction for implementation and evaluation of the model. An intensive in-person training is geared toward the implementation team members learning the key components of the GRACE model and roles of the GRACE team members, becoming familiar with GRACE assessment forms and care planning processes, and developing strategies for care coordination and transitional care. A follow-up in-person evaluation and sustainability session is offered toward the end of the 12-month period to review data and program evaluations and discuss strategic planning.

A web-based care management software program has been designed for use exclusively by GRACE programs. The software enables the GRACE Support Team to develop an individualized care plan through the selection of GRACE protocols and corresponding team suggestions (Fig. 10.4). The care plan can be downloaded, printed, and shared with the primary care physician and other providers (Fig. 10.5).

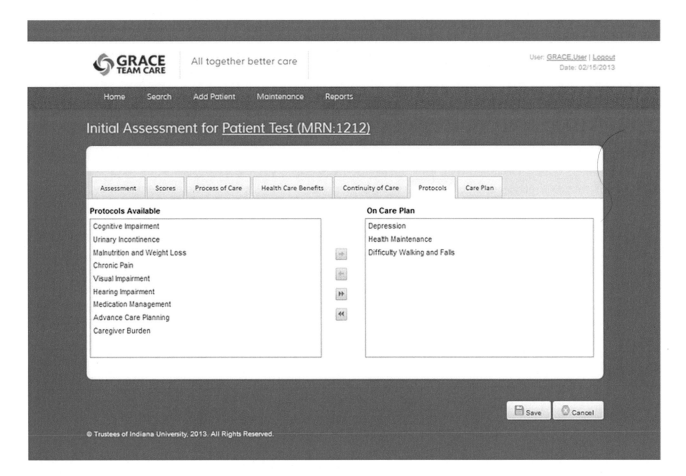

Fig. 10.4 GRACE Team Care management software (From IU Geriatrics GRACE Training and Resource Center, The Trustees of Indiana University, with permission.)

Team Suggestions Report

Depression - Priority 1		
Contributing Factors: Family Problems, Social Isolation, Infrequent Use of Anti-Depressant, Other?		
Review with PCP		
Code	Suggestion	Status
DEP-100	Review and confirm diagnosis and potential contributing causes; update problem list in computerized medical record as appropriate.	In Progress
DEP-120	Consider discontinuing the following medication that may be contributing to depression: _____ .	In Progress
DEP-122	Consider starting Sertraline.	In Progress
DEP-140	Consider Geriatrics Consult in the IU - Center for Senior Health for further evaluation and management of depression.	In Progress
CUST-29	Assist patient in re-connecting with daugther out-of-state.	In Progress
Routine Team Interventions		
Code	Suggestion	Status
DEP-200	Monitor for suicidal ideation and/or psychosis.	In Progress
DEP-201	Monitor for caregiver stress.	In Progress
DEP-221	Encourage participation in local senior center and social activities.	In Progress
DEP-	Encourage participation in volunteer activities.	In Progress

Fig. 10.5 GRACE Interdisciplinary Team care plan (From IU Geriatrics GRACE Training and Resource Center, The Trustees of Indiana University, with permission.)

The care plan can also be scanned or uploaded into the health system's EMR. The software offers a platform for the GRACE Support Team to track the implementation of the care plan including noting which interventions are "done," "in progress," "not done-patient disagrees," and "not done-physician disagrees." The ability for the GRACE team to add real-time updates to the care plan allow for the care plan to serve as a living, up-to-date tool rather than a static document. Report functions in the software assist with tracking of care plan review schedules and team member case loads.

Having the ability to connect with GRACE trainers and access tools and forms has proven to be a valuable resource to GRACE team members during program implementation.

Through the GRACE Team Care website (http://graceteam-care.indiana.edu), training participants can access the Member Forum (Fig. 10.6). The Member Forum provides participants with access to a host of tools and resources including job descriptions, implementation checklists, enrollment criteria, GRACE protocols, assessment forms, and business case materials (Table 10.11). Additionally, the Member Forum features an "Ask A Question" portal where participants can submit questions to GRACE trainers via an online bulletin board. Providing a range of training and technical assistance offerings that can be customized for each organization enable replication partners to successfully implement the GRACE model while achieving "all together better care."

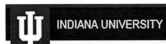
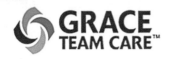
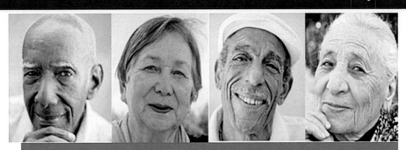

Home

About Us

Case for GRACE

Newsroom

Tools and Support

Contact Us

Member Forum

GRACE Team Care improves the health -- and lives -- of frail older adults with complex needs. Working together, a team of doctors, nurses, social workers, and pharmacists use geriatric knowledge and techniques to improve patient care -- not just in the clinic, but in the patient's home and community.

GRACE Team Care is proven to reduce costs by decreasing hospitalizations and readmissions, delaying nursing home admissions, and reducing emergency department visits.

Latest News:

Healthcare Business Today: Rethinking Care for Our Nation's Seniors

GRACE Team Care Announces Footprint in Michigan

GRACE Team Care Approach Cited Among Model Programs in New Avalere Health Study on Caring for High-Risk Seniors

Social Media:

FULFILLING the PROMISE

Fig 10.6 GRACE Team Care website home page (From GRACE Team Care [homepage on the Internet]. The Trustees of Indiana University; 2013 [updated 2015, January 12th]. Available from: http://graceteamcare.indiana.edu., with permission.)

Table 10.11 GRACE Training and Resource Center on-line tools

• Guidelines for steering committee and implementation teams
• GRACE team member job descriptions
• Implementation checklist
• Enrollment criteria (high-risk and transition)
• GRACE training manual
• Assessment forms
• GRACE protocols
• Primary care physician introduction materials
• GRACE business case guide
• Simple business case tool
• Professional development resources

From GRACE Team Care [homepage on the Internet]. The Trustees of Indiana University; 2013 [updated 2015, January 12th]. Available from: http://graceteamcare.indiana.edu, with permission

References

1. Counsell SR, Callahan CM, Buttar AB, Clark DO, Frank KI. Geriatric resources for assessment and care of elders (GRACE): a new model of primary care for low-income seniors. J Am Geriatr Soc. 2006;54:1136–41.
2. Institute of Medicine (IOM). Retooling for an aging America. Washington, DC: The National Academics Press; 2008.
3. Counsell SR, Callahan CM, Tu W, Stump TE, Arling GW. Cost analysis of the geriatric resources for assessment and care of elders care management intervention. J Am Geriatr Soc. 2009;57(8):1420–6.
4. Boult C, Wieland GD. Comprehensive primary care for older patients with multiple chronic conditions: "Nobody rushes you through". JAMA. 2010;304(17):1936–43.
5. Bielaszke-DuVernay C. The 'GRACE' model: in-home assessments lead to better care for dual eligibles. Health Aff. 2011;30(3):431–4.
6. IU Geriatrics GRACE Training and Resource Center. GRACE Team Care training manual. Bloomington, IN: Indiana University; 2013.
7. Counsell SR, Callahan CM, Clark DO, Tu W, Buttar AB, Stump TE, Ricketts GD. Geriatric care management for low-income seniors: a randomized controlled trial. JAMA. 2007;298(22):2623–33.
8. GRACE Team Care [homepage on the Internet]. Bloomington, IN: Indiana University; 2013 [updated 2015, January 12th]. http://graceteamcare.indiana.edu.
9. Counsell SR. Integrating medical and social services with GRACE. Generations. 2011;35(1):56–9.
10. Hong CS, Siegel AL, Ferris TG. Caring for high-need, high-cost patients: what makes for a successful care management program? New York, NY: The Commonwealth Fund; 2014.
11. Bodenheimer T. Strategies to reduce costs and improve care for high-utilizing medicaid patients: reflections on pioneering programs. San Francisco, CA: Center for Health Care Strategies; 2013.
12. Rodriguez S, Munevar D, Delaney C, Yang L, Tumlinson A. Effective management of high-risk medicare populations. Washington, DC: Avalere Health LLC; 2014.
13. Counsell SR, Holder CM, Liebenauer LL, et al. The acute care for elders (ACE) manual: meeting the challenge of providing quality and cost effective hospital care to older adults. Akron, OH: Summa Health System; 1998.
14. Counsell SR. Indiana University, Powerpoint Presentation.

"Guided Care" for People with Complex Health Care Needs

11

Chad Boult and Jennifer L. Wolff

Introduction

One-quarter (24 %) of Americans have two or more chronic conditions. Their health care is often fragmented, of low quality, inefficient, and unsatisfactory to them, their families, and their physicians. The Institute of Medicine has described chronic care in America as "a nightmare to navigate." People with multi-morbidity are also at high risk for generating high health care expenditures: 96 % of the US Medicare budget is spent on beneficiaries with multiple chronic conditions.

Several flaws in the infrastructure of the US health care system underlie these problems: inadequate professional education, inconsistent use of information technology, payment incentives that drive high-volume rather than high-quality or high-efficiency care, lack of financial support for inter-professional communication and patient engagement in self-care, and multiple barriers to partnering with and supporting family caregivers.

Correcting these flaws will require numerous long- and short-term initiatives. Reforming health professional education, implementing interoperable health information technology, and migrating the focus of health insurance away from fee-for-service payments toward "value-based" payments for quality and outcomes will take many years. In the meantime, however, as millions of baby boomers reach retirement age each year, near-term improvements may be achievable by developing and adopting clinical models that improve out-comes for people with multiple chronic conditions in spite of the system's current infrastructural flaws. Some such models have shown promise [1–4], while others have failed [5] or not yet been tested rigorously.

The Guided Care Model

Drawing from the chronic care model [6], guided care was designed to improve the quality of care and efficiency of resource use among older adults with complex health needs (Fig. 11.1).

In guided care, a registered nurse completes a 40-h online educational program and then works with two to five primary care physicians to meet the needs of 50–60 older patients with complex health care needs. Although the guided care nurse (GCN) supports patients across a range of institutional and community settings, the GCN is based in the primary care office to facilitate communication with the primary care physicians and office staff. The GCN's eight primary clinical activities, described below, are guided by scientific evidence and by patients' goals and priorities [7].

Patient and Family Caregiver Assessment

During an initial visit to the patient's home, the GCN begins by asking the patient to identify his or her goals and priorities for optimizing health and quality of life. Then the GCN assesses the patient's medical, functional, cognitive, affective, psychosocial, nutritional, and environmental status using standardized assessment instruments.

Care Planning

Based on the assessment results, the GCN then drafts a "preliminary care guide" that lists medical and behavioral plans for managing and monitoring each of the patient's chronic conditions to attain the patient's goals. The GCN and the

C. Boult, M.D., M.P.H., M.B.A. (✉)
Independent Consultant, 2290 N Broadview Pl,
Boise, ID 83702, USA
e-mail: chad.e.boult@gmail.com

J.L. Wolff, Ph.D.
Department of Health Policy and Management,
Johns Hopkins Bloomberg School of Public Health,
624 N. Broadway, Room 692, Baltimore, MD 21205, USA

Division of Geriatric Medicine and Gerontology, Johns Hopkins
University School of Medicine, Baltimore, MD, USA
e-mail: jwolff2@jhu.edu

Fig. 11.1 *Guided Care Elements* in the Chronic Care Model (from Boyd C, Boult C, Shadmi E, Leff B, Brager R, Dunbar L, et al. Guided Care for multi-morbid older adults. The Gerontologist. 2007;47(5):697–704 with permission)

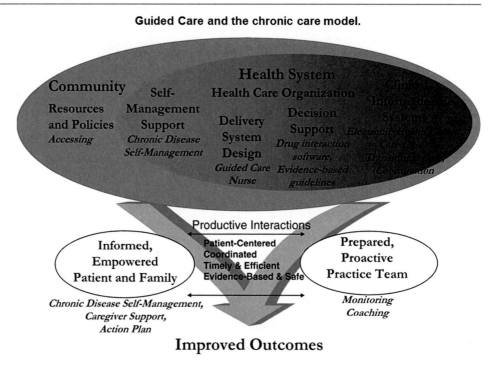

primary care physician then meet to discuss this preliminary care guide to align it with the circumstances of the patient. The GCN then discusses the preliminary care guide with the patient and the family caregiver, modifying it further for consistency with their goals, preferences, priorities, and intentions. The final care guide is a concise summary of the patient's status and care plans, which is later provided to all involved health care professionals. A patient-friendly version, called "My Action Plan," is written in lay language and displayed prominently in the patient's home. The GCN updates both documents as the patient's circumstances evolve.

Promotion of Self-Management

The GCN promotes the patient's self-efficacy in managing chronic conditions by referring him or her to a free, local, 15-h (six-session) course in "Chronic Disease Self-Management" (CDSM), if available, that is led by trained lay people and supported by the GCN. In this course, developed at Stanford University, the patient learns to refine and implement the action plan. Reinforced by simple, easy-to-read schedules and reminders, the action plan facilitates the patient's steps toward healthy eating, sleeping, exercising, and use of medication, as well as self-monitoring, using the health care system, and avoiding tobacco and alcohol abuse.

Monitoring Patients' Symptoms and Adherence

The GCN monitors each patient at least monthly by telephone to detect and address emerging problems promptly. When problems appear, the GCN discusses them with the primary care physician and takes appropriate action. In conjunction with the monthly monitoring calls, the GCN uses "motivational interviewing" to facilitate the patient's participation in care and to reinforce adherence to the action plan. The GCN expresses empathy, clarifies discrepancies between current behavior and health goals, seeks consensus, and supports self-efficacy.

Coordinating Providers of Care

Using the care guide as a communication tool, the GCN coordinates the efforts of all health care professionals involved in the patient's care across all care settings. Each patient is encouraged to share his or her care guide and action plan with their other health care providers and to inform his or her GCN of all encounters with other providers, so the GCN can track changes in plans and update the patient's care guide and action plan accordingly.

Smoothing Transitions Between Sites of Care

The GCN gives high priority to smoothing the patient's path between sites of care, focusing most intensively on transitions from hospitals to post-acute care, continually keeping the primary care physician informed of the patient's status. The GCN does not usurp the duties of other involved professionals, but instead provides each with current information about the patient, explains the GCN role, visits the patient in the hospital, and helps plan and execute post-acute care and return to the care of the primary care physician.

Supporting Family Caregivers

For the family caregivers of patients with functional impairment or difficulty with health care tasks, the GCN offers individual and group assistance: initial assessment, a free self-management course (10 h over 6 weeks), monthly support group meetings, and ad hoc telephone consultation [8].

Accessing Community Resources

The GCN facilitates access to community resources to meet the patient's and the family caregiver's needs. The GCN may suggest, for example, that the patient or family caregiver make use of a transportation service, Meals on Wheels, the Area Agency on Aging, or the local Alzheimer's Association.

Evidence That Guided Care Improves Outcomes

During 2006–2009, scientific investigators at the Johns Hopkins University conducted a matched-pair, cluster-randomized controlled trial of guided care versus "usual care" in eight community-based primary care practices operated by three large health care delivery systems in urban and suburban Baltimore, MD, and Washington, DC [9]. Six of the practices housed two teams apiece (two to five physicians per team); two of the practices, selected for their similarities, housed one team apiece. Three of the practices relied on capitated payments, while five received primarily fee-for-service payments. Additional study details are available in the scientific literature [10].

Selection of Physician Teams

Within the three delivery systems, teams of eligible physicians with panels of at least 400 patients aged 65 years or older and on-site office space for a GCN were eligible for the study. Primary care physicians within these teams were eligible to participate if they were board-certified general internists or family physicians who provided patient care at least 28 h per week. All 49 physicians within the 14 eligible teams agreed to participate.

Recruitment of Nurses

Applications from licensed registered nurses with at least 3 years of clinical experience were solicited by advertisements in local newspapers, the websites of the three participating delivery systems, and a regional nursing journal. Applicants with experience in geriatric nursing, interest in counseling patients in self-management, and comfort with interdisciplinary practice and information technology were given preference. Among the seven nurses hired, all were female, three were African-Americans, and four were Whites. The average age was 45 years (range = 32–57 years); the average nursing practice experience was 16 years (range = 4–31 years).

Recruitment of Patients

The physicians' patients were selected for initial screening if they were 65+ years old and insured through fee-for-service Medicare Parts A and B, a Kaiser Medicare health plan, or TriCare. Patients' health insurance claims from the previous 12 months were analyzed using the Hierarchical Condition Category (HCC) predictive model, which uses diagnosis codes to estimate a person's risk for generating high health care expenditures during the coming year. Patients were potentially eligible if their HCC risk scores were in the highest quartile of the population of older patients covered by their health care insurer.

High-risk patients were initially contacted by mail. A professional interviewer then called those who had not "opted out" to describe the study, answer questions, and offer an in-home enrollment meeting. At the enrollment meeting, interviewers described the study further, answered questions, and obtained written informed consent. Potential participants were deemed ineligible if they did not have a telephone, did not speak English, were planning extended travel, or failed a brief cognitive screen and did not have a proxy who could provide consent.

Randomization

Each team of physicians and their participating patients comprised a "pod." The study's statistician, blinded to the identities of the pods, used a random number generator to assign one pod from each pair (matched by practice) to the guided care group and the other to the "usual care" control group.

Results

Patients in 14 pods ($n = 13,534$) were screened, and the 2,391 (17.7 %) who were eligible and available were offered study participation [9]. Of these, 904 (37.8 %) gave informed consent and were allocated to receive either guided care ($n = 485$) or usual care ($n = 419$). At baseline, the study participants' sociodemographic, functional, and health-related characteristics were similar, except that the "usual care" control group had slightly worse finances, physical and mental health, and IADL function, but its average risk of health care utilization was lower.

More than half (56.5 %) of all guided care recipients and 48.4 % of all usual care recipients completed the final interview. Complete claims data were available for 92.0 and 95.9 % of the guided care and usual care participants, respectively.

After 32 months, the adjusted aggregate quality of chronic care was reported to be significantly higher by patients with guided care than those with usual care (difference = 0.27; 95 % CI: 0.08–0.45). Guided care recipients were also more likely to report "excellent or very good" access to telephone advice (OR = 1.66; 95 % CI: 1.02–2.73) and being "very satisfied" with the care they received from their "regular" (primary) care teams, but this difference was not statistically significant (OR = 1.50; 95 % CI: 0.77–2.82).

Guided care had no statistically significant effects on self-rated health or on scores on the SF-36 mental health or physical health subscales. Compared to the usual care group, the guided care group used home health care at a 29 % lower rate (ratio = 0.71; 95 % CI: 0.51–0.97). Reductions of 6–26 % in the guided care group's utilization of hospitals and skilled nursing facilities did not reach traditional levels of statistical significance.

Physicians' satisfaction with their communications with patients and families and their satisfaction with management of chronic care increased relative to baseline more among physicians providing guided care than among physicians providing usual care, and these differences increased over time. As compared with usual care, staff members in guided care practices were more likely to report that the care provided to patients with complex health needs was patient centered [11].

Family caregivers' reports of the quality of the chronic illness care provided to their care recipients were higher with guided care than with usual care after 18 months of follow-up (aβ = 0.40; 95 % CI = 0.14–0.67), a difference that was statistically significant ($p < 0.001$) [12].

Implementation in the Real World

Guided care improves the quality of chronic care, but the degree to which it reduces the utilization and costs of health care remains uncertain. The significant savings from reductions in the use of home health care would help to offset the costs of the intervention, but concomitant reductions (suggested, but not statistically significant in this small sample) in the use of hospitals and skilled nursing facilities would probably be necessary for the model to break even or reduce high-risk patients' net health care costs.

What lessons can we learn from this body of recent research that will help inform the next generation of comprehensive, interdisciplinary primary care for high-risk patients? Certain features are common to many of the more successful models, including systematic identification (and intensive management) of high-risk patients; primary care physicians collaborating with on-site registered nurses and other clinical staff members (all working in redefined roles "at the tops of their licenses"); health information technology that facilitates care coordination; engagement of patients and their family caregivers in self-management; easy 24/7/365 access to primary care for emerging problems; well-coordinated transitional care following hospital discharges; and the integration of community-based social and support services into health care.

Unfortunately, even models that have provided many of these features have produced only modest improvements in clinical and financial outcomes. Additional features, which have not been tested empirically but which could facilitate better outcomes in the chronic care models of the future, include well-run quality improvement processes in primary care practices; home tele-monitoring; close supervision of care managers to ensure their adherence to the model's priorities; and meaningful, risk-adjusted financial incentives for providers who provide high-quality care and achieve above-average outcomes with high-risk patients.

Accountable care organizations, comprehensive primary care providers, medical homes, and other health care delivery organizations are most likely to achieve meaningful improvements in chronic care by adopting (and judiciously adapting) care models with as many of these features as they can afford. Meanwhile, pragmatic studies of newer technologies, payment schemes, and models of chronic care will make further contributions to this rapidly evolving field. A wide range of innovations will be needed to create an economically sustainable system of health care and social services capable of meeting the rapidly growing, complex, health-related needs of the aging American population [9].

Barriers to Implementation

Practices and organizations that are interested in adopting this model need to determine whether they can meet five requirements.

1. *Panel size*: large enough to contain 50–60 patients with several chronic conditions. Panels of at least 300 Medicare patients are usually sufficient. Practices with larger panels may be able to support more than one GCN. Practices

with smaller panels could share a GCN if they were in close proximity to each other.

2. *Office space*: a small, private, centrally located office for the nurse. An ideal location is near the physicians' offices with convenient access to the practice's staff, medical records, supplies, and office equipment.

3. *Health information technology*: a locally installed or Web-based health information technology system that supports the GCN's activities.

4. *Commitment*: Practice's physicians and office staff members need to work collaboratively with the GCN. Integration of a new type of health care provider into a primary care practice is a process that requires careful planning, optimism, open communication, honest feedback, flexibility, perseverance, and patience.

5. *Supplemental revenue*: Guided care generates significant costs for the practice: the nurse's salary and benefits, office space, equipment (i.e., computer, cell phone), communication services (i.e., cell phone service, access to the Internet), and travel costs. To adopt guided care, a practice must be confident that it will receive a supplemental revenue stream that will offset these costs, e.g., risk-adjusted capitation payments.

Steps Toward Implementing the Guided Care Model

Most primary care practices can fully implement guided care in 6–9 months. There are five critical steps in implementing guided care.

1. Preparing the physicians and office staff

   It is important to introduce guided care to the physicians and the practice staff and to describe how it will work in the practice. Staff members should understand that they will need to adjust some established roles and procedures to collaborate effectively with the GCN. Some of the information that should be communicated is described in Table 11.1.

Physicians are involved in hiring, orienting, and evaluating the nurse, and are responsible for communicating regularly with the nurse about their patients and their teamwork. Table 11.2 provides a summary of the physicians' roles and responsibilities.

2. Identifying patients who are likely to benefit from guided care

   The practice's 20–25 % of patients who have the highest estimated likelihood of incurring high health care cost are identified, usually by analyzing older patients' previous 12 months of health insurance claims with a predictive model, such as the Hierarchical Condition Category [13], which is available in the public domain. Although clinicians are capable of identifying patients with multi-morbidity, electronic predictive models can identify such patients more objectively, consistently, and efficiently.

3. Hiring the nurse

   The next step is to hire a registered nurse who has completed an accredited course in Guided Care Nursing and earned a Certificate in Guided Care Nursing. To attract strong applicants, the practice should offer a salary that is competitive with local hospital and home health care employers. See Table 11.3 for required and desirable qualities of GCN applicants.

4. Integrating the nurse into the practice

   A practice leader is responsible for orienting the nurse to the people and procedures of the practice, and for orienting the physicians and other staff members to the nurse and to the operational details of how guided care will work in the practice. The goals of the orientation are for the nurse to begin to develop effective teamwork with the physicians and staff members, as well as to become familiar with office procedures and health-related resources in the local community.

   To begin building the essential nurse-physician teamwork, it is important that the nurse meet with each physician to define the many processes that they will soon conduct as a team; see Table 11.2. To build teamwork as

Table 11.1 Discussion outline for preparing physicians and office staff

Guided care introduction	Inform staff members that the practice has committed to adopting guided care
	Explain the practice's rationale for adopting guided care
	Acknowledge that change is difficult and slow, but produces benefits in the long run
	Confirm that attendees have received a written description of guided care
Describe how guided care will work in the practice	Discuss how guided care is funded
	Describe plans for hiring the nurse(s), identifying eligible patients, communicating with patients, and equipping office space
	Describe how the practice will orient the nurse and hold meetings of the GCN and the office staff
Questions	Discuss the staff's concerns and questions about guided care

Table 11.2 The physician and GCN roles and responsibilities in guided care

Nurse selection (see Table 11.3)	Each physician with whom the nurse will work should review resumes, conduct interviews, and participate in the ranking of applicants
Nurse orientation	Each physician should meet with the nurse several times during the nurse's orientation to define how they will work together to care for patients. The physicians should also introduce the guided care patients to the nurse during routine office visits and allow the nurse to observe the physician's style of interacting with these patients and their family caregivers
Building the caseload	The physician meets with the nurse for 20–25 min per patient to discuss and revise the preliminary care guide that the nurse creates following the initial home assessment
Updating each other about the status of patients	The GCN provides the physician with a current list of their mutual guided care patients
	The GCN notifies the physician of significant changes in their mutual patients' status, especially changes occurring between office visits and during care in hospitals and skilled nursing facilities
	The physician notifies the nurse of changes in their mutual patients' status, especially admissions to hospitals, visits to emergency departments, and referrals to specialists
	Depending on personal preferences, notifications could occur by e-mail, voice mail, hard copy notes, direct conversations, and/or entries in the medical record
Providing care collaboratively	The GCN and physician discuss and modify the preliminary care guides of patients who enroll in guided care
	The nurse joins the physician in the examining room during office visits, especially with patients who have acute problems or difficulty with communication, cognition, and/or adherence or who have recently received care in hospitals or emergency departments
Quality improvement processes	The GCN and the physician discuss ways to improve their guided care teamwork and the nurse attends appropriate office staff meetings

Table 11.3 Required and desirable qualities of GCN applicants

The minimum requirements for people who apply for the GCN position are:

- Current licensure as a registered nurse
- Completion of an accredited, online course in Guided Care Nursing. For information on the course, please visit https://www.ijhn-education.org/content/guided-care-nursing
- A Certificate in Guided Care Nursing. To earn the certificate, a nurse must successfully complete the Guided Care Nursing online course. The certificate could be earned between a nurse's hiring and starting to work in a guided care practice
- A minimum of 3 years of nursing experience, preferably with older patients
- Skill in using computers, the Internet, and health information technology
- Ability to travel frequently to hospitals, skilled nursing facilities, patients' homes, and other sites where patients receive care (as indicated by patients' needs)

Other desirable qualities include:

- Excellent interpersonal skills
- Flexible and creative problem-solving skills
- Good clinical judgment and decision-making skills
- Demonstrated ability to work independently and as a member of an interdisciplinary team
- Clear understanding of the role of a GCN
- Desire to learn and practice all of the position's components
- Commitment to "coaching" (rather than "teaching") patients to improve their health behaviors to attain their health-related goals
- Commitment to learning about and referring patients to health-related services in the local community
- Effective skills in oral and written communication, listening, and assertion

a new member of the office staff, the nurse meets with each office staff member to learn each person's role and the administrative relationships among them.

5. Managing guided care

The success of guided care depends heavily on the physicians' cooperation with the GCN and the GCN's consistent performance of certain essential activities. To ensure consistent performance of essential activities, the practice should participate in a system of continuous quality improvement. The GCN's supervisor should provide the GCN with a list of essential guided care activities, a performance goal for each activity, a description of how the nurse should document each activity, and a schedule of quarterly feedback and evaluation meetings. The supervisor should then manage the ongoing processes of guided care, attending watchfully to the GCN's rates of completion of monthly patient monitoring calls and visitation of hospitalized patients, both in the hospital and at home shortly after discharge. Periodic surveys to ascertain patients,' caregivers', and physicians' perceptions of the quality of care can also be used to ensure that guided care is producing the desired effects on chronic care.

Technical Assistance in Adopting Guided Care

Several forms of technical assistance are available [14] to practices that wish to adopt the guided care model.

- An implementation manual titled *Guided Care: A New Nurse-Physician Partnership in Chronic Care* provides many tools, resources, and lessons learned for adopting guided care [15].
- An accredited, online course in Guided Care Nursing is a 6-week, 40-h Web-based course and examination that lead to a Certificate in Guided Care Nursing.
- An accredited, asynchronous, online, CME-eligible, nine-module course provides physicians, practice administrators, and other practice leaders with an awareness of the competencies that facilitate effective practice within all types of medical homes.

Acknowledgments These studies of guided care were supported by grants from the Agency for Healthcare Research and Quality, the National Institute on Aging, the John A. Hartford Foundation, and the Jacob and Valeria Langeloth Foundation—and by in-kind contributions from Johns Hopkins HealthCare, Johns Hopkins Community Physicians, Kaiser Permanente Mid-Atlantic States, MedStar Physician Partners, and the Roger C. Lipitz Center for Integrated Health Care.

References

1. Counsell SR, Callahan CM, Tu W, Stump TE, Arling GW. Cost analysis of the geriatric resources for assessment and care of elders care management intervention. J Am Geriatr Soc. 2009;57(8):1420–6. Epub 2009/08/20.
2. Reid RJ, Coleman K, Johnson EA, Fishman PA, Hsu C, Soman MP, et al. The Group Health medical home at year two: cost savings, higher patient satisfaction, and less burnout for providers. Health Aff. 2010;29(5):835–43. Epub 2010/05/05.
3. Wennberg DE, Marr A, Lang L, O'Malley S, Bennett G. A randomized trial of a telephone care-management strategy. N Engl J Med. 2010;363(13):1245–55. Epub 2010/09/24.
4. Boult C, Green A, Boult L, Pacala J, Snyder C, Leff B. Successful models of comprehensive care for older adults with chronic conditions: evidence for the Institute of Medicine's "retooling for an aging America" report. J Am Geriatr Soc. 2009;57(12):2328–37. Epub 2010/02/04.
5. Peikes D, Chen A, Schore J, Brown R. Effects of care coordination on hospitalization, quality of care, and health care expenditures among Medicare beneficiaries: 15 randomized trials. JAMA. 2009;301(6):603–18. Epub 2009/02/13.
6. Wagner E. Chronic disease management: what will it take to improve care for chronic illness? Eff Clin Pract. 1998; 1(1):2–4.
7. Boyd C, Boult C, Shadmi E, Leff B, Brager R, Dunbar L, et al. Guided care for multi-morbid older adults. Gerontologist. 2007;47(5):697–704.
8. Wolff J, Rand-Giovanetti E, Palmer S, Wegener S, Reider L, Frey K, et al. Caregiving and chronic care: the guided care program for families and friends. J Gerontol A Biol Sci Med Sci. 2009;64(7):785–91.
9. Boult C, Leff B, Boyd CM, Wolff JL, Marsteller JA, Frick KD, et al. A matched-pair cluster-randomized trial of guided care for high-risk older patients. J Gen Intern Med. 2013;28(5):612–21. Epub 2013/01/12.
10. Boult C, Reider L, Frey K, Leff B, Boyd C, Wolff J, et al. Early effects of "Guided Care" on the quality of health care for multimorbid older persons: a cluster-randomized controlled trial. J Gerontol A Biol Sci Med Sci. 2008;63A(3):321–7.
11. Marsteller JA, Hsu YJ, Wen M, Wolff J, Frick K, Reider L, et al. Effects of guided care on providers' satisfaction with care: a three-year matched-pair cluster-randomized trial. Population health management. 2013. Epub 2013/04/09.
12. Wolff J, Giovannetti E, Boyd C, Reider L, Palmer S, Scharfstein D, et al. Effects of guided care on family caregivers. Gerontologist. 2010;50(4):459–70. Epub 2009/08/28.
13. Pope G, Kautter J, Ellis R, Ash A, Ayanian J, Lezzoni L, et al. Risk adjustment of medicare capitation payments using the CMS-HCC model. Health Care Financ Rev. 2004;25(4):119–41.
14. MedHomeInfo. Baltimore, MD: Johns Hopkins University. 2009. http://www.medhomeinfo.org/ (2009). Accessed 10 Aug 2014.
15. Boult C, Giddens J, Frey K, Reider L, Novak T. Guided care: a new nurse-physician partnership in chronic care. New York, NY: Springer Publishing Company; 2009.

Chronic Disease Self-Management Education: Program Success and Future Directions

12

Marcia G. Ory, SangNam Ahn, Samuel D. Towne Jr., and Matthew Lee Smith

Self-management is increasingly recognized as an essential element for improving chronic illness care in America [1]. The accumulating knowledge base provides the field with a greater understanding about the different aspects of self-management [2], an inventory of evidence-based programs for enhancing self-management behaviors [3], and guidelines of how such models can be better integrated within geriatric care programs [4].

The Stanford Chronic Disease Self-Management Program (CDSMP), the flagship CDSME program, is one of the most widely tested and disseminated self-management models. It is becoming a model for geriatric practice and increasingly being delivered to older patients with a wide array of chronic conditions [5]. This chapter addresses several questions about the application of CDSME programs designed to help older adults and their caregivers deal with chronic conditions. While the primary focus will be on the broadly disseminated small group Stanford CDSMP, it is important to note that the entire suite of Stanford self-management programs share a common philosophy and approach to self-management. Hence, basic information will be reported about the suite of programs.

Setting

While CDSMP was first developed and delivered in California [6, 7], it has now been delivered across the USA and in over 30 countries worldwide [8]. In the USA, as part of the funding for the American Recovery and Reinvestment Act of 2009 (ARRA), CDSMP has been widely disseminated through a diverse delivery infrastructure involving community and clinical sectors. In approximately 2 years, as indicated in a national review of CDSME programs [9], 100,000 participants were enrolled in 8,702 workshops in 5,586 unique implementation sites across 1,786 counties. The majority of participants enrolled in Chronic Disease Self-Management Program (CDSMP) workshops (78.4 %). Diabetes Self-Management Program (DSMP) workshops and Tomando Control de su Salud (Spanish CDSMP) workshops were also popular, accounting for 20 % of the participants. The five most common delivery sites were senior centers or Area Agencies on Aging (29.2 %), health care organizations (21.1 %), residential facilities (17.6 %), community/multipurpose facilities (9.9 %), and faith-based organizations (8.4 %). Other settings included correctional facilities, malls, RV parks, fire departments, county administration buildings, private residences, casinos, and career centers. The majority of participants attended workshops delivered in English (89.6 %) and in metro settings (79.6 %).

Consistent with the ARRA initiative goals [10], the dissemination of CDSMP placed importance on establishing better coordination between community and clinical settings and emphasized increasing referrals from primary care settings. While CDSMP is often offered in residential care facilities such as senior housing and assisted living, it is not seen as an appropriate intervention for skilled nursing facilities, given that most care recipients are cognitively impaired.

M.G. Ory, Ph.D., M.P.H. (✉)
Health Promotion and Community Health Sciences, School of Public Health at Texas A&M Health Science Center, TAMU 1266, College Station, TX 77843-1266, USA
e-mail: mory@sph.tamhsc.edu; mory@tamu.edu

S. Ahn, Ph.D.
Department of Health Systems Management and Policy, The University of Memphis School of Public Health, The University of Memphis, 133 Robison Hall, Memphis, TN 38152-3330, USA
e-mail: sahn@memphis.edu

S.D. Towne Jr., Ph.D., M.P.H., C.P.H.
Health Promotion and Community Health Sciences, Texas A&M Health Science Center, 1266 TAMU, College Station, TX 77843-1266, USA
e-mail: towne@sph.tamhsc.edu

M.L. Smith, Ph.D., M.P.H., C.H.E.S.
Department of Health Promotion and Behavior, The University of Georgia College of Public Health, 330 River Road, 315 Ramsey Center, Athens, GA 30602, USA
e-mail: health@uga.edu

M.L. Malone et al. (eds.), *Geriatrics Models of Care: Bringing 'Best Practice' to an Aging America*, DOI 10.1007/978-3-319-16068-9_12, © Springer International Publishing Switzerland 2015

Additionally, since CDSMP involves multiple interactions over time (typically six workshop sessions hosted over a 6-week period), it is also not appropriate for in-patient hospital settings.

Problem to be Addressed

Self-care or self-management is now seen as an adjunct to health care, with patient empowerment included as a major component of the National Prevention Strategy [1]. CDSMP is based on the premise that the majority of health care is what individuals do for themselves outside of traditional clinical settings. CDSMP addresses the fundamental problem of helping the growing number of individuals with chronic disease(s) gain skills and confidence to live healthier lives [11]. This is especially important given the shortage of geriatricians and other health care professionals available to treat the rapidly growing population of aging Americans [12]. While national dissemination efforts have extended to adults residing in health professional shortage areas, individuals living in more remote areas where the entire county was designated as a health professional shortage area were less likely to complete workshops (i.e., indicating less intervention dose was received) [13]. Thus, more work is needed to identify strategies to improve delivery, recruitment, and successful completion of programs to monitor national dissemination efforts.

Patients Who Benefit

Designed to accommodate a wide range of patients with a variety of chronic conditions, the generic and disease-specific versions of CDSMP have benefitted persons with multiple chronic conditions as well as those with specific conditions common in old age such as heart disease, diabetes, or arthritis [5]. Additionally, recent studies demonstrate benefits to those who are depressed or experience mental health problems [14]. Recent national studies also indicate health and health care benefits among participants from diverse socioeconomic backgrounds [15]. For example, the program attracts and benefits participants from disadvantaged educational and income backgrounds as well as those from underserved geographical areas (e.g., rural settings) or racial/ethnic groups [16]. For groups with low literacy, lay leaders can adapt classes to minimize reading. While the average age of participants in the national study was 65, younger participants also enroll and report positive outcomes [17]. The program has had more difficulties recruiting men and those from rural areas, but those who do enroll experience health improvements [15]. Given the emphasis on group interaction that includes problem solving, decision making,

and action planning, adults with marked cognitive impairment are assumed to do less well in CDSMP workshops. Hence, program developers discourage participation from those with dementia and recruitment from nursing homes and skilled nursing facilities.

Model Overview

The CDSMP is part of a larger suite of chronic disease self-management education (CDSME) programs offered by Stanford University Patient Education and Research Center [5]. Some of the programs are disease specific (e.g., diabetes, arthritis, HIV, cancer, chronic pain), while others are more general in nature (e.g., CDSMP). Programs are offered in English and Spanish (e.g., Tomando Control de su Salud, Tomando Control de su Diabetes). The format of these programs varies, with small group programs representing the vast majority. Programs are also offered via the Internet and mail.

All CDSME programs are based on Social Learning Theory [18] and emphasize skill-driven processes of problem solving, decision making, goal setting, and action planning. Small group workshops with about 10–15 participants consist of six sessions held once a week for 2.5 h each over 6 consecutive weeks. The workshops cover a range of topics intended to empower participants by helping them develop self-management skills to take care of their chronic conditions outside of traditional health care settings. Figure 12.1 illustrates the topics covered over the 6-week intervention.

The workshops are hosted by two trained facilitators, many of whom have a chronic condition themselves. Peer lay leaders use a uniform manual when hosting a workshop to ensure program consistency. Each participant also receives a book containing general information related to the session content and serves as a resource throughout the workshop [11]. Table 12.1 displays the basic elements of CDSME programs.

CDSMP utilizes a train-the-trainer model where certified Master Trainers (MTs) conduct trainings to certify lay leader workshop facilitators. The small group format provides participants with high levels of both instrumental and emotional support and holds participants accountable for completing behavioral assignments. Further, lay leaders delivering CDSMP have access to various resources and tools that can be individualized to help participants overcome barriers and remain committed to the program. MTs are typically sent to Stanford to receive Master Training, or such trainings can be held by T-Trainers at local sites (depending on the availability of T-Trainers in a given state). Once Master Trained, MTs can be cross-trained and certified to host other programs in the CDSME program suite. To grow the CDSMP delivery infrastructure, MTs can host lay leader trainings to expand

	Week 1	Week 2	Week 3	Week 4	Week 5	Week 6
Overview of self-management and chronic health conditions	★					
Making an action plan	★	★	★	★	★	★
Relaxation/cognitive symptom management	★		★	★	★	★
Feedback/problem-solving		★	★	★	★	★
Difficult emotions		★	★			
Fitness/exercise		★	★			
Better breathing			★			
Fatigue			★			
Eating well				★		
Advance directives				★		
Communication				★		
Medications					★	
Making treatment decisions					★	
Depression					★	
Informing the health care team						★
Working with your health care professional						★
Future plans						★

Fig. 12.1 Topical overview by weekly session

Table 12.1 Basic elements of the CDSME program model

Uses structured protocol that outlines content and methods
Train-the-trainer model
Emphasis on group participation, problem solving, decision making, goal setting, and action planning
2½-h group sessions that meet once per week for 6 consecutive weeks (incorporates a CD and participant book)
Uses two trained lay leaders in each workshop
Targets people with any chronic condition
Works to increase self-efficacy through skill mastery, modeling, reinterpreting symptoms, and persuasion
Fidelity monitoring protocol

the number of lay leaders in a particular community. Lay leaders can facilitate CDSMP workshops, but they cannot train others.

Program Fidelity

Maintaining fidelity during program implementation is an integral part of delivering the program successfully [19]. Translational studies especially emphasize the importance of maintaining fidelity, which can be defined as the adherence of actual treatment delivery to the protocol originally developed [20]. Failure to secure fidelity raises many questions about the validity of the intervention outcomes [21].

In recognition of its dissemination across time and space by different parties, CDSMP program developers have created multiple systems to maintain fidelity of program delivery. First, a centralized training and certification system (http://patienteducation.stanford.edu/programs/cdsmp.html) can support programmatic adherence to implementation aspects of CDSMP. As an example, certified lay leaders from organizations with licensure to operate CDSMP learn its content and structure using the standardized resource materials including CDSMP leader manual and a textbook [11]. At the same time, more detailed fidelity guidance is provided in the CDSMP Fidelity Manual (http://patienteducation.stanford.edu/licensing/FidelityManual2012.pdf). This manual provides a fidelity checklist of what should be done before, during, and after the sessions by different key players in the implementation and dissemination of CDSMP.

Barriers to Implementation

Given the diverse composition of the middle-aged and older adult population, there are many competing demands when selecting and subsequently implementing community-based health and wellness programs. With the array of Tier I evidence-based programs endorsed by the National Council on Aging [22], communities have the freedom to select programs that best match their community's needs. As such, CDSMP may not always be the obvious program choice in all communities. Often there are difficulties reaching especially vulnerable populations with chronic conditions. Individuals who are homebound or reside in remote areas may not have access to CDSMP, even when it is offered in their community. Additionally, there are licensing and delivery costs associated with CDSMP listed at http://patienteducation.stanford.edu/licensing/. The range of costs to deliver the intervention are based on whether or not the program has been delivered in the community previously (i.e., has a history and already accounted for the one-time start-up costs), the number of participants served, and the number of participants enrolled in each workshop. For some communities, the costs associated with CDSMP delivery may be perceived as too great. These communities may select other interventions without licensure requirements and lower delivery costs.

Outcomes to Be Monitored

The Stanford Patient Education Research Center [23] provides a list of standardized evaluation tools for assessing program impact. These include measures of self-management behaviors, self-efficacy, health status, and health care utilization. For use in community and clinical settings, we recommend pragmatic measurements [24] that are not burdensome to collect but that can help program administrators understand who is being reached, the extent to which participants attend the different workshop sessions, and outcomes of interest to different stakeholders. From a practice and policy point of view, it may be useful to assess the extent to which CDSMP helps achieve the triple aims of health care reform [25]. Of particular relevance to geriatric care is the extent to which there is improved coordination between different care sectors, and specifically improved doctor-patient communications.

Evidence of Benefits

CDSMP earned its evidence-based title after successfully conducting a randomized controlled trial in the late 1990s. Dr. Kate Lorig, the program developer of CDSMP, conducted a 6-month randomized controlled trial and found that CDSMP participants demonstrated improvements in exercise, cognitive symptom management, communication with physicians, self-reported health, health distress, fatigue, disability, and social/role activity limitations [6]. In her 2-year follow-up study, CDSMP participants maintained their increase in self-efficacy and decreased their health distress and emergency room (ER)/outpatient visits [7]. Nevertheless, the 10-year-old findings necessitated reexamination of the effectiveness of CDSMP, especially in light of the

widespread dissemination of CDSMP under the ARRA initiatives.

The *National Study of CDSMP* ($n = 1,170$), conducted from 2010 to 2012 among 22 licensed sites in 17 states, tested the effectiveness of the CDSMP by evaluating if CDSMPs could accomplish the *Triple Aim* goals emphasized by the Affordable Care Act [15]. Berwick and his colleagues [25] argued that improving the US health care system requires simultaneous pursuit of three goals (i.e., *Triple Aims*) including improving the experience of care (i.e., better care), improving the health of populations (i.e., better health), and reducing per capita costs of health care (i.e., better value). With regard to better care, CDSMP study participants in the *National Study* displayed improvements in communication with physicians, medication compliance, and health literacy between baseline and 12-month follow-up. In terms of better health, CDSMP study participants demonstrated improvements in self-assessed health, fatigue, pain, depression, and unhealthy physical and mental health days between baseline and 6- and 12-month follow-ups. Regarding better value, CDSMP study participants reported a 5 % reduction in ER visits between baseline and 6-month follow-up as well as another 5 % reduction between baseline and 12-month follow-up. Study participants also reported a 3 % reduction in hospitalization between baseline and 6-month follow-up. The better value component was further assessed to estimate health care cost savings. Reductions in ER visits and hospitalization among CDSMP participants could equate to potential net savings of $364 per participant and a national savings of $3.3 billion if CDSMP could reach 5 % of American adults with at least one chronic condition [26].

Buy-In from Health System Leaders and Patients

In parallel with the ARRA initiatives [5], the aging services network has provided technical assistance to help community program managers learn how to make the business case for CDSMP and more effectively reach out to health care providers [27, 28]. However, more health care leaders need to be aware of benefits of patient referral and assured that there will be a consistent delivery system for continuous referral [15]. To help communities make the business case for CDSMP, a new health care cost savings estimator was developed to facilitate understanding about the cost-effectiveness of this intervention. The cost estimator tool can be tailored by users to ensure that the details of program delivery match their specific community and/or clinical setting [26]. As a patient empowerment model of care, CDSMP reflects a patient-centered approach in which patients helped design the CDSMP model of care, are often co-facilitators, and have an active voice in when and where workshops are being held.

Program Scalability

The CDSMP presents an excellent example of a research study being transformed into a scalable best practice. From its initial origins as a tightly controlled research study in California, it flourished with support from the Administration on Aging (AoA), which propelled dissemination through the aging services network with early evidence-based disease prevention initiatives to 14 communities, beginning in 2003. With additional AoA support from 2006 to 2009, CDSMP delivery grew to reach 28,855 participants in 27 states. Based on this success, additional federal support was received to disseminate CDSMP in 45 states and two territories, reaching over 160,000 participants from 2010 to 2013. While the delivery of CDSMP expanded substantially over the past decade, additional funding is needed to support ongoing efforts to reach the millions of adults with chronic conditions.

A variety of funding mechanisms exist to further support the growth of CDSMP to new markets. A new ruling for Area Agencies on Aging to direct their Title III-D health promotion dollars toward evidence-based programs that have been shown effective is likely to help sustain and grow CDSMP programming to even larger numbers of seniors. Having Medicare reimbursement (e.g., the Diabetes Self-Management Program is now eligible for Medicare funding) will help institutionalize self-management programs in clinical settings. As another example, the NIH and CDC are supporting efforts to learn more about CDSMP delivery among working-aged individuals in workplace settings (i.e., individuals less commonly reached by CDSMP because it is delivered through the aging services network).

To facilitate the embedment of CDSMP in communities across the USA, a variety of tools and resources have been created to educate decision makers and program administrators about the benefits of each evidence-based program and for whom it is most effective [22]. Further, these resources assist communities to learn "best practices" associated with gaining partner support, embedding CDSMP in multiple community sectors, recruiting and retaining participants, and seeking/securing funding to support implementation.

Integration with the Electronic Health Record

Electronic health records (EHRs) allow for integration of patient or resident medical/health information into an easily retrievable/accessible digital format [29]. For those with multiple chronic conditions, the use of EHRs is necessary to improve care transitions [30] and facilitate the provision of high-quality and efficient care [31–33]. Coordinating health care for those with chronic conditions is an essential concept conveyed to participants during CDSMP workshops. EHRs have the potential to serve as a way for physicians and patients to monitor self-management success. For example, the use of EHRs in diabetes coordinated care has been linked with improved health outcomes, better communication between providers, and better access to data [34]. Successful integration of EHRs and chronic disease management may be effective for electronic decision support [35]. Further investigations into this potential integration will be needed to determine potential benefits. Policies that support reimbursement for CDSME programs are critical to support future integrations with EHRs. For example, CDSMP has been supported via Medicaid waivers or Medicaid state plans [36]. Policy makers will need to continue to support CDSME programs if we are to extend the benefits of CDSME programs to greater numbers of participants throughout the nation.

Future Plans

The role of CDSMP is dynamic and evolving. CDSME programs have been met with great success in improving the lives of participants, enhancing health care, and curbing medical costs. There is a continual updating and expansion of CDSME programs through Stanford's Patient Education Research Center, as evidenced by the cancer-specific program being launched in 2015. The success of CDSME programs alone may be improved with the delivery of multiple complementary evidence-based programs, such as fall prevention or hands-on physical activity programs. Adults may suffer from multiple types of chronic conditions (e.g., diabetes, heart disease), many of which may be comorbid. Thus, many adults may benefit from programs that target multiple chronic conditions in a variety of ways [37]. The delivery of multiple evidence-based programs to vulnerable populations is currently under way throughout the USA, but is still limited [38]. Additional efforts are under way to translate CDSMP for implementation in workplace settings to expand the target market [39]. Continued monitoring over time will be needed to identify long-term success in the delivery of multiple types of evidence-based programs to meet the diverse needs of our aging population.

Application to the Patient Protection and Affordable Care Act

The Patient Protection and Affordable Care Act (2010), also known as the ACA, has several provisions that target the amelioration of chronic conditions. Title IV of the ACA, Prevention of Chronic Disease and Improving Public Health, includes provisions specific to evidence-based programs and older adults. For example, Section 4202 subsection (b) ACA directs the Secretary of the Department of Health and Human Services to develop a plan for promoting healthy lifestyles and chronic disease self-management for Medicare beneficiaries.

In addition to identifying evaluations of the effectiveness of evidence-based programs for improving health outcomes, one of the underlying goals of the ACA is to identify ways to lower health care costs and provide better value. This is evident with several provisions targeting prevention and wellness programs, accountable care organizations, value-based purchasing, and provider incentives for preventing potentially avoidable hospital readmissions [40]. All of these provisions affect older adults, specifically Medicare beneficiaries, either directly (e.g., waived co-payments for annual wellness visits) or indirectly (e.g., Medicare payment policies for hospital readmissions) [40]. CDSME programs are strategically positioned to target these goals of better health outcomes, lower cost, and better value. In particular, the CDSMP has been shown to improve health outcomes and lower hospitalizations, thereby potentially reducing health care costs [15]. Thus, CDSMP is a prime example of an evidence-based program integrating several goals of the ACA and the triple aims of health care reform.

Further supporting the growth and sustainability of CDSME is the articulation of a value proposition for self-management interventions. As stated by the Self-Management Alliance [41], "Self-management interventions create and sustain behavior change that improves chronic disease health outcomes and lowers health care costs." As such, the future supports the development of an infrastructure for supporting further growth and sustainability of CDSME programs.

Acknowledgements We acknowledge partial support from the South, West, and Central Consortium: Geriatric Education Center of Texas, Grant #99-500984. We thank Jessica Smarr and Rachel Coughlin for their editorial assistance.

References

1. National Prevention Council. National Prevention Strategy. In: Services US Department of Health and Human Services, editor. Washington, D.C.: Office of the Surgeon General; 2011.
2. Brady T, Murphy L, Beauchesne D, Bhalakia A, Chervin D, Daniels B, et al. sorting through the evidence for the arthritis self-management program and the chronic disease self-management program: Executive Summary of ASMP/CDSMP meta-analysis. 2011.
3. National Council on Aging. Title III-D highest tier evidence-based health promotion/disease prevention programs. 2014.
4. Ory MG, Smith ML, Patton K, Lorig K, Zenker W, Whitelaw N. Self-management at the tipping point: reaching 100,000 Americans with evidence-based programs. J Am Geriatr Soc. 2013;61(5):821–3.
5. Kulinski K, Boutaugh M, Smith ML, Ory MG, Lorig K. Setting the stage: measure selection, coordination, and data collection for a national self-management initiative. Frontiers in Public Health. 2015. In-press.
6. Lorig KR, Sobel DS, Stewart AL, Brown BWJ, Bandura A, Ritter P, et al. Evidence suggesting that a chronic disease self-management program can improve health status while reducing hospitalization: a randomized trial. Med Care. 1999;37(1):5–14.
7. Lorig KR, Ritter P, Stewart AL, Sobel DS, William Brown BJ, Bandura A, et al. Chronic disease self-management program: 2-year health status and health care utilization outcomes. Med Care. 2001;39(11):1217–23.
8. Stanford Patient Education Research Center. Organizations Licensed to Offer the Chronic Disease Self-Management Program (CDSMP). 2014.
9. Smith M, Ory, MG, Ahn, S, Kulinski, K, Jiang L, Lorig, K. National Dissemination of Chronic Disease Self-Management Education (CDSME) Programs: an incremental examination of delivery characteristics. Frontiers in Public Health Education and Promotion. 2015. In-press.
10. U.S. Department of Health and Human Services. ARRA - Communities Putting Prevention to Work: Chronic Disease Self-Management Program, vol. 93. Washington, DC; 2009. p. 725.
11. Lorig K. Living a healthy life with chronic conditions : self-management of heart disease, arthritis, diabetes, depression, asthma, bronchitis, emphysema, and other physical and mental health conditions. 4th ed. Boulder, CO: Bull Pub. Co.; 2012. vii, 343 p. p.
12. Lee W-C, Dooley KE, Ory MG, Sumaya CV. Meeting the geriatric workforce shortage for long-term care: opinions from the field. Gerontol Geriatr Educ. 2013;34(4):354–71.
13. Towne SD Jr, Smith ML, Ahn S, Ory MG. The reach of chronic disease self-management education programs to rural populations. Frontiers in Public Health: Public Health Education and Promotion. 2:172. 2015. In-press.
14. Lorig K, Ritter PL, Pifer C, Werner P. Effectiveness of the chronic disease self-management program for persons with a serious mental illness: a translation study. Community Ment Health J. 2014;50(1):96–103.
15. Ory M, Ahn S, Jiang L, Smith M, Ritter P, Whitelaw N, et al. Successes of a national study of the chronic disease self-management program: meeting the triple aim of health care reform. Med Care. 2013;51(11):992–8.
16. Ory M, Smith ML. Evidence-based programming for older adults. Frontiers in Public Health Education and Promotion. 2015. In-press.
17. Ory MG, Smith ML, Ahn S, Jiang L, Lorig K, Whitelaw N. National study of chronic disease self-management: age comparison of outcome findings. Health Educ Behav. 2014;41(1 Suppl):34S–42.
18. Bandura A. Social cognitive theory of self-regulation. Organ Behav Hum Decis Process. 1991;50(2):248–87.
19. Mowbray CT, Holter MC, Teague GB, Bybee D. Fidelity criteria: development, measurement, and validation. Am J Eval. 2003;24(3):315–40.
20. Borrelli B. The assessment, monitoring, and enhancement of treatment fidelity in public health clinical trials. J Public Health Dent. 2011;71(s1):S52–63.
21. Frank JC, Coviak CP, Healy TC, Belza B, Casado BL. Addressing fidelity in evidence-based health promotion programs for older adults. J Appl Gerontol. 2008;27(1):4–33.
22. National Council on Aging. Advantages of Evidence-Based Programs [cited 2014 October 10]. http://www.ncoa.org/improve-health/center-for-healthy-aging/advantages-of-evidence-based.html.

23. Stanford Patient Education Research Center. Program Fidelity Manual: Stanford Self-Management Programs 2012 Update. 2012.
24. Glasgow RE, Magid DJ, Beck A, Ritzwoller D, Estabrooks PA. Practical clinical trials for translating research to practice: design and measurement recommendations. Med Care. 2005;43(6):551–7.
25. Berwick DM, Nolan TW, Whittington J. The triple aim: care, health, and cost. Health Aff (Millwood). 2008;27(3):759–69.
26. Ahn S, Basu R, Smith M, Jiang L, Lorig K, Whitelaw N, et al. The impact of chronic disease self-management programs: healthcare savings through a community-based intervention. BMC Public Health. 2013;13(1):1141.
27. National Council on Aging. Evidence-based health promotion programs for older adults: key factors and strategies contributing to program sustainability. 2012.
28. National Council on Aging. Creating a business plan for evidence-based health promotion programs.
29. Kuperman GJ. Health-information exchange: why are we doing it, and what are we doing? J Am Med Inform Assoc. 2011;18(5):678–82.
30. Coleman EA. Falling through the cracks: challenges and opportunities for improving transitional care for persons with continuous complex care needs. J Am Geriatr Soc. 2003;51(4):549–55.
31. Brailer DJ. Interoperability: the key to the future health care system. Health Aff (Millwood). 2005;Suppl Web Exclusives:W5-19-W5-21.
32. Stewart BA, Fernandes S, Rodriguez-Huertas E, Landzberg M. A preliminary look at duplicate testing associated with lack of electronic health record interoperability for transferred patients. J Am Med Inform Assoc. 2010;17(3):341–4.
33. Hamilton B. Evaluation design of the business case of health information technology in long-term care: project summary. In: Services US Department of Health and Human Services, editor. Washington, DC; 2005.
34. Branger PJ, van't Hooft A, van der Wouden JC, Moorman PW, van Bemmel JH. Shared care for diabetes: supporting communication between primary and secondary care. Int J Med Inform. 1999;53(2–3):133–42.
35. Barretto SA, Warren J, Goodchild A, Bird L, Heard S, Stumptner M. Linking guidelines to electronic health record design for improved chronic disease management. AMIA Annu Symp Proc. 2003;2003:66–70.
36. National Council on Aging AoA. Working with State Medicaid Agencies. In: National Council on Aging, http://www.ncoa.org/improve-health/center-for-healthy-aging/content-library/NCOA-AoA-Flyer-State-Medicaid-1.pdf.
37. Anderson G. Chronic care: making the case for ongoing care. Princeton, NJ: Robert Wood Johnson Foundation; 2010. p. 43.
38. Towne SD Jr, Smith ML, Ahn S, Belza B, Altpeter M, Kulinski KP, Ory MG. Delivering multiple evidence-based programs to at-risk seniors. Frontiers in Public Health: Public Health Education and Promotion 2015. In-press.
39. Wilson M, Smith ML. Putting CDSMP to work: implementation of the live healthy, Work Healthy Program. National Heart, Lung, and Blood Institute of the National Institutes of Health under Award Number R01HL122330.
40. Zuckerman S. What are the provisions in the new law for containing costs and how effective will they be? Washington, DC: Urban Institute; 2010. p. 5.
41. National Council on Aging Self-Management Alliance. Developing a Value Proposition for Self-Management Washington, DC [cited 2014 October 1]. http://selfmanagementalliance.org/why-self-management/value-proposition/#.VDV1ivldVkl (2014).

Patient Centered Medical Home: A Journey Not a Destination

Neela K. Patel, Carlos Roberto Jaén, Kurt C. Stange,
William L. Miller, Benjamin F. Crabtree, and Paul Nutting

Broad Model Overview

Brief History

The concept of the "Medical Home" has had a long period of maturation, with the introduction by the American Academy of Pediatrics (AAP) in 1967 of the concept as a single source of information for the patient [1]. Since then multiple organizations including the World Health Organization (WHO) and the Institute of Medicine (IOM) and US primary care groups

N.K. Patel, M.D., M.P.H. (✉)
Division of Community Geriatrics, Department of Family and
Community Medicine, University of Texas Health Science Center
at San Antonio, 7703 Floyd Curl Drive, MC 7784,
San Antonio, TX 78229, USA
e-mail: pateln4@uthscsa.edu

C.R. Jaén, M.D., Ph.D.
Department of Family and Community Medicine, University
of Texas Health Science Center at San Antonio, Room 610L,
Mail Code 7794, 7703 Floyd Curl Drive,
San Antonio, TX 78229, USA
e-mail: jaen@uthscsa.edu

K.C. Stange, M.D., Ph.D.
Department of Family Medicine and Community Health, Case
Western Reserve University, 11000 Cedar Avenue, Suite 402,
Cleveland, OH 44106-3069, USA
e-mail: kcs@case.edu

W.L. Miller, M.D., M.A.
Department of Family Medicine, Lehigh Valley Health Network,
School of Nursing, 1st Floor, 1628 West Chew Street,
Allentown, PA 18103, USA
e-mail: william.miller@lvhn.org

B.F. Crabtree, Ph.D.
Department of Family Medicine & Community Health, Rutgers
Robert Wood Johnson Medical School, Rutgers, The State
University of New Jersey,
1 World's Fair Drive, Somerset, NJ 08873, USA
e-mail: benjamin.crabtree@rutgers.edu

P. Nutting, M.D., M.S.P.H.
Center for Research Strategies, University of Colorado Health
Sciences Center, Denver, CO, USA

have adopted the basic tenets of the medical home under the rubric of the Patient-centered Medical Home (PCMH) [2–4]. In 2004 the American Family Medicine organizations issued the Future of Family Medicine Report [5] with a call for a new model of practice through a "proof of concept" demonstration project in typical family medicine practices. This led to the National Demonstration Project (NDP) of the PCMH that included some geriatric practices. Our team was selected as the evaluation team and published results in 2009 and 2010 [6]. Many of the lessons from the NDP guided our implementation of this project.

The Primary Care Patient-Centered Collaborative (PCPCC) was formed among employers, payers, clinicians and more than 1,200 stakeholders dedicated to "advancing an effective and efficient health system built on a strong foundation of primary care and the patient-centered medical home (PCMH)". This coalition assembles a large number of publications and analyses of demonstration projects supporting the PCMH.

In 2007 all the major primary care physician membership organizations [American Academy of Family Physicians (AAFP), American College of Physicians (ACP), American Academy of Pediatrics (AAP) and the American Osteopathic Association (AOA)] issued a consensus statement articulating the following joint principles of what came to be known as the Patient-Medical Home (PCMH) [4].

The Core Features of the PCMH are:

- Personal physician
- Physician directed medical practice
- Whole person orientation
- Care is coordinated and/or integrated
- Quality and safety
- Enhanced access
- Payment reform

As proposed by Wagner and colleagues [7], the PCMH responds to the new constellation of chronic health needs as well as of opportunities to respond to them through closely engaged community and health system resources. The final aim of the model was proposed to support productive

M.L. Malone et al. (eds.), *Geriatrics Models of Care: Bringing 'Best Practice' to an Aging America*,
DOI 10.1007/978-3-319-16068-9_13, © Springer International Publishing Switzerland 2015

Table 13.1 Mental models for primary care practice

	Old model: physician-centered	New model: patient-centered
Team care	Focused on physicians delegating tasks to others to streamline the work of the practice and make the physician more efficient	Working more collaboratively within teams at the "top of their license" focused on patients' needs
Patient orientation	Focus on advising and treating individual patients within private, face-to-face encounters	Focus expanded from individual patients to encompassing populations using channels of care such as telemedicine, electronic visits, and group visits
Key emphasis	Physician autonomy and reliance	Partnering relationship with patients and much greater transparence required

interactions between an informed, activated patient and a prepared, proactive practice team. Both the community and the health system contribute to this aim through self-management and personal skills support, delivery system design, decision support and clinical information systems. The Chronic Care Model (CCM) was later expanded to include an activated community as the end goal by adding the components of developing healthy public policy, creating supportive environments and strengthening community action [8].

Collaboration is at the heart of the PCMH. We have defined a PCMH as "a team of people embedded in a community and seeking to improve health and healing in that community. The team operates under the fundamental tenets of primary care and explores new ways of organizing practice, develop internal capabilities, and deploy health care delivery system and payment changes" [9]. The four fundamental tenets of primary health care are (1) access to care, (2) comprehensive care, (3) coordinated care and (4) care based on a personal relationship over time. Patient-centered care in the PCMH is contrasted with the old, physician-centric model in Table 13.1.

What Is the Problem That the Model Addresses?

The aging of the US population has led to a subpopulation of older adults with multiple chronic conditions. The prevalence of multi-morbidity (the coexistence of multiple chronic conditions) among older adults is estimated between 55 and 98 % [10] and requires the integrative approach of primary health care and a redesign of health care services [11]. The complexities of caring for this group have made team-based care a necessity. Most of these older adults require intensely coordinated care because of multiple chronic problems and multiple barriers to optimal care. Most primary care practices, including geriatricians' practices, often fail to deliver the care needed because these practices are not organized around the needs of the patients but rather have a focus on improving the efficiency and productivity of the individual

practitioner. Often the question is, "what can we do to make the geriatrician/clinician more efficient?" This focus is in part a response to the demands of a payment system that emphasizes production in terms of number of patients seen or relative value units (RVUs) over value-based care that is particularly relevant to the care of older people in improving patients' quality of life. This tension may lead to care that is not necessarily aligned with the needs of the patients or their family caregivers.

What Is the Setting for Our Model?

The Patient Centered Medical Home (PCMH) is a potentially useful approach for optimizing primary health care delivery to older adults. Our model is a geriatrics outpatient clinic in an academic setting in partnership with a community hospital. The clinic is adjacent to an acute care of elders (ACE) unit. The patients are seen as new patients to establish primary care and for follow-up to ensure continuity of care for chronic problems. There is same-day access if needed for acute problems. Other visit types include medication management and polypharmacy visits with pharmacists, transitions of care visits (discharges from emergency rooms, acute hospital visits, rehabilitation and skilled nursing units). Mostly focused in the ambulatory setting the clinic is well connected with community partners—local emergency rooms, ACE unit, rehabilitation facilities, home health agencies, durable medical equipment companies, Alzheimer's Association, local Area Agency on Aging and adult protective services. Thus, our clinic focuses on all the key elements of the PCMH—patient centered, comprehensive, coordinated care, access to care, and focus on quality and safety.

Older adults with multi-morbidity are heterogeneous in terms of illness severity, functional status, prognosis, personal priorities, and risk of adverse events even when diagnosed with the same conditions. Not only the individuals themselves but also their treatment options will differ, necessitating more-flexible approaches to care in this population. Older adults require high levels of care coordination because of their frequent hospitalizations, transitions to alternate levels of care, and multiple consultants taking care of individual diseases. Many lack a primary care clinician and often do not have a PCMH that coordinates care. They frequently receive redundant, wasteful, non-integrated and potentially harmful care from unanticipated effects of therapies or interventions.

Integration of geriatric services is an advantage of the PCMH. Our clinic focuses on community dwelling older adults, but we are mindful that our patients are likely to get services integrated with our ACE unit, long-term facilities, hospice and rehabilitation services. Our team helps older adults to age in place with dignity and respect. They can maintain their independence and optimize their functional status. Frail older adults and their families are most likely to benefit from a PCMH model because of the patient's severe or multiple health conditions and functional limitations, and the support services provided for families; however, all older adults could benefit from being enrolled in a PCMH.

Transformation Not Recognition Is the Goal

As the PCMH concepts are more widely accepted several organizations have entered the field to try to provide assurance that a particular practice is "PCMH recognized or certified". The National Committee for Quality Assurance (NCQA) is the most widely used recognition program. Others include the Joint Commission's Primary Care Medical Home certification, the Utilization Review Accreditation Commission (URAC)'s PCMH program, and the Accreditation Association for Ambulatory Health Care (AAAHC)'s medical home accreditation. Table 13.2 lists the standard criteria for these programs. The checklists that are required for obtaining the designation and/or accreditation are helpful in focusing the practices in important processes

that are not necessarily important in traditionally organized practices. A recent review of these programs found that they were equivalent in terms of meeting PCMH guidelines [12]. However, recognition/accreditation does not guarantee patient-centered transformation. It is possible to check all the boxes and get the highest designation and still be physician-centered.

Building a PCMH is hard work. Before a clinic can be transformed into a PCMH there are core elements that must be in place: material and human resources, and organizational structure and functional processes [13]. The core elements, including finances, technology infrastructure, facilities, space, equipment and operational processes, are a necessary initial condition for success. The next step is building the internal capabilities of the practice. A key concept developed during the NDP that helps understand the needs of the practice is adaptive reserve. By adaptive reserve we mean the features in primary care practice that enhance resilience and facilitate adaptation and development. Elements of adaptive reserve include action and reflection cycles, facilitative leadership, a learning culture, the ability to improvise, a repository of stories about change in the practice, sense-making and teamwork in the context of a dynamic local ecology and health policy. Action and reflection based on social skills are the means to strengthen teamwork and sense-making; that is, to the collective and collaborative understanding of the interactions between the patients and their families, communities and providers. The PCMH model recognizes the need for change and transformation, from established practices focusing on a critical mass of patients, clinical processes and staff, towards a paradigm shift where patient-centered and population-based care predominate, including a whole person, holistic care approach where persons are recognized as "citizens of health care neighborhoods". Change includes a total practice redesign, including space

Table 13.2 PCMH standards for recognition and/or accreditation for 4 selected organizations

2014 NCQA PCMH recognition	URAC PCMH Program V 2.0	Joint Commission 2013–2014	2013 AAAHC Medical Home Accreditation
• Patient-centered access • Team-based care • Population health management • Care management and support • Care coordination and care transitions • Performance measurement and quality improvement	• Access to services • Community services and resources • Patient registry • Comprehensive chronic care management • Wellness and health promotion • Managing tests and results • Referral process • Individual care management • Coordination of care • Self-management support • Medical home organizational core	• Patient-centered care • Comprehensive care • Coordinated care • Superb access to care • Systems-based approach to quality and safety	• Medical home patient rights, responsibilities and empowerment • Medical home governance and administration • Medical home relationship • Medical home accessibility • Medical home comprehensiveness of care • Medical home continuity of care • Medical home clinical records and health information • Medical home quality

PCMH patient-centered medical home, *NCQA* National Committee for Quality Assurance, *URAC* Utilization Review Accreditation Commission, *AAAHC* Accreditation Association Ambulatory Health Care

and office, access points, care processes, technology platforms, visit types and financial models. An identity shift is sought through Web portals, team structures and proactively planned care. Change and transformation observe a process of discontinuous improvement through time, with points when structures are "unfreezed" leading to moments of risk and uncertainty that, if successful, should be followed by rapid periods of transition and periods of "chill" prior to further acceleration. The provider payment reform options to support change and transformation towards the PCMH are enhanced fee-for-service towards performance payment, bundled episode payment and population-based global payments

Steps in Our Transformational Journey

When we started our transformational journey towards a PCMH we first engaged our team members. Table 13.3 summarizes the steps in our journey. By way of background, our clinic was physician-centered and the staff and clinicians worked as two separate teams. The staff worked for the physicians and the workflow in the clinic was different for every physician with a focus on the physicians' needs. Staff and patients expressed their frustration with the status quo and their frustration spread to the clinicians in the clinic. We vis-

ited our vision for our clinic and realized that we needed to change the way we did things. Our journey to accomplish our mission to care for frail older adults compelled us to evaluate our practice against the PCMH standards. We found wide variability in terms of how the different members of the team perceived how we met the standards. We produced a summary of the assessments and discussed at length the variations we found. This led to clarification of purpose (caring for older adults), redefining the processes and the beginning of learning cycles and team building.

This was an eye-opener and big enlightenment for the team, as we all realized that we were there for the same reason, and unanimously all said they were there for the patient. So when asked are we really there for the patient or the physician, some of them said physician, so we worked on how we could change from being physician-centered to a patient-centered focus. The staff mainly said we would need to have defined standards, processes and workflows in place that were more patient-focused rather than physician-focused and the system would be in place for the patient irrespective of who the clinician in clinic was caring for the patient. The bottom line question we asked ourselves was whether we would bring our parents and/or grandparents as patients to our clinic. By discussing our answers we were able to identify our strengths and areas in need of improvement.

Table 13.3 Steps and important questions in our journey to becoming a PCMH

Key steps	Key questions or tasks
Building a common mission and vision	Why are we all here?
	Would we bring our family here?
Process improvement	What needs to change in our clinic?
	What do we need to keep because is working well?
Time for reflection and course adjustment	Daily workflow preparation and adjustment
	Daily huddles
	Weekly "all hands" meetings
	Patient feedback review
	Frequent personal affirmation and feedback
Accountability	Defined roles and responsibilities for all team members
	What is my responsibility?
	Who does what?
	How does my work affect the work of others?
	How does it affect patients?
Safe work environment	Respect and trust for diversity of opinions and team engagement
	Are you afraid of telling it as you see it?
Electronic health record optimization	Ongoing optimization of use and integration into workflow, roles and responsibilities
	How can we best make this data useful information to benefit our patients?
Building the medical home neighborhood	Who do we need to partner with to benefit our patients and caregivers?
	Medical consultants, home health care agencies, durable medical equipment suppliers, adult day care centers, Alzheimer's associations, local area agencies for aging, adult protective services, senior networking groups (resources for care giving and transportation outside the patient's own families), local transportation agencies, hospitals, rehabilitation and long-term care units.

We then worked on building relationships, trust and respect for one another and understanding better our roles and responsibilities. We worked on building personal relationships with each other and thus built a single integrated team that included staff and clinicians. We build a supportive and safe environment for reflection and course adjustment.

With a clear understanding that all processes and changes are interconnected and at times have unintended consequences we started to make changes in our key processes of interactions with patients. We committed to meeting weekly to reevaluate and provide course correction in real time.

We prioritized the order in which to address the opportunities for improvement. We did the process and flow diagrams of the existing system for each of the opportunities. We also completed a root cause analysis to understand what the most important causes for negative outcomes were. We committed to change one or two small processes to improve workflow. We reevaluated and course corrected each intervention during our weekly meetings.

The team building and relationship building activities were icebreakers; these were only 5 min at the beginning of our weekly meetings. This step was critical to allow us to know one another better and improve communication and effectiveness. We built trust and respect for one another. The focus was with a process or system issue and not a person in particular all staff members were encouraged to bring patient-centered issues/concerns to the forefront of discussion. Meetings succeeded in engaging our team and defining roles and responsibilities for each member; including front end, back end, call center scheduling and registration. We also expanded clinician's responsibilities beyond direct patient care to virtual visits, handling patients' phone calls, and securing electronic messages. We set expectations and made each other accountable to meet all the functions of patient-centered care. Some of our staff and clinicians chose to not embrace our new approach and left the practice. Those who remained are deeply committed to transformation and share our common vision. They are instrumental in welcoming and orienting new members to our changed culture. We listened to our patients' requests and concerns regarding our care and adjusted our approach further. The results were reductions in the volume of phone calls, faxes and paperwork as we were able to address issues more promptly with the new processes and workflows. We then had more time for direct face-to-face and virtual patient care.

Improved relationships with our community partners were also critical to our transformation. They are essential for the continuity of care of our frail older patients to optimize their function and independence. We discovered that a large proportion of the paperwork and phone calls were from multiple home health agencies. We decided to partner with a select few agencies that were highly rated by our patients in terms of their perceived quality of care. They became

extended team members of our team assisting our patients to avoid hospital admission by seeing our patients the same day in their homes thereby preventing an office visit or emergency room visit.

Table 13.4 details new and expanded roles for the members of the geriatric PCMH team. A geriatrician is a facilitative

Table 13.4 Interdisciplinary team members' roles for our PCMH for older adults

Team member	Role[a]
Patient and caregiver	Self-care
	Medication adherence
	Lifestyle modification
	Assistance with access to care
Medical assistant	Scheduling
	Registration
	Intake
	Procedures
	Patient dismissal
Nurse	Phone triage
	Transition of care coordination
	Medication refills
	Population management for chronic and preventive care
Pharmacist	Medication management
	Consult for polypharmacy
	Adverse drug events
	Transitions of care from different levels of care
	Care coordination
Nurse practitioner/ physician Assistant	Same-day acute care appointments
	Transition of care
	Medicare wellness exams
	Continuity of care
	Care coordination
Clinic manager	Financial oversight
	Human resources management
	Daily workflows and improvisation
Geriatrician	Continuity of care
	Shared care with PA/NP
	Same-day acute care appointments
	New patient visits
	Consults
	Facilitative leader of PCMH
	Coordination with medical consults
Community partners: dieticians, psychologists, social workers, medical consultants, home health care agencies, durable medical equipment suppliers, adult day care centers, Alzheimer's associations, local area agencies for aging, adult protective services local transportation agencies, hospitals, rehabilitation and long-term care units	Supplement care not available within the PCMH but available in the PCMH neighborhood

[a]Engagement in quality improvement projects is expected of all members of the team

leader of the team, an internal clinical resource and a connector to other settings of care, ultimately responsible for the optimal care of the patient and creating a psychologically safe environment. Leader inclusiveness is a part of being an effective facilitative leader. Leader inclusiveness is the use of words and deeds that invite others and appreciates their coming. This is important in creating a psychologically safe environment [14].

Process Improvement Changes That We Made to Improve Workflow in the Clinic for PCMH

- *Scheduling templates*—changed several times until we got a flow that worked best for our patients to accommodate follow-up and new patient visits, same-day access, transition of care, and medication management visits. We have 30-min follow-up and 1-h new patient slots. New patients are the last patients for the session as they take a long time for comprehensive geriatric assessments.
- *Visit Types*—these were changed to reduce wait times for the patients. Polypharmacy and chronic disease management were long visits so we started consultant Pharm D and medication management visits with Pharm D, which helped reduce polypharmacy and improve chronic disease management. Another time consuming visit-type was hospital discharge and so we started transition of care sessions and visits.
- *Workflows*—defined by our grassroots and front line workers, our staff, mainly medical assistant (MA) driven clinic, MA's for front end, back end, and benefits coordinator. Nurses (LVN) for phone triage, treatment refills and transition of care medication reconciliation.
- *Increased Access*—We changed templates to accommodate same-day visits and make room for increased access. We worked with the electronic medical record to schedule follow-up and recall lists for patients, and increased access by making appointments available 8 weeks ahead. Follow-up reminders were created for patients who do need telephone call rather than office visits, thereby leaving open slots for same-day access.

Training That Could Facilitate PCMH Transformation

We found training in specific skills ranging from clinical safety and effectiveness methods, teamwork and communication, participatory leadership training, and electronic record champion training useful for our transformational efforts. These courses provide the tools to assure that the fidelity of the model is kept intact by providing ways to monitor our reports and outcomes on an ongoing basis.

Quality and Process Improvement

The Clinical Safety and Effectiveness Course (CS&E) is a University of Texas system-wide course that concentrates on Quality Improvement and Patient Safety. It is modeled after Dr. Brent James' Advanced Training Program at Intermountain Health Care, Utah. The curriculum emphasizes quality concepts and evidence-based medicine including patient safety, quality improvement, quality tools, teamwork, disclosure and crafting apologies, and return on investment. It is project-based and demonstrates use of quality concepts and tools. The majority of our clinicians in our clinic have graduated from this course. Quality and process improvement is embedded in our daily practice.

Communication and Teambuilding

Communication failures and lack of teamwork are major contributing factors to patient injury and harm. TeamSTEPPS (Team Strategies to Enhance Performance and Patient Safety) is a product of teamwork in that it is a collaborative effort by Agency for Healthcare Research and Quality (AHRQ) and the Department of Defense's Military Health System. The School of Nursing at our health science center has a federal award to train teams on TeamSTEPPS and trained our team of clinicians and staff. We now include these critical steps routinely; plan, do, study, act. These courses support our culture change efforts and provide us with tools to monitor and maintain patient-centered changes.

Facilitative Leadership

UT Medicine, the practice plan of our health science center, provided Next Level Leadership (NLL) training for all medical directors and managers. Working in partnership alongside with the participants, the NLL training focused on:
- Facilitative leadership development
- Fulfilling our vision and strategic objectives
- Aligning our culture to match our Vision
- Effective communication
- Building a high performance team

The training helped to develop an effective team by challenging our assumption related to limits in what we can become. It also made us aware of the power of relationships both in the positive and negative realms. It was instrumental in developing a learning culture, psychologically safe environment and growing facilitative leadership skills in both clinicians and staff. The course helped our practice develop our adaptive reserve.

Electronic Record Champion Training

UT Medicine invested in developing electronic health (EHR) record champion training for a few clinicians from each department. Our clinics have EpicCare EHR and these champions had intensive training followed by ongoing training. The Medical Director for our clinic (NKP) is an EpicCare Superuser and now a Champion. This knowledge allows for optimization and at-the-elbow training of others clinicians and staff.

Our EHR enables our team to record and share information on: (1) results from needs assessments for different domains (medical and social history, medications, home environment, social support, and family caregivers); (2) referrals and results from lab and radiologic tests, specialty consults, and home health and other community-based care; (3) real-time monitoring of such critical events as hospital admissions and ED visits that trigger a need for follow-up; (4) prompts and reminders regarding needed follow-up visits, chronic disease monitoring and preventive care; (5) decision-support tools for complex patient care, such as clinical care paths and guidelines; and (6) community resources lists.

We do not work in an island but are part of a larger system of care. When UT Medicine wanted to change all primary care clinics to a PCMH model of care, there was an attempt to make global changes to optimize our EHR from a top down perspective. The initial steps focused on smoothing workflows. Three different levels needed attention: (1) UT Medicine practice-wide, (2) primary care specific changes, and (3) clinic specific changes. We understood that primary care is a local endeavor that needs to respond to the patients and communities that it serves in a very unique way. One size does not fit all. In older adults this model needs to adapt to the practice team and to the patients' preferences and specific needs.

Evidence for Effectiveness

The PCPCC, previously described as a multiple stakeholder organization that promotes the PCMH, offers an extensive review of the evidence in their most recent publication [15]. This publication details reviews from 46 medical home initiatives across the USA and provides evidence that the PCMH improves quality of care and population health, and also reduces health care costs. A more recent observational report based on the experience of 5.6 million veterans receiving care at 913 Veterans Health Administration (VHA) hospital-based and community-based clinics that had implemented the Patient Aligned Care Team (PACT) initiative, their version of PCMH, found that veterans' clinics, with higher scores in their PCMH implementation measure, had higher patient satisfaction, higher performance on 41 or 48 measures of clinical quality measures, lower staff burnout, lower hospitalization rates for ambulatory-care sensitive conditions particularly for veterans 65 years old or older, and lower emergency department use [16]. The results are not surprising given what we know about systems of care that have a strong focus on primary health care in other developed countries [17].

Potential Barriers/Challenges to Building PCMH for Older Adults

Reluctance of some payers to provide blended payment for primary care, resistance from clinicians to change old medical models of practice, resistance from patients to using virtual care, lack of tools, lack of support or over-involvement from health system leaders can provide important impediments to the development of the needed transformation. In some settings another important barrier is the lack of multidisciplinary personnel to staff the clinic. A PCMH as an organic organization that needs to adapt to the resources and needs of the patients and populations it serves. In settings where pharmacists, nurses, psychologists and other professional are not available there is the opportunity to provide this care virtually through telemedicine and/or through community partnerships that extend beyond the office.

Our academic health center leaders recognized the importance of advanced primary care in the future of our health care organization and provided initial capital investment to build our PCMH. The initial investment allowed for the hiring of the additional personnel needed to provide the level of care we described. Additional sources of funding are necessary to sustain the PCMH. Some Medicare Advantage Programs are starting to pay for outcomes beyond traditional fee-for-service payments. Blended or advance payment allows investment in developing systems that proactively help meet the real needs of older adults, perhaps such as a guided-care approach [18].

Payment reform is essential to the long-term sustainability of the PCMH models. However, there is more than money needed for transformation. Practices can do a lot to improve communication, leadership, collaboration, and coordination without having to wait for payment reform to be in place. The journey of transformation begins with a first step, but it requires dedication and time.

Patient/Caregiver/Family Involvement

Patient and family feedback was instrumental in our practice redesign. At this point we do not have a formal process of patient/family involvement but are looking for ways to invite patients and families to our monthly meetings. We are convinced that their participation will accelerate our improvement processes to make them more patient-responsive.

The Future Is Bright

There is a virtual mandate from the Patient Protection and Affordable Care Act to expand the PCMH and team-based medical care. The US health care system is in a trajectory of unsustainability that requires major transformation. Older adults, particularly those frail and with multiple comorbidities, account for a significantly large proportion of health care expenditures often in patterns that are unsafe and wasteful. The PCMH approach provides a vehicle to transform how primary care can be delivered in our country. Transformation requires a focus on building a common mission and vision, a focus on process improvement, time for reflection and course adjustment, accountability to patients and staff, a psychologically safe work environment, electronic health record optimization, and partnering with members of the medical home neighborhood. It can be done with great benefit to older adults, clinicians, and staff.

References

1. American Academy of Pediatrics. Standards of child health care. Evanston, IL: American Academy of Pediatrics; 1967.
2. International Conference on Primary Health Care. Declaration of Alma-Ata. WHO Chron. 1978;32(11):428–30.
3. Institute of Medicine (U.S.), Donaldson M. Primary care: America's health in a new era. Washington, DC: National Academy Press; 1996.
4. American Academy of Family Physicians, American Academy of Pediatrics, American College of Physicians, American Osteopathic Association. Joint principles of the patient centered medical home. 2007. http://www.aafp.org/dam/AAFP/documents/practice_management/pcmh/initiatives/PCMHJoint.pdf . Accessed 22 Sep 2014.
5. Future of Family Medicine Project Leadership Committee. The future of family medicine: a collaborative project of the family medicine community. Ann Fam Med. 2004;2 Suppl 1:S3–32.
6. Crabtree BF, Nutting PA, Miller WL, Stange KC, Stewart EE, Jaén CR. Summary of the National Demonstration Project and recommendations for the patient-centered medical home. Ann Fam Med. 2010;8 Suppl 1:S80–90.
7. Wagner EH, Austin BT, Davis C, Hindmarsh M, Schaefer J, Bonomi A. Improving chronic illness care: translating evidence into action. Health Aff. 2001;20(6):64–78.
8. Barr V, Robinson S, Marin-Link B, Underhill L, Dotts A, Ravensdale D, Salivaras S. The expanded chronic care model. Hosp Q. 2003;7(1):73–82.
9. Stange KC, Nutting PA, Miller WL, Jaén CR, Crabtree BF, Flocke SA, Gill JM. Defining and measuring the patient-centered medical home. J Gen Intern Med. 2010;25(6):601–12.
10. Marengoni A, Angleman S, Melis R, Mangialasche F, Karp A, Garmen A, Fratiglioni L. Aging with multimorbidity: a systematic review of the literature. Ageing Res Rev. 2011;10(4):430–9.
11. Salisbury C. Multimorbidity: redesigning health care for people who use it. Lancet. 2012;380(9836):7–9.
12. Gans DN. A comparison of the National Patient-Centered Medical Home Accreditation and Recognition Programs. Englewood, CO: Medical Group Management Association; 2014. Available at: http://online.mgma.org/PCMH-Report?source=Rapage.
13. Miller WL, Crabtree BF, Nutting PA, Stange KC, Jaén CR. Primary care practice development: a relationship-centered approach. Ann Fam Med. 2010;8 Suppl 1:S68–79.
14. Bowers KW, Robertson M, Parchman ML. How inclusive leadership can help your practice adapt to change. Fam Pract Manag. 2012;19(1):8–11.
15. Nielsen M, Langner B, Zema C, Hacker T, Grundy B. Benefits of implementing the primary care patient-centered medical home: a review of cost & quality results, 2012. Patient-centered primary care collaborative, September 2012. http://www.pcpcc.org/guide/benefits-implementing-primary-care-medical-home#sthash.b0zLJWfr.dpuf. Accessed 24 Sep 2014.
16. Nelson KM, Helfrich C, Sun H, Hebert PL, Liu CF, Dolan E, Fihn SD. Implementation of the patient-centered medical home in the Veterans Health Administration: associations with patient satisfaction, quality of care, staff burnout, and hospital and emergency department use. JAMA Intern Med. 2014;174(8):1350–8.
17. Starfield B, Shi L, Macinko J. Contribution of primary care to health systems and health. Milbank Q. 2005;83(3):457–502.
18. Boult C, Wieland GD. Comprehensive primary care for older patients with multiple chronic conditions: "Nobody rushes you through". JAMA. 2010;304(17):1936–43.

Hospital at Home

14

Bruce Leff

Introduction

Hospital at Home is an innovative care model that provides patient evaluation and management services usually performed in the traditional acute inpatient hospital setting, in a patient's home [1]. In this chapter, we will describe the problems that Hospital at Home aims to address, define the Hospital at Home model, provide an overview of the robust underlying evidence base for Hospital at Home care, and then focus on several key issues related to developing and disseminating Hospital at Home into the US health care system.

Why Bother with Hospital at Home Care? The Problems Addressed by Hospital at Home

Hospital Care Is Expensive

Health care is expensive and hospital care represents a significant proportion of that expense. In 2012, Medicare spent $133 billion for inpatient hospital care among fee-for-service beneficiaries [2].

Hospital Care Is Not Always Safe for Older Adults

However, despite these massive and ever increasing expenditures, the quality and safety of care provided in hospitals is concerning. The seminal reports from the Institute of Medicine, "To Err is Human, Building a Safer Health Care System" and "Crossing the Quality Chasm" highlight the challenges of providing safe, patient-centered care in the inpatient setting. These Institute of Medicine reports launched the hospital safety movement. However, recent studies suggest that the rates of hospital-associated adverse events have not changed significantly over the past 15 years [3]. Whether this is due to an inability to change the safety and quality culture of the traditional inpatient setting, the increasing use of technology, or a patient population with a higher burden or chronic illness, or some combination thereof, the need to provide safer care to acutely ill persons remains paramount.

Hospitals can be especially problematic environments for older adults. Loss or diminution of homeostatic reserve is a hallmark of the aging process. While the usual aging process may not cause problems under ordinary circumstance, the physiological stresses associated with illness, combined with the challenges posed by the hospital environment can exhaust the physiologic reserves of older patients and lead to iatrogenic complications [4, 5].

Such iatrogenic events are common in hospitalized patients. The Harvard Medical Practice Studies found that approximately 4 % of hospitalized patients suffered an adverse event; more than two-thirds of these were due to errors. These events were more common among older patients, even after adjustment for comorbid medical conditions; at least 44,000 people die in US hospitals each year due to medical mistakes at a cost of tens of billions of dollars [6, 7].

Several iatrogenic events are especially common and troubling. Functional decline and disability is common. It affects approximately one-third of patients older than 70 and results in subsequent inability to live independently and manage basic activities of daily living. Such disability can occur even when the underlying illness that precipitated hospitalization is treated successfully. Development of disability following hospitalization is also associated with mortality. Delirium or acute confusional state is also a common complication associated with hospitalization. Although estimates vary, approximately 20–25 % of adults develop incident delirium while hospitalized; many cases go unrecognized. Symptoms of delirium may persist for months and long-term cognitive sequelae are common.

B. Leff, M.D. (✉)
Division of Geriatric Medicine and Gerontology, Department of Medicine, Johns Hopkins Bayview Medical Center, 5505 Hopkins Bayview Circle, Baltimore, MD 21224, USA
e-mail: bleff@jhmi.edu

M.L. Malone et al. (eds.), *Geriatrics Models of Care: Bringing 'Best Practice' to an Aging America*,
DOI 10.1007/978-3-319-16068-9_14, © Springer International Publishing Switzerland 2015

Additional common iatrogenic events include incontinence, pressure sores, nosocomial infections, and falls. In addition, preventable adverse events also occur during the transition from hospital to home at hospital discharge, the result of deficiencies in health system design and poor communication [8–10].

Trends That Favor Alternatives to Traditional Hospital Care

Several key trends have begun to favor alternatives to traditional hospital care, especially since the passage of the Affordable Care Act. The expectation of patients as consumers of health services for more personalized and safer care is accelerating and pushing the health care marketplace to be more consumer-friendly. Advances in the development of safe portable advanced hospital-type technologies allows health care providers to provide services and technologies that were previously available only in hospitals. In the context of increasing interest in approaches to population health, there is increased recognition on the importance to move care out of facilities such as hospitals, and into the community. Finally, payers of health care services are increasingly interested in models that are provide high-quality care at lower cost, and have been experimenting with new payment models such as traditional capitation, bundled payments, and functional capitation models, such as the case with accountable care organizations [9, 11].

What Is Hospital at Home?

A variety of health care delivery models have been included under the rubric of Hospital at Home in the international literature; some models substitute entirely for an inpatient hospital admission, while others, by providing ongoing hospital-level services in the home, facilitate early discharge from the acute hospital. Some models have targeted patients with medical conditions and others have focused on patient's following surgery or those needing rehabilitation services. In most models, nurses deliver much of the care. Relatively few models have included substantial physician inputs. Some models have focused on distinct populations such as children or on patients with psychiatric conditions. This variety of models may reflect the evolution of Hospital at Home models that have been developed chiefly in countries with single payer systems where Hospital at Home models fill a particular clinical niche [9].

In the context of the US health care delivery system there are two main models of Hospital at Home care to consider. The first is "substitutive" Hospital at Home that delivers acute hospital-level care in a patient's home in lieu of acute hospital admission. In this model, patients who require acute hospital care and appropriate for Hospital at Home are usually identified in the emergency department or ambulatory setting and taken directly home to receive Hospital at Home care. If the underlying rationale for Hospital at Home is to avoid hospital-associated complications, honor patient wishes regarding care, and reduce health care costs, the substitutive model, by avoiding the inpatient environment completely, best satisfies that rationale [12].

The other main Hospital at Home model described in the literature goes by term "early-discharge" Hospital at Home. This is unfortunate nomenclature as it implies that the patient no longer requires hospital-level care. In the US context, this terminology risks the model being confused with patients who are discharged from the hospital who no longer require hospital-level services but who are discharged and receive skilled home health services following discharge to facilitate a smooth discharge transition.

A more appropriate name for this model would be a "transfer" model of Hospital at Home. Much in the same way that patients who are hospitalized in an intensive care setting may be transferred to a regular medicine ward bed once their clinical condition is stabilized, a patient who is in a regular medicine ward bed, but who still needs hospital-level care and services, may transfer to a Hospital at Home bed and receive those services in the home. Once discharged from Hospital at Home such a patient may require and receive post-acute skilled services in the home.

Substitutive Hospital at Home and "transfer" Hospital at Home models are consistent with the previously defined "Clinical Unit" model of Hospital at Home. In the Clinical Unit model, Hospital at Home operates as a distinct or virtual, but integrated ward of a hospital, but without the usual bricks and mortar surrounding the hospital bed. Thus, in this construct, Hospital at Home provides treatment at home of an acute condition of a severity that normally requires hospitalization and provides treatment that requires hospital-type technologies or hospital-level care. The hospital or health system retains responsibility for the acute care episode, and Hospital at Home patients retain inpatient status. Funding, provision of pharmaceuticals, diagnostic, radiology, therapeutics, and other services are delivered according to standards commensurate with inpatient status and appropriate to the patient's level of medical acuity. Direct nursing care is provided at home with 24-h coverage. Physician care is provided by Hospital at Home doctors, with 24-h coverage. Hospital at Home care is provided in a coordinated manner similar to an inpatient hospital ward and patients consent to treatment [9].

The Hospital at Home Model

Conditions and Patients That Can Be Treated in Hospital at Home

Hospital at Home care is appropriate for certain conditions and for certain patients with those conditions. Suitable conditions for Hospital at Home treatment may vary between substitutive and transfer Hospital at Home models. For substitutive Hospital at Home-appropriate conditions a key feature is that the condition is one that can be diagnosed with high degree of certainty at the time of hospital admission either in the emergency department or ambulatory site. In the substitutive model, the patient will move from the emergency department or ambulatory site directly to the home. Thus, it is critical to know with a high degree of certainty what condition the patient is suffering with, as this will be the major driver of the plan of care. In addition, for both substitutive and transfer type of Hospital at Home patients, the condition occurs relatively frequently in order to provide the needed patient volume to support a Hospital at Home program. Further, the treatment of the condition is relatively well defined and can be feasibly provided to the patient in a safe and efficient manner in the patient's home.

A number of medical conditions meet these conditions and have been treated in Hospital at Home. Hospital at Home models have addressed community-acquired pneumonia, chronic obstructive pulmonary disease, chronic heart failure, cellulitis, sepsis due to urinary tract infection and complicated urinary tract infection, ischemic cerebrovascular accident, pulmonary embolism, deep venous thrombosis, pancreatitis, Parkinson's Disease, volume depletion and dehydration, febrile neutropenia, ulcerative colitis, decompensated liver disease, multiple sclerosis, acute pancreatitis, and infections requiring long-term antibiotics such as endocarditis, osteomyelitis, infected prostheses. Hospital at Home has also been employed as a substitute for facility-based rehabilitation and as a transfer model for surgical conditions such as total knee arthroplasty, total hip arthroplasty, and vascular surgery procedures. In addition, Hospital at Home has been used for psychiatric conditions [9, 13].

Selecting appropriate patients with the above noted conditions is critical to the success of Hospital at Home in terms of ensuring safe and high-quality care. Patient selection should focus on the construct of selecting patients with the Hospital at Home-qualifying condition that can be safely cared for in the home. Such patients should have a relatively low risk of unanticipated decompensation requiring transfer to the traditional acute inpatient hospital environment and should be able to receive an appropriate course of treatment without a high need of hospital-based high-tech types of treatments. For example, if heart failure is to be treated in Hospital at Home, selection criteria should identify heart failure patients who are not having active cardiac ischemia and who are not likely to need cardiac diagnostic or therapeutic procedures that are impossible or difficult to accomplish in the home, such as percutaneous coronary intervention.

Such Hospital at Home eligibility criteria have been described in the literature for certain conditions such as community-acquired pneumonia, exacerbations of heart failure or chronic obstructive pulmonary disease, and cellulitis. These eligibility criteria can be used in real time with the clinical dataset that is commonly obtained in the emergency department or ambulatory setting allowing for a patient selection process that does not impede the usual clinical workflow of the those care sites [14].

A key issue is that Hospital at Home care should only be provided to patients who truly require hospital-level care. Patients who are admitted to a substitutive model of Hospital at Home are those that but for the ability to provide Hospital at Home care, would have been admitted to the traditional acute care hospital, and not sent home from the emergency department with a prescription for an oral antibiotic, a recommendation to increase the dose of a diuretic, or other clinical recommendation or plan. In the context of a transfer Hospital at Home model, but for the existence of Hospital at Home, the patient would be staying in the acute care hospital and would not be discharged to home.

Over time, as Hospital at Home becomes an increasingly mainstream care delivery model, and as mobile and telemedical technologies improve, the scope of conditions and the severity of illness that can be safely cared for in the home will continue to expand.

How the Hospital at Home Model Works

In substitutive Hospital at Home, a patient with a Hospital at Home-qualifying condition (detailed above), who requires admission to the hospital for that condition, is identified in the emergency department or ambulatory site, or at home, e.g., by a house call physician or home care nurse. The patient eligibility for Hospital at Home care is assessed. In the example below, we focus on a patient admitted from the emergency department, the most common pathway in most programs. A first pass assessment of Hospital at Home medical eligibility can usually be made by an emergency department physician using broad Hospital at Home eligibility criteria that they would have been previously instructed in. The final assessment of eligibility, using the full set of eligibility criteria, is made by a Hospital at Home staff asset, usually a nurse.

At this point, the patient's home environment is also assessed through a brief series of questions that assure that the home is a suitable environment for care provision. This assessment focuses on general level of cleanliness, whether appropriate needed climate control is present, i.e., air conditioning in the event of warm weather, heat in winter, as well as presence of running water and basic household infrastructure. It is not necessary for the patient to have phone service; disposable cell phones can be provided at low cost to a patient if needed. Once the patient's eligibility is confirmed, the patient is offered treatment in Hospital at Home and consented for treatment in Hospital at Home.

Once the patient consents to Hospital at Home care, Hospital at Home staff mobilizes the full Hospital at Home team and initiates orders for needed medications, durable medical equipment, and providers that will be needed to provide care. These may include oral and intravenous medications (antibiotics, corticosteroids, antiviral, anticoagulation, blood products, chemotherapy), basic radiology (chest and abdominal radiographs, echocardiogram, ultrasound, venous Doppler), oxygen, nebulizer equipment, wound care supplies, assistive devices, bedside commode. Hospital beds are rarely required.

All health care is local; the specifics of how the Hospital at Home system will be set up in a particular health system depend greatly on how that particular health system has decided to implement Hospital at Home in the context of the available health care assets in its local environment. For instance, patients treated in Hospital at Home often require intravenous medications. There are a variety of ways to provide intravenous medications in the home. Such medications could come from a hospital pharmacy, an infusion pharmacy of a home health agency affiliated with the health system, an independent contracted home infusion pharmacy, among others. The specific choice made by a health system to implement this important piece of the Hospital at Home model will depend greatly on the characteristics of the local health care market in which Hospital at Home is implemented, and on payment practices in the particular context of the Hospital at Home implementation.

As these arrangements are being made and coordinated, the patient may be evaluated in the emergency department briefly by the Hospital at Home nurse or physician, depending on some of the details of staffing, as well as the relationship between the emergency department and the Hospital at Home program. In some systems, this initial non-emergency department evaluation may be made by a hospitalist associated with the Hospital at Home program. The patient is then sent home. Transportation is usually accomplished by an ambulette, especially if the patient requires oxygen during transfer. Ambulance transfer is usually not required. Transportation for some patients can be accomplished by the patient and their family, e.g., a patient being admitted to Hospital at Home for cellulitis may be taken home by the patient's family member by car.

The patient arrives at home and is met by the Hospital at Home nurse, who begins to implement the care plan. In some Hospital at Home research studies in the USA, the Hospital at Home nurse was required to stay with the patient continuously for the first 24 h of care [15]. This was found not to be necessary. In fact, many patients did not like having a nurse present for such an extended period of time. In more recent Hospital at Home implementations, the Hospital at Home nurse conducts in initial extended visit that lasts between 2 and 4 h. The nurse completes a full evaluation of the patient and the home. The nurse ensures that all ordered equipment is delivered to the home. In addition, the nurse educates the patient and, if present, family, on the Hospital at Home care model and what to expect in terms of how care will be provided, how to communicate effectively with the care team, and how to notify the care team in the case of urgent or emergent events.

The Hospital at Home physician visits the patient at home and performs her assessment of the patient and refines the care plan with the Hospital at Home nurse. Plans for ongoing intermittent nursing visits are made based on the patient's condition and care plan needs. The Hospital at Home physician will then visit the patient at least daily. The Hospital at Home nurses will usually visit the patient at least daily. Illness-specific care plans guide the provision of care. The Hospital at Home team is available at all times in the event that the patient requires urgent or emergent evaluation and or treatment.

Treatment in Hospital at Home proceeds and, as the patient improves, discharge planning begins. The acute phase of Hospital at Home is designed to be a brief intervention. Average lengths of stay are in the 3–4 day range, similar or slightly less than the length of stay in the traditional acute care hospital. However, discharge from Hospital at Home offers advantages over traditional hospital discharge. The relationship between Hospital at Home staff and the patient and family members and the teaching and education that was provided to the patient during the Hospital at Home admission contribute to robust patient understanding of their condition and issues related to self-management. The knowledge obtained by the Hospital at Home staff, by being in the patient's home for several days can help optimize discharge planning and the planning for any post-discharge services such as skilled home health care. This and the ability to perform medication reconciliation in a patient's home "at the kitchen table" may contribute to a smoother care transition.

The physician's role in Hospital at Home has varied widely. As noted, early discharge models usually involve physicians in supervision at a distance; substitutive Hospital at Home models also report varied physician roles. In some substitutive models community-based general practitioners are available for home visits to Hospital at Home patients but make few visits. Other models require that physicians visit the patient at home every day on the premise that Hospital at Home patients require the same care that they would have received inside hospital walls. There appears to be a relationship between clinical benefits obtained and the degree of physician participation in providing Hospital at Home care.

The role of caregivers has varied in different Hospital at Home models. Some models will only accept patients into Hospital at Home if a caregiver is present in the home and may use the caregiver to supervise the patient or deliver care. Other programs have not maintained such a requirement on the theory that it may not be appropriate to shift the burden of care provision to the patient's family. Such programs will also accept patients who live alone for Hospital at Home admission. If a patient who lives alone requires assistance with activities or additional supervision, then a nurse aide can be provided to that patient. As will be noted below, caregiver strain and stress has been found to be lower in Hospital at Home compared with usual hospital care, even in Hospital at Home models where caregivers provide some level of care to the patient.

Outcomes of Hospital at Home: The Evidence Base

Hospital at Home is one of the best-studied care delivery models in the medical literature; the evidence base is robust and several meta-analyses have been performed. We review the meta-analytic data and then focus on several programs in detail.

The meta-analyses of Hospital at Home have focused on different Hospital at Home model types and have used somewhat varying definitions for study inclusion.

Shepperd et al. conducted the most recent systematic review that focused on admission avoidance Hospital at Home, i.e., substitution Hospital at Home. They included randomized controlled trials that compared programs aimed at avoidance of admission through provision of hospital care at home with inpatient care in acute care hospitals for patients 18 years and older. Hospital at Home care had to substitute for care that would have required inpatient admission, i.e., if the Hospital at Home program had not been available, the patient would have been admitted to the acute care hospital. Early discharge Hospital at Home was excluded, as were pediatric, obstetric, and mental health patients. Ten randomized controlled trials met the study definition with total of 1,327 patients studied across the ten trials. Seven of the trials were eligible for meta-analysis of individual patient data. Of the ten trials, two trials focused on patients with chronic obstructive pulmonary disease, two recruited patients with acute stroke, three recruited patients with acute medical conditions who were mainly elderly, one for patient with cellulitis, one for patients with community acquired pneumonia,

and one for frail patients with dementia. There was a non-significant reduction in mortality at 3 months favorable to Hospital at Home (hazard ration 0.77, confidence interval 0.54, 1.09) and a significant reduction in mortality favorable to Hospital at Home after 6 months (HR 0.62, CI 0.45, 0.87). Patients receiving Hospital at Home care reported greater satisfaction with care than those who received care in the traditional acute care hospital across a range of medical conditions. Clinical outcomes such as bowel or urinary complications, delirium, and others, when reported, were favorable to Hospital at Home. Length of stay was generally shorter for Hospital at Home patients, and Hospital at Home was less expensive than traditional care [16].

A Cochrane systematic review and meta-analysis of early discharge Hospital at Home identified 26 trials ($N=3,967$). The trials were of adults aged 18 and older; obstetric, pediatric, and mental health Hospital at Home trials were excluded. If the early discharge Hospital at Home were not available, the patient would not have been discharged from the hospital and would remain on the acute care unit of the hospital. The types of conditions that these models focused on included: patients following surgery for hernia varicose veins, coronary artery bypass grafting surgery, hip fracture, or total knee replacement. Other target conditions included patients recovering from stroke, patients with a mix of acute medical conditions such as chronic obstructive pulmonary disease and others. For patients recovering from stroke and elderly with a mix of medical conditions, there was insufficient evidence of a difference in mortality between groups (HR 0.79, CI 0.32, 1.91). Readmission rates were higher for Hospital at Home elderly patients with a mix of conditions (HR 1.57, CI 1.10, 2.24). For patients recovering from stroke (HA 0.63, CI 0.40, 0.98) and elderly patients with a mix of conditions (HR 0.69, CI 0.48, 0.99), fewer Hospital at Home patients were admitted to nursing home care at follow up. Patients reported greater satisfaction with early discharge Hospital at Home. Evidence on cost savings was mixed [17].

In 2012, Caplan et al. published a systematic review of "hospital in the home." They adopted a definition of Hospital at Home that "significantly substitute for in-hospital time" and hypothesized that replacing inpatient care with home-based care for at least 7 days or for at least 25 % of the duration of the control hospital admissions would produce different clinical outcomes such as mortality, readmission rates, patient and carer satisfaction, and lower costs of care. This broader model definition encompassed substitution and early discharge type models. This systematic review reported on 61 randomized controlled trials and included medical, surgical, rehabilitation, and psychiatric models. Overall, care at home, compared with usual hospital care, resulted in reduction in mortality at 6 months (odds ratio 0.81, CI 0.69, 0.95), readmission rates (0.75, CI 0.59, 0.95), and reductions in costs. Patient satisfaction was higher in Hospital at Home, as was carer satisfaction. Carer burden was lower compared with usual hospital care. The authors suggested that these outcomes were likely to be generalizable given the range of types of studies and patient populations examined [13].

In the USA, development of Hospital at Home was spearheaded by investigators at Johns Hopkins. They focused on development of a substitutive model of Hospital at Home with a robust physician component. Initial work focused on the identification of acute medical conditions that were appropriate for Hospital at Home care. Clinical eligibility criteria to select appropriate Hospital at Home patients were developed and validated [14]. The initial set of Hospital at Home conditions were community acquired pneumonia, chronic heart failure, chronic obstructive pulmonary disease, and cellulitis. Pilot studies demonstrated clinical and economic feasibility of this Hospital at Home model [18]. Because of a lack of payment mechanisms for Hospital at Home in fee-for-service Medicare, larger studies were performed in integrated healthcare delivery systems such as Medicare managed care and the Veterans Affairs health systems. The model studied by Hopkins in its research phase employs continuous nursing care, followed by intermittent nurse visits, and at least daily physician home visits. A randomized controlled trial was forbidden by the Center for Medicare and Medicaid services because of regulations governing Medicare managed care plans. Using a quasi-experimental design with a conservative intent-to-treat analysis, Hospital at Home care was shown to be feasible and efficacious. Patients received timely hospital-level care at home that met quality standards. Compared with patients treated in the acute hospital, those treated in Hospital at Home suffered fewer important clinical complications including mortality, sedative medication use, chemical restraints, and incident delirium [19]. Patient and family member satisfaction was higher [20]. Although patients were not required to have a caregiver (30 % lived alone), caregiver stress was lower [19]. Hospital at Home patients improved in the ability to perform IADLs compared with usual care patients [21]. Health care provider satisfaction with the model was high [22]. The average amount paid for Hospital at Home patients was lower; savings resulted from reduced use of laboratory and high tech procedures [23].

Dissemination of Hospital at Home

Everett Roger's framework for diffusion of innovations is useful to consider in the context of Hospital at Home. Rogers described several features of the innovation that favored adoption and dissemination. These are: (1) relative advantage of the innovation compared to current practice; (2) compatibility of the innovation with the values, beliefs, needs, and culture of the adopter; (3) complexity of the innovation—the simpler the better; (4) trialability, or how the inno-

vation can be tested easily before investing in the innovation; and (5) observability, that is, the ability of an adopter to see others try it first with visible benefit

In this Rogerian framework, several key recent trends are working in favor of Hospital at Home dissemination. There has been growing awareness of the hazards of hospitalization (especially for older adults), the high costs of health care for older adults, and the robust evidence base for Hospital at Home, establishing properties of relative advantage for Hospital at Home. The rapid evolution of the US health care system in the wake of the Affordable Care Act into a system that is capitated or functionally capitated has elevated the compatibility of Hospital at Home significantly with regard to payment, a key driver in health service adoption and dissemination. As health systems try to move care to less expensive cost centers, i.e., the community, and community-based systems of care improve, and as the capacities of technologies such as telehealth improve, Hospital at Home has and will continue to become a less complex model to develop

Dissemination Experience to Date

Implementing the Hospital at Home model at a hospital or within a health system, at a high level, requires alignment of the payer, hospital, health care providers (including those who will provide care to the patient in the home as well as key hospital-based providers, notably hospital emergency department personnel and, sometime, hospitalists), and home health service delivery assets. In the current health care environment to date, the environments in which it is easiest to create such alignment have been in integrated delivery systems, Medicare managed care, and the Veterans Affairs (VA) health system [24].

To date, Hospital at Home has been adopted by several VA medical centers and integrated delivery systems. In each case, substitutive Hospital at Home care is provided; adopters have also implemented early discharge, i.e., transfer type Hospital at Home, as well. VA adoptions of Hospital at Home have used their robust home-based primary care model as a substrate on which to build Hospital at Home.

For example, the Portland, Oregon VA medical center adopted Hospital at Home as a service offering after participating in the Hopkins Hospital at Home National Demonstration. Portland adapted the model to the VA environment; rather than focus exclusively on older adults, they allowed adults aged 18 and over to receive care. They implemented an early discharge, i.e., transfer component to the model, as well. Portland has had substantial success with the model. In 2008, Portland reported a case series on their experience with 290 patients; 23 % were admitted to Hospital at Home directly from the emergency department, 23 % were admitted directly from outpatient clinics or home care, and

56 were transfers from the inpatient service. Hospital at Home was integrated into the VA electronic medical record. The average length of stay was 3.2 days, 37 % of patients were under the age of 65, and 30 % lived alone. The program produced cost savings by diverting patients to the lower cost Hospital at Home; they estimated that the program needed to save 235 inpatient bed days of care per year to cover the costs of the Hospital at Home infrastructure, which included a 0.5 full-time equivalent physician, 1.0 full-time equivalent home care registered nurse, and 0.5 full-time equivalent clerical support, on top of the standard home-based primary care infrastructure [25]. The VA has also implemented Hospital at Home in New Orleans, LA, Honolulu, HI, Philadelphia, PA, and Cincinnati, OH.

In the Medicare managed care and integrated delivery system context, Presbyterian Health Systems (PHS), in Albuquerque, NM, adopted Hospital at Home. PHS is the largest health care system in NM. Hospital at Home was adopted in the context of capacity issues at their main hospital and a culture that was open to disruptive innovation. PHS developed and made Hospital at Home available to patients insured by their Medicare Advantage product, insuring cost savings to their system. In addition to providing in-person daily physician visits, the PHS version of Hopkins Hospital at Home also included a telehealth component in which nurses provided additional remote support by monitoring for important clinical changes via daily telehealth encounters. The telehealth unit consists of a blood pressure monitor, stethoscope, oximeter, glucometer, and video connection allowing communication for assessments and teaching. In 2009 and 2010, the program experienced 323 admissions, patients had similar or better clinical outcomes, satisfaction with Hospital at Home was better than for similar patients admitted to their traditional acute care hospital, and Hospital at Home saved 19 % costs when compared to similar inpatients. The savings were derived principally from lower average length of stay and use of fewer lab and diagnostic tests compared to similar inpatients [26].

Dissemination of Hospital at Home into the traditional Medicare fee-for-service environment has been difficult, as there is no established payment mechanism for it. Certain services provided in the context of Hospital at Home can, in theory, be paid for under various established Medicare payment codes. For example, physician home visits can be reimbursed under Medicare Part B evaluation and management payment codes. Certain home health services can be provided under Medicare Part A skilled home health care prospective payment. However, certain services, such as infusion services are difficult to obtain reimbursement for, and the intensity of services provided in Hospital at Home do not allow for Hospital at Home full costs to be covered appropriately by current mechanisms.

There have been some recent developments in developing a payment model for Hospital at Home in fee-for-service Medicare. In 2014, Mount Sinai Medical Center, New York, received a 3-year Innovation Challenge Grant from the Center for Medicare and Medicaid Innovation of the Center for Medicare and Medicaid Services [27]. The goal of this work will be to implement the Hospital at Home model at hospitals in the Mount Sinai system and to develop data to inform the development of a 30-day bundled payment model for Hospital at Home that could be implemented in the Medicare fee-for-service system. If such a payment model could be developed and implemented, it would likely spark substantial dissemination of the Hospital at Home model in the US health care system.

Barriers to Dissemination

In addition to the payment and structural challenges noted above, several additional barriers to Hospital at Home dissemination are worth considering. Health system leaders are often concerned about the risk for malpractice lawsuits and litigation with Hospital at Home. To date, litigation has been relatively non-existent in Hospital at Home. The malpractice literature suggests that lack of effective patient/family–physician communication is a basic cause of many malpractice actions. There are reasons to believe that in Hospital at Home, as in other home-based models, communication between providers and patients, in general, may be more effective and of higher quality than that which occurs in the hospital or other facility-based care. By virtue of being present and a guest in a patient's home, providers must communicate well, enhancing trust between patients and health care providers, thus reducing the risk of malpractice litigation. Further, to date, admission to Hospital at Home, to date, has always been a choice made by a patient, which also mitigates risk.

Currently, Hospital at Home lacks a regulatory home. It provides hospital-level care in the home, but does not entirely replicate the hospital environment. It provides a level of care significantly more intense and timely than that provided in typical skilled home health care. To date, most adopters have situated Hospital at Home within their home health administrative structure, sitting under the larger umbrella of the hospital and health system. If Hospital at Home does become more widely disseminated, it will need to develop a quality regimen more appropriately specific to its needs. Some programs, to date, have been accredited under the home health realm of The Joint Commission.

Attitudinal barriers and clinical inertia can also be substantial barrier to Hospital at Home dissemination. Hospital at Home is one of the best studied health service delivery models; the evidence base is robust, but dissemination has been modest. Stein et al. reported on the modest response in translation to home management of deep venous thrombosis despite the demonstration of the safety and efficacy of such home treatment. They hypothesized that attitudinal barriers may be one of several factors inhibiting widespread dissemination of the model [28].

The Future State

There are examples of Hospital at Home models that have scaled. In Victoria State, Australia, Hospital at Home has been reimbursed at the same rate as traditional hospital care since the mid-1990s. By 2009, Hospital at Home accounted for 2.3 % of all inpatient admissions, 5.3 % of all multiday admissions, and 5 % of all hospital bed days. There was high satisfaction with the model. But for the existence of Hospital at Home, health authorities note that they would have had to build another 500-bed inpatient facility [29].

Changes in health service delivery and payment occurring under the Affordable Care Act will likely serve to promote Hospital at Home adoption and dissemination. Medicare managed care in the form of Medicare Advantage plans continue to grow and will provide a favorable payment environment for Hospital at Home. The development and increasing presence of Affordable Care Organizations will also provide a permissive environment for Hospital at Home. Improvement in telehealth and other remote monitoring and service delivery technology will make home-based care safer and easier to administer. The demographic trends associated with an aging population, an increase in the prevalence of chronic illness, and trends towards the increasingly high-tech environment of the traditional acute hospital will put pressure on health systems to move more care to the community as hospitals become cost centers, rather than profit centers.

References

1. Montalto M. Hospital in the home: principles & practice. Victoria, Australia: ArtWords Pty Ltd; 2002.
2. MEDPAC. A data book: health care spending and the medicare program. Washington, DC: Medicare Payment Advisory Commission; 2014.
3. Landrigan CP, Parry GJ, Bones CB, Hackbarth AD, Goldmann DA, Sharek PJ. Temporal trends in rates of patient harm resulting from medical care. N Engl J Med. 2010;363(22):2124–34. doi:10.1056/NEJMsa1004404.
4. Creditor MC. Hazards of hospitalization of the elderly. Ann Intern Med. 1993;118(3):219–23. doi:10.7326/0003-4819-118-3-199302010-00011.
5. Mills WR, Landers SH. Home is where the heart of the ACO is. J Am Med Dir Assoc. 2013;14(7):527. doi:10.1016/j.jamda.2013.04.002.
6. Brennan TA, Leape LL, Laird NM, Hebert L, Localio AR, Lawthers AG, et al. Incidence of adverse events and negligence in hospital-ized patients. N Engl J Med. 1991;324(6):370–6. doi:10.1056/NEJM199102073240604.
7. Leape LL, Brennan TA, Laird N, Lawthers AG, Localio AR, Barnes BA, et al. The nature of adverse events in hospitalized patients. N Engl J Med. 1991;324(6):377–84. doi:10.1056/NEJM199102073240605.
8. Covinsky KE, Pierluissi E, Johnston C. Hospitalization-associated disability: "she was probably able to ambulate, but I'm not sure". JAMA. 2011;306(16):1782–93. doi:10.1001/jama.2011.1556.
9. Cheng J, Montalto M, Leff B. Hospital at home. Clin Geriatr Med. 2009;25(1):79–91. doi:10.1016/j.cger.2008.10.002.
10. Inouye SK, Schlesinger MJ, Lydon TJ. Delirium: a symptom of how hospital care is failing older persons and a window to improve quality of hospital care. Am J Med. 1999;106(5):565–73. doi:10.1016/S0002-9343(99)00070-4.
11. Landers SH. Why health care is going home. N Engl J Med. 2010;363(18):1690–1. doi:10.1056/NEJMp1000401.
12. Leff B, Montalto M. Home hospital—toward a tighter definition. J Am Geriatr Soc. 2004;52(12):2141. doi:10.1111/j.1532-5415.2004.52579_1.x.
13. Caplan G, Sulaiman N, Mangin DA, Ricauda N, Wilson A, Barclay L. A meta-analysis of "hospital in the home". Med J Aust. 2012;197(9):512–9.
14. Leff B, Burton L, Bynum JW, Harper M, Greenough W, Steinwachs D, et al. Prospective evaluation of clinical criteria to select older persons with acute medical illness for care in a hypothetical home hospital. J Am Geriatr Soc. 1997;45:1066–73.
15. Leff B, Burton L, Mader SL, Naughton B, Burl J, Inouye SK, et al. Hospital at home: feasibility and outcomes of a program to provide hospital-level care at home for acutely ill older patients. Ann Intern Med. 2005;143(11):798–808. doi:10.7326/0003-4819-143-11-200512060-00008.
16. Shepperd S, Doll H, Angus RM, Clarke MJ, Iliffe S, Kalra L, et al. Avoiding hospital admission through provision of hospital care at home: a systematic review and meta-analysis of individual patient data. CMAJ. 2009;180(2):175–82. doi:10.1503/cmaj.081491.
17. Shepperd S, Doll H, Broad J, Gladman J, Iliffe S, Langhorne P, et al. Early discharge hospital at home. Cochrane Database Syst Rev. 2009;1, CD000356. doi:10.1002/14651858.CD000356.pub3.
18. Leff B, Burton L, Guido S, Greenough W, Steinwachs D, Burton JR. Home hospital program: a pilot study. J Am Geriatr Soc. 1999;47(6):697–702.
19. Leff B, Burton L, Mader SL, Naughton B, Burl J, Koehn D, et al. Comparison of stress experienced by family members of patients treated in hospital at home with that of those receiving traditional acute hospital care. J Am Geriatr Soc. 2008;56(1):117–23. doi:10.1111/j.1532-5415.2007.01459.x.
20. Leff B, Burton L, Mader S, Naughton B, Burl J, Clark R, et al. Satisfaction with hospital at home care. J Am Geriatr Soc. 2006;54(9):1355–63. doi:10.1111/j.1532-5415.2006.00855.x.
21. Marsteller JA, Burton L, Mader SL, Naughton B, Burl J, Guido S, et al. Health care provider evaluation of a substitutive model of hospital at home. Med Care. 2009;47(9):979–85. doi:10.1097/MLR.0b013e31819c93fc.
22. Leff B, Burton L, Mader SL, Naughton B, Burl J, Greenough WB, et al. Comparison of functional outcomes associated with hospital at home care and traditional acute hospital care. J Am Geriatr Soc. 2009;57(2):273–8. doi:10.1111/j.1532-5415.2008.02103.x.
23. Frick KD, Burton LC, Clark R, Mader SI, Naughton WB, Burl JB, et al. Substitutive Hospital at Home for older persons: effects on costs. Am J Manag Care. 2009;15(1):49–56.
24. Leff B. Defining and disseminating the hospital-at-home model. Can Med Assoc J. 2009;180(2):156–7. doi:10.1503/cmaj.081891.
25. Mader SL, Medcraft MC, Joseph C, Jenkins KL, Benton N, Chapman K, et al. Program at home: a Veterans Affairs Healthcare

Program to deliver hospital care in the home. J Am Geriatr Soc. 2008;56(12):2317–22. doi:10.1111/j.1532-5415.2008.02006.x.

26. Cryer L, Shannon SB, Van Amsterdam M, Leff B. Costs for 'Hospital At Home' patients were 19 percent lower, with equal or better outcomes compared to similar inpatients. Health Aff. 2012;31(6):1237–43. doi:10.1377/hlthaff.2011.1132.

27. Health Care Innovation Awards to provide better health care and lower costs. Icahn School of Medicine at Mount Sinai:

U.S. Department of Health & Human Services. 2014. http://www.hhs.gov/news/press/2014pres/07/20140709b.html.

28. Stein PD, Hull RD, Matta F, Willyerd GL. Modest response in translation to home management of deep venous thrombosis. Am J Med. 2010;123(12):1107–13. doi:10.1016/j.amjmed.2010.07.016.

29. Montalto M. The 500-bed hospital that isn't there: the Victorian Department of Health review of the Hospital in the Home program. Med J Aust. 2010;193(10):598–601.

Home-Based Primary Care Program for Home-Limited Patients

Peter A. Boling and Jean Yudin

Historical Recap: Home Medical Care in Past Times

Back in the day, the house call was the principal setting for most of primary care in the U.S. Physicians had few effective tools and patients were less mobile, so it made sense. In 1850, physicians in Philadelphia reportedly made 30 home visits a day—likely seeing families as a group in smaller communities without traffic. And in the early 1900s Richmond, Virginia hired four physicians who made daily rounds in horse drawn carriages treating accidental injuries and infections, and rendering the earliest forms of palliative care. Concurrently, in the first half of the twentieth century voluntary parish nurses and public health workers in some urban settings offered the precursor of care now rendered by modern home health agencies. These nurses provided care at home, much of which was counseling and supportive care since technical services were still limited.

Then, as technologic revolutions in medical care drove health care into hospitals in the mid-1900s, physicians organized their work in office settings. Despite innovations like the 1950 Montefiore chronic illness care program in New York City led by Bluestone and Cherkasky which provided physician care, including subspecialty services, to chronically ill adults at home, house calls dropped from 40 % of primary care visits in 1930 to 1 % in 1980. Relative inefficiency of home visits in a fee-for-service world with inadequate reimbursement per visit, and the lack of physicians' now familiar office support team and access to quick

diagnostics combined to relegate house calls to an occasional social service from a bygone era, offered only to longstanding patients and often only when they were dying.

Contributing to home visits' decline was the rapid growth of home health agency care, authorized in the 1965 Medicare legislation. This law states that Part A home health care is available to patients who meet a specific definition of homebound (able to leave home infrequently other than for medical care and religious worship, and then with difficulty), plus needing defined skilled professional services on a part-time, intermittent basis, and finally having a physician's order. By the mid-1990s, Medicare home health agency care expenses were $18 billion and growing 17 % annually. Though intermittent, this model provided the bulk of in-home health care for sick patients. While Medicare home health agency care required physician authorization, the typical care process became disconnected from the ordering physician and has largely remained so. Many of these sick patients who are functionally homebound see physicians far less often than similarly ill patients managed in any other setting, and have less physician's input on the evolving care plan. The presence of a professional care option (home health agency care) for the sicker patients, at least for a short interval, probably made it easier for physicians to step aside. These immobile patients then simply dropped out of view of the medical community.

Through the 1990s, operating under cost-based reimbursement, home health agency care episodes extended to 6 months in many cases and almost half of the visits were made by home health aides who were in the home for several hours per day; this was becoming a chronic care service which was not what was intended when the law was created. Medicare home health agency care growth was then abruptly constrained by the 1997 Balanced Budget Act and the Interim Payment System (1997–2000) which cut services in half and put thousands of agencies out of business. Skilled home care slowly rebounded under the home health care Prospective Payment System (implemented in 2000), that pays agencies on a 60-day case rate that is adjusted to patient condition. This business is again approaching $20 billion in

P.A. Boling, M.D. (✉)
Department of Internal Medicine, Virginia Commonwealth University, 1300 East Marshall Street, Richmond, VA 23298, USA
e-mail: pboling@mcvh-vcu.edu

J. Yudin, G.N.P.-B.C.
Division of Geriatric Medicine, Department of Medicine, University of Pennsylvania Health System,
3615 Chestnut Street, Philadelphia, PA 19104, USA
e-mail: yudin@mail.med.upenn.edu

M.L. Malone et al. (eds.), *Geriatrics Models of Care: Bringing 'Best Practice' to an Aging America*,
DOI 10.1007/978-3-319-16068-9_15, © Springer International Publishing Switzerland 2015

annual expenses with more than 11,000 Medicare certified home health agencies in the US Home health aide visits are almost entirely gone, professional visits per episode have dropped by half and episodes themselves now average only 35 days. This care model is fragmented, limited more than ever by the short-term nature of Medicare home health benefits, and it still fosters frequent use of emergency services and hospitals when illness worries patients and families. The rate of hospital care during a 60-day home health episode has remained in the 25–30 % range since 1985.

What has happened with the medical component of health care of these patients? After decades of steep decline, primary care in the home is now experiencing a gradual and accelerating renaissance. The rebirth was initially sparked in the 1970s by visionary academic geriatrician leaders like Phillip Brickner, whose lead article in the 1975 Annals of Internal Medicine was titled, "the homebound aged: a medically unreached group,"; and Knight Steel and John Burton, who recognized the inherent value of seeing people at home, along with clinician advocates who felt the need for more direct physician involvement in home care. In the mid-1980s, a new generation of leaders forged the American Academy of Home Care Physicians—now the American Academy of Home Care Medicine. With a dual focus on education and advocacy, the Academy grew and pushed the agenda to enhance the Medicare fee schedule for home and domiciliary visits between 1996 and 2001. Under these new drivers, Medicare home visits almost tripled, resulting in some large and sustainable (though volume-dependent) clinical programs.

Finally, with the 1997 Balanced Budget Act, advance practice nurses (APNs, most of whom are nurse practitioners or NPs) could be reimbursed for services provided within their "scope of practice," regardless of site, and subject to state regulations. Not requiring the collaborating physician to be physically present led to rapid growth in NP home-centered medical practice ; by 2006 the fraction of 3.8 million Medicare home visits billed by physician assistants (PAs) and NPs rose from 15 to 26 % [1].

This recap sets the historical stage for in-home medical care. We now move into an era of managing chronic illness, heavily influenced by the demography of 78 million baby boomers. Further, we provide care in the context of the successes of biomedical care in preventing rapid death when people develop serious health problems, including organ system failure and advanced cancers. These challenges have both clinical and economic implications.

House Calls

Let us consider why house calls are compelling. Clinicians who are familiar with office, hospital or nursing home settings and then start making house calls have a shared realiza-

tion that several things are unique to the home setting. One was formally studied by Joe Ramsdell at San Diego whose team observed 1.6 new findings during home geriatric assessment after comprehensive clinic-based assessment, while noting that individuals with moderate cognitive impairment performed on average 5 points better on the Mini-Mental State Exam when seen at home. The provider in the home quickly gains important insights about the patient's needs and care processes that are difficult or impossible to obtain otherwise. Beyond getting a more accurate assessment, more efficiently, the provider is also better able to calibrate the care plan to the preferences, capabilities and constraints of the home after doing environmental assessment, safety assessment, and medication reconciliation.

Moreover, one of the most important values of the home visit is that it engenders trust and places the provider on the patient and family's turf, thus altering the power dynamic in the therapeutic relationship. This promotes a more effective care process with greater opportunity for patient empowerment, and fosters outcomes that are aligned with patient and family preferences including peaceful death at home when that is best.

In addition to providing better information and building trust, house calls overcome a major barrier to care access which is immobility. Whether immobility derives from physical limitations, dependence on poorly portable technology like ventilators, or neuropsychological problems including dementia, patient immobility leads to many misadventures in health care caused by the lack of timely access and the discontinuity. Once we started making house calls, it never seemed right that a frail patient would be pulled from home, sometimes from bed, to endure arduous transport to the provider's office for a brief visit on the provider's turf and schedule, often not matched to patient need, and then returned home where they would report needing some days to recover from going to see the doctor!

Now, in the context of reducing avoidable acute care episodes with their related risks and costs, a unique value of mobile medical care is the provider's ability to respond to immobile patients' urgent or emergent needs in a timely manner that is often simply not achievable using the office care setting.

Along with increasing pressure to reduce reliance on hospitals with their risks to vulnerable patients and cost, the past decade has witnessed rapid advances in portable technology including lab testing at the point of care, X-rays, ultrasound, electrocardiograms, and electronic records; many technical limitations of home visits that concerned office-based providers in the 1980s are in the past.

Paralleling these changes to medical care in the home, there has been a steady presence of various social supports in the community available to subsets of patients as they qualify based on low income or other factors. Most notable is

Fig. 15.1 Subpopulations that use home care in different ways

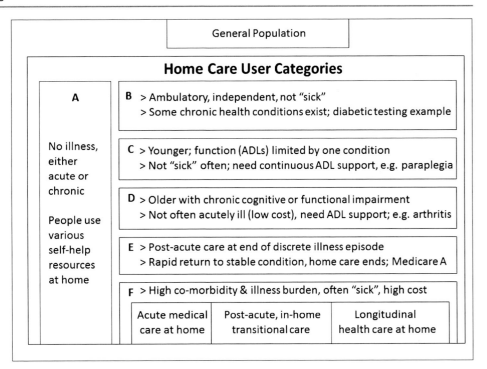

General Population

Home Care User Categories

A

No illness, either acute or chronic

People use various self-help resources at home

B > Ambulatory, independent, not "sick"
> Some chronic health conditions exist; diabetic testing example

C > Younger; function (ADLs) limited by one condition
> Not "sick" often; need continuous ADL support, e.g. paraplegia

D > Older with chronic cognitive or functional impairment
> Not often acutely ill (low cost), need ADL support; e.g. arthritis

E > Post-acute care at end of discrete illness episode
> Rapid return to stable condition, home care ends; Medicare A

F > High co-morbidity & illness burden, often "sick", high cost

| Acute medical care at home | Post-acute, in-home transitional care | Longitudinal health care at home |

Medicaid-funded personal care for those with very low incomes and who have documented clinical needs for daily activity support. Personal care is also an option for those who can afford $20 per hour for the service or who have private long-term care insurance. Personal care aides play an important role in helping people stay at home.

Other support services, which vary greatly from community to community, are also important in keeping people safely at home. Among those has been a constant and important role of adaptive technology that is needed for care at home. Figures 15.1 and 15.2, respectively, show common home care user categories and related payment sources for services to meet the patients' needs. In our discussion here, we would include population groups C through F.

Payment for services creates much of the fragmentation. Figure 15.2 partially demonstrates this complex issue, featuring the most common services and payment mechanisms.

Epidemiology and Scope of Need for Home-Based Primary Care

An important consideration for health policy-makers in relation to home-based medical care is the size of the population needing home-based medical services, among the groups demonstrated in Fig. 15.1. This book presents many models of in-home medical care, from highly acute (hospital at home), short-term transitional care when acutely ill, longitudinal care, and palliative care. Some longitudinal home med-

ical care models incorporate the full range of acute, post-acute, and chronic care services. Patients who need and should benefit from medical care at home have heterogeneous needs and clinical indications. Let us start with those who are largely home-limited on a chronic basis.

Most patients and families prefer living at home over institutional care. Using a prevalence estimate derived from national surveys for community-dwelling persons, among the 65+ age group there are about 7 % with chronic dependency in 3 or more ADLs (3 million), and about 1 % have bed-to-chair or bedfast status. Eleven percent (3.7 million) of older Medicare enrollees received personal care services in 1999. Over three million elderly are now homebound due to physical and cognitive impairments that make it difficult for them to leave their home [2]. Comparing children and younger adults with older persons, there are lower but still noteworthy rates of advanced ADL limitation. In all, there are probably three million people who are chronically home-limited and [3] can leave home only with considerable difficulty. This number will grow rapidly with the baby boom.

And, while less chronic care is now supported by Medicare, the proportion of Medicaid funding used for institutional long-term care relative to home-based care has dropped from 80 to 62 % by 2009, a shift that increased both the available supports and the functional dependency levels in the community. These vulnerable individuals require and are supported by a network of services, often coordinated through an Area Agency on Aging, of which there is one for nearly every U.S. community. Those states that have invested in community supports have lower nursing home use.

Fig. 15.2 Common home care services and major payment sources

Home Care Silo's & Payment Sources

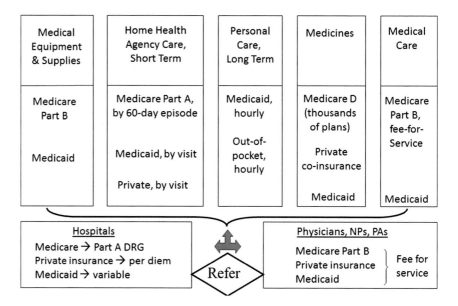

The numbers of persons who need short-term mobile medical care during a year are at least twice that of chronically immobile persons, but many in this short-term group recover mobility and no longer need home medical care, or die; in all the approximate total numbers of persons needing home visits remains manageable, annually in the 5–6 million person range. Many of these individuals reside in clusters, in senior apartment buildings and other new residential options such as assisted living communities, which also permits greater efficiency when delivering mobile medical care.

How does this translate to the need for home visits? For many chronically immobile individuals, medical service encounters are needed about once a month or more on average, some more and some less, to maintain stability and avoid reliance on hospitals and nursing homes when urgent problems appear. If you add in people who need only acute and post-acute care in-home care, as well as those who receive end-of-life and hospice care, groups where the need is usually limited to a few months of medical home visits, you complete the picture of need for house calls.

Combined, the need for mobile medical visits probably exceeds 20 million visits annually, which contrasts with the 3.8 million visits recorded by Medicare now. Estimates for physician in-home services from national surveys in 1985 [4] and 2003 [5], suggest that less than half of office-based primary care providers make house calls and then infrequently. By 2003, 18 % of US physicians had made house calls, and those who did averaged fewer than 5 per week. An analysis from 2012 Medicare billing data showed 10,773 providers (MDs, DOs, NPs, and PAs) with house call and

domiciliary visit bills, of whom 3,891 providers had at least 250 visits [6].

It Takes a Village: The House Call Team and the Home-Based Primary Care Model

To use an overused expression, if you have seen one house call program, you have seen one house call program. Most share an understanding of the core value of taking medical care to frail patients at home. Past that, there are many variations. Some are concentrated in group living settings and have formal relationships with residential communities. Some use medical technicians as drivers and assistants to the medical providers. Some own and deploy technology including imaging services, tele-monitoring, and other diagnostic tools such as remote cardiac impedance testing. Some are more comfortable with delivering an acute care or emergent care response while others prefer rendering primary care. Some serve technology-dependent patients like those on home ventilators; others do not. The degree of medical complexity in a given practice varies considerably. Some are rural rather than urban and suburban. Some charge a substantial per-visit travel fee, not covered by insurance. Some are concierge programs that do not accept Medicare. Some are hospital-based and supported while others are completely independent of medical centers. Some are closely affiliated with a home health agency or hospice and may even have an integrated agency or hospice organization. Some are small with 1–3 providers while others are multi-state organizations with hundreds of employees and substantial administrative infrastructure. Central administrative support is likely to include billing and business management, plus support services including triage and dispatch, routing programs to support providers, and advanced information systems. Most programs now use EHRs. Medical malpractice is not a major issue in home care to this date. Lexus Nexus searches reveal very few lawsuits, probably because of the favorable relationship with patients and the poor clinical prognosis.

The daily operations of house call teams also vary. Some programs have weekly team meetings. Others rely on distance communication and EHRs to maintain connections. In our experience managing very complex patients, a team meeting is important because of the need to get multiple perspectives on a difficult case, and to update the team on regulatory and other community-level changes. Provider visit volumes can range as high as 12–14 visits a day and as low as 3–4 a day, depending on the clinical model and circumstances. For program efficiency as programs grow it is essential to have personnel in the office with clinical credentials to answer phone calls (nurses, for example), to perform triage provide support, and help route providers. Grouping visits and patient panels by geography is common.

In most programs, home-centered medicine is a team effort. Though many programs serve younger adults or children, a core concept arises from geriatric care: the importance of the interdisciplinary team, where each member plays a vital role. A house call program needs an extended team with partners from community-based programs. Typically there is a network of resources that are familiar to providers: pharmacies that deliver medications, social service agencies, preferred home health agency and durable medical equipment providers, adult homes and assisted living settings. These networks are critical to effectively managing this population. A recent review [7] described elements of home-based primary care practices which were successful in improving clinical outcomes (hospitalizations, costs, hospital or nursing facility days of care). Key strengths noted were: interdisciplinary teams, frequent contact among team members, and 24/7 access for patients.

When the full context of supporting frail elders in the community is considered, including both medical and social supportive services, the scope of need to be addressed becomes apparent. Comprehensive care plans require the skills of social workers, therapists, pharmacists, psychiatrists, psychologists, nurses, technologists (lab and radiology) as well as the core medical team (physician, nurse practitioner, or physician assistant), service coordinators, and often individuals who provide daily ADL support when patient and family are not able.

Small private home medical practices may consist of a physician or nurse practitioner who make home visits 2 days a week and see patients in other settings on other days. Their team may include a home health agency and an office staff that handles phone calls, scheduling, and paperwork. A larger practice may consist of several physicians, nurse practitioners, and physician assistants who provide routine and urgent home visits. A larger house call practice may also support a social worker, a registered nurse, and support staff.

Visit frequencies vary. Commonly patients served in this model average 10–15 visits a year. Some patients only need a few visits and others may be seen weekly because they are so sick. A typical day in a practice that is not focused on congregate living may include 5–6 visits per provider, with space held for acute visits or new patients. In practices with both NPs and physicians, some have the physician make the initial visit, while in others nurse practitioners have this role. Occasional team visits are effective, as several disciplines focus on a particularly complex situation.

Providing medical care at home requires a distinctive set of provider attributes. These include: (1) confidence in one's decision-making and clinical skills, (2) higher tolerance for uncertainty, (3) willingness to use time as a diagnostic tool, (4) respect for teammates and their contributions to the patient's care, (5) willingness to practice in less than pristine circumstances, and (6) comfort working with patients and families around difficult issues, some of which cannot be resolved.

Looking Forward, Finances, and Specific Care Models

To deliver in-home medical care in an optimal manner there must be sufficient funding. Medicare payments are insufficient to pay for advanced care coordination, or for employing the other team members needed by the core medical providers, such as social workers, triage nurses, or pharmacists. Reliance on fee-for-service revenue unfortunately skews the model away from patient needs and limits the team's potential to do the work needed to keep patients out of hospitals or nursing homes. Unless the fee-for-service team has a sponsor to defray the extra costs, the focus must be on volume to cover provider salaries and the bottom line, which ultimately take priority over societal value.

Value-based purchasing requires alternative payment strategies, aligned with the goals of advanced clinical models. This can occur in several ways. An Accountable Care Organization (ACO) or other health system with a large-scale risk contract might choose to include house call services, though to date most have not. A payer might contract directly with house call services for primary care or transitional care, potentially under a risk contract, and might also consider innovative options like gain-sharing. In the latter regard, help from actuaries who understand risk adjustment in this frail population is necessary to assure accurate determination of "expected costs" in the absence of an intervention so that gain-share calculations will be fair. Creating alternate payment models and aligning incentives requires a forward-thinking and innovative management team. The organization taking the risk must be aware of what in-home care can do. That organization will make the investment and the necessary changes in administrative processes to manage the finances. Specific examples are discussed below.

Department of Veterans Affairs Home-Based Primary Care (HBPC)

HBPC is a major component of the VA's strategy to shift care from institutional to community settings. Between 2000 and 2012, the number of veterans aged 85 and older tripled and the HBPC census increased from 7,300 to 30,000 while the VA-provided nursing home care census rose only 20 % from 30,700 to 36,000. HBPC is delivered by a broad interdisciplinary team. The program targets veterans with multiple chronic diseases and complex challenges. The program functions as an intensive patient-centered medical home for these most vulnerable veterans. In VA terminology, patient-centered medical homes are Patient Aligned Care Teams (PACTs) and HBPC is a Specialty PACT. Since 1972 with six sites, HBPC has expanded to all 139 VA medical centers by 2012. Since 2006 over 60 new programs have been added, while maintaining fidelity of the intervention and clinical outcomes [8]. In 2007, a new setting was added—the Medical Foster Home where veterans who would otherwise require a nursing facility for safety live in the home of a foster caregiver, with care coordinated by the HBPC team.

The HBPC team consists of a nurse, physician, nurse practitioner, social worker, rehabilitation therapist, dietitian, pharmacist, and psychologist. Some programs also have psychiatrists, chaplains, or recreation therapists as core personnel. Programs that paired an NP or PA with a physician used less institutional care than teams that relied exclusively on physicians. Through a consensus process, recommended HBPC caseloads are: 30–40 patients per nurse; 75–100 patients per NP, and 100–125 patients per therapist.

HBPC is tasked to care for individuals where "clinic-based care is not effective," Most of these individuals have chronic, complex disabling disease, and mortality averages 20 %–25 % annually. Veterans trust this type of care, attributing prevention of avoidable and unwanted hospital and emergency care to HBPC. In qualitative studies, HBPC characteristics that correlate with fewer hospital readmissions of Medicare beneficiaries include better adherence to medication management, individual involvement in healthcare decisions, early recognition of exacerbation of symptoms, and family caregiver support. On the VA's 2007 National Patient Satisfaction Survey, 83 % of veterans rated HBPC care as very good or excellent, the highest overall satisfaction rating among VA programs.

HBPC teams cover a wide geography, including rural areas. Strategies to overcome barriers related to travel time include dissemination of satellite HBPC teams to community-based outpatient clinics [CBOC], and tele-medicine, ranging from electronic reminders for chronic disease management to comprehensive video for remotely conducting a physical exam.

HBPC's effects have been studied repeatedly. The core team is expensive, costing $10,000–$13,000 per beneficiary year. All analyses demonstrate improved caregiver and patient satisfaction, improved caregiver function; importantly, analyses also consistently demonstrate reduced hospital and nursing facility days, hospital admissions, hospital readmissions, and total costs. In a 2002 longitudinal pre–post analysis of 11,334 individuals, HBPC enrollment was associated with 24 % total VA cost reduction. In a similar 2007 analysis, HBPC enrollment was associated with reductions in VA hospital bed-days of care (59 %), nursing home bed-days of care (89 %), and 30-day hospital readmissions (21 %). Because the VA is an integrated system, it has been able to establish benchmarks for team performance, following hospital days of care, hospital admissions, and hospital readmissions from the 6 months before admission to the 12 months after admission. As HBPC expanded during 2006–2013, hospitalization rate declined to 6 hospitalizations per 100 veteran months, and hospital days dropped 50–60 % in more than 85 % of the programs [8]. A recent analysis [9] demonstrated that the VA HBPC programs reduced total costs to both Medicare and to the VA by 11 % compared with prospectively estimated cost benchmarks that were carefully risk-adjusted. Targeting is essential. It is hard to prevent hospitalizations among veterans who do not use the hospital.

ElderPAC

Patients who are eligible for both Medicare and Medicaid are among the frailest, least educated and most expensive Medicare beneficiaries. These eight million dual-eligible individuals generate 46 % of Medicaid and 25 % of Medicare expenditures. More than a quarter have 3 or more ADL dependencies and 11 % have 5 or more chronic conditions. Their social and medical needs are complex. Current arrangement of health care in service settings that are separate silos creates inefficiencies, duplication, and gaping holes that can result in long-term institutional care.

To fill these gaps, for 15 years the University of Pennsylvania Health System has operated an integrated, interdisciplinary team called ElderPAC, linking a house calls team and a home health agency with staff from the local Area Agency on Aging (AAA), and serving frail low income elderly

Fig. 15.3 ElderPAC community survival and costs. *EPAC* elder partnership for all-inclusive care, *NH* nursing home, *HCBC* home and community-based care, *Waiver* control patients selected from Aging Waiver, *Waiver-c* control patients residing in the community

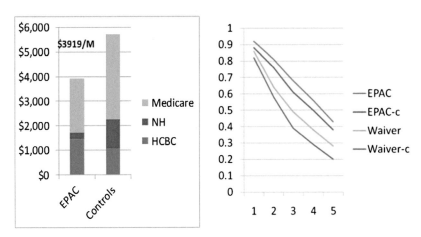

ElderPAC Outcomes

COSTS ($per month)   Community Survival

consumers. Before ElderPAC formed, 3 nurse practitioners caring for 180 patients had to work with 39 case managers at the AAA while each case manager at the AAA worked with 50 different providers. This inhibited formation of productive relationships and effective teamwork. The cement for ElderPAC initially was weekly team meetings; using telecommunications, a shared electronic medical record and a unified care plan, the team now meets monthly. Two evaluations of ElderPAC have addressed the potential to prolong community survival for frail elders, and reduce Medicaid nursing home costs and total Medicaid costs by providing more and better home and community-based care [10].

The initial ElderPAC cohort of 50 patients was matched with 50 consumers from the Pennsylvania low income service programs that were not managed by an integrated team. Patients were followed for 5 years to track community survival. Medicare costs were compared for the initial 2 years (1997–1999). Matched controls were randomly picked from low-income community long-term care service consumers. Medicare costs were estimated from Hierarchical Condition Category (HCC) scores and Medicaid costs were obtained from the State of Pennsylvania. Deaths were obtained from state vital records. Community service costs were measured from the local care plan system and Medicaid files. Functional status scores came from the common intake assessment. Primary outcomes were community survival time (alive and residing outside an institution), nursing home use, mortality, and costs.

The second cohort of 92 patients had 4,360 beneficiary-months of observation and very high risk scores for institutional care need. The control cohort overall had 300 consumers, with 6,910 waiver months of observation.

Among 92 ElderPAC consumers, mean age was 82, and 86 % were female. Mean HCC score was 3.55, compared with the mean PACE HCC of 2.33; these patients have very high disease burden. ElderPAC participants had 3.7 ADL impairments, with 48 % having 5–6 impairments. The community comparison group was somewhat less impaired—biasing against finding a favorable impact.

The first ElderPAC cohort demonstrated a 60 % reduction in annual Medicare spending compared to matched controls, from an annual $47,015 to $18,808 per beneficiary in 2,010 dollars. As a further control, annual Medicare costs of the 1999 National Long Term Care Survey participants who had 3+ ADL dependencies and were receiving home health care were over $49,681. In the second cohort, HCC-based expected costs were reduced by approximately 50 % ($24,000 vs. $51,000).

In the second cohort, the ElderPAC group had 3.8 hospitalizations/100 beneficiaries compared to 7.2/100 among the control group. Long-term nursing home use over the 5 years was less (5.9 % vs. 24.9 %), while the care plan costs for community care were greater ($1,942±1,117 vs $1,084±477). ElderPAC patients had a mean survival of 44.3 months in the community, and 46.8 months overall, while for HCBS comparison consumers community survival was 24.2 months, and 31.9 months overall (Fig. 15.3). There was 76 % less time in nursing homes: 7.7–2.5 months. Using Medicaid claims, average monthly expenditures for ElderPAC patients was $20,640 compared to $27,084 for control consumers, with the major difference being in the costs spent on NH care (24 % reduction). Thus, integrated care is a dominant strategy, providing greater health (survival) at lower cost.

Nurse Practitioner-Led Programs

There are notable house call programs where the main workforce is nurse practitioners (NPs), and some that are primarily operated by NP leaders. These programs engage physicians as consultants, but function in states with strong independent practice regulations where nurse practitioners can evaluate patients, diagnose, order and interpret diagnostic tests, initiate and manage treatments—including prescribing medications—under the exclusive licensure authority of the state board of nursing. There are now nearly 20 states with a full practice regulatory environment. Some programs operate in states with more limited practice regulations, where state licensure law limits the ability of nurse practitioners to undertake some elements of NP practice. Some of these programs are physician operated, but rely exclusively on NPs to provide the primary care at home, while others are owned by nurse practitioners. Other programs, given the complexity of their homebound patients, use a collaborative model, rather than a consultant physician model, with both providers caring for the patient; nurse practitioners are often the primary providers and do 75 % or more of the visits.

Independence at Home Demonstration

Section 3024 of the 2010 ACA created the Independence at Home (IAH) demonstration, to test the house calls team model in the context of Medicare fee-for-service. IAH enrollment requires sick patients, who have been in the hospital within the past 12 months, have used post-acute care (skilled home health care, skilled nursing facility (SNF) care, inpatient rehab in that same period); have two or more serious chronic conditions; and two or more persistent ADL deficits. The law prescribes a 3-year demonstration with a cap of 10,000 Medicare beneficiaries. There are 18 sites involved in this demonstration, including 2 consortium groups. The demonstration is in its third year. There are several quality measures, designed to insure that patients receive good care and to insure timely response by the IAH teams in the face of acute problems. The payments are standard Medicare payments—patients use their Medicare and other insurance benefits as they always have—plus payments to the IAH team based on a share of residual savings, calculated by subtracting actual costs from calculated expected costs, after a minimum 5 % savings is retained by Medicare. Excellent, timely, continuous care of very sick patients across the care continuum should result in less hospital and nursing home and generate savings. The demonstration includes a variety of programs and is being evaluated by federal contractors.

A recent paper using case–control methods describes successful results from a cohort of 722 patients treated before the IAH demonstration started, and cared for by one program that is participating in the IAH demonstration. Overall savings were reported to be 17 % over 2 years [11], and by using a subset of patients that met IAH administrative enrollment criteria, savings are estimated to have been 31 % over two years. This clinical team provides physician and nurse practitioner home visits, has strong social work support, nurse triage, pharmacy consultation, and a network of social services that are affiliated. Most of the inpatient care is managed by the core team at one hospital.

Academic Programs

Much of the developmental work with house calls models and the renaissance of the field have arisen from organized programs that now exist across the country at dozens of academic medical centers. Ultimately, this will also be where the future leaders and the workforce will be trained. Generally these programs are smaller than private practices in the community and may have institutional support to help sustain multifaceted missions that include teaching, research, and helping hospitals manage readmissions plus other risks. There are some larger academic programs such as those of the Boston University home medical service that has operated for 130 years, Mount Sinai visiting physicians and the Cleveland Clinic house call program that carry a census around 1,000 patients. Like Boston University and Mount Sinai, the program at Virginia Commonwealth University (VCU) supports a mandatory house call experience for all 211 medical students in each class as well as other learner activities. The VCU initiative [12] includes a Naylor model transitional care program that has shown consistently positive impacts for 14 years and is integrated across the continuum of care with clinic, inpatient care, chronic house calls, nursing home, and hospice. VCU is also participating in one of the IAH demonstration consortia along with the Washington Hospital Center and the University of Pennsylvania.

Evidence-Based Care

Until recently there have been relatively few formal studies of the in-home primary care model. A small randomized controlled trial (RCT) in the late 1970s showed improved satisfaction and probable cost savings in the final months of life. An early randomized controlled trial of VA HBPC with 16 sites from the early 1980s did not show savings, but it was evident that the model was not faithfully implemented in many centers during those earlier years. However, combining newer evidence from the revamped and structured VA HBPC, Hospital at Home, the Washington Hospital Center program, the Naylor transitional care program, the GRACE trial and others, there is a growing, substantial body of support for the home-based care model. In fact, the evidence for cost savings from in-home care that focuses on complex patients is substantially stronger than what has come from disease-focused strategies, and other models of care that are now being discussed as central strategies for health care redesign. It also makes good sense to care for people where they live, whether in a nursing home or in their own home. This home-centered care should continue indefinitely, if needed, following support during a short-term period of instability and transitional care.

The Future

Health care systems change in an organic manner, variously influenced by exemplary practices, published evidence of benefit, market forces, health policy and insurance changes, patient and provider preferences, entrepreneurial efforts, local culture, and workforce development. The pace of change can be remarkably fast: witness the rise of hospitalists or statin usage, and the stoppage in use of estrogen replacement on the heels of the Woman's Health Initiative Study. Change can be agonizingly slow in the case of developing the model of home-based primary care to serve the vulnerable populations in our community that need those services. Given the growing evidence of efficacy and cost-effectiveness plus clear consumer preferences, and basic common sense, we should align incentives so that market forces can complete the transformation which has begun in caring for home-limited persons. The need is clear: home-based primary care is the right thing to do.

References

1. Moran. Data source: physician/supplier procedure summary (PSPS) master record file for medicare part B summary data (2005–2012). Physician/Supplier Procedure Summary (PSPS) Master File-2012.
2. Boling PA. Physicians in home care: past, present and future. Caring. 1998;17:10–5.
3. Kaye HS, LaPlante M, Harrington C. Do non-institutional long term care services reduce medicaid spending. Health Affairs. 2009;28(1):262–72. doi:10.1377/hlthaff.28.1.262.
4. Boling PA, Ellis J, Retchin SM, Pancoast S. The influence of physician specialty on housecalls. Arch Intern Med. 1990;150:2333–7.
5. Cheerie DK, Burt CW, Woodwell DA. National ambulatory medical care survey: 2001 summary. Adv-Data. 2003;11:337.
6. Sowislo R. US medical management, personal communication.
7. Stall N, Nowaczynski M, Sinha S. A systematic review of outcomes from home-based primary care programs for homebound older adults. J Am Geriatr Soc. 2014;62(12):2243–51. doi:10.1111/jgs.13088.
8. Kinosian B, Edes T, Becker P. Expanding VA's Home Based Primary Care (HBPC) while improving performance: 2006–2012. J Am Geriatr Soc. 2014;62 suppl 1:S136.
9. Edes T, Kinosian B, Vuckovic NH, et al. Improved access and cost for clinically complex veterans with home based primary care. J Am Geriatr Soc. 2014;62(10):1954–61. doi:10.1111/jgs.13030.
10. Yudin J. Sewing an all-inclusive quilt from Home and Community Services for Frail Elders: a community-academic housecall program partnership. Geriatr Nurs. 2013;34:162–5.
11. De Jonge KE, Jamshed N, Gilden D, Kubisiak J, Bruce SR, Taler G. Effects of home-based primary care on medicare costs in high-risk elders. J Am Geriatr Soc. 2014;62(10):1825–31. doi:10.1111/jgs.12974 (advanced e-publication).
12. Boling PA, Chandekar RV, Hungate B, Purvis M, Selby-Penczak R, Abbey LJ. Improving outcomes and lowering costs by applying advanced models of in-home care. Cleve Clin J Med. 2013;80(Electronic Suppl 1):eS7–14. doi:10.3949/ccjm.80.e-s1.03.

Outpatient Geriatric Evaluation and Management

Thomas R. Hornick and Laurence Rubenstein

As individuals age, debility from the accumulation of illness combined with the age-related loss of physiological reserve leads to increasing functional decline and resultant disability. While aging cannot be reversed, and most chronic illnesses cannot be cured, a pragmatic approach based on health and function can improve the quality of life of the older person. This approach—comprehensive geriatric assessment (CGA)—is a multidimensional, usually interdisciplinary, diagnostic process designed to determine a frail elderly person's medical, psychosocial and functional capabilities and problems with the intention of developing an overall plan for treatment and long-term follow-up [1]. Teams that provide CGA and then perform the management (e.g., interdisciplinary primary care) derived from that evaluation are often termed geriatric evaluation and management (GEM) teams. The terms are often used interchangeably in practice, and in this chapter we will use both, CGA being the more general term. CGA has been implemented most frequently by interdisciplinary professional teams in various settings, and targeted at older patients with complex medical conditions and need for caregiver support. This chapter will specifically detail team-based CGA/GEM in the outpatient setting.

CGA is central to the practice of geriatricians (and those in training) and is predicated on the idea that a thorough and systematic evaluation of problems in an older frail person will lead to better quality of life and better outcomes. In the treatment of older individuals with complex problems, CGA remains a useful means of guiding care.

The differences between CGA and a good history and physical are important to detail. A thorough history and physical by a trained provider is aimed at discovery, prevention, and treatment of medical problems. The assumption behind the full medical evaluation is that improving the care of the medical conditions of the patient will thus improve or maintain patient physical functioning and quality of life. For the healthy and well-functioning patient, this assumption remains valid. For the old-old and/or frail individual, with multi-morbidity and geriatric syndromes, this assumption does not apply. Due to their nonspecific symptoms, many of the geriatric syndromes may not be obvious during a routine medical history and physical. In contrast, CGA places a major focus on the functioning (psychosocial and physical) of the individual, identifying issues that may be paramount but are not necessarily medically based. Difficulties with activities of daily living (ADLs) and instrumental activities of daily living (IADLs) in older individuals may stem from other than medical problems: cognitive decline, poor social supports, medication non-adherence, polypharmacy, and co-morbid conditions among others. Focusing on the functioning difficulties will uncover these issues and open avenues for their treatment.

A common example is an 85-year widower with degenerative arthritis (DJD) of the knee. Medically this is straight forward, with treatment focusing on pain control and exercise, often with eventual knee replacement. In both young and healthy old patients, this is likely all that is necessary to provide optimum care. Focusing on function, a CGA is performed by a team of geriatric specialists, in this case a nurse, a geriatrician and a social worker. The evaluation determines that the knee arthritis may be contributing to social isolation, with resultant decreased food intake and a reactive depression from being housebound. Urinary frequency with occasional urinary incontinence (due to the inability to reach the bathroom in time due to knee pain) also contributes to the social isolation. Each of these issues will need to be addressed to improve the quality of life of the patient. Given that DJD is not easily controlled with medical interventions, addressing the social isolation may be the most important part of the intervention. Many of these issues will not be obvious on

T.R. Hornick, M.D. (✉)
Geriatric Research Education and Clinical Centers, Louis Stokes Cleveland VAMC, 10701 East Blvd, Cleveland, OH 44106, USA
e-mail: Thomas.hornick@va.gov

L. Rubenstein, M.D., M.P.H.
Reynolds Department of Geriatric Medicine, University of Oklahoma Health Sciences Center, HSC, 1122 NE 13th Street, ORB 1200, Oklahoma City, OK 73117, USA
e-mail: laurence-rubenstein@ouhsc.edu

M.L. Malone et al. (eds.), *Geriatrics Models of Care: Bringing 'Best Practice' to an Aging America*,
DOI 10.1007/978-3-319-16068-9_16, © Springer International Publishing Switzerland 2015

routine examination and will not be brought up as difficulties unless sought after.

Who Should Be Referred for CGA?

Given the intensity of the evaluation, CGA is targeted toward those most likely to benefit. The frail elderly are the most likely population to be helped by CGA (Table 16.1). Targeting criteria other than age include functional status, presence of geriatric syndromes, social isolation, mood disorders, chronic disease burden, and/or those at risk for transitioning to a higher level of care.

Those who are too young and too healthy and who are functioning well in their environment are not as likely to benefit. Conversely, those who are too sick and too disabled may not benefit substantially either, especially where there is minimal room for improvement. This would include those requiring long-term nursing home care due to dependence, those with terminal illness, or those with severe dementia. While generally aimed at the older individual (geriatric age), the definition of "older" is generally qualified by several factors. Older to a teenager is anyone over 30, for most it is any over the retirement age. For CGA, old generally focuses on those above 80 because the prevalence of age-related conditions is highest.

Table 16.1 Who will benefit from Comprehensive Geriatric Assessment?

Community living patients > 65 likely to benefit from Comprehensive Geriatric Assessment
Functional loss
ADL decline
(bathing, dressing, toileting, transfer, feeding, continence)
IADLs loss
(cooking, cleaning, shopping, finances, medications, telephone, driving)
Geriatric syndromes
Cognitive decline (dementia/delirium)
Falls
Incontinence
Frailty
Polypharmacy
Weight loss
Depression
Chronic debilitating disease
CHF
Dementia
Parkinson disease
COPD
Transitioning to a different level of care
Community living to assisted living
Assisted living to long term care
Nursing home to community living
Caregiver stress
Frequent admissions to the hospital
New diagnosis of cancer before chemotherapy
Preoperatively prior to major surgery
Community living patients > 65 unlikely to benefit from CGA
Too well
Fully functional with no geriatric syndromes
Independent in ADLs/IADLs
Cognitively intact
Good social supports
Too impaired
Dependent in ADLs and requiring full-time care
Severe dementia
Those already in long-term care

Function

Under normal conditions, older individuals should be able to maintain their independence in the community with minimal assistance. If difficulties arise, then a close investigation of why should ensue. For evaluation purposes, independence is quantified using an activities of daily living (ADL) instrument [such as the Katz ADLs scale that includes bathing, dressing, toileting, transferring, feeding and continence] [2]; and an instrumental activities of daily living (IADL) measure [such as the Lawton IADL scale that included cooking, cleaning, driving, finances, shopping, taking medications, and telephoning [3]]. Change in ability to live independently should trigger an investigation into the causes, with the goal to reverse or ameliorate the debility through medical, functional, or social means.

Geriatric Syndromes

These syndromes interfere with function and impact caregivers and patients alike. Often the causes are multifactorial and irreversible requiring a multifaceted approach to treatment. The geriatric syndromes that tend to most benefit from the multifaceted investigation include dementia, delirium, depression, falls, gait difficulties, weight loss, incontinence, and frailty.

Chronic Illness

In older individuals with severe or multiple chronic illness, the ability to self-manage these illnesses may be impaired and lead to an overall loss of function. The multifaceted evaluation of CGA can identify ways to reduce the burden. This can be especially useful in those with multiple hospital admissions, given that the reason for readmissions often is the interaction between the illness and the individual's ability to manage it in their home environment.

Specialty Uses of CGA

CGA has proven useful in caring for older adults in several other specialty settings. For example, CGA is useful in oncology—increased life expectancy has led to an increased number of older individuals with cancer, with a need for appropriate disease- and age-specific management. The CGA can estimate the impact of cancer and chemotherapy on the psychosocial functioning of the patient, help with chemotherapy decisions [4], and determine whether there is underlying cognitive impairment or geriatric syndromes which are likely to be exacerbated during the treatment phase or impact prognosis.

Preoperative CGA has been more recently used for much the same reasons as in oncology to better predict postoperative complications and issues which may complicate recovery [5, 6]. Specialized geriatric orthopedic services have demonstrated improved outcomes over traditional care for older patients with hip fracture or those undergoing joint replacement. Other areas trialing CGA include patients before dialysis and those with congestive heart failure.

When to Refer the Patient for CGA

Many of the functional problems and geriatric syndromes noted may not be evident in routine office practice. However, simple screening assessments can be performed by primary care providers. Many tools exist for screening cognition, function, mood, geriatric syndromes, and social supports. Simple screens in office-based practices could include short cognitive screens [e.g., Mini-cog [7], Montreal Cognitive Assessment (MOCA) [8]], Mini-mental State Evaluation (MMSE) [9], depression screens [e.g., PHQ-2 and 9 [10], GDS short form [11]], gait/balance screens [e.g., measured gait speed, Tinetti's Performance Oriented Mobility Assessment (POMA) [12], or the Timed Up-and-Go test [13]], fall risk [e.g., history of falls, CDC STEADI instruments [14]]. Older patients who screen positive with these tools could be considered appropriate referrals to a team for CGA.

The Model of CGA

The health care needs of an older individual are often complex, and any successful treatment will require more than medical management of disease. The evaluation of multiple domains of health may be necessary, including medical, physical function, cognition, mood, social, and financial. CGA uses a systematic evaluation by an interdisciplinary team of health professionals to identify treatable health problems, thereby leading to better health outcomes.

Interdisciplinary Team

For a frail older person, the ability to follow and or carry through a medical plan of care, however well thought out, may be impossible due to functional and psychological circumstances. Travel issues, financial issues, caregiver issues, personal mobility issues, cognitive issues all may render good medical care ineffective. A team of geriatric providers with areas of expertise in these areas is invaluable for the assessment of these issues. Each team member evaluates and develops a plan to overcome or at least address the barriers/

health issues of the patient. The plans are then discussed and combined for the overall plan for the patient.

For the purpose of CGA, it is useful to distinguish between multidisciplinary and interdisciplinary teams. Multidisciplinary teams bring together members with diverse training with the purpose of sharing information, and this can often be done by meetings, through chart notes (greatly aided by electronic records) or individual or group communication. Interdisciplinary teams are similarly skilled but are focused on a group process for problem solving, which requires team interaction and derivation of a group assessment which incorporates the individual assessments and plans. In-person (or virtual) meetings are necessary for the problem solving function of this team. Although either model works well, for complex older patients the interdisciplinary meeting will derive more thorough patient-centered plans.

Therefore, a key feature of the CGA model is the interdisciplinary team meeting. Traditionally done in person, evaluations are presented and an overall plan of care is arrived at, incorporating medical, social, psychological and functional plans of care. The team is often led by the geriatrician. The value of the in-person meeting of all members is to ensure that social, psychological and functional aspects of care are not overlooked, as these may be key to improving the patient's quality of life. In a multidisciplinary model, the medical evaluation might overshadow the psychosocial aspects, since the physician is often the point of contact person for the patient evaluation and follow-up. Problems encountered that are psychosocial in nature might be overlooked.

The core assessment team generally consists of nursing, social worker and geriatrician, but may include other members depending on the population being served. Many teams include other members depending on the patients served and the setting: psychologists, occupational or physical therapist, pharmacist (or PharmD), and nutritionist (Table 16.2). These members may see all patients or are brought in depending on the need.

The outcome of the CGA is a written care plan, which lists and addresses all problems (functional, medical, psychosocial), action plans for interventions and future care, including resources such as the need for support services, and further evaluation and/or follow-up. This plan includes a summary plan of care as well as the recommendations of the team members. This document should serve as a guide for the providers caring for the patient as well as for the patient and their family/caregivers. Patient and family caregiver involvement is vital to the success of many of the interventions, and it is recommended that they are engaged throughout the process. In many practices, it is ideal to perform a team meeting with the family and patient to review the complete plan.

CGA programs exist both as a consultant team to primary care and also as a bridge to geriatric primary care practice. In the consultative model, the patient is referred back to their primary care providers to complete the plan. For the GEM model, the CGA team generally performs the majority of the recommendations, as many of the plans generated are not fully implemented after referral back to primary care. The team plan should detail responsibilities for follow through on individual items. The success of implementation of the plans should be monitored, with modification of the plan to ensure that problems identified are adequately addressed. This monitoring can be carried out by a team member using phone follow-up with the patient and or family caregiver, and/or reassessed on follow-up visits.

Roles of the Team Members

Many of the roles of the team members overlap, and experienced teams find that streamlining evaluations to avoid duplication is necessary for smooth functioning, and often teams will distribute screening tools on the basis of skills, needs or time for evaluation. Prescreening can often improve the efficiency of the evaluation since known resources can be gathered beforehand. Many geriatricians feel that they can perform the CGA without team members, given their training in functional assessment, knowledge of social services, ability to perform cognitive evaluation, and polypharmacy assessments. However, geriatricians working with teams usually attest to increased efficiency through utilization of team member's multiple skill sets and benefit as well through increased opportunity to communicate during the CGA. The broad range of skills and experience of the team will cast a wide "net," evaluating functional deficits and developing fruitful avenues for improvement.

Geriatrician

A geriatrician is often the center of an interdisciplinary team, if not always the leader. Geriatricians are trained in internal medicine or family practice with fellowship training in geriatrics, giving them skill in the evaluation and treatment of the ailments of the frail elderly. Geriatrician evaluations will focus on diagnosed and undiagnosed problems, pain, medications (medication reconciliation, age appropriateness), and age-related syndromes. The key evaluations include medical diagnostics, medication review (the "brown bag of medications"—customarily patients are asked to bring in all the medications they have, including over-the-counter medications, in a bag), and integration of the medical plan with the other members of the team.

Table 16.2 Roles of the members of the interdisciplinary team

Team member	Evaluations
Geriatrician	Thorough medical evaluation/development of problem list
	Differential diagnosis of functional impairments
	Evaluation of geriatric syndromes: Falls, incontinence, frailty, cognitive impairment, etc.
	Medication review/reconciliation
	Integration of medical plan with other team members
Nurse	ADLs
	IADLs
	Common screening instruments: Frailty, falls, cognitive, depression etc.
	Caregiver stress
Social work	Social connectedness
	Informal supports/availability of help
	Caregiver stress
	Community resources
	Financial evaluation
Psychology	Cognitive evaluation and diagnosis
	Mood/anxiety screening and treatment
PharmD	Medication review and education
Nutrition	Dietary history
	Evaluate access to nutritional foods
	Medical diet recommendations
Physical therapy/occupational therapy	Fall/gait evaluation and treatment
	ADL/IADL recommendations

Nurse

The nurse in the geriatric assessment team frequently brings advanced training in gerontology, and often a wealth of experience. The key elements of the RN evaluation consist of the functional evaluation of the frail elder. What can they do for themselves and what do they need help with? Can they get through a single day without help—basic ADLs; can they get through a week without help: IADLs. Other major evaluations include the determination of who is providing help during the week, a complete compilation of medications (assembling the brown bag of medications for MD/PharmD review), and often psychological/cognitive screening (e.g., MOCA, MMSE or Mini-cog, GDS, PHQ). Allergies, alcohol use, smoking, and "illicits" are often determined during the nursing screening.

Social Work

Social workers typically have a master's degree in social work with training in gerontology. They perform a key aspect of the evaluation—determination of the social connectedness of the patient, reviewing what professional and nonprofessional help they are receiving. Home assessments are invaluable, but the in-office assessment can often substitute and give a picture of how the patient is functioning in their environment. Recommendations for available services based on need and location are vital pieces of assessment recommendations. Often the "how" of the CGA recommendations falls squarely on the creativity and skill of the social worker.

Psychology

Gero-psychologists can be a valuable member of the CGA team, although given their rarity, they are often not present. Gero-psychologists have an advanced degree in psychology and have typically done a clinical fellowship in gero-psychology. Their expertise is in the diagnosis and treatment of disorders in the elderly, most frequently depression, dementia, and anxiety disorders. Neuropsychologists can fulfill this role as well, although their greatest utility is in diagnostics based on detailed neuropsychological testing. Most often, gero-psychologists and neuropsychologists serve a consultative role for patients with unusual or difficult to diagnose cognitive/psychosocial disorders. Determination of capacity is an often overlooked but vital function for the care of elders with poor social supports in need of more stable living conditions. The psychologist role is to evaluate cognitive/psychological disorders, and in the team meetings will often discuss probable diagnosis and recommend necessary further evaluations/treatments to clarify diagnosis.

Pharmacy

PharmDs with training in geriatrics often function in a consultative role in the CGA. In instances where polypharmacy is a major issue, the PharmD evaluation of the medical regimen for indications and interactions can be invaluable.

Nutrition

Licensed dietitians with gerontological experience or training can bring great expertise to bear on patients' problems, and when available are active members of the assessment team. The problem of under-nutrition is frequent in the frail elderly and has myriad causes, including medical, social, cognitive, psychological factors. Nutritional evaluations are time-consuming and recommendations need to be tempered by the medical social and psychological needs of the patients. Additionally, medical diets such as for diabetes need to be adapted to the patient and their unique situation.

Physical/Occupational Therapy

Therapists are often available for consultation in the outpatient setting and can be invaluable for physical performance evaluations, gait training, prescription of assistive devices for ambulation and ADL assistance. Sometimes, geriatricians and therapists collaborate in dedicated falls and balance clinics that provide specialized gait training and fall prevention interventions.

Goal of CGA

The evaluation of the patient is multidimensional, examining medical, psychosocial, and functional problems/strengths of the patient. The goal is to develop a comprehensive plan to improve quality of life and maximize function. Patient-centered goals will be important in order to determine the direction of the care plan and the patient's goals of care, including advance directives and end of life wishes. The evaluation that flows from these goals therefore takes a predictable and logical direction: determination of functional status, current medical illnesses and their functional impact, polypharmacy/medication review, gait and balance assessment, fall risks, cognitive status, evaluation of mood, frailty assessment, social supports/social network, nutritional status, vision/hearing screening, goals of care (Table 16.3).

Functional status is quantified by examining the ability to perform those activities that enable independent living at home: the ADLs and IADLs. As a focal point for evaluation, the determination of the ability/inability to perform these activities is fundamental to developing a patient-centered plan. Acute and chronic physical illnesses frequently impair ADLs and IADLs, and helping the patient adapt will greatly improve quality of life. Patients with cognitive impairment will have difficulty with IADLs, especially finances and medication adherence. Functional evaluation serves as a practical point of entry for problem solving to improve quality of life. A memorable patient of one of the authors was a 91-year-old man with severe congestive cardiomyopathy who had dyspnea on minimal exertion. Although he was admitted frequently with fluid overload, he claimed adherence to his medications, constantly adapting dosing of diuretics to his weight. Among other things, CGA determined that he was having increasing difficulty with bathing and dressing, and food shopping was getting too difficult. The social worker implemented a home health service for 2 h on 2 days/week to maintain home cleanliness and perform shopping chores. Within 2 months he had shed most of his extra fluid, achieved a stable dose of diuretics, and was not admitted for the next 2 years. In retrospect, he admitted that he was getting over-fatigued with household chores and was too fatigued to shop for appropriate food. The home health aide allowed him to use his limited energy to eat better food—leading to a better outcome. GEM teams have the advantage of following change in function over time as reassessments are made during ongoing care. This change in function over time can be used to evaluate response to interventions, and develop long-term plans of care.

Current Medical Illness and Functional Impact

The evaluation and treatment of underlying disease is an important aspect of the medical part of the geriatric evaluation. With age, disease burden often increases. CGA thoroughly evaluates the disease burden of the patient, reevaluates present treatment and ensures that progressive and impairments are addressed.

Polypharmacy/Medication Review

Although time-consuming, a thorough medication review is an important feature of the CGA. Patients accumulate large numbers of medications, many outdated and un-discarded. It is important that all medications, both prescribed and over-the-counter, be brought in for evaluation. A medication review will often uncover errors in self-administration, and use of medications that should be used cautiously in the older

Table 16.3 Domains of evaluation and screening tools for geriatric assessment

Domain	Purpose	Useful scales
Function: activities of daily living	Ability to maintain self for a day without outside help	Katz ADL [2]
Function: instrumental activities of daily living	Ability to maintain self for a week without help	IADL [3]
Social	Availability of help, informal (including family) and professional	Lubben Social Network Scale [15]
	Social connectedness	Older Americans Resources and Services, Social Resources Section [16]
Gait and balance	Evaluate mobility and risk for falls	Tinetti's Performance Oriented Mobility Assessment (POMA) [12]
		Timed Up-and-Go Test [13]
		CDC STEADI instruments [14]
Cognition	Evaluate cognitive function	Mini-mental State Evaluation (MMSE) [9]
		Mini-cog [7]
		Montreal Cognitive Assessment (MOCA) [8]
Mood/anxiety	Evaluate for depression anxiety disorders	Geriatric Depression Scale [17, 18]
		PHQ-2 and 9 [10]
		GDS short form [11]
Nutrition	Adequate nutritional access/intake	Nutrition Screening Initiative Checklist [19]
		Mini Nutritional Assessment [20]

patient due to age or age disease interactions [21]. Polypharmacy evaluation is a term frequently invoked for this process, and while the term polypharmacy means too many medications, operationally it means an inappropriate medication regimen. Appropriateness of the regimen is determined by matching medications to diagnosed disease, evaluation of regimen for potential interactions, including age and disease-based interactions, and under- and/or overtreatment of disease. In complex cases of polypharmacy, the inclusion of a PharmD on the interdisciplinary team is invaluable.

Gait and Balance Assessment

Gait can be a key factor for functional independence and gait speed is predictive of future disability and mortality [22, 23]. Gait and balance assessment can reveal risk for falls and can trigger referral for physical therapy for gait safety and falls evaluation. Various scales have been used, from the Timed Up and Go (TUG), to the more extensive Tinetti POMA scale [12].

Fall Risk

Fall risk assessment incorporates gait and balance, but other important features include visual and hearing acuity, determination of sitting and standing blood pressure, and medications [24]. The prevalence of orthostatic hypotension is high among older individuals, leads to an increase risk of falling,

and is affected by diet and medications. It is often silent, so direct determination will help guide care.

Cognitive Status/Mood

Direct screening for cognition/mood status is recommended given the prevalence of cognitive and mood disorders older age and the tendency to cover them up. Cognitive impairment is frequently unrecognized by providers [25], thus formal cognitive screening is recommended with follow-up diagnostic assessments for those with evidence of neurocognitive impairment. Patients may retain independent functioning with early dementia by use of adaptation of their habits, reliance on external memory aids, family supports, etc. Many will not admit to increasing difficulties for fear of diagnosis, fear of loss of function, removal from home, or loss of driving privileges. Implementation of the CGA plans must be tempered by the cognitive capabilities of the patient and their caregiver.

Advance Directives/End of Life Decisions

With family present, discussion of advance directives and end of life decisions can be discussed. Optimally, this discussion can occur during the initial evaluation, but due to time constraints may be delayed for a follow-up discussion. The written CGA plan of care should incorporate these as indicated.

Effectiveness of Outpatient CGA/GEM

Research on models of care has given mixed evidence of the efficacy of CGA in the outpatient setting. While many early studies suggested efficacy of the CGA in the outpatient arena, later studies were more neutral. Comparison of studies of CGA is made difficult by the use of slightly different models and targeted patients, and the degree to which the interventions were implemented. Studies of GEMs, e.g., where the CGA team both craft and carry out the interventions, tend to show better outcomes than programs that only make assessments and then give recommendations to other providers to implement [26]. A randomized clinical trial of GEM in a community hospital showed less functional loss, less health-related restriction in activity, and less depression than controls [27]. There was no difference in health care utilization or Medicare costs. In a large systematic review of the evidence [28], there was a slight reduction in nursing home admissions, improved physical function, lower risk of hospital admissions, and no change in mortality. A large randomized trial in the Department of Veterans Affairs (VA) found that outpatient GEM (with 1 year of ongoing care) was associated with better medication management, fewer adverse drug effects, and more appropriate therapy for identified conditions [29].

Financial Considerations

CGA represents a significant investment of time and effort of multiple professionals to create an informed plan for an individual patient. Medicare fee for service does not reimburse all team members, and team meetings are generally not covered. Therefore, most CGA programs exist under the auspices of hospital systems where the increased cost of the full team is absorbed on the premise that the coordination of the care saves costs elsewhere.

There are many positive effects of CGA or GEM for hospital systems. While hospitals frequently boast about the high quality and comprehensive care offered by CGA geriatric services, there are other real benefits to the hospital systems. The CGA program as part of a hospital outpatient system serves as a focus for the referral of frail older individuals who will need a spectrum of services. These patients tend to be high utilizers and the presence of a CGA or GEM program allows focused management and care coordination. CGA programs also serve as excellent training sites for geriatric personnel, from medical students, residents, trainees, social worker students and professionals, nurse, nurse practitioners, psychologists, etc. Referrals from geriatric services tend to be high and these patients remain active in the hospital system. As Medicare payments shift to reimbursement based on quality and less on episodic care/admissions for care, these teams can be a focus for quality and improvement of post hospital care for complex patients. Other areas of focus that benefit the hospital system include coordination of care for difficult patients with community services such as Adult Protective Services.

The use of the electronic medical record enhances the utility of the geriatric assessment implementation. Once in the electronic chart, the team assessment and plan is available to all providers coming into contact with the patient. It will save on redundant evaluations, serve as a record of the medication review, and document the functional status and social supports, all of which can aid in other sites of care. For example, hospital discharge plans can be more precise, e.g., the admitting/discharging cardiologist will get a clear picture of the functioning of the patient with CHF prior to the admission, and a clear idea of all the medications that are being used including OTC, and the interventions to assure adherence to medications and diet. The referral to home care will have a clearer idea of the goals of the functional interventions and support. Other outpatient providers consulting on chronic disease will likewise have detail on the functioning of patient to make better informed therapeutic decisions.

As the Affordable Care Act shifts away from Medicare fee-for-service toward value/quality-based reimbursement, the potential value of CGA programs will grow. The focus on improving quality of life, function, and appropriate medication/medical care will maintain their importance. As cost containment measures increase, the coordination of care that can be provided will serve to maintain quality of care in the vulnerable aging population.

The largest healthcare system in the country, the VA, has supported GEM both for inpatient and outpatient care. Within this large capitated payment system, the GEM programs have thrived. The multi-site GEM study by Cohen and colleagues evaluated both inpatient and outpatient GEMs, and concluded that there were improvements in mental health for the outpatient GEM patients at 1 year without an increase in cost to the system [30]. Serious adverse drug events were reduced by 35 % by the outpatient GEMs compared to usual care [29] with overall improvement in drug regimens. The GEMs have served as sites for quality improvement, clinical trials, and clinical demonstrations for testing of novel programs of care for older veterans. The GEM programs in the VA are often the focus of academic geriatric sections, and have served as invaluable training sites for geriatrics. As a testament to their training value, they have trained many of the practicing geriatricians in the USA today, as well as many medical students, medicine and family practice residents, psychologists, nutritionists, and PharmDs.

Conclusion

CGA/GEM is a widely used model of assessment and care of frail older individuals. It addresses the complex interplay of health, disease, loss of physiological reserve with age, and function through systematic evaluation and treatment by an interdisciplinary team of geriatric experts. While developed for frail elderly, it is being adapted for specialty populations, especially for cancer, orthopedic and preoperative patients, and also is being trialed for patients approaching dialysis, and patients with chronic respiratory or cardiac disease. CGA/GEM has been widely adopted as a model of care in the United States, and CGA programs remain a major site of training in geriatrics.

References

1. Stuck AE, Siu AL, Wieland GD, Adams J, Rubenstein LZ. Comprehensive geriatric assessment: a meta-analysis of controlled trials. Lancet. 1993;342(8878):1032–6.
2. Katz S, Ford AB, Moskowitz RW, Jackson BA, Jaffe MW. Studies of illness in the aged: the index of ADL: a standardized measure of biological and psychosocial function. JAMA. 1963;185(12):914–9.
3. Lawton MP, Brody EM. Assessment of older people: self-maintaining and instrumental activities of daily living. Gerontologist. 1969;9(3):179–86.
4. Chaïbi P, Magné N, Breton S, Chebib A, Watson S, Duron J-J, et al. Influence of geriatric consultation with comprehensive geriatric assessment on final therapeutic decision in elderly cancer patients. Crit Rev Oncol Hematol. 2011;79(3):302–7.
5. Liang C-K, Chu C-L, Chou M-Y, Lin Y-T, Lu T, Hsu C-J, et al. Interrelationship of postoperative delirium and cognitive impairment and their impact on the functional status in older patients undergoing orthopaedic surgery: a prospective cohort study. PLoS One. 2014;9(11):e110339.
6. Ommundsen N, Wyller TB, Nesbakken A, Jordhøy MS, Bakka A, Skovlund E, et al. Frailty is an independent predictor of survival in older patients with colorectal cancer. Oncologist. 2014;19(12):1268–75.
7. Borson S, Scanlan J, Brush M, Vitaliano P, Dokmak A. The mini-cog: a cognitive "vital signs" measure for dementia screening in multi-lingual elderly. Int J Geriatr Psychiatry. 2000;15(11):1021–7.
8. Nasreddine ZS, Phillips NA, Bédirian V, Charbonneau S, Whitehead V, Collin I, et al. The Montreal Cognitive Assessment, MoCA: a brief screening tool for mild cognitive impairment. J Am Geriatr Soc. 2005;53(4):695–9.
9. Folstein MF, Folstein SE, McHugh PR. "Mini-mental state". A practical method for grading the cognitive state of patients for the clinician. J Psychiatr Res. 1975;12(3):189–98.
10. Kroenke K, Spitzer RL, Williams JB. The PHQ-9: validity of a brief depression severity measure. J Gen Intern Med. 2001;16(9):606–13.
11. Hoyl MT, Alessi CA, Harker JO, Josephson KR, Pietruszka FM, Koelfgen M, et al. Development and testing of a five-item version of the Geriatric Depression Scale. J Am Geriatr Soc. 1999;47(7):873–8.
12. Tinetti ME. Performance-oriented assessment of mobility problems in elderly patients. J Am Geriatr Soc. 1986;34(2):119–26.
13. Podsiadlo D, Richardson S. The timed "Up & Go": a test of basic functional mobility for frail elderly persons. J Am Geriatr Soc. 1991;39(2):142–8.
14. CDC - STEADI - Older Adult Falls - Home and Recreational Safety - Injury Center [Internet]. Accessed on 2015 Jan 8. Available from: http://www.cdc.gov/homeandrecreationalsafety/Falls/steadi/index.html?s_cid=tw_injdir1
15. Lubben JE. Assessing social networks among elderly populations. Fam Community Health. 1988;11(3):42–52.
16. Fillenbaum GG, Smyer MA. The development, validity, and reliability of the Oars Multidimensional Functional Assessment Questionnaire. J Gerontol. 1981;36(4):428–34.
17. Sheikh J, Yesavage J. Geriatric Depression Scale (GDS): recent evidence and development of a shorter version. Clin Gerontol. 1986;5:165–73.
18. Yesavage JA, Brink TL, Rose TL, Lum O, Huang V, Adey M, et al. Development and validation of a geriatric depression screening scale: a preliminary report. J Psychiatr Res. 1982–1983;17(1):37–49.
19. Posner BM, Jette AM, Smith KW, Miller DR. Nutrition and health risks in the elderly: the nutrition screening initiative. Am J Public Health. 1993;83(7):972–8.
20. Kaiser MJ, Bauer JM, Ramsch C, Uter W, Guigoz Y, Cederholm T, et al. Validation of the Mini Nutritional Assessment short-form (MNA®-SF): a practical tool for identification of nutritional status. J Nutr Health Aging. 2009;13(9):782–8.
21. American Geriatrics Society 2012 Beers Criteria Update Expert Panel. American Geriatrics Society updated Beers Criteria for potentially inappropriate medication use in older adults. J Am Geriatr Soc. 2012;60(4):616–31.
22. Cesari M, Kritchevsky SB, Newman AB, Simonsick EM, Harris TB, Penninx BW, et al. Added value of physical performance measures in predicting adverse health-related events: results from the Health, Aging And Body Composition Study. J Am Geriatr Soc. 2009;57(2):251–9.
23. Studenski S, Perera S, Patel K, Rosano C, Faulkner K, Inzitari M, et al. Gait speed and survival in older adults. JAMA. 2011;305(1):50–8.
24. Panel on Prevention of Falls in Older Persons, American Geriatrics Society and British Geriatrics Society. Summary of the Updated American Geriatrics Society/British Geriatrics Society Clinical Practice Guideline for Prevention of Falls in Older Persons: AGS/BGS CLINICAL PRACTICE GUIDELINE FOR PREVENTION OF FALLS. J Am Geriatr Soc. 2011;59(1):148–57.
25. Chodosh J, Petitti DB, Elliott M, Hays RD, Crooks VC, Reuben DB, et al. Physician recognition of cognitive impairment: evaluating the need for improvement. J Am Geriatr Soc. 2004;52(7):1051–9.
26. Totten A, Carson S, Peterson K, Low A, Christensen V, Tiwari A. Evidence brief: effect of geriatricians on outcomes of inpatient and outpatient care. VA Evidence-based Synthesis Program Evidence Briefs [Internet]. Washington (DC): Department of Veterans Affairs (US); 2011. Accessed on 2014 May 28. Available from: http://www.ncbi.nlm.nih.gov/books/NBK98020/
27. Boult C, Boult LB, Morishita L, Dowd B, Kane RL, Urdangarin CF. A randomized clinical trial of outpatient geriatric evaluation and management. J Am Geriatr Soc. 2001;49(4):351–9.
28. Beswick AD, Rees K, Dieppe P, Ayis S, Gooberman-Hill R, Horwood J, et al. Complex interventions to improve physical function and maintain independent living in elderly people: a systematic review and meta-analysis. Lancet. 2008;371(9614):725–35.
29. Schmader KE, Hanlon JT, Pieper CF, Sloane R, Ruby CM, Twersky J, et al. Effects of geriatric evaluation and management on adverse drug reactions and suboptimal prescribing in the frail elderly. Am J Med. 2004;116(6):394–401.
30. Cohen HJ, Feussner JR, Weinberger M, Carnes M, Hamdy RC, Hsieh F, et al. A controlled trial of inpatient and outpatient geriatric evaluation and management. N Engl J Med. 2002;346(12):905–12.

Stepping On, a Community-Based Falls Prevention Program

Jane Mahoney, Lindy Clemson, and Meryl Lovarini

Introduction

Stepping On is a group-based fall prevention program for older people living in the community. Developed in Australia, the program now has been implemented successfully in the United States. In this chapter we describe Stepping On, discuss the implementation of the Stepping On model, and outline current initiatives focusing on how this model can be delivered effectively and sustained by organizations into the future.

The Stepping On Model

Background

For older people, a fall can result in injury, a loss of confidence and activity restriction. It is known that approximately 30 % of older people living in the community fall each year. Of these, 20–30 % of people who fall suffer moderate to severe injuries including lacerations, sprains, fractures, or head trauma [1]. In 2012, there were 2.4 million emergency department visits for fall injuries among older adults in the United States [2]. The average Medicare cost for a fall in 2012 ranged from $13,797 to $20,450. In addition to direct

J. Mahoney, M.D. (✉)
University of Wisconsin School of Medicine and Public Health, 310 N. Midvale Boulevard, Suite 205, Madison, WI 53705, USA
e-mail: jm2@medicine.wisc.edu

L. Clemson, Ph.D.
Faculty of Health Sciences, University of Sydney, East Street, Lidcombe, NSW 2141, Australia
e-mail: lindy.clemson@sydney.edu.au

M. Lovarini, Ph.D., M.H.Sc.
Discipline of Occupational Therapy, Ageing, Work and Health Research Unit, The University of Sydney, Cumberland Campus, 75 East Street, Lidcombe, NSW 2141, Australia
e-mail: meryl.lovarini@sydney.edu.au

costs related to hospitalization, nursing home care, doctor's office visits, rehabilitation, medical equipment, prescription drugs, changes made to the home, and insurance processing, indirect costs include long-term effects such as disability, dependence on others, lost time from work and household duties, and reduced quality of life. By 2020, direct and indirect costs of fall-related injuries are estimated to reach $54.9 billion dollars [3]. The prevention of falls therefore is vital to achieving the health care triple aim of improving population health and patient experience, and decreasing per capita cost.

The Stepping On program offers older people a way of reducing their falls risk and increasing their self-confidence. The program allows older people to identify issues that are personally relevant, to determine their risk of falling and gain knowledge about safety practices. The program uses adult learning principles and is built on a sound conceptual basis to facilitate decision-making, self-efficacy, and behavior change. In the program, participants explore options and strategies to reduce their falls risk. In this way, the older person can take control, explore different coping behaviors, and utilize appropriate strategies in everyday life [4].

Stepping On was developed in Australia and effectiveness has been evaluated in a randomized controlled trial [5]. Compared to a randomized control group, participation in Stepping On led to a 31 % reduction in falls as well as improved self-confidence in mobility and greater use of protective behaviors. The cost-effectiveness of Stepping On is similar to group-based falls prevention exercise programs [6]. Stepping On has been recommended as an effective fall prevention intervention for use in the US [7] and was introduced into the US in 2006. The Centers for Disease Control and Prevention (CDC) have provided funding to develop and test the Stepping On model for US national dissemination.

Setting

Stepping On is conducted in community settings. In the US, the program has been sponsored by aging units, health care providers, senior retirement apartment complexes, parks and recreational services, and other community-based organizations. The program is held at places convenient to older people such as community centers, libraries, senior centers, health clinics, and retirement complexes.

Participants

The program is aimed at older people who have fallen or have a fear of falling. Participants must be cognitively intact, live independently in the community, and be able to ambulate without assistance from another person. Use of an assistive device does not preclude participation, but older adults who require a walker for indoor walking are not included as they may be too mobility impaired to participate in the group exercises. These individuals would benefit from an individualized approach instead. While medical clearance is not required, prior to participation, participants are encouraged to talk with their physician about the program and their fall history.

Content and Delivery

The program uses a small-group approach plus individualized follow-up. The ideal group size is 8 to 12. The workshop includes topics such as falls and risk, strength and balance exercises, home hazards, safe footwear, vision and falls, safety in public places, community mobility, coping after a fall and understanding how to initiate medication reviews [4]. The content is delivered over seven weekly sessions. A booster group session is conducted at 3 months to review achievements and provide ongoing support. In the original study, after the workshop, individualized support was provided through a home visit to facilitate follow through of preventive strategies, and through a phone call at 6 months to help sustain gains. In the US, for feasibility of adoption by organizations, the home visit typically does not occur. Instead, leaders cover many of the same concepts by phone call. The workshop is facilitated by a group leader along with invited guest presenters. In the US, group leaders have a range of backgrounds including: occupational therapists, registered nurses, physical therapists, social workers, fitness experts, other gerontology professionals, and health educators. Volunteer guest presenters include a physical therapist, low vision expert, pharmacist, and community safety expert who have knowledge on pedestrian safety. In the US, a peer leader, who has been recruited from previous Stepping On participants, assists the leader to facilitate the workshop.

Evaluation

Quick and simple measures can be used to evaluate program impact. A frequently used evaluation is the program attendance records, where 80 % attendance at five of seven sessions is considered the benchmark. Attendance that falls short of that may indicate the need to evaluate the leader's fidelity to program delivery. Other evaluation measures include the Falls Behavioural Scale [FaB] [8] and the timed Get Up & Go test [9], with measures assessed pre and immediately post workshop. Lastly, self-report of falls in the past 6 months and falls behavioral risk by the FaB can be assessed by questionnaire at baseline and 6 months after the end of the workshop.

Implementing the Stepping On Model

Need for Effective Implementation

The implementation of community-based fall prevention programs is complex and many factors can influence program success [10]. Early experiences in implementing Stepping On in the US were associated with poor program effectiveness outcomes initially. In 2006, five county aging units in Wisconsin trained leaders via a self-study group. Leaders included RNs, other health professionals, and directors of community-based aging services. The self-study group met with Dr. Clemson several times by phone to discuss questions. From 2006 to 2008, 363 older adults participated in Stepping On workshops. There was no reduction in falls from the 6 months prior to the 6 months after the workshop neither in the sample with complete data ($n=151$), nor in the complete sample using multiple imputation [11]. From 2008 through the first half of 2010, with funding from the Centers for Disease Control and Prevention, we identified key elements of Stepping On using a Delphi Consensus, refined the US version of the Stepping On program package [4], trained one new leader, and monitored fidelity with each session of that leader's first workshop. We identified substantial fidelity lapses. Root cause analysis resulted in the identification of causes and mapping of solutions to improve fidelity of implementation. From these activities, changes were made in how program leaders were selected, trained and coached, how program participants were identified and recruited, how the workshops were implemented, and how organizations were prepared to adopt the program. For example, fidelity tools were developed based on the key elements. Trainers observed fidelity at one session of each new leader's first workshop. Insights from the fidelity observations were recorded on fidelity tools and became a focus for reflection and feedback following the session. As changes to the program package were made, they were disseminated to existing leaders via new manuals, monthly phone calls, and group emails, and were incorporated into all new leader trainings. Outcomes were evaluated for 2018 participants involved in 253 workshops between 2008 and 2011. Compared to 6 months before the workshop, the rate of falls was reduced 50 % in the first 6 months after the end of the workshop (95 % CI 45–56 %), and 48 % in the second 6 months (95 % CI 41–54 %) [11]. These findings, showing improvement in effectiveness simultaneous with improvements in the program package to maximize fidelity, suggested that elucidation of key elements, and training and support to achieve them are essential for program effectiveness.

Training, Resources, and Support

The Wisconsin Institute for Healthy Aging (WIHA) (www.wihealthyaging.org) provides training and resources to support program implementation in the United States and Canada.

Training

Training is required for all new leaders. To be eligible to be trained as a leader, individuals must be: (1) retired or current health professionals (e.g. physical therapist, registered nurse, occupational therapist) or other professionals who provide services to older adults (e.g., fitness instructor, senior center activity director, social worker); (2) have professional experience working with older adults, (3) have group facilitation experience with adults, (4) have basic falls prevention knowledge, and (5) be affiliated with a sponsoring organization that is covered by a Stepping On license. New leaders must commit to facilitating at least one Stepping On workshop yearly. Leaders view a brief pre-training webinar, attend a 3-day training taught by two certified master trainers, take two quizzes (key elements and falls prevention knowledge) and demonstrate competency in facilitating both small group discussion and exercise practice. Following training, a master trainer monitors fidelity (in person or by video) at one session of a new leader's first workshop, and gives feedback regarding areas for improvement. After having conducted two workshops and received a satisfactory fidelity check, a leader may receive an additional half-day training provided by WIHA's lead trainer to become a Master Trainer.

Resources

Stepping On leaders receive the Stepping On Leader Manual and supporting materials as part of their 3-day training. Supporting materials include: slides, DVDs, handouts for participants, publicity materials, participant registration forms, the list of key elements, a checklist for workshop set-up and more. Master trainers receive a Master Trainer manual and supporting materials including slides, registration forms and publicity materials for Leader trainings, quizzes for new leaders, and fidelity monitoring tools for Stepping On sessions.

Support to Sponsoring Organization

A sponsoring organization is one that ensures that resources can be committed to facilitate successful adoption of the workshops. The sponsoring organization, leader, and other partners divide the work of implementation (e.g. coordination, finding a site, recruiting participants, finding guest experts, and so on). The sponsoring organization typically commits funding to pay the leader, provide an honorarium to an older adult peer leader, and cover snacks and other supplies. WIHA provides a CDC-approved Site Implementation Guide for interested organizations available at https://wihealthyaging.org/stepping-on. WIHA also provides consultation as needed before and during start-up to ensure successful adoption and implementation by new organizations.

Licensing

WIHA issues 3-year licenses to organizations that are implementing Stepping On. The purpose of the license is to protect the fidelity of Stepping On. Licensees may be state, community, or health care organizations. The license may be held by one organization (e.g., health care organization, local community organization), or by an entity that oversees Stepping On implementation by a number of other organizations (e.g., state office on aging or state office of injury prevention). The license covers workshops implemented by the leaders under their umbrella. The first license is included with leader training; subsequently they are renewed for a fee every 3 years. WIHA trains the first set of leaders for a newly licensed organization, but licensees are encouraged to have at least two leaders under their umbrella who become trained as master trainers, so they may continue to train new leaders within the organization.

In summary, comprehensive services have been developed by WIHA to facilitate program implementation and to assist leaders and organizations in addressing any challenges that may arise. These services include coaching for sponsoring organizations, trainings for leaders and master trainers, a website containing support materials, leader listserv, newsletters, leader coaches, and an annual summit for program stakeholders.

Gaining Buy-in from Health System Leaders

Stepping On is implemented in both community and health care settings. Sponsoring organizations may be health care systems or community-based organizations. However, even if community organizations host the workshops, health system engagement is key to maximize reach. Referral from health care providers is an important avenue for identifying and referring at-risk individuals for the workshops. The CDC STEADI (Stopping Elderly Accidents, Deaths, and Injuries) intervention recommends that older adults at risk for falls be referred to community-based exercise and fall prevention programs [12].

The Affordable Care Act (ACA) offers new incentives to health care providers to focus on preventive health care measures and has as its core the "triple aim" of "Better Health, Better Health Care, and Better Value (i.e., lower costs)." The ACA includes incentives for health care practices to become accredited by the National Committee for Quality Assurance as a "patient-centered medical home," a way of organizing primary care that emphasizes care coordination and communication to transform primary care into "what patients want it to be." Standard 4 for accreditation requires a medical provider to assess patient/family self-management abilities and to work with the patient to develop a self-care plan and provide tools and resources, including community resources. The ACA also includes a provision that allows Medicare to reward health care organizations with a share of the savings that would result from improving care and reducing costs for their Medicare members. Health care organizations that want to participate can apply to Medicare to be designated as Accountable Care Organizations (ACOs). ACOs have strong incentive to implement prevention programs such as Stepping On to reduce fall injuries and costs. Another part of the ACA is the annual wellness visit, which is covered for all patients on Medicare. This visit, with its focus on prevention, can serve as a venue in which to ask about history of falls and refer patients at risk to Stepping On. Medicare has also instituted quality improvement incentives that reward practices for screening older adults for fall risk, and for those at risk, assessing risk factors and developing treatment plans. For those at risk, referral to Stepping On should be an integral part of the treatment plan. The electronic medical record can be configured to facilitate screening and referrals to Stepping On. The CDC is working with several large electronic medical record vendors to develop screening and referral algorithms that include community resources such as Stepping On. However, each health system must identify local community resources and the most efficient path to accessing those.

Apart from providing referrals, health care organizations can support Stepping On directly, either by sponsoring workshops or by reimbursing participants to attend workshops in their communities. Models for such arrangements have been successful with other evidence-based community health programs and are beginning to be developed for Stepping On. WIHA is actively working with several large health care organizations to explore various partnerships to support Stepping On.

Insurers may also have a vested interest in supporting the workshops in order to decrease costs of fall injuries. Stepping On has a 59 % return on investment, meaning a net benefit of $125.27 per participant in prevented fall injury costs [13]. A recent evaluation of 177 participants in Stepping On in Wisconsin supports the potential for decreased costs, with fall-related ER visits decreasing from 4 per 100 participants in the 6 months pre workshop to 0 for the 6 months post workshop ($p = 0.046$).

Bringing Stepping On to Scale

The Wisconsin Institute for Health Aging (WIHA) has been established to foster successful dissemination of evidence-based health promotion programs and to facilitate local and national dissemination of Stepping On. Since 2006, Stepping On programs have been implemented in four-fifths of Wisconsin's counties and 19 other states with over 7,000 older adults participating to date. Our experience shows that participants enjoy the workshop, retain falls prevention behaviors up to a year post workshop, and recommend the workshop to their friends. Guest experts, all of whom are volunteers, enjoy the experience and most return to present in subsequent workshops.

Adoption and start-up are the most difficult aspects of implementation. WIHA has evaluated a coaching intervention to help organizations in the first year of start-up. In a randomized, controlled pilot study, eight counties in Wisconsin receiving the coaching intervention had an average increase of 1.38 workshops per year compared to 0.5 per year in the eight wait list control counties ($p = 0.056$). The coaching intervention focuses on identifying partner organizations, developing participant referral sources, and identifying committed leaders, peer leaders, and funders.

Future Initiatives

Despite the success of the Stepping On model, some implementation and sustainability challenges remain. Program implementation with older people from African-American, Hispanic tribal and other cultures in the United States has been limited, although the program has been successfully implemented with different cultural groups in Australia [14]. In the latter, there was a preference for program leaders who were health workers or therapists from the participants' cultural group, and often close associations with local cultural organizations provided enriched potential for partnership and support for venues and recruitment. Many of the Stepping On handouts are now available in different languages. Work is currently underway in the US on an adaption of Stepping On, "Pisando Fuerte" for Spanish-speaking older people.

WIHA is currently working with other Wisconsin counties to implement and evaluate a sustainability model that engages triads of community organizations (typically county aging unit), health care partners, and insurers to support Stepping On. Collaborative partnerships between program stakeholders have been identified as a potential strategy to facilitate the sustained implementation of community-based fall prevention programs [15]. Triad stakeholders collaborate to ensure that the tasks of workshop coordination, participant referral, and financial support for leaders can be sustainably accomplished. Such triads can help communities scale up the number of workshops to reach more at-need individuals.

Challenges and Promising Approaches

Financial limitations remain a significant challenge. Title III-D of the Older Americans Act provides minimal funds for the aging network to administer evidence-based health promotion programs. There is no direct reimbursement (yet) through fee-for-service Medicare or Medicaid for the program. Non-physician health care professionals potentially may bill Medicare for reimbursement under group exercise and patient self-management codes, however interpretation of Medicare regulations varies from carrier to carrier, so organizations should check with their Medicare carrier first. Medicare Advantage Plans are one financial model currently being used in some health systems for either fully subsidizing or paying a significant portion of costs involved in Stepping On. In these Plans the insurance carrier receives a lump sum of money to manage an older adult's health, similar to an HMO model. To date there has been little investment from private insurers, though such companies would have financial incentive to reduce downstream fall injury costs by reimbursing patients who enroll in Stepping On. Policy changes are needed to enable at-risk older Americans to benefit from this effective program.

Financial incentive models exist in fee-for-service clinical care for identifying fallers but typically efforts are directed toward screening for those who have fallen and less so for also managing falls [16]. This is despite the fact that the Physician Quality Reporting System (PQRS) and the Meaningful Use Incentive Program include screening and a care plan for falls. Initiatives developed under the Affordable Care Act may offer some solutions to improve falls risk screenings and referrals to Stepping On. Under this Act, "Wellness" visits to older people are covered by Medicare and could be used to identify older people at risk of falls and then refer those appropriate to Stepping On. Accountable Care Organizations (ACOs) created under this Act have a financial quality improvement incentive to accomplish falls screening, but have no financial quality improvement incentive to manage falls once patients are screened. However,

given the high cost of falls, ACOs may find it business worthy to pay physical therapists, occupational therapists, health educators, or social workers in their organization to provide the Stepping On program directly.

Better understanding and application of both financial and clinical drivers of practice change are needed [16]. Clinical practices can facilitate referral pathways to Stepping On through use of national falls clinical guidelines or the STEADI tool to guide decisions for falls management. Successful falls management requires links to evidence-based programs like Stepping On. Quality training and support for Stepping On leaders is a key ingredient in widespread adoption and at a leader level the use of fidelity tools can be critical to ensuring key elements of the program are maintained in practice.

Sustainability

Sustainability of the Stepping On program was explored in an Australian implementation study using in-depth interviews over a 3-year period [17]. Sustainability relies on three critical conditions: (1) the program must provide benefits and value; (2) committed, motivated and skilled leaders must be available, and (3) ongoing support for the program that matches the needs of the organization must be received at the time it is needed. Working in partnership and developing networks with others were key strategies used by community organizations to meet these conditions and hence sustain Stepping On over time. The "Wisconsin experience" supports this and has demonstrated how integral planning, training and collaborative partnerships are to sustainability.

Thus "Stepping On Partnerships" may offer a promising approach for sustained program delivery. Collaborations between WIHA, Medicare Advantage, insurers, ACOs, along with state and community stakeholders have the potential to lead to more sustained program co-ordination, referrals and support where costs can be recouped in terms of decreased emergency room visits, hospitalizations, and nursing home stays related to falls and injuries. Re-thinking how service providers, health care services, and insurers can work collaboratively may enable more sustained and effective delivery of Stepping On into the future.

References

1. Sterling DA, O'Connor JA, Bonaides J. Geriatric falls: injury severity is high and disproportionate to mechanism. J Trauma. 2001; 50(1):116–9.
2. Centers for Disease Control and Prevention, N. C. f. I. P. a. C. (2014b). Web-based Injury Statistics Query and Reporting System (WISQARS). Retrieved August 15, 2014.
3. Alexander BH, Rivara FP, Wolf ME. The cost and frequency of hospitalization for fall-related injuries in older adults. Am J Public Health. 1992;82(7):1020–3.

4. Clemson L, Swann M, Mahoney J. Stepping on building confidence and reducing falls. A community-based program for older people. Leader Manual. 3rd ed. Cedar Falls, IA: Freiburg Press; 2011.

5. Clemson L, Cumming R, Kendig H, Swann M, Heard R, Taylor K. The effectiveness of a community-based program for reducing the incidence of falls in the elderly: a randomised trial. J Am Geriatr Soc. 2004;52:1487–94.

6. Church J, Goodall S, Norman R, Hass M. An economic evaluation of community and residential aged care falls prevention strategies in NSW. N S W Public Health Bull. 2011;22(3–4):60–8.

7. National Center for Injury Prevention and Control. Preventing falls what works. A CDC compendium of effective community-based interventions from around the world. Atlanta, GA: Centers for Disease Control and Prevention; 2008.

8. Clemson L, Bundy A, Cumming R, Kay L, Luckett T. Validating the Falls Behavioural (FaB) scale for older people: a Rasch analysis. Disabil Rehabil. 2008;30(7):498–506.

9. Podsiadlo D, Richardson S. The timed "Up & Go": a test of basic functional mobility for frail elderly persons. J Am Geriatr Soc. 1991;39(2):142–8.

10. Child S, Goodwin V, Garside R, Jones-Hughes T, Boddy K, Stein K. Factors influencing the implementation of fall prevention programmes: a systematic review and synthesis of qualitative studies. Implement Sci. 2012;7:91. doi:10.1186/1748-5908-7-91.

11. Mahoney, J., Gangnon, R., Clemson, L., Gobel, V., & Lecey, V. (2012). Evaluation of stepping on implementation across Wisconsin. Paper presented at the Gerontological Association of America 65th Annual Meeting, San Diego, CA.

12. Centers for Disease Control and Prevention, N. C. f. I. P. a. C. (2014a). STEADI (Stopping Elderly Accidents, Deaths & Injuries). Toolkit for Healthcare Providers. Retrieved 7 August, 2014.

13. Carande-Kulis V, Stevens JA, Florence CS, Beattie BL, Arias I. A cost-benefit analysis of three older adult fall prevention interventions. Am J Prev Med. 2015;52:65.

14. Clemson L, Mathews M, Dean C, Lovarini M, Alam M. Translating research into practice: sustainability of a community-based falls prevention program in minority communities. Lidcombe, NSW: The University of Sydney; 2008.

15. Lovarini M, Clemson L, Dean C. Sustainability of community-based fall prevention programs: a systematic review. J Safety Res. 2013;47(4):9–17.

16. Schubert TE, Smith ML, Prizer LP, Ory MG. Complexities of fall prevention in clinical settings: a commentary. Gerontologist. 2014; 54:550–8.

17. Lovarini, M. (2012). Sustainability of a community-based falls prevention program: a grounded theory [Doctoral thesis]. Accessed on 18 November, 2014 from http://ses.library.usyd.edu.au/handle/2123/8044

Part IV

Emergency Department Models of Care

Geriatrics Emergency Department—The GEDI WISE Program

Ula Hwang, Mark S. Rosenberg, and Scott M. Dresden

With the aging of the U.S. population, the proportion of older adults requiring health care services will increase and the emergency department (ED) is situated at the crossroads of outpatient and inpatient care. It is positioned to be a key facilitator in transforming emergency care for the geriatric population by improving patient care coordination, reducing hospitalizations and ED visits/revisits, and reducing complications that arise from ED and hospital encounters [1]. Unfortunately, the special care needs of older adults have not been well aligned with traditional priorities of ED physical design and acute care. Geriatrics Emergency Departments that address the multimorbidity, functional, and psychosocial challenges of providing emergency care to older adults are an innovative model of care and potential solution [2]. The imperative for an alternate geriatric emergency medicine model in the coming years has become a clinical priority with national Geriatric and Emergency Medicine organizations. The recent endorsement of the Geriatric ED guidelines in 2014 [3–5] includes recommendations for enhanced expertise, educational and quality improvement expectations,

equipment, policies, and protocols. The guidelines represent the first formal, joint society and organizational attempt to develop evidence-based guidelines for the organization and care of older adults [3].

GEDI WISE (Geriatric *E*mergency *D*epartment *I*nnovations in care through *W*orkforce, *I*nformatics, and *S*tructural *E*nhancements) is a Health Care Innovations Award (HCIA) that was funded during Round 1 of the Affordable Care Act's Centers for Medicare and Medicaid (CMS) Innovations (CMMI) program (from 2012 to 2015) [6]. It incorporates most of the Geriatric ED guideline recommendations and has been implemented at three large, urban hospitals: The Mount Sinai Medical Center (MSMC) in New York City, St. Joseph's (SJ) Regional Medical Center in Paterson, NJ, and Northwestern Memorial Hospital (NMH) in Chicago, IL. GEDI WISE is an integrated, interdisciplinary approach to improving care for older adults via *workforce* education, training, and expansion; evidence-based geriatric specific clinical protocols; *informatics* support for patient monitoring and clinical decision support; and *structural enhancements* to improve patient safety and satisfaction. GEDI WISE targets ED patients 65+ years in age to improve patient care and satisfaction while decreasing hospitalizations, return ED visits, improving the transition from ED back to the community or home, and potentially reducing health care costs.

The GEDI WISE model follows Berwick's CMS "triple aim" [7] with the goals of achieving: (1) Better health care, (2) Better health, and (3) Lower (health care) costs for patients 65+ years age seen in the ED setting. The implementation of GEDI WISE interventions was a massive programmatic effort across all three programs during year 1 (July 2012–June 2013). Since SJ was the most "mature" of the three EDs (having had a Geriatric ED since 2009 (prior to participation in the GEDI WISE program)), MSMC having opened a Geriatric ED in February 2012, and NMH being the "youngest" of the three hospitals (no Geriatric ED programs in place), interventions and approaches varied at each site based on patient population needs and physical, administrative, clinical, and demographic capabilities of the hospitals.

U. Hwang, M.D., M.P.H. (✉)
Department of Emergency Medicine, Icahn School of Medicine at Mount Sinai, One Gustave L. Levy Place, Box 1062, New York, NY 10029, USA

Brookdale Department of Geriatrics and Palliative Medicine, Icahn School of Medicine at Mount Sinai, New York, NY, USA

Geriatric Research, Education and Clinical Center, James J. Peters Veterans Affairs Medical Center, New York, NY, USA
e-mail: ula.hwang@mountsinai.org

M.S. Rosenberg, D.O., M.B.A.
Department of Emergency Medicine, St. Joseph's Healthcare System, Paterson, NJ 07503, USA
e-mail: mark.rosenberg@MandLholdings.com

S.M. Dresden, M.D., M.S.
Department of Emergency Medicine, Center for Healthcare Studies–Institute for Public Health and Medicine, Northwestern University Feinberg School of Medicine, 211 Ontario St. Suite 200, Chicago, IL 60616, USA
e-mail: s-dresden@northwestern.edu

M.L. Malone et al. (eds.), *Geriatrics Models of Care: Bringing 'Best Practice' to an Aging America*,
DOI 10.1007/978-3-319-16068-9_18, © Springer International Publishing Switzerland 2015

All three sites incorporated the addition of new members to the ED clinical *Workforce* (either with expansion of existing staff and their clinical duties or the creation of new roles) to improve initial evaluation and assessment of older adults seen in the ED setting, specific evaluation of geriatric syndromes (e.g., delirium, falls risk, functional status) and psychosocial supports, care coordination, and if discharged home, patient transitions of care from the ED to community or home. MSMC and SJ took a broad approach and implemented education, protocols, and expansion of existing clinical staff and roles at all levels, inclusive of the entire workforce. This included training for all ED clinical staff inclusive of physicians (attendings and residents), nurses, pharmacists, social workers, technicians, and unit secretaries. NMH took a narrower approach with the creation of "Geriatric Nurse Liaisons" (GNLs) in the ED. The GNLs provide geriatric consultations to the general ED staff with older adult patients [8]. The implementation of *Informatics* elements also varied across sites based on site capabilities. All three sites utilize electronic health records (EHR) and were able to program documentation specific to evaluations and protocols implemented. MSMC is also part of a regional health information organization (RHIO), Healthix, that allowed the implementation of clinical event notifications (CEN) [9]. Prior to the GEDI WISE HCIA award, all three participating EDs had pre-existing *S*tructurally enhanced Geriatric ED spaces. Physical space for these EDs follows environmental recommendations outlined in the Geriatric ED Guidelines [10]. Common features across three sites also included continuous *E*ducation of ED clinical staff of not only programmatic implementation of protocols and new staff, but also geriatric-specific content. Content varied based on site-specific efforts, but commonalities include education about communicating with older adults, ageism, using the Identification of Seniors at Risk (ISAR) [11] screening tool, falls risk assessment, cognitive impairment and delirium screening, care coordination and transitions of care management, following new protocols and workflows that incorporated these enhanced assessments and procedures.

The remaining chapter will further describe site-specific GEDI WISE programs located at the three hospitals.

St. Josephs Regional Medical Center

Approximately 160,000 geriatric, adult, and pediatric patients visit Saint Joseph's Regional Medical Center (SJ) Emergency Department (ED) each year. Geriatric emergency patients have an abbreviated triage to determine their age and the seriousness of their complaint. Critically ill seniors are triaged to the ED; all seniors who do not require aggressive resuscitation are brought back immediately to the Geriatric ED, which opened in 2009. All of this is accomplished in a 24-bed Geriatric ED that is designed specifically for seniors. Every aspect of care and every part of the environment was designed with seniors in mind. The thicker mattresses on the stretchers, the adjustable lighting, the non-glare floors, the improved soundproofing all combine to make a more comfortable environment that is more conducive to senior-focused care.

In the SJ Geriatric ED, doctors, nurses, social workers and case managers perform health care screenings to evaluate physical and psychological needs and utilize case management resources to assure the best care for this vulnerable population. In St. Joseph's Geriatric ED, the patient's comfort is also a priority. There, a patient liaison, which can be a volunteer or technician level position, sees the patient and the family every 20–30 min to make sure there are no other needs even as small as adjusting the television. Hearing assist devices, reading glasses, pillows, warm blankets, coffee, tea, food and snacks are all made available by a patient liaison. These small comfort measures improve patient satisfaction and overall perception of care.

From the emergency physician's point of view, care processes in the ED continue as they do anywhere else in the ED. The patient is seen and examined, orders are written or entered into the computer and the physician proceeds to evaluate the next patient. What happens subsequent to the initial physician evaluation and decision making is what makes the Geriatric ED team (this consists of an advance practice nurse trained in geriatric patient care, a social worker, a case manager, and a Geriatric ED nurse navigator) unique for older patient outcomes and disposition. Transition of care begins with notification of the primary physician, patient's pharmacy, and other necessary services to discharge the patient to home or to admit to the hospital. The social worker attempts to identify what type of needs would be required for the patient to return home safely. The case manager identifies other aspects for a safe transition of care. The nurse navigator coordinates all aspects of care. When the emergency physician is ready to reassess the patient and determine disposition, a report from the geriatric team is provided which includes findings from multiple geriatric screenings and assessments. Screenings include dementia, delirium, depression, dietary concerns, and a falls assessment for strength and balance. Assessments may determine the needs for additional screenings, such as physical therapy and medication review. The team determines the Transition of Care—whether the patient should have a discharge or admission.

Transition of Care

The importance of Transition of Care from the ED to the home or community is essential. Goals with SJ's transitions of care include having the patient's primary care physician know of the patient's status and treatment plan, but also reiterating the goals of care to the patient at and post ED discharge. This is best accomplished by using a two-step process initiated upon discharge. The ED visit is step one. Step two involves calling the patient on Day 1, Day 3, and Day 7. The callback is done by an ED nurse who makes sure the patient understands their discharge instructions, their care plan, has made an appointment with their doctor, understands their medications and is able to take care of him/herself in the home environment. If problems are identified other resources can be made available for the patient such as meals on wheels or homecare visits. If the patient is unable to get a follow-up appointment with their primary care physician or if symptoms have worsened, the patient is given an appointment to return to the Geriatric ED. For patients requiring admission to the hospital, there is an individual Transition of Care plan communicated to the receiving care team by the Geriatric ED team.

Adjunct Programs

Another unique and innovative program at SJRMC is the "*Admit to Home*" program or Extended Home Observation. As SJ does not have an observation unit, this program was created as to provide and coordinate care for patients that could potentially avoid a hospital admission. Patients best served by these programs are those with diagnoses that can be managed as an outpatient, but also have the distinct possibility of requiring hospital admission or observation if unresponsive to therapy. This pilot program focuses on a select group of senior patients who are cognitively intact and functionally independent with ED diagnoses of cellulitis, diverticulitis, and select pneumonia cases.

In essence, the patient is discharged from the ED and "admitted" to home with a set of "admission" orders. Orders for the patient include daily instructions on care for vital signs, ambulation, nutrition, medications, and other activities or restrictions. Vital signs for a patient with cellulitis may consist of taking a temperature every 4 h, ambulation may be to keep the leg elevated, nutrition may be to continue a regular diet, and drugs would be specific to antibiotic treatment and frequency. Other instructions may include warm compresses or other adjuncts. The patient is called back at an agreed upon time the next morning and essentially telephone rounds are made with the patient. If any of the symptoms have worsened, or any status changed, the patient would be directed to come back to the Geriatric ED for admission to the hospital. In all "Admit to Home" cases, patients have a scheduled return ED visit for reassessment that may include further diagnostic testing. This is done in conjunction with their primary care physician. The majority of these patients will have a straightforward transition of care plan. On revisit,

the disposition can be determined based on the patient's response to therapy. "Admit to Home" programs combined with an observation program have the potential to save significant inpatient health care dollars.

Another ED-based palliative medicine program, known as *Life Sustaining Management and Alternatives (LSMA)* focuses on patients with serious end-of-life illnesses. Incorporating palliative care in the ED setting, the LSMA program is designed to help patients establish goals of care and at the extreme help patients and their families deal with end-of-life issues earlier in their disease. When the ED staff identifies a patient who may benefit from these services, a palliative consult is ordered. A physician and nurse coordinator are available 24/7; and a bedside consult provides information on the patient's disease, prognosis and disease trajectory.

The focus of this program is in the Geriatric ED because many seniors have terminal illness such as cancer or other conditions such as dementia, Parkinson's disease, and organ failure. Just as most EDs have resuscitation rooms, SJ also has comfort rooms designed specifically for actively dying patients and their families. These rooms allow the Transition of Care from the ED to home hospice, in-house hospice, or other care systems. Patients who are near or at their end of life are given comfort measures by the palliative medicine team and every effort is made so they may die according to their wishes, even if death should occurs in one of the comfort rooms.

Finally, another innovative aspect of GEDI WISE care at SJ includes its holistic care program. To provide a little something extra, holistic care was added to traditional medicine in the Geriatric ED that includes aromatherapy, Pranic healing, and music therapy by a harpist. When asked, patients who had Pranic healing report improved pain, decreased anxiety, and overall improved perception of care. Live harp music is played throughout the Geriatric ED, 5 days a week in the afternoons. The harpist ambulates through the hallways with a portable instrument, stopping outside of ED rooms providing music for patients, families, and staff. The patient has the option of declining or ending the music at any time. At the request of the patient, family or staff, the harpist will enter a patient room to play at the bedside. The harpist does not communicate or elicit any information about the patient or their family; the role is strictly limited to playing the harp. Those patients who have experienced live harp music relate decreased anxiety and improved perception of care.

Outcomes

Patients report the Geriatric ED decreases their anxiety and improves their overall perception of care. This results in higher satisfaction scores for patients seen in this area.

Geriatric EDs decrease admissions and improve care transitions and care coordination. Further, patients can be safely managed at home for illness previously requiring hospitalization. GEDI WISE investigators are currently evaluating how patient health is improved, how population health is improved, and how decreased cost of care will be realized by the GEDI WISE model.

Mount Sinai Medical Center

MSMC consists of the Mount Sinai School of Medicine and the Mount Sinai Hospital (MSH), one of the nation's oldest, largest, and most respected hospitals. MSH has 1,127 beds and annually has over 100,000 ED visits, of which 15 % are by patient 65+ in age. The MSMC ED is an urban, academic, tertiary care facility that provides emergency care to a demographically and socioeconomically diverse patient population. The ED has a history of innovation and process redesign to improve efficiency, having implementing an EMR in 2004 to become the first "paperless" ED in New York City [12] and the first to open a "Geriatric ED" in New York City in 2012. While sharing the common goals and approach in geriatric patient care as the SJ site whereby the entire ED staff has received training and education on geriatric special care needs, and all older ED patients are evaluated for those that would benefit most from GEDI WISE care coordination and care transitions, MSMC also has additional programs featured at its site.

Informatics

The informatics components of GEDI WISE innovation tactics include the use of electronic CDS for emergency care at all three hospitals. All three hospitals utilize electronic health records (EHRs) in their EDs. This functionality allows to be embedded in the EHR; several ED templates have already been customized with evidence-based algorithms to guide assessments and clinical decision making (e.g., ISAR score, falls assessments), and alerts placed to flag patients who are already part of the GEDI WISE cohort, with frequent ED visits, recent hospitalization, and/or other high-risk conditions. With these data, each of the hospitals is able to generate (self-monitoring) quality improvement reports that facilitate performance and tracking.

A unique feature of the MSMC site is its participation in Healthix, a regional health information organization (RHIO) in the New York Metropolitan region. Healthix was formed by the merger of two of New York State's largest RHIOs, The New York Clinical Information Exchange (NYCLIX) and the Long Island Patient Information eXchange (LIPIX). Healthix is comprised of health care organizations across the New York metropolitan area and Long Island that include 107 organization with 383 facilities, 9.2 million patients, and more than 6,500 users performing more than 10,000 patient searches monthly [9], making it the largest active RHIO in the country. The Healthix platform is a centralized hub that contains patient demographic, encounter, diagnoses, vital signs, lab reports, medications, discharge summaries, and other forms of clinical data. The hub contains a master patient index that receives real-time demographic data from participating sites and is able to conduct a cross match to determine which other sites an individual patient has visited. GEDI WISE has used Healthix's considerable capabilities to monitor the health care utilization of the MSMC GEDI WISE cohort at other Healthix member institutions. With this monitoring comes the capability to recognize the occurrence of predefined events for a specified population and send clinical notifications to appropriate subscribers [13].

Implementation of a clinical event notification service (CEN) for GEDI WISE patients begins with patients being flagged in the MSMC EHR and a daily list of these active patients automated and downloaded to Healthix twice daily as part of a subscription file of patients that are part of the CEN program. The CEN used in the GEDI WISE program includes real-time information delivery of GEDI WISE patient activities at Healthix facilities outside of the MSMC. In particular, these notifications are routed to the GEDI WISE care transitions team that consists of ED-based nurse practitioners and social workers who work collaboratively to coordinate patient care and transitions in care if the patient is discharged from the MSMC ED to home or community. More specifically, notifications are sent to the GEDI WISE nurse practitioner of the following events occurring at any Healthix hospital: (1) the arrival of a GEDI WISE patient to another ED, (2) admission to or (3) discharge from another hospital [9]. As these notifications are near real-time, they have provided the GEDI WISE care transition team the ability to reach out immediately to clinicians at other hospitals or the patients themselves after hospital discharge and communicate clinical information (e.g., diagnostic study findings that were initially completed at MSMC, pre-schedule outpatient follow-up appointments, visiting nurse care plans). More importantly, these notifications have facilitated improved care coordination, a critical goal of the GEDI WISE program.

CARE: The Care and Respect for Elders Program

The Care and Respect for Elders with Emergencies (CARE) Initiative is a MSMC ED-based volunteer program, launched in 2010 that was modeled after the Hospital Elder Life Program (HELP) [14] inpatient program. As with the HELP program that has been shown to reduce delirium and functional decline in older hospitalized patients, CARE goals are to prevent avoidable complications in elder patients visiting the ED including hospital acquired delirium, falls, use of restraints, and functional decline, thus shortening length of stay and reducing the rate of hospitalization. CARE is currently staffed by trained volunteers who engage and re-orient high-risk, older, unaccompanied individuals in the MSMC ED. "The CARE initiative stemmed from the desire to improve care of older adults, many of whom present with cognitive deficits and emotional distress in the ED, and consists of bedside volunteer interventions ranging from conversation to various short activities and tools designed to engage and reorient them" [15].

CARE volunteers receive a 7-h training program that covers topics on the clinical organization of the ED, how patient flow, ED crowding, and the chaos of the environment may impact staffing patient care abilities, the more complex needs of older adults, and the importance of having volunteers attend to older adults by providing them individual attention. Training is conducted by the CARE director who is a licensed social worker. The volunteers receive specialized training in the use of conversation, anxiety-reducing techniques, and various memory- and cognition-stimulating interventions to keep patients engaged and oriented. To ensure maximal impact, volunteers are staffed in the ED during afternoon and evening hours when ED flow and times of greatest patient and staff need [15]. The CARE program enhances support to ED clinical care by providing additional attention to older adults. This has resulted in improved satisfaction and prevention of further decline.

Northwestern Memorial Hospital

Geriatric Nurse Liaisons

As with the SJRMC and MSMC GEDI WISE goals, those of the NMH Geriatric Nurse Liaison (GNL) model are to ensure geriatric patients in the emergency department have geriatric specific needs addressed prior to discharge home, and when possible, prevent unnecessary hospitalizations. Geriatric EDs have been developed to help address the mismatch between geriatric patients' needs and the priorities in the fast-paced ED environment [2]. Some EDs have developed a separate physical space dedicated to the care of older patients. Building a dedicated physical space for geriatric patients, however, may not be feasible in many EDs. In order to be more generalizable and scalable, the GEDI NL model uses pre-existing space and personnel from the NMH ED. The intervention centers on geriatric assessments performed by specially trained ED nurses to identify older patients who are at risk for adverse outcomes, and ensure that geriatric specific needs are met prior to discharge home. Often these needs can be addressed in the ED, and hospitalization can be prevented.

Personnel

The GNL model utilizes nurses with extensive ED experience and provides in-depth training in geriatrics. Other models of comprehensive geriatrics assessments in the ED are dependent on hospital departments outside of the ED for personnel and sustainability [16–18]. The ED, however, is a unique and challenging clinical environment. It is a fast paced, sometimes chaotic environment with frequent interruptions, and sees a wide variety of patients from the worried well to the critically ill. The GNL model capitalizes on the experience of ED nurses who are comfortable and thrive in this environment and provides them with the expertise, to identify and address geriatric-specific needs that frequently go unnoticed or unaddressed in typical EDs.

Four GNL positions were created to staff the NMH ED that sees 88,000 ED visits annually (approximately 18 % are visits of older individuals). The GNLs staff the ED from 9 am to 8 pm, Monday–Friday. The hours were selected to balance availability of resources and peak ED geriatric patient volume. Additional personnel including pharmacists, social workers, and physical therapists that work with the GNLs are available "as needed" for ED consults and referrals.

The GNLs completed a multidisciplinary curriculum over 4 months which encompassed clinical, didactic, and practical components. The curriculum involved clinical rotations in geriatrics (inpatient, outpatient, and inpatient consultations), palliative medicine (inpatient consultations and simulated patient encounters), physical therapy, and skilled nursing facilities. The didactic curriculum was multi-faceted and centered on 82 h of small group discussions with emergency physicians, geriatricians, pharmacists, and social workers. GNLs also completed independent study using American College of Emergency Physicians' geriatric educational videos, a reading list including primary research articles describing the assessments used by the GNLs, and video demonstration of the GEDI assessment tests [19]. The curriculum concluded with the practical phase, and completion of a GEDI-independent project. The GNLs continue to work part time as ED staff nurses to maintain their clinical skills. During their GNL shifts they focus only on GNL interventions and do not participate in primary ED clinical nursing.

Patient Selection

The GNL model was designed for patients who have unclear dispositions from the ED. The GNL model targets patients who are medically stable enough to be discharged with appropriate measures to ensure a safe transition home. By investing dedicated time with geriatric patients in the ED, GNLs often are able to prevent hospitalizations for reasons other than acute injury or illness, or so-called "social admissions." Additionally, they are able to identify geriatric specific needs such as falls risk or mild cognitive impairment that may have been missed during a typical ED visit and could lead to an adverse event if the patient were discharged from the ED.

The GNL intervention may also be expanded to geriatric patients in the ED who are likely to be hospitalized. The assessments performed by the GNLs are not routinely performed in the inpatient setting, and may provide clinicians with valuable information while caring for patients in the hospital and for discharge planning. The results of the GNL assessments can be communicated to inpatient physicians, nurses, social workers, physical therapists, and pharmacists to ensure that the issues raised in the ED are addressed prior to discharge from the hospital. Performing this assessment at the very beginning of the hospital stay may help to start the discharge planning process, so that delays in PT and social work assessments are prevented. Additionally, the GNL assessment may highlight issues that are best addressed with a geriatrics or palliative care consult during the patient's hospitalization.

To prioritize which patients may benefit most from an in-depth GNL assessment, the Identification of Seniors at Risk (ISAR) score is used as a screening tool for all geriatric patients in the ED [11]. This assessment is performed by the patient's primary nurse during their initial nursing assessment. Patients who have an ISAR score 2 or less are felt to be less likely to benefit from a GNL assessment because they have lower risk for adverse outcome if discharged from the ED when their medical complaint is adequately addressed. On the other end of the spectrum, patients who are critically ill are also unlikely to benefit from the GNL intervention. They may be unable to participate fully in the assessments, and their clinical condition may change dramatically from initial evaluation in the ED to discharge from the hospital. These patients may be candidates for geriatrics consult after stabilization of their critical illness. GNL interventions may also be requested by clinicians in the ED regardless of ISAR score.

Intervention

During the GNL intervention, multiple short, validated tests are preformed to assess for: cognitive function (Short Portable Mental Status Questionnaire) [20], delirium (Confusion Assessment Method) [21], functional status (Katz Activities of Daily Living) [22], falls risk (Timed Up and Go test) [23], care transitions (Care Transitions Measure-3) [24], and caregiver strain (Modified Caregiver Strain Index) [25]. Depending on the results of the assessments, the GNL may consult social work, pharmacy, physical therapy, geriatrics, palliative care, and hospice. The GNL

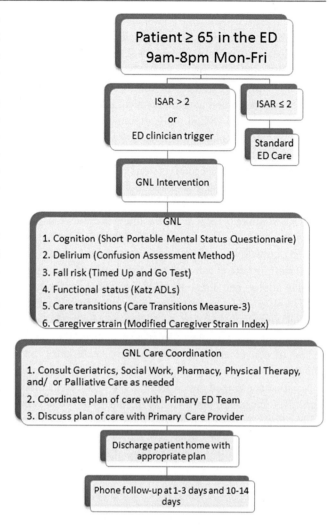

Fig. 18.1 Geriatric Emergency Department Innovations Nurse Liaison (GNL) intervention protocol (from Aldeen AZ, Mark Courtney D, Lindquist LA, Dresden SM, Gravenor SJ. Geriatric Emergency Department Innovations: Preliminary Data for the Geriatric Nurse Liaison Model. J Am Geriatr Soc. 2014 Aug 12 with permission)

discusses his or her recommendations with the primary care team. The GNL later performs follow-up phone calls at 1–3 and 10–14 days to ensure effective transition from the ED or hospital if the patient was admitted (Fig. 18.1) [8].

Outcomes

Continuous measurement of processes and outcomes with the assistance of informatics-based electronic medical records and a data monitoring dashboards are important to quantify improvements in care and identify issues and potential pitfalls. Monitoring the hourly geriatric patient volume, the frequency and time of day consults are made with pharmacy, social work, and physical therapy, can inform optimal GNL and consultant availability. ED length of stay (LOS), discharge, observation, and inpatient admission rate, inpatient length of stay, 30-day hospital readmission rate, and 72-h ED repeat visits are key outcomes that are monitored monthly and quarterly to assess the effects of the GNL program.

Preliminary results from the initial GNL site are promising. GNL patients are more likely to be discharged from the hospital than patients who did not receive the GNL intervention. When these results are stratified by acuity, there is a significant decrease in the hospitalization rate of GNL patients with higher acuity—emergency severity index (ESI) [26] scores of 2 or 3 (on a scale of 1–5, 1 is most acute)—compared to patients who did not receive the GNL intervention. For patients with lower acuity (ESI 4), the results are reversed. GNL patients are more likely to be hospitalized than non-GNL patients. There is no statistically significant change in 30-day readmission rate or 72-h repeat ED visit rate. ED length of stay, however, appears to increase for GNL patients [8]. While more data are needed to make definitive conclusions, the initial results suggest that the GNL assessment has been successful in assisting with safe discharges home for higher acuity patients. However for perceived low acuity patients, the GNL assessment may be uncovering underlying problems that normally would have gone untreated in the ED. Further, the overall increased discharge rate for GNL patients has not resulted in adverse outcomes such as hospital readmission or repeat ED visits.

The Business Case for a Geriatrics ED

The primary function of a geriatric ED is to deliver quality emergency care to the community; yet entry into the Geriatric ED world is often hampered by financial constraints and concerns. Minor changes, such as a larger font in discharge instructions and comfort issues targeting older patients can be implemented with minimal cost. It may not be prudent or feasible to build "bigger and better" structural "geriatric EDs" when budgets are limited. Furthermore, the Geriatric ED guidelines do not require this type of investment.

The GEDI WISE programs described here of the three hospitals may seem unattainable or unnecessary depending upon the specific population and community served. In particular the program at SJ, the most mature of the three, has evolved since 2009 and has been constantly adjusting to meet the changing needs of the senior population within the context of an evolving health care system. As part of continuous quality improvement initiatives and self-monitoring, there have been many trials and errors through the days and months of finding the "right" blend of services with all three programs. For some of the sites this has included surveying older patients and their families when they use emergency services; running pilot programs; consulting with various medical specialties; reviewing the literature and collaborating with colleagues with similar programs. The key point is that the Geriatric ED has a solid foundation, as well as the flexibility to meet the needs of the individuals whom they serve.

Making the Case

In making the business case for a Geriatric ED, one of the first questions to be answered is: "Why does the hospital and community need a Geriatric ED?" For example, the need to focus on the geriatric emergency population in the SJ community was identified in 2002; however, the Geriatric ED did not open until 7 years later as a 14-bed unit serving approximately 60 patients per day. The conceptual model was introduced at MSMC in early 2005, however its Geriatric ED did not open until 2012. Identification of the population and its needs along with progressive buy-in and support of hospital leadership, clinical services, and administrative support are necessary.

It is essential for a hospital considering a geriatric ED to define program specifics at the earliest planning stages so the resources and space can be better allocated. This includes defining the patient population that will be using these services. To accomplish this, multiple meetings with staff, geriatricians, and the community are needed. The initial discussions need to include financial constraints; potential physical locations for emergency services including the feasibility of structural modifications and the identification of an advocate or champion (physician or nurse) to attain and sustain initiatives.

Administrative support is vital to the implementation and ongoing success of the program. Potential benefits to discuss with hospital leadership include increased patient satisfaction scores; more appropriate admissions; decreased return visits; and increasing visits from patients outside of the catchment area. It may also be prudent to discuss a range of options to be implemented over time to determine the value of the program and individual hospital metrics to monitor progress. Programs may begin with existing ED staff and infrastructure along with ongoing education of all staff members in the ED about geriatric-specific issues. From a quality of care perspective, implementing geriatric-specific protocols helps ensure that best practices are incorporated into practice.

The Cost

Cost for the Geriatric ED can be divided into three areas: (1) structural enhancements, (2) service enhancements, and (3) personnel. Structural enhancements can span a wide range, are not a necessity, and do not need to break the budget. The only time a new structural ED is necessary may be based on total patient volumes and the age of existing infrastructure. A recent internal cost analysis at SJRMC, improvements such as mattresses, room painting, non-glare floor coatings, soundproofing, switching lights to dimmers can cost as little as $1,500 per room. A ten-bed area can be renovated to meet the needs of senior patients for less than $20,000.

Enhancements of already existing clinical services such as social work, case management, physical therapy, and pharmacy are feasible. Redesigning workflows to provide services in a Geriatric ED (or targeting older adults in any ED) can be done without relying on additional resources. An example would be case management. Most hospitals have case managers that focus on admitted patients. Instead of having case managers focused those admitted on the inpatient floor, their efforts could be shifted earlier to target admitted patients when they are in the ED. Since the majority of unscheduled hospital admissions arrive through the ED, care coordination can begin at the time of admission in the ED; and those who are being discharged from the ED may collaterally benefit with these services now potentially available to them. This is a reasonable and feasible shifting of already existing services to engage the same patient population, but at an earlier time point in the care continuum, thus potentially shortening lengths of stay.

The third area where cost needs to be analyzed is in personnel. Every geriatric program must have a champion or advocate. For the three GEDI WISE programs, all included staff with specific responsibilities to assess patients at risk and provide targeted care coordination and transitions of care that currently do not exist for older patients seen in traditional EDs. Such personnel (SJ's nurse navigator, MSMC's care transitions NP, NMH's GNL) can be identified within existing staff, based on how the program is designed. A significant benefit of the GNL model is that it can be implemented without developing a separate space. It is an individual hospital's choice what positions they will support as well as what personnel they will need to hire to create a Geriatric ED.

Finally, and most importantly, ongoing personnel education is essential to the success of any Geriatric ED program. Although nursing and physician education programs already exist online, all staff members, from the point of entry into the ED through disposition, require geriatric specific education and awareness of changes to patient approach and protocols in the care of older individuals.

Revenue

In medicine today, the financial complexities of the hospital business are in constant flux. As the industry transitions from a fee-for-service model to one more consistent with health care reform, a shift in financial priorities will evolve. Decreasing cost for a set group of patients will become more important than increasing admissions in a fee-for-service environment. The GEDI WISE experience at the three participating hospitals has been encouraging. Geriatric volume has continued to increase; there will be changes in quality metrics including door to doctor time, the duration of the patient stays in the ED, and decisions to admit. Patient satisfaction has improved. Each of these metric changes will need to be translated and interpreted to a dollar value for the health care organization, and to Medicare. Each hospital will need to look at their market share and evaluate their competitive environment and decide if a geriatric ED makes sense for their community. The Geriatric ED creates opportunities for cost savings as well. Geriatric EDs have the potential to decrease avoidable admissions to the hospital and improve Transitions of Care. It is unclear at this point in time, what impact Geriatric ED may have on hospital readmissions.

Summary

The contemporary ED has evolved in response to conditions and pressures of the health care system. Additional savings may be realized from a hospital-wide global perspective, with a timely geriatric evaluation. The benefit to medical staff, patients, and families may be measured in time needed to complete an outpatient assessment and treatment plan. During the ED visit, appropriate comprehensive assessments with labs, imaging, and consultations can provide a diagnosis and plan of care, thereby creating an otherwise nonexistent safety net for this vulnerable population. This is an example of the EDs response to the changing needs of its patients and the demands of health care reform.

Disclosure

This publication of GEDI WISE was made possible by Grant Number 1C1CMS331055-01-00 from the Department of Health and Human Services, Centers for Medicare & Medicaid Services. The contents of this publication are solely the responsibility of the authors and do not necessarily represent the official views of the U.S. Department of Health and Human Services or any of its agencies.

References

1. Hwang U, Shah MN, Han JH, Carpenter CR, Siu AL, Adams J. Transforming emergency care for older adults. Health Aff. 2013;32(12):2116–21.
2. Hwang U, Morrison RS. The geriatric emergency department. J Am Geriatr Soc. 2007;55:1873–6.
3. Carpenter CR, Bromley M, Caterino JM, Chun A, Gerson LW, Greenspan J, et al. Optimal older adults emergency care: introducing multidisciplinary geriatric emergency department guidelines from

the American College of Emergency Physicians, American Geriatrics Society, Emergency Nurses Association, and Society for Academic Emergency Medicine. Acad Emerg Med. 2014;21(7):806–9.

4. Carpenter CR, Bromley M, Caterino JM, Chun A, Gerson LW, Greenspan J, et al. Optimal older adults emergency care: introducing multidisciplinary geriatric emergency department guidelines from the American College of Emergency Physicians, American Geriatrics Society, Emergency Nurses Association, and Society for Academic Emergency Medicine. Ann Emerg Med. 2014; 63(5):e1–3.

5. Carpenter CR, Bromley M, Caterino JM, Chun A, Gerson LW, Greenspan J, et al. Optimal older adults emergency care: introducing multidisciplinary geriatric emergency department guidelines from the American College of Emergency Physicians, American Geriatrics Society, Emergency Nurses Association, and Society for Academic Emergency Medicine. J Am Geriatr Soc. 2014;62(7):1360–3.

6. Centers for Medicare and Medicaid Innovation. Health Care Innovation Award project profiles [Internet]. Washington DC. 2012. Accessed on 2014 August 18. Available from: http://innovation.cms.gov/Files/x/HCIA-Project-Profiles.pdf, http://innovation.cms.gov/initiatives/Health-Care-Innovation-Awards/New-York.html

7. Berwick DM, Nolan TW, Whittington J. The triple aim: care, health, and cost. Health Aff. 2008;27(3):759–69.

8. Aldeen AZ, Courtney MC, Lindquist LA, Dresden SM, Gravenor SJ. Geriatric emergency department innovations: preliminary data for the geriatric nurse liaison model. J Am Geriatr Soc. 2014;62(9):1781–5.

9. Gutteridge DL, Genes N, Hwang U, Kaplan B, GEDI WISE Investigators, Shapiro JS. Enhancing a Geriatric Emergency Department Care Coordination Intervention Using Automated Health Information Exchange-Based Clinical Event Notifications. eGEMs (Generating Evidence & Methods to improve patient outcomes). 2014;2(3):Article 6.

10. American College of Emergency Physicians, American Geriatrics Society, Emergency Nurses Association, Society for Academic Emergency Medicine. Geriatric Emergency Department Guidelines. 2014. Accessed on 2014 June 25. Available from: http://geriatrics-careonline.org/ProductAbstract/geriatric-emergency-department-guidelines/CL013/?param2=search

11. McCusker J, Bellavance F, Cardin S, Trepanier S, Verdon J, Ardman O. Detection of older people at increased risk of adverse health outcomes after an emergency visit: the ISAR screening tool. J Am Geriatr Soc. 1999;47(10):1229–37.

12. Baumlin KM, Shapiro JS, Weiner C, Gottlieb B, Chawla N, Richardson LD. Clinical information system and process redesign improves emergency department efficiency. Jt Comm J Qual Patient Saf. 2010;36:179–85.

13. Moore T, Shapiro JS, Doles L, Calman N, Camhi E, Check T, et al. Event detection: a clinical notification service on a health information exchange platform. AMIA Annu Symp Proc. 2012;2012:635–42.

14. Inouye SK, Bogardus ST, Charpentier PA, Leo-Summers L, Acampora D, Holford TR, et al. A multicomponent intervention to prevent delirium in hospitalized older patients. N Engl J Med. 1999;340:669–76.

15. Sanon M, Baumlin K, Kaplan S, Grudzen C. The Care and Respect for Elders with Emergencies (CARE) Program. J Am Geriatr Soc. 2014;62(2):365–70.

16. Mion LC, Palmer RM, Anetzberger GJ, Meldon SW. Establishing a case-finding and referral system for at-risk older individuals in the emergency department setting: the SIGNET model. J Am Geriatr Soc. 2001;49(10):1379–86.

17. Sinoff G, Clarfield AM, Bergman H, Beaudet M. A two-year follow-up of geriatric consults in the emergency department. J Am Geriatr Soc. 1998;46(6):716–20.

18. Miller DK, Lewis LM, Nork MJ, Morley JE. Controlled trial of a geriatric case-finding and liaison service in an emergency department. J Am Geriatr Soc. 1996;44(5):513–20 [Clinical Trial Controlled Clinical Trial Research Support, Non-U.S. Gov't].

19. Morrison RS, Siu AL. A comparison of pain and its treatment in advanced dementia and cognitively intact older patients with hip fracture. J Pain Symptom Manage. 2000;19:240–8.

20. Erkinjuntti T, Sulkava R, Wikstrom J, Autio L. Short Portable Mental Status Questionnaire as a screening test for dementia and delirium among the elderly. J Am Geriatr Soc. 1987;35(5):412–6 [Comparative Study Research Support, Non-U.S. Gov't].

21. Inouye SK, van Dyck CH, Alessi CA, Balkin S, Siegal AP, Horwitz RI. Clarifying confusion: the confusion assessment method. A new method for detection of delirium. Ann Intern Med. 1990;113(12):941–8 [Research Support, Non-U.S. Gov't].

22. Katz S. Assessing self-maintenance: activities of daily living, mobility, and instrumental activities of daily living. J Am Geriatr Soc. 1983;31(12):721–7 [Research Support, U.S. Gov't, Non-P.H.S. Research Support, U.S. Gov't, P.H.S. Review].

23. Podsiadlo D, Richardson S. The timed "Up & Go": a test of basic functional mobility for frail elderly persons. J Am Geriatr Soc. 1991;39(2):142–8.

24. Parry C, Mahoney E, Chalmers SA, Coleman EA. Assessing the quality of transitional care: further applications of the care transitions measure. Med Care. 2008;46(3):317–22.

25. Thornton M, Travis SS. Analysis of the reliability of the modified caregiver strain index. J Gerontol B Psychol Sci Soc Sci. 2003;58(2):S127–32 [Research Support, U.S. Gov't, P.H.S.].

26. Wuerz R, Milne L, Eitel D, Gilboy N. Reliability and validity of a new five-level triage instrument. Acad Emerg Med. 2000;7:236–42.

The Kindred Healthcare Model of Post-acute Care

Sally Brooks and Lauren Williams

Introduction

The passage and implementation of the Patient Protection and Affordable Care Act (ACA) in 2010 set the stage for the ongoing evolution and changing landscape of healthcare delivery. The ACA laid the platform for penalties to hospitals with high readmission rates. It also created health insurance exchanges, requiring that all individuals have health insurance, and expanded the Medicaid program.

Healthcare reform was the first step in transitioning from the historic disparate, fee-for-service, volume-based system to one that is value-based. The National Quality Strategy was established in 2011 by the Agency for Healthcare Research and Quality on behalf of the U.S. Department of Health and Human Services. The goal is to provide high quality, affordable healthcare that is "patient-centered, reliable, accessible and safe." [1] also described as the "Triple Aim." This term was coined by Donald Berwick while President and CEO of the Institute for Healthcare Improvement to describe the goals of "improving the experience of care, improving the health of populations, and reducing per capita cost of health care." [2]

As a next step in reform, Congressional leaders recognized that post-acute care providers play an important role in the full continuum of patient care. As healthcare reform is moving forward, a focus on effective care transitions is evolving in the field of post-acute care. One example of this trend is the creation of the Care Transitions Intervention, led by Eric Coleman, MD, MPH, and described as "a patient-centered coaching intervention to empower individuals to better manage their health." A 2014 study of the program concluded that "… the CTI [Care Transitions Intervention] generates meaningful cost avoidance for at least 6 months post-hospitalization, and also provides useful metrics to evaluate the impact and cost avoidance of hospital readmission reduction programs." [3]

For payors, the volume-to-value-based trend is also progressing. A 2014 survey of Blue Cross insurers found that companies are "experimenting with new formulas for reimbursing doctors and hospitals, slowly moving away from the traditional approach of basing payments on the numbers of tests and procedures performed" [4]. According to the survey, $1 out of every $5 of reimbursements is being paid for improvement of care and lowering of costs. $65 billion a year is being spent in new value-based payment models [5].

Meeting the Challenges of Healthcare Reform: The Kindred Case Study

Over the course of Kindred Healthcare's 30-year history, the company has sought to diversify its business model and service offerings to encompass the entire post-acute spectrum to better meet the needs of patients. Beginning as a provider of long-term acute care hospital services, expansion included the addition of skilled nursing facilities, acute rehabilitation facilities and units, comprehensive contract rehabilitation therapy services, home health, and hospice. This enables the company to provide care and recovery for patients in the continuum of settings after discharge from a traditional hospital. However, early in the evolution, the individual services, organized in separate divisions, were operating in silos. Efforts were disconnected from one another in an existing fee-for-service environment. An early adopter of the value-based model, Kindred supports collaboration across sites and services and espouses care coordination as the foundation for future innovative models.

The organization has a national scope with more than 103,000 Kindred employees taking care of over 1 million patients and residents every year in more than 2,800 locations in 47 states. In June 2014, the majority of patients served were Medicare beneficiaries with approximately

S. Brooks, M.D. (✉) • L. Williams, B.A., M.A.
Kindred Healthcare, 680 S. Fourth Street, Louisville, KY 40202, USA
e-mail: sally.brooks@kindred.com; lauren.williams@kindred.com

M.L. Malone et al. (eds.), *Geriatrics Models of Care: Bringing 'Best Practice' to an Aging America*, DOI 10.1007/978-3-319-16068-9_19, © Springer International Publishing Switzerland 2015

68 % of patients cared for in Kindred's hospitals and nursing centers being 65 or older, with 17 % over 85.

Today's Kindred includes about 100 transitional care hospitals (licensed as acute care hospitals and certified as long-term acute care hospitals), 90 nursing and rehabilitation centers, 100 acute rehabilitation units, and about 2,300 RehabCare sites of service. There has been significant growth in the home health, private duty, and hospice sector. Many of the above services are aligned in 16 integrated care markets. These markets feature strategic partnerships with physicians and health systems and some include care transitions managers to facilitate effective patient-centered care management.

Strategic Realignment to Provide Patient-Centered Care

Kindred Healthcare has evolved from a company operating individual businesses to one with a patient-centered focus, providing services across the continuum. Creating integration between sites and services helps ensure the best patient outcomes. To align with healthcare reform and accomplish Kindred's 2014 5-year strategic plan, a focus on the delivery of care in integrated care markets is designed to increase value for patients, payors, and employees. In an integrated market, the full spectrum of post-acute care services is provided as patients move through the continuum. The strategy includes realignment of services requiring aggressive growth in rehabilitation, home health, assisted living services, oversight by a care management team, and partnerships with payor sources and ACOs. As healthcare evolves, more care will be delivered in the home. Home is where patients want to receive care with a coordinated, communicative clinical team [6]. The strategic plan strives to meet the challenges of that changing healthcare environment.

An Interdisciplinary Team Approach

Although the interdisciplinary team (IDT) is a familiar concept with geriatricians, the Kindred model deploys IDT concepts across, yet unique to, the individual care settings. IDT is active in each of Kindred's divisions and is a critical component of patient-centered care. Dependent upon setting, there are differences in process. In the transitional care hospital setting, representatives from each discipline providing care for a patient are included. This team is composed of physicians, nursing, pharmacy, therapy (PT, OT, ST, RT), dietary, wound care, social work, and case management. As is typical of an IDT, they meet and formulate treatment plans based on the patient's goals, along with medical and functional needs. Patient and family involvement is critical to success.

The IDT in the Nursing Center Division is similar. The team meets 72 h post-admission with the patient and family to discuss goals and care plans. After the initial meeting, the team meets again in 21 days, monthly, and then quarterly for long-term residents until the patient is discharged.

Nursing leaders have shared that the IDT process serves as validation that the care provided is aligned with the patient and caregiver goals. A key success factor is to budget time to accommodate the IDT in the daily workflow. In home care, IDT takes place weekly to discuss new patient admissions and assure all patients are meeting their individual goals. Discharge planning commonly includes a social worker to arrange community services while assessing financial limitations that impact access to care.

Within hospice, regulatory and accrediting bodies guide the IDT format and content. The IDT's formal process includes physicians, nurse practitioners, nurses, social workers, bereavement counselors, chaplains and therapists.

IDT has a unique role in the RehabCare services. There are regulatory standards that govern the IDT process in most inpatient settings, providing guidance about the involvement of therapists in care planning. The therapy team members may be the first to notice a change in condition based on their frequent patient interactions.

In an inpatient rehabilitation unit, each member of the care team attends a bi-weekly conference led by the unit's medical director. In most instances, the patient's family and caregivers are engaged to assure ongoing rehabilitation continuity after discharge. Partly because of this family involvement, research reveals that there are continued functional independence gains at 95 days post-IRF discharge for stroke patients [7].

In discussions with physicians, they find an interdisciplinary team model to be especially valuable for geriatric patients. With the growing aging population, the complexity of care increases drastically. The IDT provides the benefit of more than one pair of eyes watching the patient, more than one pair of hands on the patient, and more than one mind considering the totality of the patient's care. For example, it may be the physician who orders a diuretic for a patient, but it is often an observant therapist who realizes this patient has suddenly become orthostatic, or an attentive nurse who realizes the patient can no longer sleep soundly due to frequent trips to the bathroom. An interdisciplinary team shifts care from disease-centered to person-centered—a shift that is sorely needed in modern healthcare.

Geriatricians can play an important role in caring for patients in post-acute sites and lead these IDTs focused on functional improvements in the growing aging and chronically ill population.

Creation of a Care Transitions Program

Kindred incorporated several care transition principles into development of its Care Transitions Program in Boston, Cleveland, Dallas, Las Vegas, and Indianapolis. Patients served are those with specific diagnoses and risk factors. The Care Transitions program is evidence-based and is the foundation in achieving the "Triple Aim." A Care Transitions Manager (CTM) shepherds high-risk patients throughout their stays at Kindred facilities—or at home with Kindred at Home—until 35 days post-hospital discharge. CTMs meet with the patients within 72 h of admission, at least weekly after that, and within 24 h of each transition. This is to help ensure continuity of care by providing a "warm" and written handoff to the receiving provider, with updated patient information. When the patient transitions to home, the CTM visits the patient within 24 h to minimize the risk of re-hospitalization during this vulnerable time. Patients who transition to a non-Kindred provider receive phone calls 24–48 h post-discharge.

It is important that the CTM does not replace any other member of the care team. It is a unique role filled by a nurse, social worker, or therapist. Close collaboration and information sharing with the patient's primary care provider is paramount. Key to enhancing the patient's successful transitions is availability of information. This includes pertinent healthcare records, discharge summary, medication lists, and upcoming physician appointments. In addition, assessing the patients' health literacy and engaging the patient is crucial to the plan of care.

Some of the responsibilities of the CTM include:

- Training in all relevant electronic health record systems
- Attending IDT meetings
- Ensuring that the PCP appointment is made within 7 days of transition home
- Sending a letter to the PCP with each transition
- Referring high-risk patients to Transitional Care Pharmacists where available

"I Pass the Baton" is an evidence-based tool developed by the U.S. Department of Health and Human Services and used by the CTMs to achieve improved outcomes:

*I*ntroduction (Transitional Care Nurse name and cell number); *P*atient; *A*ssessment; *S*ituation; *S*afety Concerns; *T*he; *B*ackground; *A*ction; *T*iming; *O*wnership; *N*ext [8].

Early data from the 2013 Care Transitions pilots served as the impetus to scale the program to additional integrated markets. In the Boston pilot, patients who received the intervention had a 6.3 % hospital readmission rate, 30 days post-discharge from any Kindred site of care, as compared to 16.1 % in the control group. The control group included patients with the same eligibility criteria who received usual care. Patient satisfaction was calculated on a 1–4 scale (4 being the highest), with the intervention group score of 3.98

exceeding the control group score of 3.16. The average length of stay (LOS) for the intervention group in long-term acute care hospitals, skilled nursing facilities and home health combined was 19.2 days, compared to 25.7 days for the control group.

In Indianapolis, early program data demonstrate similar success. Over a 6-month period from January 1, 2014 through July 31, 2014 [$n = 148$], the all-cause, hospital readmission rate (within 30 days or less after admission) was 6.84 %. The market achieved 95 % compliance with securing a PCP appointment for patients within 7 days of discharge.

Implementation of the Care Transitions Program has not been without challenges. One of the program's leaders acknowledges that the organization has to accept upfront costs in order to build a better bridge for a coordinated, patient-centered approach. In the current volume-based models, these investments are not reimbursed. In addition, it takes time and transparent communication to gain the buy-in of facility-based care managers with similar, yet distinct, roles.

Building a Care Management Division

In 2013, Kindred created a Care Management Division to ensure adequate resources support and advance integrated care market strategies. Existing market resources were inadequate to drive consistent development and implementation of a cohesive care management approach, especially given the day-to-day workload of the existing clinical work force. The goal is to enhance capabilities for seamless patient care in the right place, at the right time and for the right cost.

Rehabilitation as the Thread That Binds

Kindred's 2011 acquisition of RehabCare Group, Inc., the country's largest contract manager of rehabilitation services, represents a calculated recognition of the role that rehabilitation plays in augmenting and complementing the spectrum of post-acute care services. The ability to provide patient rehabilitation services and metrics, across the care spectrum, ensures care continuity and positions the organization for value-based payment arrangements.

With this expansion of rehabilitation services, current RehabCare capabilities include provision of rehabilitation services for skilled nursing facilities, care in freestanding inpatient rehabilitation facilities (IRFs), management of hospital-based inpatient rehabilitation units, and contracts to provide hospital inpatient and outpatient programs. For its skilled nursing facility partners, RehabCare provides access to an advanced technology platform, best practice clinical programs, and a strong therapist labor pool. The SMART TX™ system with iTouch capability tracks real-time patient outcome data to assess Functional Improvement Measures (FIM), discharge location, and hospital readmissions. For the inpatient settings, the capabilities include efficient patient throughput and clinical outcomes tracking based on best practice programs. These programs include diagnoses such as stroke, brain and neurologic disorders, orthopedic, cardiac, and pulmonary rehabilitation. Rehabilitation services provide a common thread to create value for communities by providing standardized recovery care protocols throughout the care episode.

In 2013, RehabCare delivered intense, medically necessary therapies to more than 500,000 patients in approximately 1,800 distinct service locations. Outcomes exceeded the national average in several areas. In freestanding inpatient rehabilitation hospitals (IRFs) and acute rehabilitation units in host hospitals, FIM gain efficiency exceeds the national rates and the "discharge to community" rate is higher with lower re-hospitalization rates than the national average [Fig. 19.1].

Data also show that RehabCare stroke patients are discharged to the community more frequently than the national average—71.9 % versus 70 % [9].

Evolving Care Delivery Models

A strategic decision was made in 2014 to acquire a home-based primary care practice. The rationale was to scale and replicate care delivery models shown to enhance quality and reduce unnecessary costs for chronically ill, homebound individuals. Recent research reveals that home-based primary care models lead to lower costs to Medicare—17 % lower over a mean 2 years of follow-up, with no difference between cases and controls in mortality [10]. Additional peer-reviewed research has shown that home-based delivery of primary care services reduces hospitalizations, re-hospitalizations, and skilled nursing facility placements [11]. Building this capability allows Kindred to create and expand "pre-acute" strategies.

Deploying Best Practices, Measuring Care and Service Quality Outcomes

One of Kindred's earliest efforts to integrate services and develop value-based care is reflected in its adoption of the INTERACT program https://interact2.net/. The INTERACT program provides tools and processes to enable nursing center staff to recognize, evaluate, communicate, and document acute changes in condition and manage them in place whenever safe, appropriate, and feasible. The INTERACT program helps centers reduce unplanned emergency room visits, hospitalizations, and hospital readmissions. Kindred's Nursing Center Division implemented key components of

the INTERACT program in early 2010. Since this time, the division has reduced its unplanned hospital readmissions by 15 % [Fig. 19.1]. Other types of Kindred care sites have incorporated key INTERACT methods to achieve similar results, such as implementing the quality improvement process. This process engages key members of the IDT who examine opportunities for improvement following an unplanned ER or hospital transfer.

The INTERACT program is thought to be most effective if it is combined with cross-setting teams that involve staff from nursing centers, hospitals, and other post-acute care providers meeting to discuss root cause analysis of potentially preventable transfers and other adverse events.

Care Quality

Identifying outcome metrics to assure program success is crucial to achieving organizational goals. For example, Kindred collaborated with a Las Vegas health plan as the preferred post-acute provider for its members. The goal was to move patients through the care continuum assuring efficient, effective care. Data revealed that the average length of stay (LOS) for these health plan members (14.4 days) in Kindred Hospitals was lower than Medicare fee-for-service (FFS) patients (26.6 days). Other metrics revealed lower hospital readmission rates (16.8 %) for the health plan members in Kindred Subacute care facilities, as compared with Medicare FFS patients (23.5 %).

Certain quality outcome and cost-effective metrics are shared across Kindred's portfolio. These metrics include: patient discharge destination, LOS, hospital readmission rates, patient satisfaction, and site-specific quality measures [Fig. 19.1].

Service Quality

A key pillar of "Triple Aim" is to enhance patient experience, and it is especially critical to engage and retain staff with experience in caring for the older, chronically ill population. In that vein, a pilot project was implemented in two long-term acute care locations and one inpatient rehabilitation hospital in the Dallas Integrated Care Market. The pilot program tested the efficacy of a values-driven culture.

The leaders recognized the need to show employees how much the organization valued their opinion and services before they could expect them to devote their talents and passion for patients and families.

The market leaders borrowed a page from Zappos.com, sending staff to attend Zappos' 3-day "boot camp." This is a program designed to transform any company's culture to "improve employee engagement, increase productivity, promote brand loyalty, and enhance financial performance"

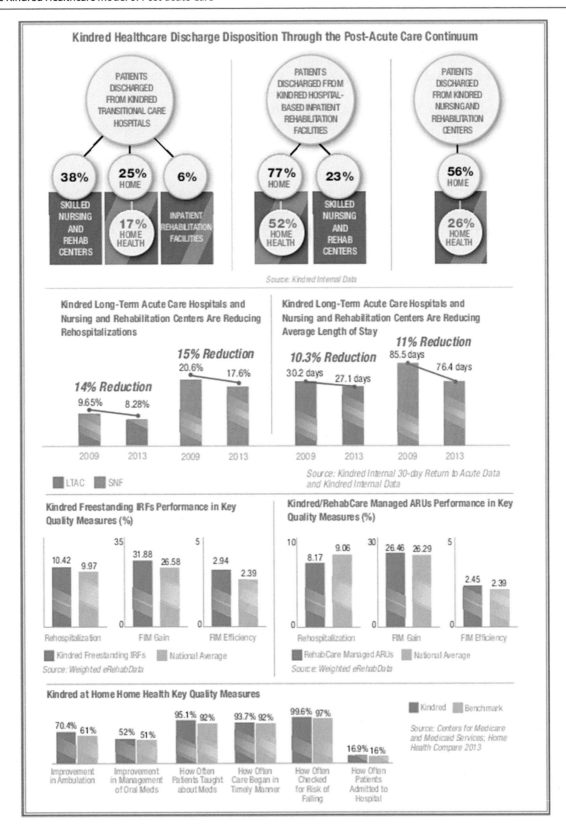

Fig. 19.1 Kindred healthcare discharge disposition through the post-acute care continuum

[12]. The leaders engaged a team that evaluated the current service culture, finding that the current culture did *not* represent what Kindred aspires to be. They implemented a program that empowered employees to set the values of the organization.

The employees re-defined "teamwork" to a term that resonated with them: "respect individuality to create the team." Other common values evolved and were redefined, including "compassion, integrity, respect and fun."

Management was trained on servant leadership, built on the premise of empowering employees. Values and servant leadership were then infused into four key areas: hiring, family involvement, performance management, and recognition. The results for the three pilot hospitals demonstrated an increase in employee engagement, patient satisfaction, patient access and thus, revenue. Importantly, decreases in employee turnover, employee performance issues, and malpractice claims were also achieved. Two of the three facilities demonstrated significant reduction in employee turnover of 26 % and 32 %, respectively. Clinical quality index scores went up 85 % for those same facilities.

Information and Technology Investment

Kindred Healthcare has allocated significant resources to develop electronic health records to coordinate healthcare and achieve improved outcomes. Due to the variability in the regulatory environment and care delivery needs, each division has a unique system. However, these unique systems are being connected through an "internal" health information exchange (HIE) [Fig. 19.2]. This technology will allow a patient care summary to be viewed at the next point of care, whether it is another Kindred facility, a non-Kindred facility, or home. Kindred also participates in regional and statewide HIEs.

Collaborations

Kindred has collaborated with several health systems to assure continuity of care and desired outcomes. The foundation for system integration includes good communication and trust. Good communication pillars include: providing direct access to medical information; use of the SBAR (Situation, Background, Assessment, Recommendation) tool to assure nurses completely communicate changes in condition to physicians; transparent metric sharing and collaboration on best practice programs.

Trust requires responsive versus defensive collaboration, integrated services, and willingness for each organization to allocate resources.

Identifying potential partners is the first step in forming Joint Quality Committees that work, followed by the establishment of mutual objectives and articulation of those goals in a formalized charter. Assuring physician engagement and alignment involves education, training, and gaining buy-in. Communication protocols must be established and complementary clinical capabilities facilitate the process. Sharing transparent outcomes, with mutually developed quality and operating measures, quantify the success of the committee.

Examples of collaborations are as follows. Kindred has established a Joint Quality Committee with the University of Washington with the mission of providing "oversight of the relationship and to review quality, operational and outcome indicators on patients transferred from UW Medicine to Kindred hospitals," according to the shared charter. Shared quality indicators include: total admissions, total discharges, discharge dispositions, unplanned readmissions to the hospital, average LOS, nosocomial infection rates, ventilator wean rates, and patient satisfaction.

In Indianapolis, Kindred has formed a collaborative relationship with the Franciscan Alliance Pioneer Accountable Care Organization (ACO). According to recent estimates, the number of patients receiving care from ACOs is expected to be more than 130 million by 2017 [13]. This relationship is particularly relevant because of the role ACOs will play in the evolution of healthcare reform.

Kindred was one of the first post-acute care providers chosen to be a preferred provider for the ACO. Skilled in-network providers are eligible for CMS waivers for the qualifying 3-day length of stay. ACO preferred providers participate in: attendance at ACO meetings and committees; weekly ACO interdisciplinary calls; monthly quality metric reporting; utilization of the INTERACT tool; and shared root cause analysis on opportunities. Kindred offers the St. Francis transitional care nurses access to facilities to visit patients on any shift. Committees include: clinical quality, medication reconciliation, advanced care planning, an end-stage renal disease (ESRD) program, behavioral health, and shared educational opportunities.

Kindred Healthcare is taking the lead in national health innovation by participating in the Bundled Payment Care Improvement (BPCI) initiative and forming an ACO partnership.

The organization was chosen by the Centers for Medicare & Medicaid Services (CMS) to participate in a BPCI pilot project in Cleveland, and has made investments in the resources needed to form Joint Quality Committees with collaborating organizations involved in that project. An ACA program, the (BPCI) initiative pilots innovative payment and care delivery models to assure higher quality and coordinated care at lower cost [14]. Results are pending, however,

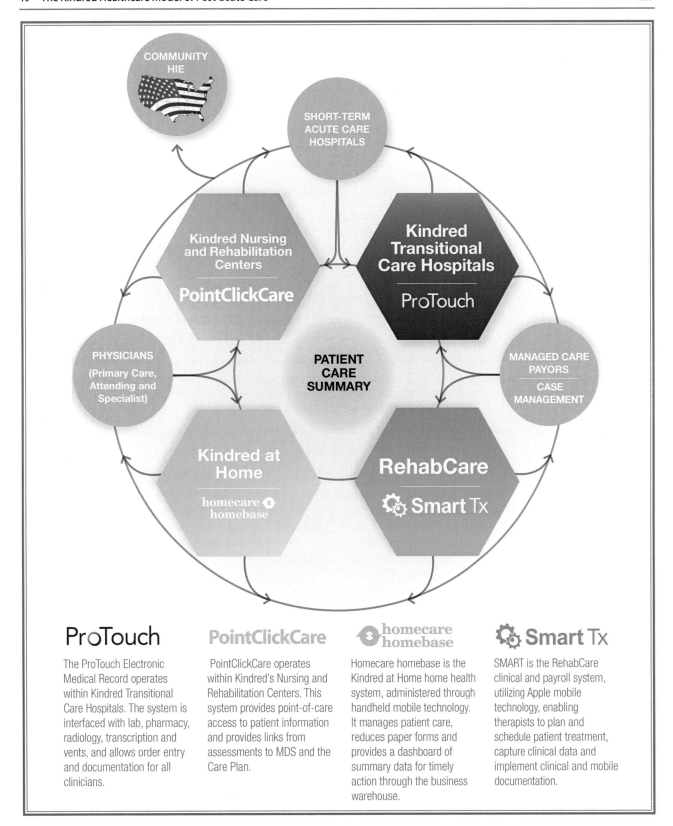

ProTouch

The ProTouch Electronic Medical Record operates within Kindred Transitional Care Hospitals. The system is interfaced with lab, pharmacy, radiology, transcription and vents, and allows order entry and documentation for all clinicians.

PointClickCare

PointClickCare operates within Kindred's Nursing and Rehabilitation Centers. This system provides point-of-care access to patient information and provides links from assessments to MDS and the Care Plan.

homecare homebase

Homecare homebase is the Kindred at Home home health system, administered through handheld mobile technology. It manages patient care, reduces paper forms and provides a dashboard of summary data for timely action through the business warehouse.

Smart Tx

SMART is the RehabCare clinical and payroll system, utilizing Apple mobile technology, enabling therapists to plan and schedule patient treatment, capture clinical data and implement clinical and mobile documentation.

Fig. 19.2 Continuum of the Kindred care services

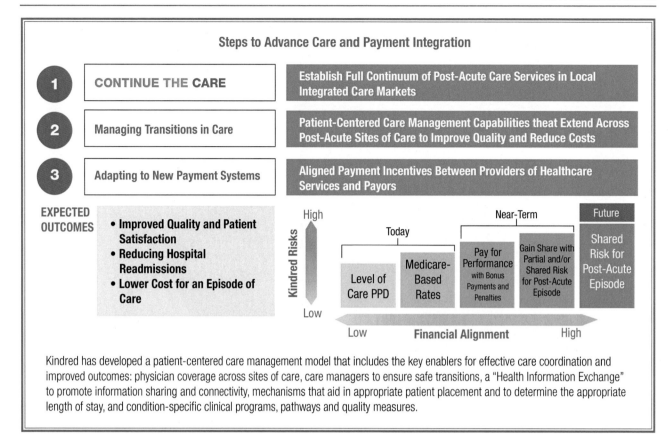

Fig. 19.3 Steps to advance care and payment integration

and program implementation has uncovered many opportunities for process improvement.

In addition, in the spring of 2014, Kindred became a strategic partner in the Silver State Accountable Care Organization in Las Vegas, Nevada. Formed in 2013, Silver State was approved by CMS as a "shared savings" ACO to serve Medicare fee-for-service patients in Southern Nevada. The ACO is a collaborative effort with independent doctors, physician groups, and affiliated healthcare providers. Silver State has secured the participation of approximately 150 primary care physicians and other healthcare providers covering approximately 10,000 lives. Silver State will partner with Kindred's Care Management Division to more effectively manage the patients' experience across the entire episode of care through a population health model.

Platform for the Future

In summary, key capabilities of a successful post-acute care model are:

One: Offer the full continuum of post-acute services in local healthcare delivery markets

Two: Provide "care management" services to patients throughout an entire post-acute episode of care

Three: Test and implement "pay for value" and risk-based payment models

As policy development continues, integrated post-acute care providers are well suited to deliver desired outcomes. Developing integrated post-acute care services requires an investment in the capabilities and innovation necessary to meet the needs of patients throughout an entire episode of care. Collaboration across health systems and with payors for innovative care delivery and payment models will better serve patients with chronic conditions, including the growing dual-eligible population [Fig. 19.3].

References

1. http://www.ahrq.gov/workingforquality/nqs/nqs2011annlrpt.htm
2. Berwick DM, Nolan TW, Whittington J. The triple aim: care, health, and cost. Health Aff. 2008;27(3):759–69.
3. Gardner R, Li Q, Baier RR, Butterfield K, Coleman EA, Gravenstein S. Is implementation of the care transitions intervention associated with cost avoidance after hospital discharge? J Gen Intern Med. 2014;29(6):878–84.

4. Abelson, Reed. Health insurers are trying new payment models, study shows. The New York Times 10 July 2014: B3. Print

5. Blue Cross and Blue Shield. (2014). Blue Cross and Blue Shield Companies Direct More Than $65 Billion in Medical Spending to Value-Based Care Programs [Press release]. Accessed from http://www.bcbs.com/healthcare-news/bcbsa/bcbs-companies-direct-more-than-65b-in-medical-spending-to-value-based-care-programs.html

6. Hughes SL, Weaver FM, Giobbie-Hurder A, Manheim L, Henderson W, Kubal JD, Ulasevich A, Cummings J, Department of Veterans Affairs Cooperative Study Group on Home-Based Primary Care. Effectiveness of team-managed home-based primary care: a randomized multicenter trial. JAMA. 2000;284(22): 2877–85.

7. Graham JE, Granger CV, Karmarkar AM, Deutsch A, Niewczyk P, Divita MA, Ottenbacher KJ. The uniform data system for medical rehabilitation: report of follow-up information on patients discharged from inpatient rehabilitation programs in 2002–2010. Am J Phys Med Rehabil. 2014;93(3):231–44.

8. http://www.ipasshandoffstudy.com/

9. Stroke Recovery IRF Setting, Kindred data. www.eRehabData.com (2013).

10. De Jonge KE, Jamshed N, Gilden M, Kubisiak J, Bruce S, Taler G. Effects of home-based primary care on medicare costs in high-risk elders. J Am Geriatr Soc. 2014;62:1825. doi:10.1111/jgs.12974.

11. Wajnberg A, Wang KH, Aniff M, et al. Hospitalizations and skilled nursing facility placements before and after the implementation of a home-based primary care program. J Am Geriatr Soc. 2010;58: 1144–7.

12. http://www.zapposinsights.com/training/3-day-culture-camp

13. http://www.parksassociates.com/blog/article/chs-2014-pr4

14. Bundled Payments for Care Improvement (BPCI) Initiative: general information. Centers for Medicare and Medicaid Services. http://innovation.cms.gov/initiatives/bundled-payments/

The UCLA Dementia Care Program for Comprehensive, Coordinated, and Patient-Centered Care

David B. Reuben, Leslie Chang Evertson,
Michelle Panlilio, Jeanine Moreno, Mihae Kim,
Katherine Serrano, Lee A. Jennings, and Zaldy S. Tan

Background

In the USA, an estimated 5.2 million persons are affected by Alzheimer's disease [1]. Moreover, the total burden of dementia is even higher as Alzheimer's disease accounts for only 60–80 % of cases of dementia. The clinical manifestations of dementia are protean and devastating, including cognitive impairment, immobility and falls, swallowing disorders and aspiration pneumonia, urinary and fecal incontinence, and behavioral disturbances (e.g., agitation, aggression, depression, and hallucinations) leading to caregiver stress, burnout, and medical illnesses.

As a result, older persons with dementia have three times as many hospital stays as others their age as well as higher medical provider, nursing home, home health, and prescription drug costs. In 2014, the direct costs of caring for patients with Alzheimer's disease will total $214 billion, including $150 billion to Medicare and Medicaid [1]. In 2010, the attributable costs of dementia to Medicare, after adjusting for other diseases, were $2,752 per person and the yearly monetary cost per person that was attributable to dementia was either $42,000 or $56,000 depending on how the value of informal care is calculated [2]. Nationwide in 2013, an estimated 15 million caregivers provided 17.7 billion hours of unpaid care worth $220.2 billion [1].

D.B. Reuben, M.D. (✉)
Division of Geriatrics, David Geffen School of Medicine at UCLA,
Los Angeles, CA, USA
e-mail: dreuben@mednet.ucla.edu

L.C. Evertson, M.S.N. • M. Panlilio, M.S.N.
J. Moreno, M.S. • M. Kim, M.S.N. • K. Serrano, B.A.
L.A. Jennings, M.D, M.S.H.S. • Z.S. Tan, M.D., M.P.H.
Division of Geriatrics, UCLA, 10945 Le Conte Ave.,
Suite 2339, Los Angeles, CA 90095, USA
e-mail: levertson@mednet.ucla.edu; mpanlilio@mednet.ucla.edu;
jemoreno@mednet.ucla.edu; dementia@mednet.ucla.edu;
kserrano@mednet.ucla.edu;
ztan@mednet.ucla.edu

Setting

The UCLA Alzheimer's and Dementia Care (UCLA ADC) program provides comprehensive, coordinated, patient-centered care for patients with Alzheimer's disease and other dementias. The program primarily serves a fee-for-service Medicare population where care is provided by primary care physicians in a highly competitive market, and is based in an academic health care system and partners with community-based organizations (CBOs). Patients are seen in three sites in Santa Monica, Westwood, and Thousand Oaks, California.

Generally, the entry point into the program is referral as an outpatient although some patients are referred during hospitalizations. Once a patient has been enrolled in the program, care is provided in outpatient, inpatient, in-home, and nursing home settings.

Problem That the Model Is Addressing

Busy physicians, including geriatricians, have neither the time nor, in some cases, the skills to adequately manage many aspects of dementia, including coordinating social as well as medical care, instructing caregivers, and counseling families. As a result, the quality of care for dementia is poor compared to other diseases that affect older persons [3–5]. Community resources (e.g., the Alzheimer's Association) can help improve the quality of care, especially by providing patient education and support for caregivers [6]. However, these organizations are underutilized and are poorly integrated with the health care system.

The goals of the UCLA ADC program are to provide comprehensive, coordinated care spanning between the health care system and community to maximize patient function, independence, and dignity; minimize caregiver strain and burnout; and reduce unnecessary costs through improved care.

Key Contextual Issues

The program has been developed with several major contextual issues including:

- The need for coordinated services that are provided both in health care facilities and community-based settings
- The inadequacy of the work force including physicians who do not have the time to provide high-quality dementia care, an inadequate supply of nurse practitioners who can fill the roles of Dementia Care Managers, and a largely untrained work force of formal (paid) and informal (unpaid) caregivers
- The lack of funding stream for non-face-to-face services to traditional Medicare Fee-For-Service payment structures
- The absence of case management software in most electronic health records

Which Patients Will Be Best Served by the Intervention? Are There Patients Who Should Be Excluded from This Model?

Patients with all stages of dementia who are living in the community may benefit from the program. Those who have early dementia may benefit from receiving education about the disease and being able to participate in advance care planning and mobilizing resources for their inevitable decline. Caregivers of patients at all stages of dementia can benefit from learning to better navigate the health care system, access community-based resources, manage behavioral and psychological complications with behavioral approaches, and receive caregiver support and respite. Persons who are already institutionalized in nursing homes are less likely to benefit because many of the interventions are based in the community and aimed at keeping people with dementia in their homes as long as possible.

Model Overview

Key Components

The UCLA Alzheimer's and Dementia Care (UCLA ADC) program consists of six key components:
- Patient recruitment and a dementia registry
- Structured needs assessments of patients in the registry and their caregivers
- Creation and implementation of individualized dementia care plans based on needs assessments
- Monitoring and revising care plans, as needed

- Facilitating transitions in care
- Access 24/7, 365 days a year for assistance and advice [7]

A description of each of these components and a summary of progress since the program began are described below.

Recruitment of Patients to the Program and UCLA Dementia Registry

Generally, the entry point into the program is referral as an outpatient. Patients who are already living in nursing homes are not eligible for the program because the anticipated benefit would be less. The program has two other requirements for eligibility. First, patients must have a diagnosis of dementia and second, they must have been referred by a UCLA physician. The latter requirement is because the program does not assume primary care. Rather, it is co-management program with a dementia care manager and the partnering physician.

Patients were originally recruited into the program through two methods: (1) referrals from the UCLA primary care and geriatrics practices, the psychiatry and neurology Memory and Dementia clinics, or direct inquiries from patients or families, and (2) identification of potential participants by billing codes (ICD-9 diagnosis codes 290.0, 290.1, 290.2, 290.3, 290.4, and 331.0). With the switch to an EPIC-based electronic health record, billing codes have been replaced by electronic health record problem lists, both for inpatients and outpatients, to identify potential participants for the program. Additionally, to promote recruitment, the program has made presentations to practice groups, approximately twice a month to generate referrals and increase awareness about the program.

Conduct Structured Caregiver/Care-Recipient Needs Assessments of Patients in the Registry

The UCLA ADC begins with an in-person visit with the dementia care manager (DCM) including the patient and at least one family member or caregiver. To prepare for the visit and make it most efficient, patients (if early stage) and/or family/caregivers are asked to complete a structured pre-visit instrument that includes medical, functional, and psychosocial information about the patient and the caregivers.

The assessment is scheduled as a 90-min in-person session during which additional information is obtained through semi-structured interview and examination. In this manner, the DCM assesses the patient and family's needs as well as the resources, human and financial, available to meet these needs. The assessment can be supplemented by phone calls and follow-up assessments if more information is needed. At the end of the visit, the patient and family/caregiver are given a binder with information about the program, patient information (e.g., medication lists and advance directives) and specific information about referrals to community-based organizations, and, if needed, management of behavioral symptoms.

Develop and Implement Individualized Dementia Care Plans Based on Needs Assessments

Based on these initial assessments, the DCM (often with input from a physician dementia specialist) works with the patient and family to create a draft personal care plan, which is sent to the referring physician for approval or modification. This interaction with the physician is aimed at ensuring continuity of care and also providing education about the care of the patient with dementia. To be efficient and succinct, the care plan is transmitted through the physicians in-basket in the electronic record and is divided into medical recommendations that referring physician is asked to respond to and social and behavioral recommendations that the DCM implements independently. When the DCM has received a response from the referring physician, the assessment note is finalized and uploaded to the electronic health record. The patient/family then receives a phone call from their DCM to discuss the final recommendations and receives a written copy of the care plan.

All patients and their families receive dementia care management by a nurse practitioner supervised by a physician dementia specialist, which may include:

- In-person sessions at which patient and family members' specific questions about problems, resources, and implementing care plans are answered
- Telephone follow-up to monitor implementation of dementia care plans
- Facilitation of appointments with consultants when the treatment plan needs to be reassessed (e.g., new behavioral complications)
- Teaching dementia management skills to caregivers through individual counseling including information on legal and financial planning with referral to community services, behavioral techniques to avoid/manage behavioral problems, and coping strategies for caregivers.

Because patients enrolled in the UCLA ADC program vary in terms of stages of evaluation, severity of dementia, and nature and extent of resources and needs, the other components of the care plan are tailored to the individual and can include:

- *Consultation with neurology, geriatric psychiatry, psychology, or geriatrics*. When needed, patients are referred for additional diagnostic evaluation, discussion of treatment options, and planning appropriate follow-up.
- *Support groups at UCLA hospitals, the Patti Davis "Beyond Alzheimer's" support program*. These are held twice weekly at no cost and are co-led by former President Reagan's daughter and a psychologist.

- *Caregiver education through a community lecture series*. Lectures are held monthly, initially in person and now by webinar, and include topics such as "What is Dementia," "Communicating with Dementia Patients," Resources for Families," and Medical Management of Memory and Psychiatric Problems in Dementia." Caregivers can also access archived lectures through the program's website http://dementia.uclahealth.org/.
- *Hospitalization, when needed, on the Santa Monica-UCLA Geriatrics Special Care Unit or Geriatric Psychiatry Unit at the Neuropsychiatric Hospital*. The Santa Monica-UCLA Geriatrics Special Care Unit is multidisciplinary and patient centered with services aimed at the frail elderly, including those with dementia. Patients with dementia with severe behavioral problems (e.g., aggression and psychosis or profound mood disorders) are referred for admission to the dementia unit on the Geriatric Psychiatry floor at the Neuropsychiatric Hospital, which is multidisciplinary and focuses on a therapeutic milieu as well as expert geriatric psychiatry and geriatric medicine care.
- *Referral to the Mary S. Easton Alzheimer's Disease Research Center (ADRC) at UCLA for appropriate clinical trials*. Through its ADRC, UCLA has access to investigational treatments that are commercially unavailable.
- *Referral, when appropriate, to the California Southland chapter of the Alzheimer's Association or other community-based organizations* (Jewish Family Services, Leeza's Place, Optimistic People In a Caring Atmosphere [OPICA] Adult Day Care & Caregiver Support Center, Wise & Healthy Aging, and other community-based organizations). When appropriate, patients are referred to community-based organizations for services such as support groups with or without respite care, caregiver referrals, delivered meals, adult day care, care/case management, counseling, and transportation assistance. A key function of the CBOs is to provide caregiver training through evidence-based programs such as the Savvy Caregiver [8, 9], and Powerful Tools for Caregivers [10]. As part of the program, these CBOs have established formal relationships with UCLA. Referrals are made at the time of the assessment or at any time they are needed. The CBOs are notified that the referral has been made by e-mail or telephone. If the patient/family has signed a HIPPA release, a copy of part or all of the care plan is often e-mailed to the contacts at the CBOs.

Monitoring and Revising Care Plans

Patients in the program receive active monitoring and support of the caregiver's emotional and physical health. Patient acuity has been indicated by red, yellow, or green alert indicators and criteria for determining the acuity and transitioning to new levels of acuity have been determined (Table 20.1).

All patients are called at a minimum frequency of every 3 months and seen at a minimum of yearly. More frequent

Table 20.1 Criteria for acuity status and levels of intensity

	Criteria	Level of intensity
Green	• No acute crisis • No behavioral issues • No medication compliance issues • Low NPI-Q, MCSI, PHQ9 scores • No serious social or medical issues	• Patient and caregiver contact 2 weeks after initial visit, by phone or e-mail. Discuss dementia care plan, recommended services, and community-based organizations. • Regular check-in with patient and caregiver 3 months thereafter, by phone.
Yellow	• Mild to moderate caregiver stress (stabilizing) • Recently controlled behavioral issues • Hospitalizations in the past 3 months	• Patient and caregiver contact 2 weeks after initial visit, by phone or e-mail. Discuss medication changes, hospitalizations, and ED visits. • Patient and caregiver contact every 1–2 months by phone or e-mail until patient is "green."
Red	• Caregiver is extremely stressed • ED/hospitalizations in the last 30 days • Active psychosis • Adult protective service referral • Safety concerns • Medication recommendation that was acted upon	• Patient and caregiver contact 2 weeks after initial visit, by phone or e-mail. Check-in with caregiver about their stress level. Discuss any hospitalizations, ED visits, medication changes, or referrals. • Patient and caregiver contact every 2 weeks until stabilized and "yellow."

NPI-Q neuropsychiatric index questionnaire, *MCSI* modified caregiver strain index, *PHQ-9* patient health questionnaire-9 item

contacts are determined by the initial care plans and revisions needed as a result of progression of disease, the emergence of complications, acute exacerbation of comorbid conditions resulting in hospitalizations, and caregiver distress. Throughout the program, the electronic health record (CareConnect) is the primary method of communication with primary physicians. The DCMs enter their notes into CareConnect using program-developed templates for the initial and follow-up electronic medical record notes.

Facilitating Transitions in Care

When patients in the program are hospitalized, the DCMs make a visit with the patient/caregivers in the hospital and connect with the inpatient team. Within 3 days after hospital discharge, patients and/or their caregiver are contacted by the DCM. During this contact, the DCM:

– Reviews d/c summary and discharge meds with caregivers and answers any questions.
– Identifies any needs (e.g., additional help at home) and helps arrange for these.
– Ensures timely follow-up appointment with the primary care physician and/or specialists.
– Identifies barriers (e.g., transportation) for their follow-up appointment.
– Refers to social workers and care coordinators as needed.
– Writes telephone note on EPIC and copies the partnering physician.

Access 24/7, 365 Days a Year for Assistance and Advice

By providing full-time access, pressing questions can be answered in real time and crises can be managed to avoid unnecessary emergency department (ED) utilization and hospitalization. Daytime calls come into a dedicated phone

number with triage to the DCM, when indicated, and nights and weekend calls are managed by UCLA geriatricians who are skilled in management of dementia.

Training

To date, all nurse practitioners recruited to the program have had specific gerontologic training or expertise. Specific training for the program includes an apprenticeship period with existing dementia care managers, review of printed materials, and observed performance of assessments. In addition, during the training period, all cases are presented to the geriatrician Medical Director.

Fidelity

Fidelity to the model is maintained through several mechanisms including weekly case discussion meetings of all DCMs with the Medical Director as well as periodic "summits" to establish protocols and rules. In addition, weekly meetings with the Program Director, Medical Director, all DCMs, and support staff are held to ensure that protocols are being followed. Finally, the Dementia Care Management Software allows the performance of DCMs to be monitored and compared.

Barriers to Implementation

The major barriers to implementation have been recruiting and credentialing nurse practitioners to become DCMs, establishing relations with CBOs to ensure that appropriate services are provided, and developing software that can serve several functions including case management, data collection, and communication with CBOs. Moreover this software needs to be compatible with the electronic health record to receive data that are needed to monitor the program's progress in meeting its objectives.

Role of Interdisciplinary Team Members

The linchpin of the program is the nurse practitioner DCM. However, a variety of other health professions are involved in the program including primary care physicians, psychologists who lead support groups, and social workers to whom the program refers.

Geriatrician's Roles

The geriatricians' roles have included serving as primary care physicians for many patients referred to the program, Medical Director of the program, and overall Program Director. In addition, geriatricians assist the program by performing evaluations on patients who have complaints of memory impairment whose primary care physician would like assistance with evaluation for dementia. A geriatrician evaluates these patients to determine whether they are appropriate for entry into the program.

Outcomes to Be Monitored

The program is evaluating outcomes that reflect the Center for Medicare and Medicaid Services (CMS) triple aim of better care for individuals, better health for populations, and lower costs [11]; the program will need to be evaluated on each of these components (Table 20.2).

Evidence That the Model Will Improve Outcomes

At this point, data from the UCLA program are still preliminary. However, some insights into the program's effectiveness can be drawn from the Indiana University Wishard Health System Aging Brain Center, which many of the components of the UCLA program are modeled after and which uses a dementia care manager to tailor and facilitate delivery of non-pharmacological and pharmacological care process components to individual patients in collaboration with the primary care physician. That program implemted in a safety net population has demonstrated effectiveness on quality measures and patient outcomes (reduced behavioral symptoms and caregiver stress by half at 12 months)

[12, 13]. Moreover, there is some evidence that the Indiana program may be cost saving as a result of reducing ED visits, inpatient hospitalizations, and 30-day readmission by almost half [14].

Buy-In from Health System Leaders and Business Plan

To obtain buy-in from health system leaders and other academic departments, a series of meetings was held with the Medical Center CEO and leaders of all the clinical and research programs that focused on Alzheimer's disease and other forms of dementia. A Steering Committee and seven working groups (Assessment, Outcomes, Communication, Community-based Organizations [CBOs], Software, Media and Marketing, and Development) were established to implement the program.

The program serves 1,000 patients and their families enrolled over 2½ years. To meet this need, the program employs four full-time DCMs, a Medical Director initially at 0.25 and then at 0.5 FTE, and a program manager initially at 0.5 and then at 1.0 FTE. All of the clinical support services (e.g., scheduling, encountering, and billing) are built into the overhead of the Department of Medicine Practice Group. The Health System has provided support for media and marketing services, a part-time development officer, and funding for one of the support group leaders.

The optimal caseload for the DCMs is still being determined. Although the original intent was 250 patients, the work load does not appear to be sustainable at this level with the original care processes. Accordingly, we have added a bachelor's level dementia care manager assistant to help with tasks such as:

- Maintaining contact with patient families and scheduling telephone or in-person appointments with the dementia care managers, as appropriate
- Documenting under the supervision of the dementia care managers in the electronic medical record
- Identifying families in crisis and following protocols to ensure that their needs are met

The current financial model to support the program relies on three sources of income. First, the DCM generates clinical income from in-person visits including initial assessments. All other components of the program are provided free of charge. Second, a Centers for Medicare & Medicaid Services Healthcare Innovations Challenge Award has supported expansion of the program to the intended 1,000 patients within approximately 2 years, a more rapid expansion than originally planned. Third, the program has been successful in obtaining philanthropic support. Patients' families have recognized the gaps in current care for dementia and have been generous in making contributions ranging from $10 to over $1 million.

Table 20.2 Assessment domains, instruments, and timing

Outcome domain and measure	Instrument	Data collection	Baseline	Month 6	Month 12	Month 18	Month 24	Month 30
Better care								
Process of care[a]	ACOVE and PCPI quality indicators for dementia	Medical records	First 3 months		X			
		Dementia care software			X		X	
Caregiver rating of care[a]	Caregiver survey	Pre-visit questionnaire	X		X		X	
Better health								
Neuropsychiatric complications[a]	NPI-Q, patient and caregiver	Pre-visit questionnaire	X		X		X	
Function	Functional assessment quest and ADL and IADL scales	Pre-visit questionnaire	X		X		X	
Depression	Cornell depression scale	During visit	X		X		X	
(Cognition)	MMSE	During visit	X		X		X	
Caregiver burnout[a]	MCSI	During exam	X		X		X	
Caregiver depression[a]	PHQ-9	During exam	X		X		X	
Caregiver self-efficacy[a]	Caregiver survey	Pre-visit questionnaire	X		X		X	
Less utilization								
Institutionalization[a]	–	Care manager database, CMS, MG			X		X	X
(Mortality)	–	Care manager database, CMS, MG			X		X	X
Emergency department use[a]	–	Care manager database, CMS, MG			X		X	X
Hospital use[a]	–	Care manager database, CMS, MG			X		X	X
Nursing home use[a]	–	Care manager database, CMS, MG			X		X	X
Overall utilization	–	CMS						X
Informal caregiver effort[a]	–	Pre-visit questionnaire	X		X		X	
Quality of dementia program								
Caregiver rating of care	Caregiver assessment	4 weeks after visit	X		X		X	
Primary care physician care rating	Physician assessment	4 weeks after visit	X		X		X	

NPI-Q neuropsychiatric index questionnaire, *MCSI* modified caregiver strain index, *PHQ-9* patient health questionnaire-9 item, *ACOVE* assessing care of vulnerable elders, *PCPI* physician consortium for performance improvement, *(Domain)* measured but not an outcome, *CMS* Centers for Medicare & Medicaid Services, *MG* medical group data for managed patient population

[a]Primary outcome

Without grant support and philanthropy, the program would not be sustainable under fee-for-service Medicare funding. Under managed care reimbursement, the program could be directly supported as a member benefit. If the return on investment is high (e.g., cost savings based on reduced hospitalization and emergency department use), the program could potentially be supported through a start-up case management fee, which could be paid to accountable care organizations with continuation of payment dependent on shared savings to Medicare that offsets the payment, or through a redesign of the Medicare benefit. Another possibility would be to directly charge patients for the service, which would amount to approximately $1,400 per year per patient, less than $4 per day.

Older Adult Patient/Family Caregiver Involvement

Since the inception of the program, we have had a variety of stakeholders, including patients and families and community-based organizations, involved in the planning and implementation of the program including serving on the Steering Committee.

Bringing the Model to Scale

To support this program, precise protocols, educational materials, and stand-alone dementia case management software were developed. The software system allows each DCM to view a calendar (synchronized with their Outlook calendars) and linkages to patient's task lists (e.g., follow-up phone calls, annual reevaluations) with respect to the UCLA ADC. In addition, a novel voucher system was developed to reimburse community-based organizations for services provided.

Integration into the Electronic Medical Record

Early on, the UCLA ADC program worked with the leadership implementing EPIC as the electronic health record for UCLA. It was determined that case management functions were not available in EPIC and that many data elements that were collected outside of EPIC could not be imported. Hence, the decision was made to build stand-alone software that would be compatible with EPIC and other electronic health records but only receives data and does not enter information directly into the electronic medical record. Instead, the DCMs use templates to document their assessment notes as well as other features such as telephone follow-ups. The dementia care software also has a portal to permit easy back-and-forth communication with community-based organizations.

Future Planning

Although the rapid expansion of the program was facilitated by a component of the Affordable Care Act (i.e., a Center for Medicare and Medicaid Services Innovations Challenge Award) and CMS has the authority to implement successful programs under this initiative without congressional legislation, the most likely effect of the ACA on implementation would be the uptake by accountable care organizations.

Medicare Fee-for-Service Payment for the Program

Because the majority of the program's services are not face to face, they are not reimbursable under traditional fee-for-service Medicare. Moreover, the new Care Coordination code requires coordination of care for all chronic conditions rather than for a specific disease.

Conclusion

The UCLA Alzheimer's and Dementia Care program has been designed to help every patient with this disease maintain independence and functioning to the highest degree possible and maintain dignity always. The program has been successfully implemented in a competitive, predominantly fee-for-service Medicare population. If it succeeds in its goal of providing improved quality of care and better health for patients and caregivers, the program has the potential to become a national model for comprehensive dementia care.

References

1. http://www.alz.org/alzheimers_disease_facts_and_figures.asp. Accessed 31 Aug 2014.
2. Hurd MD, et al. Monetary costs of dementia in the United States. N Engl J Med. 2013;368:1326–34. doi:10.1056/NEJMsa1204629.
3. Chodosh J, Mittman BS, Connor KI, Vassar SD, Lee ML, DeMonte RW, Ganiats TG, Heikoff LE, Rubenstein LZ, Della Penna RD, Vickrey BG. Caring for patients with dementia: how good is the quality of care? Results from three health systems. J Am Geriatr Soc. 2007;55(8):1260–8.
4. Belmin J, Min L, Roth C, Reuben D, Wenger N. Assessment and management of patients with cognitive impairment and dementia in primary care. J Nutr Health Aging. 2012;16:462–7.
5. Wenger NS, Solomon DH, Roth CP, MacLean CH, Saliba D, Kamberg CJ, Rubenstein LZ, Young RT, Sloss EM, Louie R, Adams J, Chang JT, Venus PJ, Schnelle JF, Shekelle PG. The quality of medical care provided to vulnerable community-dwelling older patients. Ann Intern Med. 2003;139(9):740–7.
6. Reuben DB, Roth CP, Frank JC, Hirsch SH, Katz D, McCreath H, Younger J, Murawski M, Edgerly E, Maher J, Maslow K, Wenger NS. Assessing care of vulnerable elders–Alzheimer's disease: a pilot study of a practice redesign intervention to improve the quality of dementia care. J Am Geriatr Soc. 2010;58(2):324–9. Epub 2010 Jan 26. Erratum in: J Am Geriatr Soc. 2010;58(8):1623.
7. Reuben DB, Evertson LC, et al. The University of California at Los Angeles Alzheimer's and dementia care program for comprehensive, coordinated, patient-centered care: preliminary data. J Am Geriatr Soc. 2013;61:2214–8.
8. Ostwald SK, Hepburn KW, Caron W, Burns T, Mantell R. Reducing caregiver burden: a randomized psychoeducational intervention for caregivers of persons with dementia. Gerontologist. 1999;39(3):299–309.
9. Ostwald SK, Hepburn KW, Burns T. Training family caregivers of patients with dementia: a structured workshop approach. J Gerontol Nurs. 2003;29(1):37–44.

10. Savundranayagam MY, Montgomery RJ, Kosloski K, Little TD. Impact of a psychoeducational program on three types of caregiver burden among spouses. Int J Geriatr Psychiatry. 2011;26(4):388–96. doi:10.1002/gps.2538. PubMed.

11. Berwick DM, Nolan TW, Whittington J, Aim T. The care, health, and cost. Health Affairs. 2008;27(3):759–69.

12. Callahan CM, Boustani MA, Weiner M, Beck RA, Livin LR, Kellams JJ, Willis DR, Hendrie HC. Implementing dementia care models in primary care settings: the aging brain care medical home. Aging Ment Health. 2011;15(1):5–12. PubMed PMID:20945236, PubMed Central PMCID: PMC3030631.

13. Callahan CM, Boustani MA, Unverzagt FW, Austrom MG, Damush TM, Perkins AJ, Fultz BA, Hui SL, Counsell SR, Hendrie HC. Effectiveness of collaborative care for older adults with Alzheimer disease in primary care: a randomized controlled trial. JAMA. 2006;295(18):2148–57.

14. Boustani MA, Sachs GA, Alder CA, Munger S, Schubert CC, Guerriero Austrom M, Hake AM, Unverzagt FW, Farlow M, Matthews BR, Perkins AJ, Beck RA, Callahan CM. Implementing innovative models of dementia care: The Healthy Aging Brain Center. Aging Ment Health. 2011;15(1):13–22. PubMed PMID: 21271387, PubMed Central PMCID: PMC3077086.

The Indiana Aging Brain Care Project

Catherine A. Alder, Michael A. LaMantia,
Mary Guerriero Austrom, and Malaz A. Boustani

Background

Over the last two decades, scientists from the Indiana Center for Aging Research (IUCAR) have led or participated in two randomized clinical trials testing comprehensive care models for older adults suffering from dementia and depression. Both studies were conducted in a primary care practice within Eskenazi Health (Eskenazi) [formerly Wishard Health Services], an urban safety net hospital system primarily serving a racially and ethnically diverse population of vulnerable adults [1, 2]. The findings from these two trials provided the justification and the foundation for the Indiana Aging Brain Care Project.

The IMPACT study demonstrated the effectiveness of the collaborative care model in reducing symptoms of depression and improving physical function and health-related quality of life [1]. The key component of the intervention was a care coordinator who worked with the patient's primary care provider to deliver an individualized care plan including antidepressant medications and problem-solving therapy within the primary care setting [1]. Building on the success of the IMPACT intervention, IUCAR scientists designed the PREVENT intervention to improve the treatment of dementia in primary care [2]. Similar to the IMPACT model, a care coordinator assumed a central role in the

PREVENT intervention, serving as a liaison connecting the patient and caregiver to the primary care provider, a panel of geriatric and psychiatric expert consultants, and resources in the community. Results of the PREVENT study demonstrated the effectiveness of the model in reducing the behavioral and psychological symptoms of dementia for both the patient and the informal caregiver.

While both models showed improved health outcomes and quality of care, they have not been widely implemented, primarily because the translation of research-based models into cost-effective clinical programs requires substantial additional resources and expertise in the implementation process. In collaboration with community partners, IUCAR scientists have developed this expertise and applied it locally in the implementation efforts of the Aging Brain Care Project (ABC Project). Now in its eighth year, the ABC Project has produced two distinct yet integrated aging brain care programs and represents the successful implementation of research results into real-world clinical practice. This chapter describes the development, organization, and operations of both programs, identifies lessons learned to date and discusses plans for sustainability of the project.

The Healthy Aging Brain Center

The ABC Project began in late 2007 when IUCAR scientists first undertook the challenge of translating the PREVENT model of dementia care into a real-world memory care clinic at Eskenazi [3]. The development of the memory clinic was previously described in detail [3] and the following pages summarize the history, key components, and operations of the Healthy Aging Brain Center (HABC), the first clinical program of the project. The first step in this process was to assemble a team of experts representing each of the disciplines providing dementia care at Eskenazi. The implementation team included a primary care physician, three geriatricians, a nurse provider, a social worker, two neuropsychologists, a social psychologist, a

C.A. Alder, J.D., M.S.W. (✉)
Eskenazi Health, 720 Eskenazi Avenue, Indianapolis,
IN 46202, USA
e-mail: catherine.alder@eskenazihealth.edu

M.A. LaMantia, M.D., M.P.H. • M.A. Boustani, M.D., M.P.H.
Indiana University Center for Aging Research and Regenstrief
Institute, 410 West 10th Street, Suite 2000, Indianapolis,
IN 46202, USA
e-mail: malamant@iu.edu; mboustan@iu.edu

M.G. Austrom, Ph.D.
Department of Psychiatry, Indiana University School of Medicine,
Goodman Hall Neuroscience Center, 355 W. 16th Street,
Suite 2800, Indianapolis, IN 46202, USA
e-mail: mguerrie@iupui.edu

clinic administrator, and a representative from the local Alzheimer's Association. Utilizing the principles of complex adaptive theory and the reflective adaptive process, the team began meeting biweekly with the goal of adapting the PREVENT model to the unique needs of clinical care at Eskenazi while maintaining the critical components of the study intervention. Within 4 months, the implementation team delivered the minimum specifications for the HABC and on January 7, 2008, the innovative new clinic opened its doors and began serving patients [3].

As previously described, the HABC program comprises two multicomponent phases—the *initial assessment phase* and the *follow-up phase*. In each phase, care is delivered by a multidisciplinary team that includes a physician, two care coordinators [a registered nurse (RN) and a social worker], a medical assistant, and a research assistant with specialized training in the administration of neuropsychological testing [3].

The HABC intervention is designed to support the primary care clinician in the specialized diagnosis and management of cognitive impairment by delivering individualized care aimed at improving the knowledge, dementia management skills, and coping behavior of both the patient and the informal caregiver. The goal of the program is to improve health care outcomes by providing a state-of-the-art diagnostic evaluation and personalized management beginning with the patient's diagnosis and continuing throughout the course of the disease. All patients aged 55 years and older are eligible for referral to the HABC. Referrals may be initiated by primary care providers, specialty providers, informal caregivers, and even patients themselves [3].

Initial Assessment Phase

Before the patient's first appointment, the care coordinator conducts a structured, comprehensive needs assessment during a telephone interview with the patient's caregiver. This interview includes an assessment of the patient's symptoms and functional status and a brief medical and social history. During the first clinic visit, the HABC physician performs a complete diagnostic evaluation including a medical assessment, a structured physical and neurological examination, and blood work and brain imaging as needed. Effort is directed to identifying reversible causes of dementia as well as factors that might be contributing to cognitive impairment. In addition, the research assistant administers a battery of neuropsychological tests to the patient. After all test results are returned, the HABC physician makes the memory diagnosis and the team develops an individualized care plan taking into account the diagnosis and the specific needs of both the patient and the caregiver. The physician and the care coordinators then meet face to face with the patient and

family during a second visit to the clinic (family conference visit) to disclose the diagnosis, answer any questions, and initiate the plan of care [3].

Follow-Up Phase

The frequency of follow-up appointments in the HABC varies based on the diagnosis, the care plan, and the emergent needs of the patient and caregiver. Follow-up visits may be scheduled anywhere from once a month to once a year. Patients and caregivers are encouraged to initiate telephone contact with the team in between visits whenever they need information or assistance. During all follow-up contacts, the HABC team assesses for cognitive, functional, behavioral, and psychological symptoms of the patient and caregiver stress. The team may modify the care plan at any time with a goal of reducing, managing, and preventing these symptoms in the future [3].

Although the content of the care plan varies from patient to patient, the seven main components are described below:
1. *Patient and Caregiver Education, Self-Management, and Support.* The HABC program uses standardized educational materials, self-management strategies, and supportive services to help manage, reduce, and prevent problematic symptoms and the physical and psychological burden on the caregiver. This component of the program begins during the initial assessment phase but is provided continuously throughout the course of the disease. Prior to the family conference visit, a care coordinator prepares a package of informational materials tailored to meet the needs of the patient and family. These materials are presented as a guidebook to help the family navigate through the disease process and may include information about the patient's diagnosis, specific behavioral techniques to help manage the patient's problem behaviors [4], coping strategies to maintain the physical and emotional health of the caregiver, and dementia care resources in the community. The guidebook is reviewed with the family during the family conference visit. Following the family conference, the HABC team continues to provide information and support during subsequent clinic visits and by telephone consultation in between appointments. The guidebook may be revised or augmented at any time as necessary to address the family's evolving needs for information and disease management strategies. In addition, caregivers are encouraged to participate in a monthly support group and to utilize the other resources available through the local chapter of the Alzheimer's Association. Finally, the HABC physician and the primary care physician may jointly decide to refer more complex patients for specialty evaluation and comanagement.

2. *Periodic Needs Assessment and Evaluation of Care Plan.* The HABC team uses the caregiver and self-report versions of the HABC Monitor to continuously assess the cognitive, functional, behavioral, and psychological symptoms of patients and the caregiver stress. The monitor is administered during the initial assessment and during each clinic visit throughout the follow-up phase. It may also be administered during telephone contact. The HABC Monitor contains 31 items to measure change over time and to identify specific care areas (including dangerous behaviors) where behavior management techniques or coping strategies may be utilized [5]. Once these care areas are identified, the HABC team works with the primary care physician (and other providers) to initiate a plan to minimize and manage the patient's symptoms and caregiver stress. This may also require the team to work with the caregiver's primary care physician. HABC protocols emphasize non-pharmacologic interventions at the outset followed by pharmacologic treatment where appropriate.

3. *Prevention and Treatment of Comorbid Conditions in the Context of Dementia Management.* The HABC team uses the pre-visit structured needs assessment in conjunction with information collected during the clinic visits to identify depression, delirium, and psychosis superimposed on the underlying diagnosis of cognitive impairment. The HABC team uses the Patient Health Questionnaire (PHQ-9) to continuously assess the patient's symptoms of depression throughout the follow-up phase of care. The HABC standardized non-pharmacological interventions are utilized to manage the symptoms of these comorbid syndromes and the resulting caregiver burden. In addition, the HABC physician may initiate pharmacological interventions including stopping or reducing dosages of psychotropic or anticholinergic medications.

4. *Medication Management.* Using the Anticholinergic Cognitive Burden Scale developed by the scientists at IUCAR [6, 7], the HABC physician works with the primary care physician to balance the benefits and harms of both over-the-counter and prescribed medications taken by the patient with a specific focus on medications with definite anticholinergic properties. In addition, the HABC physician consults with the patient and family about the indications and expected benefits of using FDA-approved medications for Alzheimer's disease and related disorders and prescribes these medications when indicated.

5. *Managing Vascular Risk Factors.* The HABC physician works with the primary care physician to identify vascular risk factors such as hypertension, hyperlipidemia, and diabetes and utilizes both pharmacological and non-pharmacological interventions to manage and reduce the vascular burden.

6. *Identification and Management of Excess Disability Due to Comorbid Medical Conditions.* Most patients seen in the HABC are complex patients with multiple comorbid chronic conditions. Effective management of these conditions typically requires adherence to complex medication regimens and self-management strategies as well as regular follow-up. Cognitive impairment interferes with the patient's ability to follow these recommendations. The HABC team works with the primary care physician to simplify the medical regimen, to assist the patient and caregiver with self-management, and to insure consistent monitoring of these conditions. It is not the intention or goal of the HABC team to "take over" the primary care of the patient, but rather to provide additional support to the primary care physician in caring for cognitively impaired patients and their caregivers.

7. *Coordination of Care Among Care Providers Within the Health Care System and the Community.* A major responsibility of the care coordinator is to serve as the liaison connecting the patient and caregiver to all of the health care providers and community agencies involved in their care. This facilitator role is critical to the effective management of the patient's symptoms and caregiver stress [3].

Within the first year of operation, the HABC successfully implemented the content of the PREVENT collaborative care model and demonstrated a positive effect on the quality of dementia care within Eskenazi. Yet despite the early success, the impact of the program was limited as a result of several factors:

- First, the clinical setting limited the number of patients that could be served not only because of the limited capacity of the clinic, but also because of the need for patients and caregivers to present at the clinic [8]. Despite referral from primary care, many patients failed their initial visit. Other patients completed the initial assessment phase but did not reliably return for follow-up visits. Reasons for failed visits include transportation problems, complex social situations, concern about the stigma of being labeled with dementia, and a general distrust of health providers and the health care system.

- Second, although collaboration with the primary care provider is a fundamental component of the HABC model, the integration of the HABC specialized services within the primary care system was incomplete [8]. The physical location of the HABC outside of primary care was a barrier not only to patient access but also to communication and collaboration with primary care physicians.

- Third, an analysis of first-year data revealed that depression was a comorbid condition for 55 % of the HABC patients [3]. Effective management of both depression and memory impairment requires attention to both conditions because either one could be the cause of the patient's symptoms. While the person-centered approach of the HABC model includes treatment of depression, limited time and resources often resulted in referral of patients with a primary diagnosis of depression to psychiatry.

In 2009, as a first step in addressing the limitations of the HABC, Eskenazi assembled a new implementation team with a goal of expanding the HABC model beyond the clinical setting and developing a new collaborative care program for both late-life depression and dementia, fully integrated within primary care. The implementation team responded by delivering the minimum specifications for the Aging Brain Care (ABC) Medical Home (ABC Med Home), the second clinical program of the project. The development of the original ABC Med Home model was previously described in detail [9] and the following pages summarize the conceptual framework of the program.

The Aging Brain Care Medical Home

In December of 2009, the ABC Med Home was implemented as a small pilot within Eskenazi. Patients were enrolled in the pilot program following an acute care event resulting in a hospitalization. Initially, a geriatric nurse practitioner served as the care coordinator for the program and the sole clinical provider; the nurse practitioner was supported by a physician medical director with specialized training in the care of older adults with dementia and depression. In October of 2011, after approximately 300 patients were enrolled in the program, a social worker care coordinator was added to the care team. While the core components for delivery of dementia care were borrowed from the HABC [9], the new model included several additional components:

1. The ABC Med Home targeted depression as well as dementia patients and the care coordinators were trained in the IMPACT model of depression care.
2. The ABC Med Home utilized the concept of a "mobile office" to deliver care beyond the traditional clinical setting. The mobile office allowed the ABC care coordinators to spend time in the primary care offices and to develop relationships with the primary care physicians as well as the clinical and administrative staff. In time, the ABC care coordinators were accepted as comanagers of the patients and recognized as members of the primary care team. The mobile office also allowed the ABC care coordinators to take into account the physical, emotional, and psychological comfort of patients and caregivers when scheduling appointments. Mobile office sites included the patient's or caregiver's home, any of the primary care or specialty clinics, the hospital or ER, and a variety of locations within the community [9].
3. Each member of the ABC Med Home team was supported by a variety of information technology tools

including a cell phone, laptop computer with wireless access to the Internet, and the eMR-ABC, a Web-based electronic tracking system designed to facilitate care coordination [9]. The eMR-ABC created a registry of all patients enrolled in the program, tracked visits, monitored the current symptoms of the patients and informal caregivers, and recommended individualized care protocols based on current symptoms [10].

The pilot program successfully eliminated the need for patients and caregivers to come into the clinic, fully integrated the intervention within primary care, and expanded the model to include standardized, evidence-based depression care; however, the program was not yet scalable.

In 2012, the ABC Med Home was chosen to receive a Health Care Innovation Challenge Award from the Centers for Medicare & Medicaid Services (CMMI). With the support of CMMI funding, the ABC Med Home was successfully expanded to serve more than 1,500 patients across the entire system of community health centers at Eskenazi and was simultaneously converted to a scalable population health management program [8]. We have previously described the structure, preliminary results, and lessons learned from the CMMI project [8] and the following pages summarize the growth and operations of the "new" ABC Med Home developed with the support of the CMMI award.

A key component of the expansion was the development of a new type of care worker—the care coordinator assistant (CCA). The CCA serves as liaison between the patient and family caregiver in the home and the collaborative care team. The CCAs have at least a high school degree and were trained in the job-specific competencies necessary for the care of older adults with dementia and depression [8, 11]. The structure of the CCA position relies heavily on the concept of "task shifting." Tasks that require less training and expertise are provided by less expensive members of the care team under the close supervision of the clinical professionals. The CCAs are responsible to assist the care coordinators in scheduling and performing patient and caregiver visits, administering the bio-psychosocial needs assessment, delivering care protocols, monitoring medication adherence, and managing data entry [8, 11].

CCAs were hired utilizing an innovative interviewing and recruitment process designed to quickly identify individuals with the qualities and skills necessary to be successful in the new position. Applications were reviewed by Eskenazi Health Human Resources to identify those who met the basic requirements for employment. A subset of those candidates were invited to participate in preliminary screens that included assessments of experience with and attitudes toward the elderly along with the traditional Eskenazi team and skill-focused questions. Selected candidates were then invited to participate in a six-station Multiple Mini Interview (MMI) process developed to simulate challenging scenarios likely to be encountered in real home visits. Actors trained to play the roles of older adults and their caregivers interacted with the candidates while interviewers observed and evaluated the interaction. Immediately following the process, interviewers met together to discuss, rank candidates, and identify those candidates to whom an offer of employment would be made [11].

Successfully hired CCAs received an intensive 10-day training program to prepare them to deliver the intervention within a multidisciplinary care team. The training included:

- Interactive sessions with imbedded didactic lectures covering a variety of dementia care topics, video sessions, role playing, reflective reading and writing, and team building
- Clinical immersion—shadowing HABC clinic visits and home visits and preliminary training on the eMR-ABC
- Two half days of simulation training with standardized patients in the Medical Education Simulation Center

In addition, all CCAs have received training in the IMPACT model of depression care [1] and specialized palliative care training preparing them to discuss and assist with advanced care planning issues.

As previously described, the ABC Med Home includes two care teams, each one serving approximately 750 patients [8]. Each team is led by an RN (1.0 FTE) and a social worker (0.75 FTE) who serve as the care coordinators and supervise five care coordinator assistants (CCAs) [8]. Four team members (one social worker and three CCAs) are employed by CICOA Aging & In-Home Solutions, Indiana's largest Area Agency on Aging (CICOA). These employees have received specialized training in "options counseling" and serve as liaisons between the ABC Med Home and the resources facilitated by CICOA (Fig. 21.1).

To be eligible for enrollment in the ABC Medical Home, a patient must be a Medicare or Medicaid beneficiary aged 65 and older, must have had at least one visit to one of Eskenazi's primary care practices within the last 2 years, and must have at least one dementia or depression ICD-9 diagnosis code. In addition, the patient and/or the family caregiver must agree to enrollment in the program. Eligible patients were initially identified from Eskenazi's billing records and administratively enrolled (by inclusion in the eMR-ABC) with the consent of the primary care physician. It is important to note that not all patients enrolled in the program with a diagnosis of depression were clinically depressed at the time of enrollment; however, given that depression is a chronic illness, these patients were included in the program with a goal of relapse prevention. Enrolled patients remain in the program unless discharged because (1) the patient dies or moves to long-term care or (2) the patient, family, or primary care physician requests that the patient no longer be contacted by the program. Patients who are discharged may be replaced by eligible patients referred to the program by

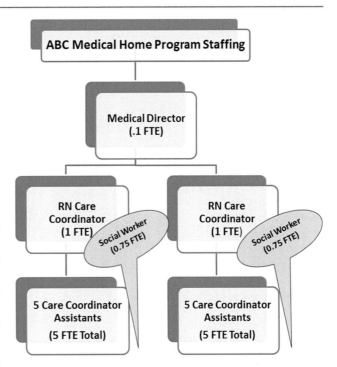

Fig. 21.1 ABC Medical Home Program Staffing

primary care providers, practitioners at the Healthy Aging Brain Center, or other specialists. Patients may also be enrolled in the program by referral from their informal caregivers or self-referral.

Similar to the HABC, the ABC Med Home delivers care in multicomponent phases: the *initial assessment phase*, the *follow-up phase*, and the *acute care transition phase*, a third phase of care triggered whenever an ABC patient is hospitalized or visits the emergency room (ER).

Initial Assessment Phase

Following enrollment in the program, the CCA contacts the patient and/or caregiver by phone (or in person during a physician visit), explains the purpose of the ABC Med Home and the patient's eligibility, and schedules the first in-person visit. The initial visit is conducted at the patient's home or another location selected by the patient or caregiver. During the initial visit, the CCA completes multiple assessments to determine the severity of the patient's dementia and/or depression and the needs of the patient and caregiver including (1) the Mini-Mental State Examination, (2) the PHQ-9, and (3) the caregiver and self-report versions of the HABC Monitor. The CCA also reviews and documents the patient's over-the-counter and prescribed medications and performs a home safety evaluation. Following the initial visit, the CCA meets with the RN and social worker care coordinators to present the results of the initial assessment and to develop an

Table 21.1 Tools of the ABC Med Home

Tools of the ABC Med Home
Multiple Mini Interview
Training Curriculum
eMR-ABC Tracking Software
"Mobile Office"
Cell phone
Laptop computer
Wireless access to the Internet
PHQ-9
HABC Monitor—Caregiver Version
HABC Monitor—Self-Report Version
Mini-Mental State Exam
Individualized care plan including:
• Medications
• Non-pharmacological dementia and depression care protocols
• Self-management educational materials
• Coordination with community resources

individualized care plan taking into account the diagnosis and the specific needs of both the patient and the caregiver. If deemed necessary by the RN care coordinator (after consultation with the medical director), the patient may be referred to the HABC or a mental health specialist for a more extensive evaluation. Within 1 month of the initial assessment, the CCA schedules another in-person visit with the patient and family to review and initiate the individualized care plan. The care plan may include a variety of tools available to address the needs of both the patient and caregiver. These tools (Table 21.1) were developed and/or utilized in the collaborative care research models for dementia and depression and in the HABC program and include medications (prescribed by the primary care provider after consultation with the RN); self-management educational materials and non-pharmacological protocols; behavioral activation and relapse prevention; and coordination with community resources.[8]

Follow-Up Phase

Similar to the HABC, the frequency of follow-up visits varies based on the emergent needs of the patient and caregiver, but the CCAs are required to provide an in-person visit to each patient (1) at least once a month for the 3 months following the initial assessment and (2) at least once every 3 months thereafter. During the follow-up contacts, the care coordinators and CCAs will continuously measure and monitor the patient's response to treatment using the PHQ-9 and the HABC Monitor. Medications will also be reviewed and recorded at each visit. Each clinical team meets weekly to discuss patient care, problem solve issues related to patient and caregiver needs, and make any necessary revisions to the plan of care [8].

With the support of CMS funding, the eMR-ABC has been modified to serve as a population health management tool. New functionalities include multiple improvements to data collection and self-monitoring features. The enhanced software allows the team to monitor the health outcomes of the entire population and then quickly shift focus to examine the status of an individual patient. This functionality allows the team to quickly identify patients with poor outcomes and adjust the plan of care to reallocate program resources where needed most. New reports have been developed to assist in tracking fidelity to the intervention and assessing the performance of individual staff members; problems with adherence can now be identified and addressed quickly. The eMR-ABC also has a new scheduling function to assist the CCAs in identifying those patients who require a visit either (1) to meet the minimum number of visits required by the program or (2) because the scores on the patient's clinical assessments indicate a need for intervention.

Acute Care Transition Phase

The eMR-ABC is now connected to the Indiana Network for Patient Care which sends a message to the eMR-ABC when ABC patients are admitted to a hospital or emergency room in any hospital located within the state of Indiana. When an ABC patient is hospitalized, a member of the ABC staff contacts the hospital team to provide them with information concerning the patient's health and social support to aid in decisions about the patient's care and discharge plan. Patients who are hospitalized will receive a home visit from the RN care coordinator within 72 h after discharge from the hospital. During that visit, the RN conducts medication reconciliation and coordinates the post-hospital discharge care plan. Patients who have an emergency room (ER) visit that does not result in a hospitalization will receive a home visit within 1 week after discharge from the ER. The post-ER visits are the responsibility of the RN care coordinator but may be conducted by any member of the ABC Med Home team as directed by the RN [8].

Lessons Learned

Many times during both the development and the operation phases of the project, the clinical and administrative staff as well as the project leadership have been asked to reflect on the successes of the project and the challenges faced along the way. Several common "lessons learned" emerged from this exercise. First, building relationships is critical to the success of our intervention. Stories from the CCAs repeatedly highlight the need to build the trust necessary to engage the patient in an open and honest conversation about care.

Second, the enthusiastic support of our hospital system's leadership was an important first step in engaging the primary care providers in this project. This support is rooted in a partnership between Eskenazi and IUCAR that began more than two decades ago and has transformed the way older adults are cared for at Eskenazi. Third, patient engagement can be challenging even with widespread support from leadership and the primary care providers. Staff members have developed innovative ways to successfully contact patients and caregivers and have worked very hard on the method and style of introducing themselves and explaining the services of both programs. Fourth, management and measurement must go hand in hand. The eMR-ABC links our measures of success to an electronic tracking system that allows us to continuously monitor outcomes so that we can make the timely adjustments in care plans required to improve results [8]. Finally, feedback from patients and caregivers is essential for future program development and quality improvement. The ABC Med Home consumer advisory board (comprising patients, families, and their advocates) is convened every 6 months to provide valuable feedback and suggestions to improve the experience of patients and caregivers. Information collected from this group has been helpful to identify outcomes of interest, unmet needs, and other concerns of patients and caregivers. This information will be used to inform decisions regarding potential modifications or additions to the intervention.

Plans for the Future

The success of the ABC Med Home will be judged on its ability to improve care and health outcomes while simultaneously lowering the cost of care through improved quality. The initial data on performance of the ABC Med Home demonstrate significant progress toward improving the health outcomes of older adults with dementia and depression. Recent work also demonstrates the financial sustainability of the care processes implemented in the HABC (and incorporated in the ABC Med Home model) based on cost savings achieved through reduced inpatient medical expenditures combined with reduced emergency department and related outpatient care expenditures [12]. The current system of medical reimbursement, however, does not incentivize such cost reduction [12, 13]. Furthermore, reimbursement processes favor procedure-specific and volume-based activities that do not include the types of services required to meet the complex needs of patients with dementia and depression [12].

CMS will allow awardees to develop a business model for financial sustainability that contemplates alternative methods of reimbursement. A reimbursement approach that realigns incentives by allowing providers to share in the cost savings generated by these programs offers the best promise both for sustainability of the ABC Project and for answering the challenges posed by our nation's rapidly aging population.

Acknowledgments The project described was supported by Grant Number 1C1CMS331000-01-00 from the Department of Health and Human Services, Centers for Medicare & Medicaid Services. The contents of this publication are solely the responsibility of the authors and do not necessarily represent the official views of the US Department of Health and Human Services or any of its agencies. MG Austrom is also supported in part by the Indiana Alzheimer's Disease Center funded by NIA P30AG10133.

References

1. Unützer J, Katon W, Callahan CM, Williams JW, Hunkeler E, Harpole L, et al. Collaborative care management of late-life depression in the primary care setting. JAMA. 2002;288(22):2836–45.
2. Callahan CM, Boustani MA, Unverzagt FW, Austrom MG, Damush TM, Perkins AJ, et al. Effectiveness of collaborative care for older adults with Alzheimer disease in primary care: a randomized controlled trial. JAMA. 2006;295(18):2148–57.
3. Boustani MA, Sachs GA, Alder CA, Munger S, Schubert CC, Guerriero Austrom M, et al. Implementing innovative models of dementia care: The Healthy Aging Brain Center. Aging Ment Health. 2011;15(1):13–22.
4. Guerriero Austrom M, Damush TM, Hartwell CW, Perkins T, Unverzagt F, Boustani M, et al. Development and implementation of nonpharmacologic protocols for the management of patients with Alzheimer's disease and their families in a multiracial primary care setting. Gerontologist. 2004;44(4):548–53.
5. Monahan PO, Boustani MA, Alder C, Galvin JE, Perkins AJ, Healey P, et al. Practical clinical tool to monitor dementia symptoms: the HABC-Monitor. Clin Interv Aging. 2012;7:143–57.
6. Campbell N, Boustani M, Limbil T, Ott C, Fox C, Maidment I, et al. The cognitive impact of anticholinergics: a clinical review. Clin Interv Aging. 2009;4:225–33.
7. Boustani M, Campbell N, Munger S, Maidment I, Fox C. Impact of anticholinergics on the aging brain: a review and practical application. Aging Health. 2008;4(3):311–20.
8. LaMantia MA, Alder CA, Callahan CM, Gao S, French DD, Austrom MG, Boustany K, Livin L, Bynagari B, Boustani MA. The aging brain care medical home: preliminary data (Editor's note prepared for) J Am Geriatr Soc. 2015.
9. Callahan CM, Boustani MA, Weiner M, Beck RA, Livin LR, Kellams JJ, et al. Implementing dementia care models in primary care settings: The Aging Brain Care Medical Home. Aging Ment Health. 2011;15(1):5–12.
10. Frame A, LaMantia M, Reddy Bynagari BB, Dexter P, Boustani M. Development and implementation of an electronic decision support to manage the health of a high-risk population: the enhanced Electronic Medical Record Aging Brain Care Software (eMR-ABC). eGEMs (Generating Evidence & Methods to improve patient outcomes). 2013;1(1):8.
11. Cottingham AH, Alder C, Austrom MG, Johnson CS, Boustani MA, Litzelman DK. new workforce development in dementia care: screening for "Caring": preliminary data. J Am Geriatr Soc. 2014;62(7):1364–8.
12. French DD, LaMantia MA, Livin LR, Herceg D, Alder CA, Boustani MA. Healthy aging brain center improved care coordination and produced net savings. Health Affairs (Project Hope). 2014;33(4):613–8.
13. Colla CH. Swimming against the current—what might work to reduce low-value care? N Engl J Med. 2014;371(14):1280–3.

The INTERACT Quality Improvement Program

22

Joseph G. Ouslander and Jill Shutes

Introduction

Federal health care reform in the USA is focused on the "triple aim" of improving care, improving health, and making care more affordable. The federal "Partnership for Patients" has two goals: reducing hospital-acquired conditions, and reducing hospital readmissions. Unnecessary hospitalizations and hospital readmissions of vulnerable long-term care (LTC) patients/residents can cause hospital-acquired complications, morbidity, mortality, and excess health care expenditures. Estimates suggest that a substantial percentage of these hospitalizations can be prevented, and result in billions of dollars in Medicare and Medicaid savings over the next several years. Some of these savings could be shared with providers to further improve care through accountable care organizations (ACOs) and other similar strategies [1–4].

The triple aim affords geriatric health care providers a golden opportunity [5]. Health care professionals who work in LTC are especially well positioned and skilled to improve our system of care, provide leadership in new models of care, and benefit from shared savings. The Centers for Medicare and Medicaid Services (CMS) has funded a major initiative that is based on this principle, supporting seven sites and close to 150 nursing homes to improve quality and reduce unnecessary hospitalizations.

Several care transition interventions can help seize the opportunities that arise from health care reform. The American Medical Directors Association has made important contributions by crafting and disseminating its Transitions in Care Clinical Practice Guideline [6], and other resources directed at reducing unnecessary hospitalizations. Models of care that engage advanced practice nurses to bridge the gap between the hospital and LTC setting such as the Transitional Care Model [7] or to work in teams with physicians have proven effective in reducing hospitalizations [8]. Adaption of the hospital-based project RED (Re-Engineered Discharge) [9] in the nursing home and a palliative care consult service [10] have also shown promise in reducing hospital readmissions.

INTERACT (Interventions to Reduce Acute Care Transfers) is a quality improvement program that has been adopted by many nursing homes throughout the USA, and is also being used in other countries, including Canada, the United Kingdom, and Singapore. Active implementation of the INTERACT program has been associated with up to a 24 % reduction in all-cause hospitalizations of nursing home residents over a 6-month period [11]. A reduction of this magnitude would result in over $100,000 in Medicare savings annually in each nursing home that could effectively implement and sustain the program. Similar to any quality improvement initiative in the LTC setting, INTERACT requires support of the interprofessional leadership team, including directors of nursing, administrators and medical directors, as well as buy-in from primary care clinicians (including physicians, nurse practitioners, and physician assistants) in order to be maximally effective.

Development of the INTERACT Program

INTERACT was first developed in a project supported by a CMS contract to the Georgia Medical Care Foundation, the Medicare Quality Improvement Organization in Georgia. A detailed analysis of the frequency, causes, and factors associated with hospitalizations of Georgia nursing home residents [12] and an expert panel process were used to develop a toolkit which was pilot tested in three nursing homes with high hospitalization rates. The toolkit implementation was well accepted and, with the regular guidance of a project nurse practitioner, was associated with a 50 % reduction in hospitalization rates, as well as a 36 % reduction in the proportion

J.G. Ouslander, M.D. • J. Shutes, M.S.N. (✉)
Department of Integrated Medical Sciences, Charles E. Schmidt College of Medicine, Florida Atlantic University, Bldg 71, 777 Glades Rd., Boca Raton, FL 33431, USA
e-mail: jousland@fau.edu; jbannis1@fau.edu

of hospitalizations rated as avoidable through systematic record review by an expert clinician panel [13]. With the support of the Commonwealth Fund, the INTERACT toolkit was refined through review by experts nominated by several national organizations as well as input from focus groups of nursing home providers, and then tested in a collaborative quality improvement project involving 30 nursing homes in three states (Florida, New York, and Massachusetts). Among the 25 homes that completed the project and for which baseline and intervention hospitalization rate data were available, there was a 17 % reduction in all-cause hospitalizations; among the 17 homes rated by the project team (masked to hospitalization rates) as "engaged" the reduction was 24 % [11]. These data must be interpreted with caution, because these studies were not randomized or controlled, environmental forces of health care reform were at work, and the nursing homes were volunteers who were probably motivated early adopters with relatively high baseline hospitalization rates. But, the data provides evidence that the program, even in the absence of strong oversight or financial incentives, is feasible to implement, and that more active program implementation is associated with higher reductions in hospitalization.

Through additional support from the Commonwealth Fund and the Retirement Research Fund, INTERACT has been further refined through a second round of input from experts nominated by national organizations, as well as ongoing input received from many direct users participating in a curriculum development project. With the support of a CMS Innovations Award, the program has been refined and has undergone usability testing for assisted living facilities and home health care programs. The resulting INTERACT program tools and related resources are now available free for clinical use at http://interact.fau.edu.

Overview of the INTERACT Program

An overview of how the INTERACT program is meant to be incorporated into everyday practice is illustrated in Fig. 22.1. The specific components of the program are described briefly in the section that follows. INTERACT has been updated from a "toolkit" to a quality improvement program that focuses on improving the management of acute changes in condition; as a result, hospitalizations are avoided in situations that can be feasibly and safely managed in the nursing home. INTERACT implementation is based on five fundamental strategies:

1. *Principles of quality improvement*, including implementation by a team facilitated by a designated champion and strong leadership support; measurement, tracking, and benchmarking of clearly defined outcomes with feedback to all staffs; and root cause analyses of

hospitalizations with continuous learning and improvement based on them
2. *Early identification and evaluation of changes in condition* before they become severe enough to require hospital transfer
3. *Management of common changes in condition* when safe and feasible without hospital transfer
4. *Improved advance care planning* and use of palliative or hospice care when appropriate and the choice of the patient/resident (or their health care proxy) as an alternative to hospitalization
5. *Improved communication and documentation*—both within the nursing home, between the nursing home staff and families, and between the nursing home and the hospital

INTERACT Program Resources and Tools

Resources for Implementation

The INTERACT website includes announcements and articles that can be downloaded, Implementation Guides, Implementation Checklists that can assist nursing homes, assisted living facilities, and home health care programs in getting started and monitoring their implementation processes, and a "Contact Us" section for questions that will be answered by a member of the INTERACT team. There are also links to a licensed printer for program materials, and an electronic interactive implementation curriculum.

The INTERACT program and tools have been designed so that they can be incorporated into electronic health records (EHRs) and other forms of health information technology (HIT), and there is a growing demand for electronic versions of programs such as INTERACT as more and more post-acute and long-term care facilities and programs embrace clinical software applications. Incorporation of INTERACT into EHRs and other forms of HIT will make it easier for direct care providers to "do the right thing at the right time," improve communication and documentation, enable timely availability of decision support, and facilitate tracking and trending of care processes and outcomes. Information on the availability of electronic applications of the INTERACT program can be obtained from the "Contact Us" section of the program website.

Quality Improvement Tools

Fundamental aspects of implementing an effective quality improvement program include tracking, trending, and benchmarking well-defined process and outcome measures, and conducting and learning from root cause analyses of events. INTERACT includes a hospitalization tracking tool that can

Fig. 22.1 Overview of the INTERACT program in everyday care. This overview illustrates the use of the INTERACT program in everyday care in the nursing home, from the time of admission to identifying a change in condition, and communicating and documenting relevant information, as well as the quality improvement components of the program at the bottom of the figure

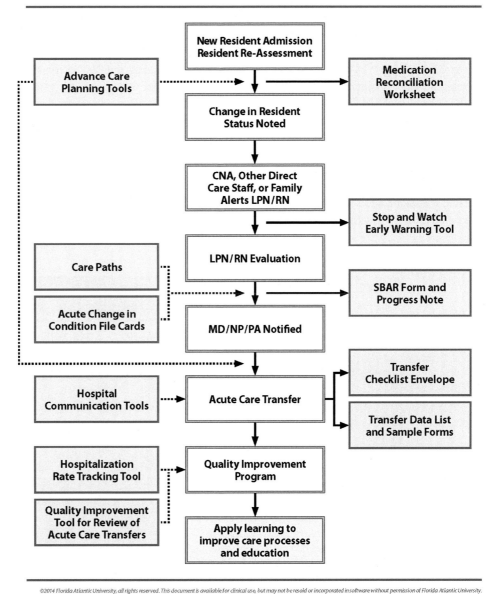

Using the INTERACT Tools
In Every Day Care

INTERACT
Version 4.0 Tool

calculate hospitalization and readmission rates consistent with anticipated CMS definitions for the 30-day readmission measure for nursing homes. A similar tracking tool is available through the Advancing Excellence Campaign at http://www.nhqualitycampaign.org/; readmission rates are also calculated by the American Health Care Association for its members, and by several private vendors that provide risk-adjusted rates. These rates are also generated by some EHRs and a quality improvement software company that have a license agreement to utilize the INTERACT program (Loopback Analytics, Dallas, TX). The *INTERACT Quality Improvement Tool* provides guidance on how to conduct a root cause analysis of an individual transfer; the *Quality Improvement Summary*

Worksheet provides guidance on how to roll up the data to target education and care process improvements. The INTERACT quality improvement tools can be used to generate "quality dashboards" such as those illustrated in Fig. 22.2, which are capable of tracking, trending, and benchmarking a variety of care processes and hospitalization outcome measures.

Communication Tools

INTERACT includes tools designed to improve communication and documentation within the organization, as well as between the organization and hospital. The focus of

INTERACT is the management of an acute change in condition. The "*STOP and WATCH*" *Tool* was developed based on the evidence that an "early warning" instrument for certified nursing assistants (CNAs) might be helpful in identifying acute changes in condition [14]. The STOP and WATCH Tool uses simple language to identify common, but nonspecific changes in condition, and has been adapted for use not only by CNAs, but also by other direct care staff (e.g., housekeeping, dietary, rehabilitation) and by families. Completion of a STOP and WATCH Tool is meant to be a clinical alert for a licensed nurse to determine if further evaluation is necessary. When it is, INTERACT provides an "*SBAR Communication Form and Progress Note*," which is meant to guide the licensed nurse through a structured evaluation of the change in condition, as well as prepare them for and structure communication with primary care clinicians. It is based on the "Situation, Background, Assessment,

Recommendation" method that is used in many health care settings. The language in the tool has been adapted to accommodate the fact that in many states "assessment" is beyond the scope of practice of licensed practical nurses based on their state Nurse Practice Act. The tool is intended to prevent the call from an unprepared nurse that "Mrs. Smith looks bad"; without adequate information, such calls often result, understandably, in transfer to the emergency room for further evaluation. Experience thus far with the INTERACT SBAR tool has demonstrated its value in improving communication as well as the overall professional relationship between nursing staff and medical care providers.

INTERACT tools for improving communication with acute hospitals include a checklist of key transfer documents, lists of critical data for inter-facility communication at the time of transfers, examples of forms to document these data in easily readable formats, and a tool to assist in medication

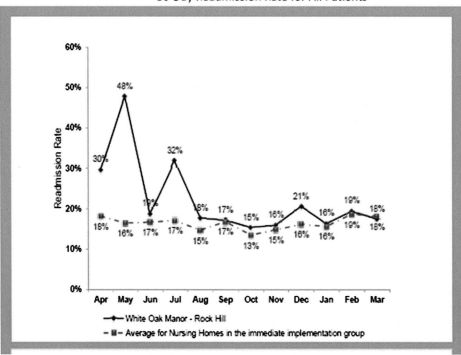

Fig. 22.2 Example of an INTERACT quality improvement dashboard. This is one example of the type of quality improvement data that can be generated from the INTERACT program. (**a**) Illustrates how 30-day readmission rates can be tracked, trended over time, and benchmarked against a group of nursing homes. (**b**) Illustrates how data from the root cause analyses of transfers using the INTERACT Quality Improvement Tool can be summarized to highlight areas for education and care pro-

cess improvements. In this example summarizing close to 5,000 transfers, the most common changes in condition associated with transfers were abnormal vital signs, altered mental status, uncontrolled pain, and shortness of breath; 22 % were transferred after being in the facility <7 days; 19 % went to the Emergency Department and were sent back to the nursing homes without hospital admission; and 23 % of the transfers were rated as potentially preventable by the facility teams

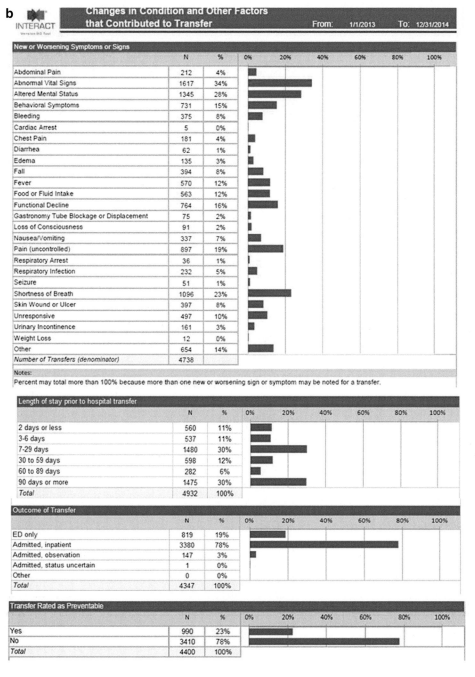

Fig. 22.2 (continued)

reconciliation at the time of admission to the facility or home health care program. The transfer forms have been vetted repeatedly by emergency department nurses and physicians as well as post-acute and long-term care health professionals in order to insure that it includes the information they need to make an informed decision about evaluation and management of the transferred patient/resident. The *"Hospital to Post-Acute Care Transfer Form"* contains critical time-sensitive information essential to provide care in the first 48–72 h after transfer. Discharge summaries, while helpful,

are usually not available in time; even when available, they often do not contain critical details that, if not attended to, can result in complications and rapid hospital readmission. The INTERACT data lists were created in recognition that many states and coalitions have their own universal transfer forms; the data lists are meant to be helpful in insuring that data in these forms are complete. Many groups are working on electronic "Continuity of Care Documents" that will include these data, and federal (e.g., HL-7) data standards that will be required on such forms are currently evolving.

The INTERACT *Medication Reconciliation Worksheet* is intended to provide guidance for the critical process of medication reconciliation. Polypharmacy and unclear medication orders are a recipe for disaster that require meticulous attention and collaboration between nurses, pharmacists, and medical care providers in order to prevent adverse drug events that can precipitate hospital readmission. The worksheet is meant to guide the thought process and first structure examination of the hospital medication list in order to identify clarifications needed, including unclear diagnosis or indication, uncertain dose or route of administration, stop date, hold parameters, lab tests needed for monitoring, dose different than before hospitalization, and medication duplications. The second part of the worksheet guides evaluation of medication the patient/resident was on before hospitalization in order to insure that one or more medications, which may have been appropriately stopped or changed in the hospital, are resumed when appropriate.

The INTERACT tools for communicating with hospitals have proven popular and helpful. But, there is no substitute for in-person communication via phone, secure e-mail, or other more individualized strategy. Not only does this insure timely communication of critical information, but it also fosters mutual professional understanding and respect. When patient safety is at stake, INTERACT or other similar tools are not adequate—there is no substitute for an in-person "warm handoff" to communicate the critical information.

Decision Support Tools

The INTERACT decision support tools are central to the INTERACT program and play a critical role in the management of patients/residents with acute changes in condition and in communication between nurses and primary care clinicians. The tools are intended to help guide decisions about further evaluation of changes in patient/resident condition, when to communicate with primary care clinicians, when to consider transfer to the hospital, and when to provide suggestions on how to manage some conditions without hospital transfer when it is safe and feasible. While the INTERACT *Change in Condition File Cards* and *Care Paths* are consistent with established clinical guidelines published by several national professional organizations, most are based on expert opinion as opposed to definitive scientific clinical trials. The Change in Condition File Cards concept was originally described in 1990 [15]. Subsequently AMDA developed a clinical practice guideline on acute change in condition [16] and has made guidance available to nurses ("Know It All Before You Call"); both provide much more detail than the

INTERACT tools, which are meant to be readily usable at the bedside. An example of an INTERACT Care Path is illustrated in Fig. 22.3.

The recommendations in the INTERACT Change in Condition File Cards and Care Paths are not meant to be fixed in stone. These tools are meant to guide clinical decision making, not dictate it. The systematic, clearly defined approach to symptoms and signs, combined with agreement on explicit criteria for communication, is more important than the specific recommendations in these tools. Clinical teams or corporations may therefore choose to modify specific criteria and recommendations for facility or corporate policies and procedures. In order for these decision support tools to be effective in everyday practice, the medical director and all primary care clinicians, including those who cover after hours, must be familiar with and support the use of these tools.

Advance Care Planning Tools

One of the most common reasons cited by expert clinicians in rating hospitalizations of nursing home patients/ residents "potentially avoidable" is that among patients/ residents with severe end-stage illness, the risks of hospitalization outweigh the benefits. Moreover, family insistence on transfer to the hospital is a commonly cited reason for not attempting to manage changes in condition in the nursing home. Research has clearly shown that such care transitions can be burdensome in this population, and that implementation of advance care planning interventions can result in positive outcomes [17]. While an increasing number of older patients have advance directives, the process of advance care planning and updating the advance directives at critical times may not be optimal. As suggested in Fig. 22.1, advance care planning should be undertaken, regardless of whether advance directives are already in place, at the time of admission or readmission to the facility or home health program, at regular intervals (for example at quarterly care planning meetings in nursing homes), and at the time of changes in condition. Patients/residents and families may change their mind about advance care plans and directives in these situations. Thus, INTERACT Care Paths suggest updating the advance care plan as a key component of managing changes in condition, and the INTERACT Quality Improvement Tool asks about the role of advance care planning in transfers.

INTERACT advance care planning tools include a variety of tools for education of staff and patients/residents. A fundamental theme underlying these tools is that advance care planning is a team endeavor and not just the

Fig. 22.3 Example of an INTERACT care path. The INTERACT care path for symptoms of lower respiratory illness is one of nine that provide guidance on evaluation and management of common conditions precipitating hospital transfers. All have been made consistent with expert recommendations; the care path shown is based on one proven to reduce hospital admissions by Loeb and colleagues in Canadian nursing homes [20]. Clinicians may elect to use alternative specific criteria in the care paths and change in condition guidance, but working with nursing staff on common approaches, language, and explicit criteria for alerts is critical to the effectiveness of the INTERACT program

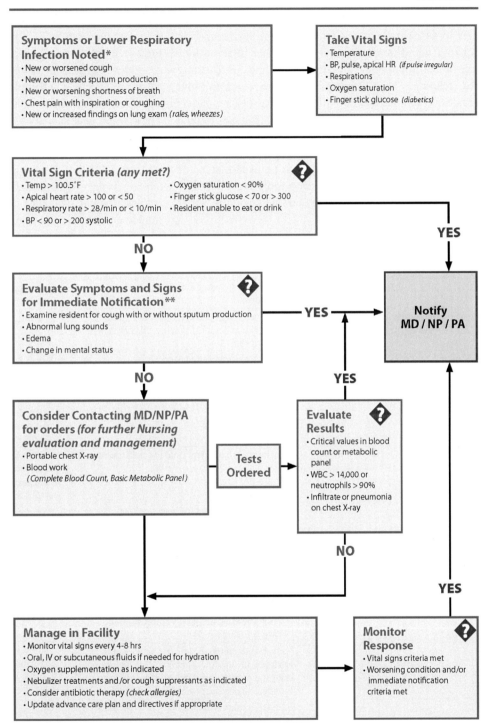

CARE PATH *Symptoms of Lower Respiratory Infection*

INTERACT
Version 4.0 Tool

Symptoms or Lower Respiratory Infection Noted*
- New or worsened cough
- New or increased sputum production
- New or worsening shortness of breath
- Chest pain with inspiration or coughing
- New or increased findings on lung exam *(rales, wheezes)*

Take Vital Signs
- Temperature
- BP, pulse, apical HR *(if pulse irregular)*
- Respirations
- Oxygen saturation
- Finger stick glucose *(diabetics)*

Vital Sign Criteria *(any met?)*
- Temp > 100.5°F
- Apical heart rate > 100 or < 50
- Respiratory rate > 28/min or < 10/min
- BP < 90 or > 200 systolic
- Oxygen saturation < 90%
- Finger stick glucose < 70 or > 300
- Resident unable to eat or drink

YES

NO

Evaluate Symptoms and Signs for Immediate Notification**
- Examine resident for cough with or without sputum production
- Abnormal lung sounds
- Edema
- Change in mental status

YES

Notify MD / NP / PA

NO

YES

Consider Contacting MD/NP/PA for orders *(for further Nursing evaluation and management)*
- Portable chest X-ray
- Blood work *(Complete Blood Count, Basic Metabolic Panel)*

Tests Ordered

Evaluate Results
- Critical values in blood count or metabolic panel
- WBC > 14,000 or neutrophils > 90%
- Infiltrate or pneumonia on chest X-ray

NO

YES

Manage in Facility
- Monitor vital signs every 4-8 hrs
- Oral, IV or subcutaneous fluids if needed for hydration
- Oxygen supplementation as indicated
- Nebulizer treatments and/or cough suppressants as indicated
- Consider antibiotic therapy *(check allergies)*
- Update advance care plan and directives if appropriate

Monitor Response
- Vital signs criteria met
- Worsening condition and/or immediate notification criteria met

* Refer also to the INTERACT Shortness of Breath Care Path
** Refer also to other INTERACT Care Paths as indicated by symptoms and signs

responsibility of the primary care clinician. The *Communication Guide* is based largely on publications by Quill and colleagues [18, 19] and is meant for staff education, including role playing. Other INTERACT tools have been carefully constructed to be simple and illustrative in order to assist patients/residents and families in making decisions about hospital transfer and other interventions such as cardiopulmonary resuscitation and gastrostomy tube feeding. The *Comfort Care Interventions* tool includes a sample set of palliative care orders and is intended to be helpful in situations where hospices (which generally have similar order sets) are either not available or not desired by the resident or family. Many other similar resources that can complement or be used instead of INTERACT advance care planning tools are available; links to many of these resources can be found at http://interact.fau.edu.

Keys to Successful Implementation and Overcoming Common Barriers

There are three general characteristics shared by facilities that have successfully implemented the INTERACT Quality Improvement Program: executive leadership support for the program; engagement of direct care staff by the facility-based INTERACT champion(s); and what can best be described as a culture dedicated to quality improvement. These same characteristics also provide the foundation for successfully overcoming common barriers to implementation. A sample of specific strategies used by executive leaders and INTERACT champions as well as examples of nursing facility culture that supports quality improvement are described in Table 22.1. More details are provided in the Implementation Guides available on the program website.

Table 22.1 Keys to successful INTERACT implementation

	Examples of successful implementation strategies	Examples of common barriers to implementation and how they are overcome
Executive Leadership Support for the INTERACT Quality Improvement Program	Articulates vision and commitment regarding the purpose and goals for using INTERACT to the entire staff.	*Internal resistance to change:*
(Executive Leaders include Executive Directors, Administrators, Directors of Nursing, Corporate Leaders if applicable, Medical Directors, Clinical Pharmacists)	Demonstrates commitment by:	Works with multidisciplinary team to evaluate systems and processes already in place to ensure that INTERACT tools do not duplicate other tools already in place; to determine how best to incorporate new tools and to try to "Add one tool and remove two" when possible to reduce redundant work for staff.
	• Allocating sufficient time for staff training	Recognizes that organizational improvement takes time and takes the lead in sustaining focus by keeping INTERACT as agenda item at all staff and quality meetings.
	• Attending relevant training sessions	*"We are in our survey window":*
	• Promoting formation of multidisciplinary team to plan/deliver/and sustain inclusion of INTERACT into standards of care for facility	Promotes ongoing training and use of tools throughout survey window and encourages staff to use the opportunity to share their improvement efforts with surveyors during the survey.
	• Participating in review and discussion of data including acute care transfer rates and summary of Quality Improvement Review Tools	*"Too many things going on at once":*
	Uses data to motivate staff internally and to articulate the unique value that their facility brings to cross continuum partners in efforts to reduce unnecessary acute care transfers	Develops quality agenda that includes sequential rollout of initiatives and minimizes rollout of more than one major initiative at a time.
	Initiates contact with local hospitals to establish relationship and promote collaboration	
Engagement of Direct Care Staff by INTERACT Champion(s)	Criteria for the role of INTERACT champion(s):	*"Not enough time to do the training"*
(Selection of a champion is one of the most important decisions to be made. Successful implementation depends on the right person(s) in this role.)	Is able to motivate staff to attend training sessions and to try new tools	Builds training sessions around times that work for staff and minimizes long time off unit for all staffs when possible.

(continued)

Table 22.1 (continued)

	Examples of successful implementation strategies	Examples of common barriers to implementation and how they are overcome
	Has experience providing training and education	Uses "just-in-time" learning on units with clinical situations that are relevant to staff to deliver training.
	Has formal or informal authority to drive/influence change in staff behavior and practice	Delivers training according to time available; starting on one unit at a time with one tool at a time if needed.
	Provides training and directs process improvement using NON-PUNITIVE approach	*"We have no control over who goes out to the hospital … families and doctors insist"*
	Agrees or volunteers to be champion	Includes family members in program by sharing advance care planning tools with them on admission and when there is a change in condition and encouraging use of the Stop and Watch tool by families as a method to enhance communication. Families can also be educated using the facility Capabilities Checklist as to what can be done in the facility.
	Activities of effective champions:	Provides medical director, MDs, NPs, and PAs with data regarding acute care transfer rates and summary of quality improvement reviews on regular basis and seeks input on strategies to improve care relative to findings of data collection.
	• Visible on the units daily	
	• Communicates enthusiasm for the program	
	• Reminds staff to use tools	
	• Makes tools visible and accessible for everyday use	
	• Seeks and responds to staff input on how to use tools most effectively	
	• Collaborates with key staff members on the evening/night/weekend shifts to promote consistent use of the INTERACT program on all days/shifts	
Facility Culture Dedicated to Quality Improvement	The INTERACT program is an integral component of the facility's quality improvement activities and QAPI program	*"This is the project of the month"*
	INTERACT training and implementation are delivered using a non-punitive approach	INTERACT training is integrated into new hire orientation and annual competency evaluations for all staffs.
	When avoidable hospitalizations are identified, a spirit of inquiry by the multidisciplinary team seeks improvement, not blame	INTERACT tools are incorporated as standard practice in the facility.

Conclusion

INTERACT is a publicly available quality improvement program that focuses on improving the identification, evaluation, and management of acute changes in condition of patients and residents in post-acute and long-term care. The program includes clinical practice, communication, decision support, educational, and quality improvement tools and strategies to implement them. Effective implementation has been associated with substantial reductions in hospitalization of nursing home patients/residents, which could result in fewer hospital-acquired conditions and billions of dollars in savings over the next several years. Versions of the INTERACT program are also now available for assisted living facilities and home health care agencies. By using the INTERACT program, nursing homes, assisted living facilities, and home health care agencies can prevent unnecessary hospitalizations and their related complications and costs, and thereby become attractive partners for hospitals, health care systems, managed care plans, and accountable care organizations. In addition, effective INTERACT implementation will assist providers in meeting regulatory requirements for quality improvement activities. Embedding INTERACT into electronic health records will enhance its effectiveness, and provide real-time assistance for health care professionals in their efforts to provide high-quality care to a growing vulnerable population of older adults requiring post-acute and long-term care.

Acknowledgement This chapter is based on a review article published in the Journal of the American Medical Director's Association (JAMDA 15:162–170, 2014).

Dr. Joseph Ouslander is a full-time employee of Florida Atlantic University (FAU) and has received support through FAU to conduct research evaluating the INTERACT program from the National Institutes of Health (1R01NR012936), the Centers for Medicare & Medicaid Services, the Commonwealth Fund, the Retirement Research Foundation, PointClickCare, Medline Industries, and PatientOrderSets.

Dr. Ouslander and his wife have ownership interest in INTERACT Training, Education, and Management ("I TEAM") Strategies, a business that has a license agreement with FAU for use of INTERACT materials for training and management consulting.

Jill Shutes, GNP serves as a contractor to conduct educational and consulting services for I TEAM Strategies.

Work on this chapter and other projects are subject to terms of Conflicts of Interest Management plans developed and approved by the FAU Division of Research Financial Conflict of Interest Committee.

References

1. Walsh EG, Wiener JM, Haber S, et al. Potentially avoidable hospitalizations of dually eligible medicare and medicaid beneficiaries from nursing facility and home-and community-based services Waiver programs. J Am Geriatr Soc. 2012;60:821–9.
2. Ouslander JG, Maslow K. Geriatrics and the triple aim: defining preventable hospitalizations in the long term care population. J Am Geriatr Soc. 2012;60:2313–8.
3. Spectror WD, Limcangco R, Williams C, et al. Potentially avoidable hospitalizations for elderly long-stay residents of nursing homes. Med Care. 2013;51:673–81.
4. Ouslander JG, Berenson RA. Reducing unnecessary hospitalizations of nursing home residents. N Engl J Med. 2011;365:1165–7.
5. Ouslander JG. The triple aim: a golden opportunity for geriatrics. J Am Geriatr Soc. 2012;61:1808–9.
6. http://www.amda.com/tools/clinical/toccpg.pdf. Accessed 3 Aug 2014.
7. Naylor MD, Brooten DA, Campbell RL, et al. Transitional care of older adults hospitalized with heart failure: a randomized, controlled trial. J Am Geriatr Soc. 2004;52:675–84.
8. Konetzka RT, Spector W, Limcangco MR. Reducing hospitalizations from LTC settings. Med Care Res Rev. 2008;65:40–66.
9. Berkowitz RE, Fang Z, Helfand BKI, et al. Project ReEngineeing Discharge (RED) lowers hospital readmissions of patients discharged from a skilled nursing facility. J Am Med Dir Assoc. 2013;14:736–40.
10. Berkowitz RE, Jones RN, Rieder R, et al. Improving disposition outcomes for patients in a geriatric skilled nursing facility. J Am Geriatr Soc. 2011;59:1130–6.
11. Ouslander JG, Lamb G, Tappen R, et al. Interventions to reduce hospitalizations from nursing homes: evaluation of the INTERACT II Collaborative Quality Improvement Project. J Am Geriatr Soc. 2011;59:745–53.
12. Ouslander JG, Lamb G, Perloe M, et al. Potentially avoidable hospitalizations of nursing home residents: frequency, causes, and costs. J Am Geriatr Soc. 2010;58:627–35.
13. Ouslander JG, Perloe M, Givens J, et al. Reducing potentially avoidable hospitalizations of nursing home residents: results of a pilot quality improvement project. J Am Med Dir Assoc. 2009;9:644–52.
14. Boockvar KS, Lachs MS. Predictive value of nonspecific symptoms for acute illness in nursing home residents. J Am Geriatr Soc. 2003;51:1111–5.
15. Ouslander J, Turner C, Delgado D, et al. Communication between primary physicians and staff of long-term care facilities. J Am Geriatr Soc. 1990;38:490–2.
16. http://www.amda.com/tools/cpg/acoc.cfm. Accessed 1 Dec 2013.
17. Molloy DW, Guyatt GH, Russo R, et al. Systematic implementation of an advance directive program in nursing homes: a randomized controlled trial. JAMA. 2000;283:1437–44.
18. Quill TE, Arnold R, Back AL. Discussing treatment preferences with patients who want "everything". Ann Intern Med. 2009;151:345–9.
19. Casarett DJ, Quill TE. "I'm Not Ready for Hospice": strategies for timely and effective hospice discussions. Ann Intern Med. 2007;146:443–9.
20. Loeb M, Carusone SC, Goeree R, et al. Effect of a clinical pathway to reduce hospitalizations in nursing home residents with pneumonia—a randomized controlled trial. JAMA. 2006;295(21):2503–10.

Optum™ CarePlus: In-Place Clinical Delivery for Nursing Home Residents

23

Ronald J. Shumacher

Patients who struggle with multifaceted, difficult-to-manage complex chronic conditions typically represent only 5 % of the healthcare population; yet they can drive up to 50 % of total clinical expenditures [1]. This is due, in significant part, to the fact that traditional healthcare delivery models—particularly fee-for-service mechanisms—consistently underserve medically complex and chronically ill patients.

An unwieldy healthcare system seeking to avoid unnecessary costs and reform quality of care must focus aggressively on these chronically ill, medically complex patients. A solution that addresses critical factors at the core of high-utilization, high-cost medical care has the potential to create meaningful improvement.

Compelling theories and strategies arise to meet the challenge of managing high-risk populations. As with every important initiative, medically complex healthcare being a prime example, the fundamental challenge is *execution*.

How do we progress beyond theory to repeatable implementation and performance? One compelling care model is firmly in place and driving change among permanent nursing home residents. It has helped pioneer high quality care in nursing homes since the late 1980s.

Nursing home residents typify a high-risk population offering significant opportunity for pragmatic care delivery and management addressing patients with high likelihood of overutilization dominated by high-cost events like emergency room visits, acute hospitalizations, and readmissions.

Among the frail elderly, Optum CarePlus is an authentically resident-centric path to higher care quality, improved resident health, and significant cost reduction. The treat-in-place care and care management approach focuses specifically on helping higher utilization nursing home residents avert acute care transitions while promoting maximum function, comfort, and quality of life.

The History of Optum CarePlus

Optum CarePlus is an established, multistate clinical delivery model with a widely studied implementation history and proven track record addressing gaps in primary and preventative care for aging, vulnerable, and medically complex individuals.

The clinical care delivery methodology, which employs nurse practitioners (NPs) teamed with residents' primary care physicians (PCPs) and nursing home staff, began taking shape almost three decades ago. The philosophy emerged from the vision of two dedicated NPs from Minnesota who saw the need to substantively change how the frail elderly in nursing homes receive long-term care. RuthAnn Jacobson, NP, and Jeannine Bayard, NP, knew from first-hand experience that when people enter a nursing home it often is difficult for their doctors to see them regularly. In addition, families face expanded challenges attempting to coordinate a more complicated degree of care. As a result, the two NPs observed, residents move in and out of hospitals—or present at emergency rooms—with a frequency that exacts debilitating physical, financial, and emotional costs. Both resident and family feel the hardships.

In 1987, Jacobson and Bayard developed the CarePlus model (initially known as Evercare) to help nursing home residents protect their health, expand access to healthcare resources and services, and receive clinical care in a more personalized and responsive way. The NPs used a dual focus to anchor their novel approach: (1) prevention and early detection of new diseases or complications from existing conditions, and (2) timely, coordinated, and intensive treat-in-place medical care management to reduce the incidence of traumatic and costly emergency room visits, hospitalizations, and readmissions.

In 1995, following several years of increasing implementation and momentum within nursing homes, the Centers for Medicare and Medicaid Services (CMS) accepted the program as a demonstration project. Addressing nursing home

R.J. Shumacher, M.D., F.A.C.P., C.M.D. (✉)
Complex Population Management, Optum, 800 King Farm
Boulevard, Suite 600, Rockville, MD 20850, USA
e-mail: rshumacher@optum.com

care proved a strong fit with CMS initiatives to identify creative approaches that improve healthcare quality and reduce costs by transitioning from fee-for-service models to pay-for-performance and incentivized outcome improvement. CMS extended the original, six-state pilot multiple times.

Ultimately, the treat-in-place care delivery model became a permanent "special needs" Medicare plan as part of the Medicare Modernization Act of 2003. At this writing, a broad range of Medicare, Medicaid, and private long-term care delivery and coordination programs under Optum CarePlus address the complex health needs and quality-of-life circumstances of more than 46,000 elderly and disabled individuals in 33 states.

It should be noted here that Optum, as the healthcare services platform under UnitedHealth Group, provides the CarePlus clinical delivery model for a wide array of payers. The UnitedHealthcare (UHC) Institutional Special Needs Plan offering, known as the UHC Nursing Home Plan, has delegated an assortment of clinical services to Optum and represents Optum's largest customer for the CarePlus Institutional program.

A Delivery Model Attuned to the Population

When chronically ill, difficult-to-manage nursing home residents intersect with traditional healthcare delivery, efforts to improve care are commonly faced with a set of well-defined obstacles that undermine quality, patient outcomes, and cost management.

- Medically complex residents frequently present with multiple chronic conditions, cognitive issues, and psychosocial complications that render them high risk.
- Multiple providers and polypharmacy produce disjointed, confusing, and sometimes contraindicated care plans.
- Traditional in-office medical care delivery is insufficient—in time and quality—to establish the patients' perspective as well as the relationship depth that medically complex members require.
- Under traditional care delivery, primary provider and specialist practices are not structured or equipped to provide the urgent, 24/7 response known to be critical in preventing chronic illness escalation and exacerbation.
- The resulting gaps in care leave members vulnerable to frequent escalations and exacerbations. These, in turn, devolve into excessive medical crises requiring ER visits, acute hospitalizations, readmissions, and unnecessary medications.

The issue is not that high-needs nursing home residents lack access to excellent doctors or committed skilled nursing caregivers. Optum CarePlus in-place visits do not replace residents' visits with their PCPs or specialists. The needs of this segment simply require heightened care team collaboration and coordination—along with specialized infrastructure

and systems—tailored to disease processes that place residents in chronically high-risk, catastrophic, and terminal categories.

Realities within this population leave residents vulnerable to care transitions that are inherently adverse. Hospital admissions are highly stressful for the frail and chronically ill receiving long-term nursing care, and can result in complications that range from disorientation and the addition of psychotropic and other medications to heightened infection risk and increased overall frailty [2]. Placement in unfamiliar medical settings also causes nursing home residents to experience significantly higher rates of falls, catheterizations, skin breakdown, fluid and electrolyte abnormalities, adverse medication reactions, and chronic condition exacerbations.

At the same time, research indicates that at least 35 % of emergency room visits and hospitalizations involving nursing home residents are unnecessary [3, 4].

The Optum CarePlus model provides a higher level of primary and preventive care aimed at decreasing the complexity of and need for transitions among levels of care, especially by reducing preventable hospitalizations.

Under the treat-in-place, direct care, and care management model, Optum provides specialized NPs who go to the resident. These in-place providers—who work almost exclusively in skilled nursing facilities and are trained to work collaboratively with PCPs, specialist providers, and nursing home staff—support the multidimensional needs of medically complex nursing home residents.

Optum NPs monitor a resident's medical, behavioral, environmental, and social conditions and, in doing so, provide more intensive primary care and early intervention for any significant change in condition. In some instances, their reacting in real time to even the most elemental measures can drive profound care quality outcomes simply by identifying trigger events, managing risk factors, and implementing self-management techniques.

Analytics-Driven Insight Informs Patient Care

The disproportionate impact of a high-risk, high-utilization nursing home population underscores the importance of using strategic, specialized care management to treat chronic disease in a manner that helps mitigate functional decline.

One of the greatest drivers causing otherwise avoidable hospital admissions and unnecessary emergent care is the lack of real-time clarity regarding a resident's disease progression. This underdeveloped "health literacy" on the part of all stakeholders—residents, caregivers, and family—causes inappropriate utilization, increases cost, and reduces the member's quality of life. As a result, the core principle in improving care for the medically complex is delivering the right care, to the right residents, at the right time.

Generally speaking, a nursing home resident eligible for enrollment in Optum CarePlus:

- Has been a long-term resident of a participating skilled nursing facility for 90 days, with no active discharge plans
- Cannot have end-stage renal disease (ESRD) at the time of enrollment
- Must be eligible for Part A, and enrolled in Part B (enrollment does not affect Medicaid benefits)

Model Overview and Main Tenets

An initial, comprehensive Optum CarePlus assessment drives care planning based on a thorough, complete inventory of diagnoses. Next, an Optum NP and the resident's PCP develop the care management plan. During the course of care delivery and management, an electronic medical record gives all Optum providers access to the care plan. The care management infrastructure includes components such as an auto-fax feature that automatically distributes care plan changes, updates, interventions, and nursing home visit notes to the PCP.

Direct care visits by an Optum NP, specially trained in geriatric care and experienced in the skilled nursing setting, reflect a resident's acuity. Scheduled visits occur at a minimum of once per month with unscheduled visits taking place as needed to achieve care goals and address unanticipated issues. Face-to-face care management and coordination that is critical to symptom monitoring also facilitate resident/family education.

Finally, taking a holistic approach to care extends beyond managing chronic conditions. The care plan also includes a focus on relevant preventative services and guideline-driven treatment (e.g., flu shot, pneumonia vaccination) to avoid unnecessary hospitalization.

The Optum CarePlus care delivery and management structure enables a collaborative care team to fill gaps that traditional primary visits and fee-for-service models typically cannot address thoroughly and consistently within nursing home populations. The program emphasizes four key foundational components to provide long-term residents with a high level of personal, timely, and intensive care management.

Provider-Led, In-Facility, and Intensive Clinical Care Management

A certified NP provides care for chronic, acute, and urgent problems as well as routine care and preventive care man-

agement. Scheduled monthly visits and 24/7/365 virtual-office access provide timely provider availability to avoid emergency admissions for non-emergent conditions. This includes requesting an urgent nursing home visit. The urgent-response commitment is a visit from the resident's direct care team within the same day or by that evening. Optum CarePlus has the ability to initiate a Part A skilled benefit without requiring the preceding 3-day hospital stay. In addition, CarePlus makes available reimbursement to the skilled nursing facility for intensive service delivery which occurs in lieu of a hospitalization.

NPs also follow residents during recovery after an illness or hospitalization. In addition to time spent in while direct patient care, Optum NP's devote another 25 % to resident-specific communication with families, PCPs, and nursing home staff complementing the work of the primary physician [5]. The Optum NP is critical in the success of integrating all stakeholders—97 % of family members say that they are satisfied and would recommend the program to others [6].

Care Team Integration and Collaboration

In a treat-in-place partnering model (Fig. 23.1) that supplements care provided by PCPs and nursing facility staff (at no cost to the facility), NPs coordinate primary care, proactively identify health status triggers, and manage conditions to avoid unnecessary hospitalizations. The NP's frequent presence in the nursing facility, in addition to developing relationships with staff, enhances preemptive care that improves early identification of health decline signs and symptoms.

Regular Interaction, Observation, and Training/ Mentoring That Drive Personalized, More Intensive Care

In addition to focusing on effective communication with PCPs and nursing home staff, Optum CarePlus NPs meet regularly with residents and their families to set care goals and identify medical, behavioral, social, and environmental conditions that can trigger avoidable hospitalizations.

Optum CarePlus providers also manage advanced-illness discussions that enable residents and their families to establish care goals and create advance directives. Regular contact with the nursing home staff allows NPs to conduct formal and informal in-service training in specialized aspects of geriatric care. Nursing staff access to on-site, specially trained NPs is a critical factor in how nursing home administrators view Optum CarePlus. Survey results indicated that 93 % of nursing home directors said that the plan exceeded their expectations, and 92 % would recommend the model to other nursing homes [6].

Fig. 23.1 Optum provides a patient-centric, treat-in-place clinical model led by clinicians to coordinate and enhance quality of care for nursing home residents

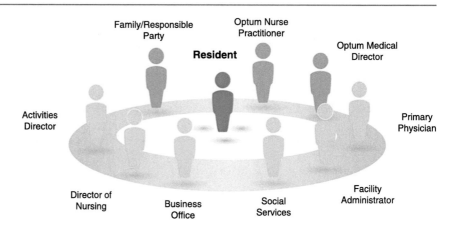

Coordination with Medicare Health Plans

Optum CarePlus provides enrolled nursing home residents with care coordination on behalf of Medicare Advantage health plans, such as the UnitedHealthcare Nursing Home Plan (UHC NHP). The UHC NHP receives payment from Medicare on a per-member-per-month (PMPM) basis, and has the ability to waive the Medicare 3-day qualifying stay requirement for coverage of skilled nursing facility care. This enables a seamless transition for residents between custodial and skilled-care levels within a facility, based on a resident's health needs.

An Experience-Driven Record of Outcomes

Acute hospitalizations represent one of the most compelling opportunities to affect the quality of residents' lives and contain an unsustainable long-term cost incurred by skilled nursing residents (Fig. 23.2).

Optum-coordinated treat-in-place experiences, systems, and processes—applied to nursing homes—benefit significantly from the model's parallel, broad-based in-home implementation. Today, many health plans around the country have implemented the Optum CarePlus community-based services program as the in-home intervention or visiting-provider model supporting the multidimensional needs of medically complex health plan members in private residences and group homes.

This clinical delivery specialization and scale form a knowledge base for improving the primary and preventative care of nursing home residents with complex and/or chronic conditions. Collaboration between a resident's NP, PCP, specialist, and nursing home staff draws on deep experience across all Optum CarePlus populations in 33 states, including:

- 450,000+ provider interventions
- 3,648,000 unique treat-in-place visits annually
- 2,500+ clinicians delivering hands-on care
- 16 years of health plan partnerships

Optum CarePlus implementations conducted since 1998 across all medically complex Medicare and Medicaid populations have been shown to [7]:

- Reduce overall healthcare costs by 42–52 % compared to non-managed at-risk members
- Reduce hospital inpatient admissions by 64 %
- Reduce hospital readmissions by 33 %
- Reduce healthcare costs in the last 6 months of life by 61 %

Today, Optum CarePlus provides treat-in-place care and care management for approximately 38,000 nursing home residents around the country. According to the study by Kane and colleagues (2003), the reduction in acute inpatient hospitalizations is 50 % [8]. These results are consistent with findings from a CMS-mandated evaluation following the model's earlier demonstration pilot.

During 2003, as part of the CMS demonstration to analyze the effectiveness of the clinical delivery model, CMS contracted with Dr. Robert Kane at the University of Minnesota to conduct an independent evaluation to determine if the model (known at the time as Evercare) successfully achieved the demonstration goals of improving primary and preventive care while reducing hospitalizations for nursing home residents. Nursing home population data was derived from five skilled nursing demonstration sites in Georgia, Maryland, Massachusetts, Colorado, and Florida [9]. The study compared plan enrollees in the five sites with two sets of control groups. One control comprised long-stay residents in Evercare-participating homes who did not enroll in the plan (enrollment was voluntary). The second control group was composed of long-stay residents from nursing homes who did not participate in the plan.

The study measured service utilization data for approximately 2 years, identifying patterns of use by calculating the monthly use rate for each group and aggregating to form annual rates. Usages included hospital admissions and days, emergency room visits, therapy services, mental health services, and podiatry. Additional surveys, case studies, and structured interviews were also conducted to assist in interpreting the quantitative results.

Fig. 23.2 Avoidable inpatient services among nursing home residents. The conservative estimate of the potential cost savings from reducing avoidable acute care hospital stays among nursing home residents is $4.5 billion (data from Webcast by Joseph G. Ouslander, MD, Florida Atlantic University, January 19, 2011. http://www.avoidreadmissions.com/wwwroot/userfiles/documents/43/ouslander-interact-presentation-for-ny-ipro-webcast-jan-19-2011.pdf)

Assume:
among
1.5 million
NH residents
in the U.S.,
~1/3 will be
hospitalized
in one year

= 450,000
hospitalizations
The cost of each
hospitalization is
~$6,500 for a
hospital DRG
payment, plus a
30 day SNF stay
for **1/3** of those
hospitalized at
$350/day

= $10,000
per
hospitalization
How much
can be saved to
reinvest in quality?

Total cost:
$4.5 billion

The evaluation concluded that the clinical delivery model achieved these *hospital use* results [10]:

- Reduced hospitalizations by 45 %, with no change in mortality: The incidence of hospitalizations was twice as high in control residents as in plan residents (4.6 and 4.7 per 100 enrollees per month vs. 2.43).
- Reduced emergency room visits by 48–55 % (3.3 visits per 100 enrollees in the model vs. 6.3 and 7.3 in the control groups).
- Reduced average hospital days by 57 % (13.5 days per 100 enrollees vs. 31.2 and 31.3).

The same pattern held for the *preventable hospitalization* rate, with residents in the (Evercare) plan experiencing 0.28 admissions per 100 enrollees vs. 0.80 and 0.86 for the control groups. Thus, each NP successfully treating residents in a skilled nursing facility—instead of admitting them to hospitals—correlated with avoiding approximately $103,000 in unnecessary inpatient costs each year [10].

Implications for Skilled Nursing Facilities

In 2013, Optum conducted an evaluation to determine the impact of the CarePlus model on nursing home facilities. The analysis of facilities participating in the UnitedHealthcare Nursing Home Plan (UHC NHP) [11] assessed emergency department and acute care hospital utilization, skilled and custodial nursing facility utilization, other services provided within a facility, and the financial impact of UHC NHP participation. By examining the impact of the UHC NHP for a 1-year period following a resident's admission to long-term care, they compared 6,922 UHC NHP residents' medical costs and utilization to a matched group of residents from the Medicare fee-for-service program.

Consistent with previous studies, the UHC NHP residents experienced fewer inpatient admissions, readmissions, emergency room visits, and skilled nursing facility admissions.

As a result, the total annual medical cost for these residents was also lower than the matched group of Medicare fee-for-service residents.

The evaluation identified several important findings that affect participating nursing homes:

1. *Residents spend more days in the nursing home.* Residents spending fewer days in the hospital results in higher, more consistent nursing home occupancy. Because Medicaid pays the majority of custodial nursing home care, payment amounts vary by state. Residents in the Optum study spent an average of 2.68 more days per year in a custodial bed in the nursing home compared to the control group. Based on an average 2010 Medicaid payment of $174.13 [12], a nursing home received an additional payment of $467 per resident each year. If an average Optum CarePlus population for a skilled nursing facility is 60, this equates to more than $28,000 each year. (This does not consider the impact of any potential Medicaid bed-hold payment policies, which are steadily decreasing due to Medicaid budget constraints.)

   Additionally, in order to support nursing homes caring for highly complex residents, Optum CarePlus developed an Intensive Service Day (ISD) level of care. Care teams use this level when a resident is clinically complex, unstable, and at risk for hospitalization. The ISD component supports the treat-in-place model by reimbursing for more clinically complex cases treated within the facility rather than transferred to an emergency department or hospital. In addition, the ISD care level does not count toward a resident's 100-day skilled nursing facility (SNF) benefit.

2. *Residents require fewer Part A skilled days.* Optum CarePlus, provided through UHC NHP or another plan, waives the Medicare requirement that patients spend 3 days in an acute hospital before becoming eligible for Part A skilled nursing facility benefits. As a result, the care team can shift a resident from a custodial status to skilled

nursing status—without admission to the hospital—as clinical needs require. Resident status can shift back to custodial care as needs diminish. The ability to trigger Part A events within the facility supports the early intervention model of care. Detecting condition changes earlier, and beginning clinical interventions sooner, helps avoid a status decline that may ultimately require hospitalization.

Optum CarePlus residents had approximately the same number of SNF admissions as those in the control group (0.70 vs. 0.74), but had fewer days at a skilled level (7.43 vs. 12.19). The average Medicare-allowed amount per skilled day for fee-for-service long-stay residents in the study was $376, and the amount collected by facilities was $291. By comparison, the actual amount paid per day of skilled nursing care for Optum CarePlus residents was an increase of 43.6 % over the paid amount from traditional Medicare [11].

Triggering skilled events and providing onsite care without the need for a transfer to the hospital provide for increased days in participating facilities, reducing the number of days with diminished or no revenue due to state-specific bed-hold policies. Additionally, unlike standard Medicare, participating nursing homes do not risk resident transfer to an alternative facility (such as a hospital-owned or other competing SNF) if additional skilled care is necessary following hospitalization.

3. *Nursing homes earn quality incentive program payments.* The UHC NHP, for example, offers dividend and shared-savings programs to participating nursing homes. A nursing home receives such payments when the facility successfully implements the clinical model and meets predetermined quality metrics. Throughout the Optum study period, 140 of the 189 (74 %) participating nursing homes received more than $8 million in quality incentive payments. (Quality incentive payments were not included in the payments described in the previous section.) The average payment was $452 per resident per year, or approximately $30,000 per year for a facility with 60 Optum CarePlus residents [11].

4. *Nursing homes receive enhanced reimbursement outside of traditional Medicare.* The UHC NHP reimbursement methodology reduces a facility's expense for Part A residents by paying separately for items generally included in Part A per diem payments received from traditional Medicare. The study considered a select number of enhanced reimbursement opportunities. Additional payments included but were not limited to:

   • *Blood glucose monitoring.* A service not traditionally billed to Medicare by facilities. UHC NHP provides reimbursement for all blood glucose monitoring services provided.
   • *Therapy screenings.* UHC NHP covers a limited number of physical and occupational therapy screenings on an annual basis.

• *Part A laboratory and radiology services.* Medicare skilled nursing facility payments include the cost of additional services, such as laboratory and imaging services. For UHC NHP members, laboratory and radiology providers bill the health plan directly for both Part A and Part B services. This reduces the facility's expense for Part A residents compared to traditional Medicare.

Other benefits include:
• More stable census
• Increased custodial days in the facility
• Opportunities to earn quality recognition payments
• Enhanced reimbursement for services typically not available to nursing homes

Finally, the Optum CarePlus model benefits nursing homes in several other tangential or indirect ways. Nursing home staffs receive additional training and mentoring that increases the skill level of the facility, enabling the treatment of more complex residents. This enhances a facility's viability as a partner to local hospitals for short-stay admissions. These factors, along with fewer transitions of care, can serve to improve public perception and marketability of the nursing home within the community.

Looking Forward with Optimism

I have been involved in medicine and healthcare for more than 25 years. Having witnessed, as all providers do, the dramatic clinical advances that science and innovation make possible, it is clear that we are overdue to dramatically advance how our medically complex elderly *experience* clinical care. Not simply what we can do, but how compassionately and intensively we do it.

The perfect storm where our aging US population intersects the incessant battle against chronic, multiple-comorbidity illness certainly demands it. The total US healthcare spend, dominated by acute care costs incurred in the later stages of life, is unsustainable and threatens substantive restraints on the effort to improve healthcare quality.

While we apply our best medical selves scientifically and technologically, let's be certain to spend equal resources working smart enough *to do no harm.* Considering everything negative that attends hospitalization within the nursing home population, are we truly focused on the best course of action for the resident?

As a medical resident in a major teaching hospital and during my time as an attending physician and a long-term care Medical Director, I witnessed many residents who were transferred from a nursing facility to an acute care setting. These residents often presented with ambulatory-care-sensitive conditions, meaning that their conditions required treatments that could have been provided at the nursing home, such as IV fluids, antibiotics, or oxygen.

It took little time to comprehend that frail older adults living in nursing homes can struggle as much from jarring care transitions as they do from the clinical changes that traditionally result in seemingly automatic hospitalization, even when inpatient care provides no value over what in-facility care can accomplish without exposing residents to middle-of-the-night ambulance transfers.

The ability to place a control on unnecessary inpatient services is complicated by intransigent policies, business systems, and even care-delivery structures that generate one complexity on top of another. The reality receiving the most attention in nursing homes is the tendency toward fragmented, non-coordinated care. But there is equal—perhaps greater—reverse momentum due to the lack of incentives to avoid hospitalization. From a patient experience perspective, reform-minded healthcare simply is fighting itself when Medicare and Medicaid payment systems incentivize hospitalization rather than treating members in the nursing care facility.

Despite the clarity about these and other causal factors—and the magnitude of progress urgently needed—discussions about improved care quality and cost reform seem more prevalent than actual, substantive, and permanent change. Optum CarePlus is a proven, collaborative, and treat-in-place care delivery and management model that transcends the obstacles of an overburdened healthcare system, as well as challenges inherent in caring for medically complex nursing home residents.

References

1. Stanton MW. the high concentration of U.S. Health Care Expenditures. Research in Action Issue 19. AHRQ Publication No. 06-0060, June 2006. Agency for Healthcare Research and Quality, Rockville, MD. http://www.ahrq.gov/research/ria19/expendria. html.
2. Palmer RM. Problems due to hospitalization. Merck Medical Manual; February 2009.
3. Caffrey Christine, CDC. "Potentially Preventable Emergency Department Visits by Nursing Home Residents: United States, 2004" NCHS Data Brief, No. 33, April 2010. http://www.cdc.gov/nchs/data/databriefs/db33.pdf.
4. Saliba D, Kington R, Buchanan J, Bell R, Wang M, Lee M, Herbst M, Lee D, Sur D, Rubenstein L. J Am Geriatr Soc. 2000;48(2):154–63.
5. Kane RL, Keckhafer G, et al. How Evercare nurse practitioners spend their time. J Am Geriatr Soc. 2001;49:1530–4.
6. Optum. Customer loyalty survey. Member Research Program; 2010.
7. Optum Data Analytics. INSPIRIS CarePlus outcomes study on acute admissions, based on claims savings for the large-patient pool programs in five markets; 2011.
8. Optum. *Perspectives* presentation by Rote and Coleman, Winter 2012.
9. Kane RL, Keckhafer G, et al. The effect of Evercare on hospital use. J Am Geriatr Soc. 2003;51:1427–34.
10. Kane, RL, Keckhafer G et al. 2003.
11. Optum. White paper. The impact of Optum™ CarePlus on nursing homes and residents; 2013.
12. Elijay. A report on shortfalls in Medicaid funding for nursing center care. Report for the American Health Care Association; 2012.

Program of All-Inclusive Care (PACE) Model

24

Lynne Morishita and Eileen M. Kunz

Introduction

PACE, the Program of All-inclusive Care of the Elderly, is a community-based alternative to a skilled nursing facility. PACE believes that older adults are better off when cared for in the community. To join PACE, participants must be deemed to meet a nursing home level of care. PACE covers all Medicare and Medicaid services and additional services as determined by the PACE Interdisciplinary Team (IDT), including fully integrated medical services, rehabilitation therapies, social services, transportation, and other supportive services. Research shows that PACE has the ability to care for those with multiple chronic health needs at a high level of quality and cost-effectiveness. The key to the model is adequate oversight, knowing the participants and being able to identify changes in these participants. In this way the care model helps prevent "avoidable" visits to the emergency room, hospital, or skilled nursing facility. By reducing the use of unnecessary and higher cost care, PACE programs are able to provide a broader and more intensive array of community-based services that in turn help prevent the exacerbation of chronic conditions and slow functional decline. This is population health management at its best.

History

PACE grew from a small community effort in San Francisco to a national Medicare and Medicaid option. Interdisciplinary from the start, the program was the brainchild of two immigrants, a Swiss social worker and a Chinese public health

L. Morishita, G.N.P., M.S.N. (✉)
Geriatric Health Care, Minneapolis, MN, USA
e-mail: moris002@umn.edu

E.M. Kunz, M.P.H.
On Lok Senior Health Services, San Francisco, CA, USA
e-mail: ekunz@onlok.org

dentist. Ongoing innovation created a new financing system and reached more and more frail older people. In 2014, 104 PACE programs operated in 31 states. Table 24.1 shows history highlights.

Population Served

To be eligible for PACE, individuals must be 55 years of age or older, meet their States' Medicaid eligibility criteria for nursing home level of care, reside in the PACE program's approved service area, and be able to live safely in the community at the point of enrollment. The typical PACE participant is aged and female, has multiple chronic conditions, and needs assistance in a number of activities of daily living, such as bathing, dressing, walking, toileting, and eating. In addition, many of these participants live alone. Table 24.2 describes the characteristics of the national PACE population in terms of age and gender, eligibility for public programs, and medical diagnosis [1, 2].

The vast majority of participants nationally are dually eligible for Medicare and Medicaid. The mix varies considerably from program to program depending on local communities' demographic characteristics. For example, among California PACE programs, the percentage of participants who are only eligible for Medi-Cal (California's Medicaid program) ranges from 6 to 27 % [3]. Some PACE programs serve a small percentage of participants who are eligible only for Medicare. These participants pay a premium equivalent to the capitation payment normally paid by Medicaid. Nationally, about 3 % of those enrolled in PACE in 2014 were eligible for Medicare only; about 40 % of PACE programs had no Medicare-only enrollees, but one suburban program had 14 % [4].

In an effort to help veterans with long-term care needs and expand the availability of PACE to non-Medicaid eligibles, the National PACE Association (NPA) and the US Department of Veterans Affairs have led collaboration between PACE programs and their local VA Medical Centers

Table 24.1 PACE history

1971	Dr. William Gee and Marie-Louise Ansak see needs of low-income older adults in San Francisco's Chinatown/North Beach, pursue comprehensive services through British Day Hospital model, and create On Lok ("peaceful abode") Senior Health Services.
1973–1974	On Lok's first adult day health care center opens, gains Medicaid reimbursement for adult day health care services.
1978–1979	On Lok adds comprehensive medical services, gets 4-year Health Care Financing Administration (HCFA) grant for consolidated model of health and social services.
1983	On Lok begins testing risk-based financing system with fixed rate per participant.
1986–1987	Federal legislation allows 10 other organizations to replicate On Lok's model; Robert Wood Johnson and John A. Hartford Foundations support replication start-up and technical assistance by On Lok.
1988	Program of All-inclusive Care for the Elderly or "PACE" becomes name for On Lok national replication.
1990	PACE replication sites begin 3-year Medicare and Medicaid waiver demonstration.
1994	On Lok and first replication sites form the National PACE Association (NPA), a national membership organization committed to advancing PACE for the benefit of vulnerable older adults.
1997	The Balanced Budget Act makes PACE model a permanent Medicare provider type and State Medicaid option.
2000	Robert Wood Johnson Foundation and John A. Hartford Foundation fund NPA's "PACE Expansion Initiative," work with state Medicaid agencies.
2006	The Deficit Reduction Act of 2005 authorizes start-up funding for 15 rural PACE programs.
2009	US Department of Veterans Affairs and NPA launch the "VA PACE Collaboration" to allow VA Medical Centers to purchase PACE services for Medicare only, nursing home-eligible veterans.

Adapted from National Pace Association http://www.npaonline.org/ website with permission

Table 24.2 PACE participant characteristics nationally

Age and gender	Percentage or number
Female	71 %
Average age of participants	77 years
Payor source	
Medicare and Medicaid (dual only)	90 %
Medicare only	3 %
Medicaid only	7 %
Community residence	
Participants residing at home/community	94 %
Participants residing in nursing home (permanent placement)	6 %
Acuity and frailty	
Average Medicare HCC Risk Score	2.37
Participants needing help with 3 or more ADLs	66 %
Participants needing help with 5 or more ADLs	42 %
Top 10 HCC diagnoses	*% with diagnosis*
Dementia (with and without complications)	47.2 %
Diabetes (with chronic complications and without complication)	46.1 %
Vascular disease	39.8 %
Heart failure	30.7 %
Chronic obstructive pulmonary disease	29.4 %
Major depressive, bipolar, and paranoid disorders	28.0 %
Polyneuropathy	25.3 %
Chronic kidney disease, moderate (stage 3)	23.3 %
Specified heart arrhythmias	21.6 %
CHF & renal disease (interactive diagnosis)	20.6 %

(VAMCs). As a result, 16 PACE programs had contracts with 10 VAMCs around the country in 2014. Although the relative numbers are small, this model holds promise for vulnerable individuals who can benefit from PACE but are not Medicaid eligible [5].

Pace Service Coordination and Delivery

The Interdisciplinary Team

The heart of the PACE model is the IDT. The core IDT team members include physicians, nurse practitioners (at some programs), nurses, physical therapists, occupational thera-pists, social workers, dieticians, recreation therapists and activity coordinators, home care coordinators, center managers, transportation staff, and personal care aides (also called health workers). Other disciplines, such as speech therapists and mental/behavioral health specialists, are available to the team to help address individual participant needs.

The IDT assesses the participant's needs at intake, at regular intervals, and when a significant change in condition occurs. This comprehensive assessment includes all aspects of the participants' health status and social situation, including medical conditions, functional status, and psychosocial and social support systems. The IDT then develops care plans for each participant that specify how often a participant comes to the PACE Center, how many hours of home care are given, and all other care to be received. The team tailors each plan to the person's unique needs and alters the plan quickly as conditions change. The team makes clinical decisions efficiently and does not need to receive prior authorization from an administrator. A caring, thoughtful, competent, and mature team offers the highest quality of service.

The whole continuum of care is provided in a comprehensive, integrated way. PACE offers preventive care (e.g., flu and pneumococcal vaccines), prescription drugs, over-the-counter medications, and durable medical equipment. PACE programs also contract with a full range of medical specialists (e.g., cardiologists, ophthalmologists, psychiatrists), inpatient acute care and long-term care providers, laboratory and radiology services, and emergency transportation, so these services are available when needed.

Setting

The IDT operates in a setting known as a PACE Center (a bricks-and-mortar structure housing a primary care clinic and adult day health care center) with PACE services delivered across all care settings, including the center, the participant's home, and inpatient facilities. In the PACE Center, participants receive primary care, nursing, social work, rehabilitation therapies, dietary counseling and personal care, and other services to maximize the participants' functional status and monitor chronic conditions. The PACE Center also provides recreation therapy and activity programs as well as congregate meals. In the co- located clinic area, participants can see their primary care physician, often a geriatrician, or a nurse practitioner. At some PACE Centers, specialty care such as dentistry, optometry, podiatry, and psychiatry are also available on-site. Socialization is encouraged and participants who are socially isolated and/or have dementia find this particularly helpful. The average PACE Center attendance for a participant is 2–3 days per week.

Some PACE programs also operate or contract with "alternative care settings." Alternative care settings have less than the full range of services that are required for the PACE Center; usually these are adult day care or adult day health care centers. The PACE Center IDT maintains responsibility for assessing care needs and coordinating care for participants attending alternative care settings.

When a participant needs care in the home, PACE provides a full range of in-home services, including home health care, personal care services, and home-delivered meals.

Interdisciplinary Team Operation

The IDT meets weekly for care planning purposes and during the week, in the morning, to review calls that took place the night before. The IDT's meeting is a very egalitarian discussion of care plans that are, and are not, working. For example, one morning the driver said, "Ms. Green is usually dressed and waiting, but she was not dressed today." Thus he alerted the team that "something is not right"—possibly signaling illness. The nurse practitioner took more history, examined the woman for signs of illness, and consulted the geriatrician. She treated the participant and avoided an ER visit and possibly hospitalization.

Communication is the key to positive outcomes and knowing the participants. All members of the team can make helpful observations. Knowing that they contribute to the team in this way makes their jobs more meaningful. A stable staff enables excellent, participant-centered care.

The IDT has many functions. The team educates members about the content presented; does interdisciplinary problem solving, with exchange of information from various points of view; undertakes interdisciplinary assessment of participants and problem-focused care planning; reviews cost/effectiveness of care plans; prevents duplication of interventions; assesses follow-through of plans and revises care plans; documents patient care; assures compliance with regulatory requirements; resolves conflicts; conducts ethical review of decision making; and establishes cultural competence [6].

An effective IDT has these characteristics: develops team cohesion and trust; uses limited time efficiently; clearly defines issues, interventions, and goals; follows up previous care plan; involves participants and caregivers; prepares in advance; uses concise summaries including recognition of stability; and adheres to the schedule [6].

Healthy IDT functioning is the most important part of developing PACE. Any education that maximizes team functions is useful. Practicing in an interdisciplinary fashion also requires specialized training for each member. Generally, the IDT defers to the person who has expertise in the issue. For example, if a participant has a swallowing problem, the speech therapist has the expertise and will be an essential member of the team. The role of the geriatrician is to provide pertinent medical information for the care plan and encourage team interaction. Communication on the team is usually respectful and courteous.

Case Examples

1. Mrs. Smith had some shortness of breath when lying down flat. The health worker noticed this, also observed more ankle edema than usual, and reported what he saw to the physician on call. In the morning the nurse practitioner had Mrs. Smith come to the PACE Center to be examined. The nurse practitioner noticed slight rales in the lungs and began a trial of medication to increase the pumping action of the heart and decrease heart failure; she consulted with the physician about treatment. Early observation and reporting of Mrs. Smith's symptoms avoided an expensive ER visit.

2. The social worker noted that Mrs. Romano had facial and right-sided weakness while at the PACE Center and alerted the nurse practitioner, who diagnosed a stroke and sent Mrs. Romano to the ER for emergency care. Observation of the change in condition and rapid treatment

with appropriate medical intervention may have reduced the severity of her stroke.

3. Mr. Robinson, who has dementia, was able to continue to live independently despite his cognitive impairment. He came each day to the PACE Center, where he received a meal, socialization, exercise, and medical care. Without the therapeutic community provided by PACE, he would have been forced to live in a nursing facility at more expense and with a poorer quality of life.

The PACE Center houses the IDT and having the team members "under one roof" facilitates coordination of care. Handoffs can be done well, ensuring continuity of care. As this model operates, the IDT stays informed and up to date on issues, the status of chronic illnesses, and treatment. The model works effectively because the whole team reports observations of when the "participant is not at the usual baseline self."

Although it is the personal touch that so often helps the participant, the electronic health records (EHR) can enhance the IDT communication and coordination. The EHR allows individual team members to review notes of others and develop interdisciplinary care goals more efficiently. In many systems, the individualized plan of care in the EHR is thought to be what keeps care coordination intact. In PACE, it is care providers who use tools in the EHR to keep care coordinated and hence ensure continuity of care.

Transitional Care

Transitional care is second nature for PACE staff. The IDT focuses on continuity of care at all transitions of settings. A plan of care for any transition is essential, particularly in regard to medications, and may require training of care providers. For example, if a participant being discharged from the hospital experiences disuse weakness, the physical therapy care plan and medications need to be coordinated.

PACE Funding

A key aspect of the PACE model is capitated financing with assumption of full financial risk by the PACE program for all services needed by PACE participants, including long-term nursing home care, if necessary. Capitated financing affords PACE programs the flexibility to design individualized care plans for PACE participants based on need rather than traditional Medicare and Medicaid payment rules. It also enables PACE programs to use savings achieved by preventing avoidable inpatient utilization to provide a more comprehensive and intensive range of long-term services and supports in the community, such as ongoing therapies to maintain function. PACE programs receive capitation payments from Medicare,

Medicaid, and/or individual participants based on each participant's eligibility for public programs.

The method for determining capitation payments for PACE programs has evolved as PACE has become a permanent provider, and the Centers for Medicare and Medicaid Services (CMS) and State Medicaid agencies have developed more sophisticated approaches to rate setting for Medicare Advantage and Medicaid managed care plans. From 1983 to the present, policy issues facing PACE programs have included whether Medicare and Medicaid rate-setting methodologies generate payment rates that reflect the costs of the population served, are adequate for program viability, and provide payers a cost-effective option relative to other institutional and community-based alternatives.

In 2004, CMS began phasing in its Hierarchical Condition Category (HCC) model to determine payments to PACE for Medicare Part A and B covered services. This model risk adjusts payments based on beneficiaries' diagnostic and demographic characteristics. It added considerable complexity, requiring PACE programs to submit individual-level diagnostic data to CMS. In particular, PACE physicians had to learn the intricacies of Medicare diagnostic coding to ensure the accuracy of Medicare payments to PACE programs.

The CMS-HCC model does not fully account for the variation in Medicare costs for the functionally impaired PACE population, so PACE payments include an adjustment for participants' frailty. With the phase-in of CMS-HCC, CMS implemented an organization-level PACE frailty adjustor based on the results of the Health Outcome Survey—Modified (HOS-M), administered annually to PACE participants. A total risk score, computed by adding this frailty adjustor to each participant's HCC risk score, is then multiplied by the county payment rate. In 2014, for PACE nationally, the average Medicare Parts A and B payment per member per month was $2,218 (before the 2 % sequestration reduction) [1].

Since its inception, PACE has covered over-the-counter and prescription drugs as part of the PACE benefit package. In 2006, Medicare implemented its Part D benefit and, for PACE programs, prescription drug reimbursement shifted from Medicaid to Medicare. Although CMS waived certain requirements, PACE programs had to become Medicare Part D Prescription Drug plans and adhere to numerous Part D requirements. CMS' Rx-HCC risk-adjustment model for the Medicare Part D program adjusts a portion of Part D payments paid to PACE programs. As with the CMS-HCC model, payments depend on beneficiaries' demographic and diagnostic characteristics, but the specific risk factors differ and payments have several additional components. PACE programs submit Medicare Part D bids annually with these payments subject to an annual reconciliation process.

State Medicaid agencies determine Medicaid payments for PACE, in consultation with their PACE program(s).

While CMS establishes requirements for Medicaid rate setting, states vary in their rate-setting approaches, reflecting the variation in their Medicaid programs. In general, states identify a comparable long-term care population and calculate total Medicaid per beneficiary per month costs for this population. During the PACE demonstration, the nursing home resident population provided the usual comparison since few community-based alternatives to institutional care existed. As such alternatives have increased, states have moved to a blend of nursing home residents and recipients of home and community-based services. Identifying an appropriate comparison group for rate-setting purposes has become increasingly challenging. The PACE monthly rate cannot exceed the comparison group's monthly per capita cost; the PACE rate is often substantially lower.

Despite interest in improving the accuracy of Medicaid payments, risk adjustment for Medicaid payments exists in just a handful of states. In 2014, nationally, for PACE the average Medicaid payment per member per month for dual-eligible participants was $3,557 [4]. For Medicaid-only participants, the average PACE Medicaid payment, which covers both medical care and long-term services and support, was $5,633 [4].

A participant who qualifies for Medicare and Medicaid has no co-payment or deductibles for PACE. Depending on income, they may have a share of cost to meet Medicaid eligibility. A participant not qualified for Medicaid pays a premium to cover the PACE long-term care benefit and to cover Part D for prescriptions. Participants have no deductible or co-payment for any drugs or treatment approved by the PACE IDT. If a participant needs long-term skilled nursing facility care—and 6 % do at any given time—PACE pays the bill and the team continues to coordinate care for these participants.

Regulatory Framework

During the national PACE demonstration, the PACE model used operational guidelines documented by On Lok, in collaboration with CMS and the initial PACE demonstration programs. As the first PACE replication sites prepared for implementation, CMS (then the Health Care Financing Administration) turned to On Lok to help define the central tenets of On Lok's PACE model. The resulting PACE Protocol, by design, included provisions offering flexibility: Certain requirements could be waived if variations met local needs and the spirit of the requirement. When the first PACE programs completed their demonstration periods, On Lok worked with their leaders to update the PACE Protocol. The Balanced Budget Act of 1997 referenced the updated version of the PACE Protocol, which then formed the basis for the PACE regulation promulgated in 1999.

Because PACE is a provider-based managed care organization, the PACE regulation includes administrative requirements typical for managed care organizations and operational requirements more typical for health care provider entities. Managed care requirements include enrollment and disenrollment, participant rights, grievances and appeals, provider contracting, administration, payment, and financial solvency. Provider requirements speak to minimum requirements for the PACE Center, IDT assessment, reassessment and care planning, physical environment, infection control, and quality assurance and improvement. PACE programs also must comply with Medicare Part D regulation. CMS, in conjunction with State Medicaid agencies, conducts routine audits of PACE programs to determine compliance with PACE regulatory requirements.

Many State Medicaid agencies have additional requirements for PACE. Some have contracts in addition to the three-way PACE program agreement. States are responsible for determining licensing requirements for PACE.

PACE programs have voiced concerns about the regulatory burden accompanying the transition from demonstration to permanent provider status. The 1999 PACE regulation included more stringent requirements than those in the revised PACE Protocol, putting successful PACE replication sites and On Lok, the model's prototype, in conflict with some new requirements. For example, in the mid-1990s, On Lok developed an innovative subcontracting model; it leveraged the expertise of an experienced local health care provider to expand PACE services throughout San Francisco without building an additional PACE Center. When CMS viewed this model as noncompliant with the 1999 regulations, Congress amended the PACE federal statute (as part of the Benefits Improvement and Protection Act of 2000 or BIPA) to give CMS greater authority to waive certain requirements and to grandfather operational practices in place at On Lok and the PACE replication sites. In 2002, the revised PACE regulation implemented the new statutory requirements. Since then, CMS has approved numerous BIPA waiver requests from PACE programs, e.g., to allow for use of community-based primary care physicians in place of staff physicians on the PACE IDT.

PACE Growth and Expansion

When the Balanced Budget Act of 1997 established PACE as a permanent Medicare provider and voluntary state option under Medicaid, 22 PACE programs had Medicare and Medicaid demonstration waiver authority with additional programs under development. In early 2014, 104 PACE programs were serving 31,654 nursing-home-eligible PACE participants nationally and an additional 18 new PACE provider applications were under CMS review [7]. Expansion of

PACE to rural communities has fueled some of this growth. In the last 5 years, PACE enrollment has increased by 87 %.

In the 31 states with PACE programs, the number of programs varies from 1 to 18. Pennsylvania has the most number of programs (18); 5 states have between 7 and 9; and 15 states have only 1. Sustained support and leadership by some state Medicaid agencies has been a key factor in expanding PACE. Several states, including Kansas, Louisiana, Pennsylvania, and Virginia, have used request for proposal (RFPs) processes to identify prospective PACE providers.

Since forming in 1994, NPA has represented its membership and encouraged PACE growth nationally. NPA collects data about PACE operations, helps to develop PACE, and has a range of tools and guides for development to assess the community, the capacity to develop the network needed for PACE, and financial feasibility (e.g., a potential PACE organization's access to start-up funds). In addition, PACE Medical Directors have led NPA's Primary Care Committee and created Preventative Care Guidelines and evidence-based clinical guidelines for diabetes mellitus, dementia, heart failure, chronic kidney disease, and chronic obstructive pulmonary disease (COPD).

State associations of PACE programs also have encouraged PACE growth. In 2007, the first state PACE association, CalPACE, formed in California. CalPACE has worked with the state Medicaid agency to streamline regulatory barriers to PACE growth and coordinate PACE programs on state policy issues. Between 2007 and 2014, the number of California PACE programs grew from four to ten, after 11 years without any new programs. By 2014, eight active state PACE associations existed around the country with a few more in development.

The average enrollment in a PACE program in 2014 was 325 participants, but five programs in heavily populated urban areas had more than 1,000 enrolled, the largest with 3,813. All of the larger programs operate five or more PACE Centers in their service areas, with three using alternative care settings to broaden their geographic reach and offer specialized care settings. Two have CMS-approved waivers to collaborate with community primary care physicians [8].

Of the original 14 rural PACE programs in 2008, 11 still are in operation. Rural PACE programs serve an average of about 130 participants each. Rural programs have successfully employed special waivers of the PACE regulations to use existing community resources. Six have CMS-approved community primary care physician waivers (among the other 93 PACE programs, just seven have such waivers). Rural communities have fewer individuals who are eligible to enroll in PACE, but they also have fewer other long-term services and supports. One rural program, Senior Comm Unity Care in Montrose, Colorado, serves approximately 260 individuals. It has enrolled 25 % of the potentially eligible individuals in its service area and has waivers to use community primary care physicians and alternative care settings [7].

Pace Outcomes

PACE has been recognized as an effective model of person-centered care for individuals with multiple chronic conditions, and functional and/or cognitive impairments. Positive outcomes attributed to PACE include improved health status, lower utilization of inpatient services, and high rates of consumer satisfaction. PACE also has been identified as one of the three primary care models with the greatest potential for improving the care for older adults with multiple chronic conditions [9]. Integral to PACE are all four primary care processes linked to quality and cost-effective care: (1) comprehensive assessment, (2) comprehensive care planning with proactive monitoring, (3) communication and coordination of professionals involved in care, and (4) promoting active engagement of individuals and their family caregivers in care.

The Administration of Community Living's (ACL) Aging and Disability Evidence-Based Programs and Practices and SAMHSA's (Substance Abuse and Mental Health Services Administration) National Registry of Evidence-Based Programs identify the PACE model as an evidence-based program [10, 11]. Table 24.3 summarizes the ACL/SAMHSA, 2007 and 2012, positive outcomes.

A recent study of 61 PACE programs found hospitalization rates for PACE participants substantially lower compared

Table 24.3 PACE outcomes

Outcome category	Findings
Utilization of medical services	• Lower rates of hospital use • Lower rates of nursing home use • Lower rates of emergency department use • Higher utilization of ambulatory services
Utilization of support services	• Higher use of adult day care services • Less likely to require a home visit by nurse
Health and functional status, quality of life, mortality	• Better reported quality of life and health status • Less deterioration in physical functioning • Lower mortality rate
Care management	• More likely to have advanced care directives • Less likely to have pain interference with normal activities • Fewer unmet needs in getting around and dressing
Health status, functioning, mental health	• Better reported health status • Fewer depressive symptoms
Preventative health services	• More likely to have vision and hearing screening • More likely to have influenza vaccinations

Data from Administration for Community Living (ACL) http://www.acl.gov/Programs/CDAP/OPE/docs/PACE_InterventionSummary.pdf, accessed 26 Aug 2014 and Substance Abuse and Mental Health Services Administration (SAMHSA), http://www.nrepp.samhsa.gov/ViewIntervention.aspx?id=316, accessed 26 Aug 2014

to dually eligible nursing home (NH) residents and home and community-based service (HCBS) waiver enrollees, 24 % and 43 % lower, respectively [12]. Readmission rates for PACE matched those of the general Medicare fee-for-service population, a much healthier population, and were 16 % lower than for the dually eligible population 65 years of age and older (19.3 % versus 22 %). Rates of potentially avoidable hospitalizations (PAH) for PACE compared to nursing home residents and HCBS enrollees were 44 % and 60 % lower, respectively. Rates of PAH for PACE for certain chronic conditions, COPD, heart failure, and asthma, and for urinary tract infections and dehydration were substantially lower than for the HCBS population. The provider-based nature of the PACE model, with opportunity for frequent contact, may account for these differences.

PACE succeeds in supporting the participant preference for living in the community and avoiding permanent nursing home placement. Although all PACE participants are certified as eligible for a nursing home level of care, only 6 % resided permanently in nursing homes in 2014. In addition, the vast majority of PACE participants remain enrolled in PACE for the last years of their lives.

Are PACE participants satisfied with the program? Research studies report high rates of consumer satisfaction [1, 10, 11]. PACE does not use a national consumer satisfaction survey such as CAHPS (Consumer Assessment of Health Plans), but PACE programs must conduct satisfaction surveys of their members. Some programs use state-required survey tools; and others use independently developed surveys.

In 2006, California PACE programs identified the need for a consumer survey tool that considered the integrated model of care and full spectrum of medical and long-term care services provided by PACE. CalPACE, the state association of California PACE programs, contracted with an expert in satisfaction measurement for frail, cognitively impaired populations to develop and test a satisfaction tool designed for PACE. Testing showed that face-to-face interviews were the only reliable means of assessing satisfaction for the PACE population, recognizing that many vulnerable older adults have difficulty completing mail and phone satisfaction surveys. Since 2008, California PACE programs have contracted with an independent survey firm to conduct an annual satisfaction survey. Face-to-face interviews of a sample of PACE participants at each PACE program occur in multiple languages, including English, Spanish, Chinese, and Korean, reflecting the primary languages spoken by PACE participants in California. In 2013, 91 % of participants reported being very satisfied with the program and 94 % said that they would refer a close friend or relative to the program [13]. Participants had high rates of satisfaction, too, for services not traditionally considered, such as transportation (95 %), home care (91 %), center aides (94 %), and social work (93 %), as well as for medical care services (92 %) [13].

Another important measure of satisfaction with the PACE program is voluntary disenrollment rates. Although PACE participants may disenroll from the program at any time, few do so due to dissatisfaction with the program. A 2006 study found the disenrollment rate for PACE programs to be 7.7 %, a much lower rate than is typical for Medicare managed care plans [14].

ACA Implications

The Affordable Care Act (ACA) has launched a transformation of the health care system with the goals of improving the health of communities and populations, improving the quality and satisfaction for individuals, and reducing health care costs. The ACA has expanded health care insurance coverage and launched initiatives aimed at meeting these goals.

PACE, a proven model of provider-based managed care, encompasses many of the principles included in these ACA initiatives. All PACE participants are assigned a health home responsible for providing primary care and coordinating all aspects of the participants. The PACE IDT includes the primary care physician and other professionals directly involved in the participant's care. There is a focus on prevention with close monitoring and early intervention to prevent exacerbation of chronic conditions. PACE programs are fully accountable for both the cost and quality of care which facilitates providing the right care, in the right place, and at the right time. PACE assists individuals at risk of institutionalization to maintain their independence and remain in their homes and communities as long as possible.

The ACA has expanded insurance coverage through broadening Medicaid and creating federal and state health insurance exchanges, so previously uninsured individuals can purchase insurance. The sustainability of these ACA coverage initiatives rests with reforming the health delivery system, particularly for individuals with multiple chronic conditions. PACE has demonstrated its success in improving care for this population. Expanding fully integrated primary care models like PACE will be critical to the success of the ACA in the long term.

The ACA created the Medicare-Medicaid Coordination Office and Centers for Medicare and Medicaid Innovations. CMS has launched initiatives designed to improve coordination of care for dual eligibles, particularly those needing long-term services and supports, the population that PACE serves. Some states are now implementing joint federal-state initiatives as part of the CMS' Financial Alignment Demonstration [15]. Among them, a number have at least one operating PACE program and participating states include four of the five largest PACE programs. In some, PACE is an option in the implementation of the Financial Alignment Demonstration. Additional states are moving forward with initiatives to implement long-term services and supports under managed care. PACE offers a more person-centered, provider-based managed care alternative to the large traditional managed care programs and is specifically designed to address the needs of these vulnerable populations.

Conclusion

PACE is a community-based alternative to a skilled nursing facility. This model provides integrated primary care, preventive care, acute care, and long-term services and supports via capitation payments. The key to this model is a high-functioning IDT. PACE provides health services, therapies, and social services in a coordinated way. This model provides high-quality care that is cost-effective community-based services for a particularly high-risk population. Participant satisfaction ratings are high. This proven model offers a path to better coordinated care in transforming the financing and care delivery system for vulnerable individuals and maintaining their functional status. Maintaining functional status equals high quality of life.

References

1. National PACE Association. DataPACEII Quarter 4 2013 Report, Run Date: 30 Jun 2014. The percent of PACE participants needing assistance in Activities of Daily Living (ADLs) is calculated from 2013 Health Outcome Survey-M (HOS-M), Frailty Adjustment Report for the 45 PACE organizations reporting this information to NPA. The HOS-M survey only collects data for PACE participants who are eligible for Medicare.
2. National PACE Association. Top 20 HCCs report and medicare risk scores and payments report. PACE Data Analyst Center (PDAC) report. 2014.
3. CalPACE. Outcome and quality measures for California PACE Programs. 2014.
4. National PACE Association. PACE census and capitation rate information, calendar year 2014.
5. National PACE Association. http://www.npaonline.org/website/article.asp?id=3305&title=Veterans_Administration_and_PACE. Accessed 30 Aug 2014.
6. National PACE Association. http://www.npaonline.org/.
7. National PACE Association. What role can PACE play in state and federal efforts to reform managed long-term services and supports issue brief. 2014.
8. National PACE Association. National PACE Association. PACE Census and Capitation Rate Information, PACE Waiver Survey Results. 2014.
9. Boult C, Wieland D. Comprehensive primary care for older patients with multiple chronic conditions: 'Nobody Rushes You Through'. JAMA. 2010;304(17):1936–43.
10. Administration for Community Living (ACL). http://www.acl.gov/Programs/CDAP/OPE/docs/PACE_InterventionSummary.pdf. Accessed 26 Aug 2014.
11. Substance Abuse and Mental Health Services Administration (SAMHSA). http://www.nrepp.samhsa.gov/ViewIntervention.aspx?id=316. Accessed 26 Aug 2014.
12. Segelman M, Szydlowski J, Kinosian B, McNabney M, Raziano D, Eng C, van Reenen C, Temkin-Greener H. Hospitalizations in the program of all-inclusive care for the elderly. J Am Geriatric Soc. 2014;62:320–4.
13. Vital Research. PACE participant satisfaction report, sixth reporting period. 2013.
14. Temkin-Greener H, Bajorska A, Mukamel DB. Disenrollment from an Acute/Long-Term Managed Care Program (PACE). Med Care. 2006;44(1):31–8.
15. Centers for Medicare and Medicaid Services (CMS). Financial Alignment Initiative. http://www.cms.gov/Medicare-Medicaid-Coordination/Medicare-and-Medicaid-Coordination/Medicare-Medicaid-Coordination-Office/FinancialAlignmentInitiative/ApprovedDemonstrationsSignedMOUs.html. Accessed 2 Sep 2014.

Wisconsin's Family Care Model

25

Stephanie Sue Stein and Thomas L. Frazier

Introduction

There are two conflicting and powerful messages heard by caregivers of older people. From mom, aunt, grandfather, or sister the caregiver hears, "I want to stay in my home." From physician, discharge planner, minister, and neighbor the son or daughter hears, "your mom should not be living alone."

Discerning what to do and where to get help with decision making and care is a dilemma faced by scores of family members every day. The considerations are complex and bewildering. They include respecting the wishes of a loved one, personal safety, proximity to caregivers, available resources, and in many states limited public options for long-term care.

In Wisconsin all older people and their caregivers have the availability of free and reliable information, assistance, and options counseling. In most of Wisconsin they have the option of staying at home with supports and services. We call this Family Care.

The Problem (The First Generation)

Wisconsin's Family Care program may best be described as the second generation of efforts in the state to reform or "redesign" its long-term care programs. The first generation in the early 1980s was called the Community Options Program (COP), and initially was totally funded with state General Purpose Revenue (GPR), or state tax dollars. At that time, and, still today, the Medicaid program was funded with

60 % of federal money and 40 % of state money. The big problem was that while Medicaid was the biggest and practically the only source of funding to help pay for long-term care, it would only pay for that care in a nursing home. Another problem was that in order to be eligible for Medicaid, a person had to have very little income or assets.

The COP idea was to use the state 40 % matching money to fund home and community-based long-term care services based on the premise that if a person could be supported at home for approximately the 40 % of state cost, then it was not only what was desirable by the recipient but also cost effective from the state's perspective. This worked pretty well and received some national attention for Wisconsin as a leader in long-term care reform. Eventually, the state Medicaid agency applied for federal waivers to match state funds with federal money, which would increase the total amount of funding for home and community care as an alternative to institutional care. These waivers became known as the COP-Waiver and the Community Integration Program (CIP)-Waiver.

There was, however, another major problem with the waivers; they had only a specified amount of total funding resulting in waiting lists when funds were exhausted while Medicaid funding for nursing homes remained an entitlement (i.e., if you were eligible, money was available from Medicaid to pay for nursing home care). As an entitlement, Medicaid funding for nursing home care received first draw on state tax dollars with the COP and CIP waiver programs receiving funding depending on the health of the state budget and the effectiveness of advocates to get additional money for home and community care.

But the possibility and cost-effectiveness of home and community care led advocates to call for long-term care reform. In 1995 a coalition of advocates for frail older persons and people with disabilities developed a proposal which they called "Keeping the Community Promise: A Comprehensive, Coordinated Long-Care System for Wisconsin." Their timing was good and the new Secretary of the Wisconsin Department of Health and Family Services

S.S. Stein, M.A.P.S. (✉)
Milwaukee County Department on Aging,
1220 W. Viliet, 3rd Floor, Milwaukee, WI 53205, USA
e-mail: stephanie.stein@milwaukeecountywi.gov

T.L. Frazier, B.A., M.P.A.
Coalition of Wisconsin Aging Groups (Retired), Verona,
WI 53593, USA
e-mail: TomFrazier21@gmail.com

M.L. Malone et al. (eds.), *Geriatrics Models of Care: Bringing 'Best Practice' to an Aging America*,
DOI 10.1007/978-3-319-16068-9_25, © Springer International Publishing Switzerland 2015

stated that "Long-Term Care Redesign" would be one of his top priorities. The beginning of the second generation of long-term care reform was under way.

Family Care (The Second Generation)

Long-term care redesign meant that the Department of Health and Family Services (DHFS) convened all the stakeholders, including advocates, providers, and various agency representatives, charged with coming up with recommendations for a new way of delivering Medicaid long-term care programs in Wisconsin. There was agreement about the need for change but many different ideas about how to make it happen. One major area of disagreement was over whether or not to have an integrated system including primary health care and long-term care, or to limit the redesign to only long-term care programs. Advocates for including only long-term care programs eventually prevailed.

Advocates for the frail elderly and people with disabilities wanted to create a system that would give people choices about where to receive services (in the community or a nursing home) and eliminate waiting lists for home and community care. This meant having equal access to Medicaid funds for both instead of an entitlement for one and a waiting list for the other.

After months and years of "redesigning" long-term care programs in Wisconsin, Governor Tommy Thompson included "Family Care" in his 1999–2001 state budget to be implemented as a five-county pilot project. With a few changes in the program during the budget process, Family Care began in 2000 in the counties of Milwaukee, Fond du Lac, Richland, Portage, and La Crosse.

Family Care is a federally approved Medicaid waiver program consisting of two components: an Aging and Disability Resource Center (ADRC) and a Managed Care Organization (MCO). The ADRC is a one-stop shopping center for Information and Assistance (I&A) for older persons and people with disabilities and their families regarding all programs and services that may be available to assist them. There is no cost for assistance and no income eligibility criteria.

The MCO is a managed care agency that receives a capitation rate to provide long-term care supports and services for each eligible person enrolled in the MCO (Family Care). The capitation rate is an average per member per month (PMPM) payment to MCOs from the state across the three target populations (frail elderly, physically disabled, and developmentally disabled). Some people may require more services at a higher cost than the capitation rate, but this may be offset by a person who needs fewer services and, therefore, a lower cost than the capitation rate. A person must meet Medicaid income eligibility requirements and be in need of long-term care (usually defined as a nursing home

level of care). These requirements also apply to the COP and CIP waiver programs.

An individual assessment for each Family Care enrollee determines what services they need, and may include a wide range of home and community services and nursing home care, thereby creating the same entitlement (and funding) for all services. The services depend on specific outcomes and goals of the enrollee and his/her family.

Family Care: How Does It Work and What Does It Offer

Family Care is two distinct and very different programs. In order to get the services and supports available the consumer or the consumer's family must first call or visit the local ADRC. Every county (72) in Wisconsin is served by an ADRC. Twenty-eight of them are single-county operations and 14 are multicounty. The ADRC's services are free and available to all. There are no income or eligibility requirements for any ADRC function. The basic services are as follows:

- *Information and assistance.* Includes information about any and every program or agency which serves older persons and persons with disabilities. Every ADRC has at least one person certified by the Alliance of Information and Referral Systems (AIRS) as an "I and A" Specialist. In Milwaukee all persons providing phone or walk in assistance are certified. The ADRCs all use and maintain a central database of services which is accessible to the public at the ADRC's websites. Calls to the ADRC are often easily answered, such as where is my nearest senior center or where do I apply for disability benefits. Others are complex and often begin with statements like "I am very worried about my mother, she seems to be slipping, or my son is graduating from high school and with his challenges we don't know what he will do." In 2012 the ADRCs recorded 422,052 contacts. For a complete description of contacts and a breakdown of what they mean please see the ADRC activity report for 2012 which can be accessed at http://www.dhs.wisconsin.gov/adrc/professionals/pubsstatsandother/index.htm.
- *Options counseling.* While a person is discussing issues with an I and A Specialist, it may become clear that there is a need for an in-person discussion about long-term care options. Often a referral for options counseling comes from community providers who recognize a need for more care. They may include hospital discharge planners, home health nurses, public health professionals, senior companions, or neighborhood volunteers. A social worker then calls the person who wants a visit and arranges to meet at the home, skilled nursing facility, or anywhere else the person wishes. Family members are often a part of these options counseling visits, and, if a guardian is in place, the guardian also must be there.

Options counseling is available for all persons without regard to income. One of the goals of Family Care is to help people understand all of the services and supports available in the community, the relative costs of those supports, and the availability of public support once they have spent their assets. With accurate information about all available choices, consumers can avoid the need for public support and make wise choices about their care.

If options counselors and the consumer decide they would like to enroll in publicly funded long-term care, the social worker will administer the Long-Term Care Functional Screen (LTC FS). The screen is an automated and objective way to determine eligibility. The LTC FS measures ADLs, IADLs, cognitive ability, medical diagnoses, mental health substance abuse, and behavioral issues. Persons administering the screen must become certified by passing an online exam and are periodically retested. The screen measures a person's risk for institutionalization in a nursing home. Once completed, the screener can immediately see the applicant's level of care and if they are functionally eligible.

Once eligibility is determined, the counselor can discuss financial eligibility and Wisconsin's publically funded long-term programs. Often these programs are collectively referred to as Family Care but they are in fact very unique.

The consumer must then apply for and be determined eligible for Medicaid. This function is performed by another group of public employees. Once this eligibility is determined, the consumer will again discuss options and can choose to enroll in a program. The ADRC staff then completes the forms and enrolls the person in the program or the MCO of his/her choice.

If a person is not happy with their choice he/she may disenroll and choose another program at any time. This process is also handled by the ADRC where the person receives counseling and then decides what to do.

- *Benefit specialists.* The resource centers house both Elder Benefit Specialists and Disability Benefit specialists. These specialists are available to all consumers to assist them in accessing public benefit programs like Social Security, SSI, Veteran's Benefits, Medical Assistance, and Family Care. The Benefit Specialist program is unique to Wisconsin and information about it can be found at www.dhs.wisconsin.gov/benefit-specialist/index.htm.
- *Wellness and prevention.* Evidence-based wellness and prevention programs also are offered through the ADRCs. They include Living Well with Chronic Conditions (Stanford), Living Well with Diabetes, Stepping On and A Matter of Balance (fall prevention), and Powerful Tools for Caregivers. These classes are offered in conjunction with hospital systems, senior centers, public housing, and public health departments.

The Second Part of Family Care Is the Benefit Package Provided by the MCO

Once a person chooses a program he/she will be assigned a nurse and a social worker.

The nurse, social worker, consumer, other family members, and often specialized therapists will make up that person's Family Care team. The team will discuss and agree on personal outcomes for each member. The team will then use resource allocation tools to determine a plan. The MCO will then authorize services and payment. The Family Care benefit package is extensive and unique. It includes all traditional home and community-based services such as adult day care, supportive home care, transportation, bathing services, financial management and medication management, home modification, vocational counseling, employment assistance, and much more. It includes Medicaid card services related to long-term care, including personal care; home health; physical, occupational, and speech therapy; durable medical equipment; disposable medical equipment; mental health services; and skilled nursing care in a facility. It includes the service part of residential options in assisted living, group homes, adult family homes, and supported apartments. A benefit that everyone receives is case management provided by their social worker/nurse team.

Acute and primary care services are not part of the Family Care benefit but medical coordination is part of the team's responsibility.

Family Care: 15 Years of Progress

All five pilot projects started in 2000 and were all operated by county governments. Milwaukee County initially served only frail elders while the other four counties served all three target groups. The first step in implementing Family Care was to transition everyone from the COP and CIP waivers to the Family Care waiver program. At the same time, each county began to gradually eliminate the waiting lists in their county. Initially, the phaseout of waiting lists took 2 years at which time waiting lists were completely eliminated.

Most, if not all, of the pilot counties struggled with finances under the capitation rates since it was a totally different way of operating from the old waiver programs. But, all were eventually successful in meeting the financial standards for an MCO, eliminating waiting lists, and providing consumers with choices regarding where and when to access long-term care services.

Table 25.1 Total Medicaid costs

Total Medicaid expenditures per member per month CY 2003–2004			
Service category	Family care	Comparison group counterpart	Significant difference
Non-Milwaukee Family Care	$2,656	$3,108	***
Non-Milwaukee Family Care FE	$2,227	$2,501	**
Milwaukee Family Care FE	$2,446	$2,501	*
Non-Milwaukee Family Care DD	$3,534	$4,548	***
Non-Milwaukee Family Care PD	$2,136	$2,404	**

From APS Healthcare, Inc., Family Care Independent Assessment: An Evaluation of Access, Quality and Cost-Effectiveness for Calendar Year 2003–2004, October 7, 2005, with permission
Level of significance: $*p<0.1$, $**p<0.05$, $***p<0.01$

The big breakthrough occurred in October 2005 when APS Healthcare produced the first Independent Assessment of the five Family Care pilot projects [1] The assessment not only showed improved functional outcomes and high consumer satisfaction, but, most importantly for political reasons, it showed a Medicaid cost saving of as much as $452 per member per month (PMPM). See Table 25.1.

This Independent Assessment led Governor Jim Doyle to call for the statewide expansion of Family Care in his January 2006 State of the State address. Family Care expansion was off and running. However, leaders in DHFS wanted to make some changes. They were not convinced that individual counties were up to the challenge of implementing such a complex new way of doing things, and wanted to develop regional MCOs that could implement Family Care in several counties, especially smaller counties. And, many counties were more than willing to get out of the long-term care business and avoid any financial risk associated with the capitation rates. DHFS discouraged counties from competing to be MCOs and instead encouraged applications for expansion from nonprofit MCOs that had developed by operating PACE (Program for All-Inclusive Care for the Elderly; see also Chap. 25) and the Partnership Program (similar to the PACE program).

The results of expansion have been impressive. Family Care is now operational in 57 out of 72 counties in Wisconsin with Governor Scott Walker recently announcing plans to include seven more counties in northeastern Wisconsin in the program. Rock County's Board of Supervisors passed a resolution stating its intent to transition to Family Care as soon as possible. This leaves only seven counties which continue to show little interest in Family Care with only one county (Dane) having a large population. The seven counties have a total waiting list of 755 people with Dane County having over 45 % of that total.

Evaluations and Reports on Family Care

Family Care has been one of the most studied and evaluated long-term care programs in the country. On the Wisconsin Department of Health Services website the following "Evaluations of Family Care" are listed with links to all the reports: (1) Long-term Care Expansion Report (December 2013), (2) April 2011 Legislative Audit Bureau Report: An Evaluation of Family Care, (3) Family Care Financial Evaluation (APS Healthcare 2010), (4) Family Care Independent Assessment (APS Healthcare, 2005), and (5) Family Care Implementation Process (The Lewin Group 2003, 2002, 2001, 2000). In addition, there are four External Quality Review Reports from MetaStar, Inc., Membership Satisfaction Surveys for the last 5 years, DHS Annual Reports for the last 6 years, and Quarterly Financial Summaries from 2008 to 2014.

The 2005 APS Healthcare Independent Assessment was most significant because it resulted in the decision by Governor Doyle to expand Family Care statewide. "The goal of the Independent Assessment is to describe the impact the Family Care program has had on long-term services in Wisconsin in terms of access to services, quality of services and cost-effectiveness during calendar years 2003 and 2004" according to the APS Healthcare Executive Summary. As Table 25.1 of the assessment shows, there was a total Medicaid cost of $452 less per member per month (PMPM) for the non-Milwaukee Family Care counties versus the comparison group. The Milwaukee County Frail Elderly also significantly outperformed their comparison group counterpart by $274 PMPM. The biggest cost difference was $1,014 PMPM less for people with developmental disabilities in non-Milwaukee counties than for comparable persons in non-Family Care counties [1]. (Note: In 2003 and 2004 there were only five pilot counties and Milwaukee County only

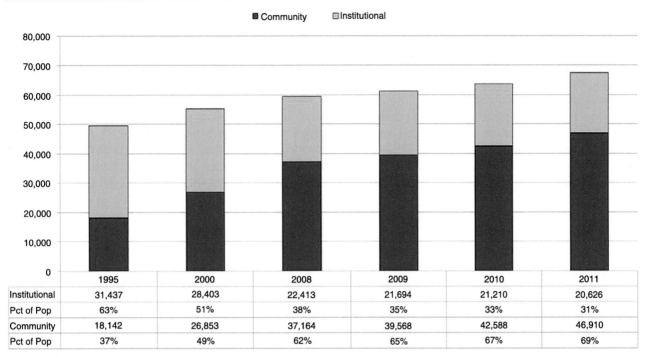

	1995	2000	2008	2009	2010	2011
Institutional	31,437	28,403	22,413	21,694	21,210	20,626
Pct of Pop	63%	51%	38%	35%	33%	31%
Community	18,142	26,853	37,164	39,568	42,588	46,910
Pct of Pop	37%	49%	62%	65%	67%	69%

* Institutional population includes managed long-term care members residing in a nursing home or ICF-IDD.

Fig. 25.1 Publicly funded adult long-term care population 1995, 2000, 2008–2011 (end of year counts) (from Wisconsin Department of Health Services, Joint Committee on Finance, Long-Term Care Expansion Report, December 13, 2013, with permission)

served the frail elderly.) Another important financial finding of the APS Healthcare IA was that Family Care also saved money on acute and primary care as well as long-term care. "The path analysis revealed that Family Care produces Medicaid savings both directly by controlling service costs and indirectly by favorably affecting Family Care members' health and abilities to function so that they have less need for services" [1].

In regard to quality of care, the APS report (2005) noted that "Overall, the Independent Assessment findings suggest that Family Care continues to improve the quality of long-term care services in its counties. Waiting lists for services have been eliminated for over three years, achievement of member outcomes remains high, and each CMO has continued to improve its cost-effectiveness through improving efficiencies and implementing innovative cost-saving measures."

In April 2011 the Wisconsin Legislative Audit Bureau (a nonpartisan legislative agency) released its evaluation of the Family Care program. The Audit Bureau noted that Family Care had expanded from 5 to 53 counties during the 5 years covered by the report, and funding for the program had increased from $248.4 million in FY 2005–2006 to $936.4 million in FY 2009–2010. Federal Medicaid Assistance funding covered 68.9 % of program expenditures in FY 2009–2010 [2]. Nearly 60 % of the 28,885 Family Care participants received care in their own homes. Most others receive residential services in small, community-based facilities or adult family homes. The report states that "In FY 2009-10, average monthly service costs ranged from $1,800

to $2,800 per participant for individuals who were physically disabled or elderly, and from $2,900 to $4,600 per participant for individuals who were developmentally disabled." One key statement in the LAB report was "Our findings indicate the program has improved access to long-term care, ensured thorough care planning, and provided choices tailored to participants' individual needs." The report recommended that DHS report back to the Joint Legislative Audit Committee on several related issues by certain dates.

During the process of adopting a state budget for 2013–2015, there was a lot of pressure on the state legislature to expand Family Care into seven northeastern counties that had been planning for expansion for several years. The Governor and the Wisconsin Legislature responded to the pressure, but, instead of including the seven counties, they called for DHS to produce another report on Family Care expansion. This report on "the long-term outlook for the Family Care program in Wisconsin" was sent to the Joint Committee on Finance on December 13, 2013.

The 2013 Expansion Report [3] noted in the executive summary "The Family Care program has demonstrated that a managed long-term care system increases quality while controlling costs." Also, it predicted that expanding Family Care to the remaining 15 counties would eliminate waiting lists for 1,600 people while reducing the growth of state spending by $34.7 million over the next 10 years. One of the most stunning developments is shown in Fig. 25.1.

As Fig. 25.1 shows, from 1995 to 2011 the percentage of the long-term care population in institutions decreased from

63 to 31 %, while the percentage receiving services in the community increased from 37 to 69 %. By 2011, the actual number of people receiving Medicaid long-term care services in the community (46,910) was more than double the number in institutions (20,626). This is an amazing turnaround in a relatively short time frame.

Also the Expansion Report demonstrated that Family Care had a positive impact on other (non-long-term care) Medicaid fee-for-service (FFS) costs. According to the report "This indicates that increased access to home and community-based long-term care services helps people to be healthier for longer and to require fewer physician visits, hospitalizations, and similar services." Acute and primary health care costs not provided by MCOs decreased 6 % from $282 a month in 2010 to $265 a month in 2012.

The report concludes that "The success of continued system reform efforts and programmatic efficiencies, as well as the analysis of benefits of managed long-term care, as presented in this report, establish that it is time to finish the statewide expansion of managed long-term care."

Finally, a recent report [4] issued by the AARP Foundation, the Commonwealth Fund, and the SCAN Foundation included Wisconsin as one of the eight states that have "clearly established a level of performance at a higher tier than other states-even other states in the top quartile." The Scorecard evaluated five performance indicators: Affordability and Access, Choice of Setting and Provider, Quality of Life and Quality of Care, Support for Family Caregivers, and Effective Transitions. While this is not specifically an evaluation of Family Care, the fact that Family Care is Wisconsin's primary long-term care program suggests that it was instrumental in the state receiving such high praise for performance.

The external quality review reports prepared by MetaStar provide some information about traditional clinical measures that are found in Performance Improvement Projects required by the state. The projects chosen over the years include such indicators as wound care, fall prevention, immunization, and diabetes management. Family Care is not a medical model; the interdisciplinary team coordinates acute and primary health care.

Family Care Today

The following "Goals of the Family Care Initiative" are listed on the Department of Health Services website:

- *Choice*. Give people better choices about the services and supports available to meet their needs.
- *Access*. Improve people's access to services.
- *Quality*. Improve the overall quality of the long-term care system by focusing on achieving people's health and social outcomes.

- *Cost-effectiveness*. Create a cost-effective long-term care system for the future. In addition, advocates for long-term care reform wanted to eliminate waiting lists, and decrease overutilization of nursing homes and use any savings to fund more people in home and community settings.

As of July 1, 2014, according to DHS website enrollment data, there were 37,790 people enrolled in the Family Care program in Wisconsin made up of 13,591 persons who are developmentally disabled, 18,003 frail elderly persons, and 6,196 people who are physically disabled. An additional 3,607 people are enrolled in other home and community-based programs (Partnership and PACE) for a total of 41,397 people. There were 20,626 people receiving institutional care. From 1995 to 2011 the number of people in institutions decreased by 10,811 persons with 85 % of the decrease coming from the frail elderly target group. While the decrease in institutionalization is good news it is somewhat offset by the fact that 58 % of frail older persons still receive long-term care services in institutions.

In dollar terms, from State Fiscal Year 2002 to SFY 2011, total Medicaid spending increased from $3.359 billion to $6.677 billion while over the same period Medicaid funding for long-term care increased from $1.775 billion to $2.889 billion. While the Medicaid funding for long-term care increased it grew at a slower rate, despite serving more people, so the percentage for long-term care compared to total Medicaid spending dropped from 53 % in 2002 to 43 % in 2011. As the numbers of people receiving long-term care services changed from more people in institutions to more people in home and community settings, the money spent on long-term care changed significantly from institutions to the community. From SFY 2002 to SFY 2011, spending for institutions, such as nursing homes, declined from 62 % of the budget to 31 %, while spending for Family Care and community services grew from 38 to 69 % of long-term care expenditures [5].

The following evidence illustrates that most, if not all, of the goals of the department and advocates have been accomplished:

- Waiting lists have been eliminated in the 57 counties that have implemented Family Care.
- The number of nursing home days paid for by Medicaid has decreased from 8.8 million in 2002 to 5.7 million in 2012, a 35 % reduction.
- Medicaid spending has shifted from nursing home care (62 to 31 %) to home and community care (38 to 69 %). The percentage of the long-term care population in institutions has decreased from 63 to 31 %, while the percentage receiving services in the community increased from 37 to 69 %.
- Family Care has proven to be cost effective even compared to other home and community-based programs (e.g., 18 % less costly than the COP and CIP waiver programs).

- The number of older persons in institutional care has decreased by over 9,000 persons under Family Care (the elderly still are being served in nursing homes at a rate of 58 % which suggests that further savings may be possible by continuing to reduce this percentage) [3, 5].

Other Consumer Options Available in Wisconsin

Public long-term care programs other than Family Care are available to consumers once their functional eligibility is determined. They include PACE (see Chap. 24), available only in Milwaukee and Waukesha counties. PACE is a fully integrated long-term care and medical care option. Coordination of care is led by a nurse practitioner. Much of the care coordination takes place in an adult day care setting. PACE enrollees only use physicians employed by or contracted to the PACE MCO.

The Wisconsin Partnership Program is available in 14 counties. Partnership is also a fully integrated program but enrollees do not have to attend the adult day care center and the Partnership MCOs contract with a wide panel of community physicians and other health care professionals. See more about Partnership at http://www.dhs.wisconsin.gov/wipartnership/.

IRIS (Include Respect I Self-Direct) is Wisconsin's long-term care self-directed option.

Participants in IRIS receive a budget based on the score of their long-term care functional screen. They have no case manager but have access to an enrollment consultant, fiscal agent, and nurse consultant. The IRIS benefit package does not include the Medicaid card services, such as home health, which are in the other options. The IRIS participants design their own care plans, purchase the services they want, and hire and supervise their own employees. It must be noted that self-directed care is also available in the Family Care benefit package for one or all services.

Home and Community-Based Care in the USA

In a National Health Forum brief entitled *THE BASICS: National Spending for Long Term Services and Supports* [6], O'Shaughnessy reports that in 2012 spending for all long-term services and supports was $219.9 billion or 9.3 % of all US personal health care spending, almost two-thirds of which was paid by the federal-state Medicaid program. She goes on to say that "A number of federal and state policy initiatives have emphasized greater use of home and community-based services, which most people prefer to institutional services" and "Medicaid supported HCBS for

3.2 million people in 2010, an increase of more than 50 percent since 2000."

Every state participates to some degree in the Centers for Medicare and Medicaid Services (CMS) home and community-based waivers. Several states have balanced their spending on home and community-based care versus nursing home care. Some states have attempted to institute aspects of managed care in their waiver programs. The newest federal effort to control cost and improve delivery of both health care and long-term care is part of the Affordable Care Act that created the Medicare-Medicaid Coordination Office. This office is funding demonstration programs that propose to serve persons dually eligible for Medicare and Medicaid under one integrated system. To date 12 states have begun these projects, 6 more are in the process of development, and 8 states, including Wisconsin, withdrew their proposals after the initial planning period.

This project is being monitored closely by policy makers and advocates to determine if the goals—better care at better costs—can be consistent with consumer rights and choice.

Wisconsin can provide some guidance in this matter relative to what choices people make when home and community-based services are an entitlement (Family Care) and there is a choice of fully integrated care (Wisconsin Partnership and PACE).

Milwaukee County reached full entitlement for persons over 60 in 2002 and full entitlement for persons aged 18–59 in 2012. Milwaukee is being used as a comparison because it has all three programs, and PACE and Partnership were available to persons aged 55 and older prior to the start of Family Care in 2000. Prior to 2000 Milwaukee County operated the COP/CIP waivers and had massive waiting lists.

In the DHS report of July 2014 the numbers are 9,932 persons enrolled in Family Care, 985 persons enrolled in Partnership, and 620 persons enrolled in PACE for a total of 11,537 enrollees. Of this number 7,396 are in the category of frail elderly who are almost all Medicare and Medicaid recipients. Only 958 (13 %) of them chose a fully integrated program.

If there is real choice in the CMS demonstrations for persons who are dually eligible, Wisconsin's experience indicates that consumers prefer the stand-alone long-term care model.

The Family Care Model: Some Concluding Remarks

The Family Care model includes the reform of Medicaid long-term care programs to provide eligible persons with an equal choice of long-term care settings, i.e., in home or community-based settings as well as nursing home care. This was accomplished through a federal Medicaid waiver that made funds an entitlement for all long-term care services, not just for nursing home care. The Family Care model does not integrate acute and primary health care, but rather coordinates health care through managed care teams of the MCOs. Evaluations of Family Care have demonstrated that this strategy has been effective in reducing acute and primary health care costs. The seven Family Care MCOs are all not-for-profit organizations that originally developed by operating PACE and Partnership programs. While they must operate as a business with sound business practices, they do not have to generate a profit of 10 % or more. In Wisconsin, a very high percentage of expenditures are for services, and it is questionable if Medicaid funding could also support a profit expense.

Extensive evaluations of Family Care have shown that it is both cost effective and meets the outcomes and goals of most enrollees. Department of Health Services' statistics show that Family Care has completely reversed the trend of overutilization of Medicaid spending for nursing home care as well as the trend of serving more people in institutions. Family Care has been successful in significantly reducing the number of older persons in nursing homes, but still more than half of the elderly receive Medicaid long-term care in nursing homes. When Family Care is available statewide in Wisconsin, all older people and persons with disabilities will have choices regarding access to and availability of long-term services and supports.

References

1. APS Healthcare, Inc. Family care independent assessment: an evaluation of access, quality and cost-effectiveness for calendar year 2003–2004. October 7, 2005.
2. Wisconsin Legislative Audit Bureau. An evaluation, family care. Department of Health Services, Report 11-5, April 2011.
3. Wisconsin Department of Health Services. Joint Committee on Finance, Long-Term Care Expansion Report, December 13, 2013.
4. The AARP Foundation, The Commonwealth Fund, and The Scan Foundation. Raising expectations, a state scorecard on long-term care services and supports for older adults, people with physical disabilities, and family caregivers. 2nd ed.; 2014.
5. Wisconsin Department of Health Services. Report to the Joint Legislative Audit Committee on Family Care, August 31, 2012.
6. The National Health Forum. The BASICS. National Spending for Long-Term Services and Supports (LTSS), 2012.

Part VII

Promising Programs

Angela Georgia Catic

Introduction

Over 5 million Americans were estimated to have dementia in 2000, a number that is expected to skyrocket to over 13 million by 2050 [1]. Of those with dementia, an estimated 1.8 million suffer from the advanced stage of the disease [2]. These individuals are commonly hospitalized for acute illnesses, despite the fact that hospitalizations are often costly, burdensome, and may have limited clinical benefit in this population [3–5].

Although research suggests that palliative care consultation improves the care of patients with other life-limited illnesses, individuals with advanced dementia have unique palliative care needs that require a specialized approach. Barriers associated with providing optimal palliative care consultation for dementia include challenges regarding recognition of it as a terminal disease, decision making regarding common complications, and education of families and medical providers regarding the expected disease course [6]. Implementation of a multidisciplinary advanced dementia consult service (ADCS) can help to address these challenges and optimize care for elders with advanced dementia.

Development

An ADCS was developed at Beth Israel Deaconess Medical Center (BIDMC) to improve the care provided to hospitalized elders with advanced dementia and reduce the risk of rehospitalization. BIDMC is a 631-bed tertiary care, teaching hospital in Boston, Massachusetts. The development and implementation of this service was a multidisciplinary effort between geriatrics and palliative care. Guided by previous work, the ADCS includes inpatient consultation, printed educational materials for surrogate decision makers, and post-discharge telephone support for families [2, 3, 7, 8]. A standardized consultation form was developed which includes important palliative care issues, components of traditional geriatrics assessment, and administrative metrics. An in-person or telephone meeting is held between the ADCS team and surrogate within 24 h of admission and focuses on understanding of the acute clinical situation and course of dementia. Other topics are addressed as appropriate to the clinical situation and include goals of care, decisions around feeding issues, caregiver needs, and palliative care and hospice. Following this encounter, ongoing daily consultation is provided as needed and recommendations are relayed to the care team through written and verbal recommendations. Recommendations are kept to five or less to improve adherence.

In addition to verbal communication, all surrogate decision makers are provided with a pocket-sized educational booklet that provides standardized information regarding advanced dementia and related issues (Fig. 26.1). It was developed using a basic decision support framework [9] and aims to (1) help proxies understand the clinical situation, care options, and possible outcomes of each option; (2) provide steps to decision making to help guide deliberation according to the patient's clinical situation, values, and preferences; and (3) promote active participation in decision making. Chapters in the book are two to three pages each and address the following topics: (1) What is Advanced Dementia?, (2) Determining the Primary Goal of Care, (3) Basic Approach to Decision Making, (4) Approach to Eating Problems, (5) Approach to Decisions about Hospitalization, (6) Approach to Treatment Decisions for Infections, (7) How Advanced Dementia Affects the Family, and (8) What is Hospice and Palliative Care?. This booklet was authored by geriatricians and a palliative care nurse practitioner. It was subsequently edited by an independent team including a palliative care physician, chaplain, geriatric nurse practitioner, geriatric physician, bioethicist, and three surrogates of

A.G. Catic, M.D. (✉)
Division Geriatrics Section, Department of Internal Medicine,
Huffington Center on Aging and the Michael E. DeBakey VAMC,
Baylor College of Medicine, 1 Baylor Plaza, Houston,
TX 77030, USA
e-mail: acatic@bcm.edu

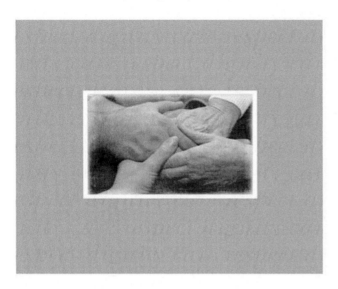

ADVANCED DEMENTIA
A Guide for Families

Fig. 26.1 Cover and index page from booklet given to surrogates of patients with advanced dementia (courtesy of Hebrew SeniorLife Institute for Aging Research)

patients with dementia. After the content was professionally translated to a sixth-grade reading level, a decision-maker reaction panel consisting of three surrogate decisions makers of patients with advanced dementia reviewed the booklet for acceptability of length, clarity, and usefulness.

Following discharge, the ADCS team provides the patient's primary care physician with a written summary of issues discussed in the consult including recommendations for symptom control, goals of care, and advanced care planning. During the study phase of the ADCS, the healthcare surrogate was contacted 1 month after discharge to review the patient's health status, advanced care planning, decision making, and caregiver needs.

Identification of Participants

Accurate, timely identification of inpatients who meet the criteria for advanced dementia is a challenging aspect of implementing an ADCS. BIDMC maintains a robust clinical computing system that includes outpatient and inpatient electronic medical records (EMR), physician order entry (POE), and administrative data. Individuals ≥65 years with a prior diagnosis of dementia based on their existing BIDMC EMR (i.e., outpatient problem lists, prior discharge diagnosis, billing codes) are automatically identified on hospital admission. For these individuals, a series of pop-ups appear

in the POE when admission orders are entered aimed at determining if the patient meets the criteria for severe dementia based on the Global Deterioration Scale (GDS) 7 [10]. The first pop-up reads, "This patient has a diagnosis of dementia. At baseline, patients with advanced dementia are: 1. Functionally mute (e.g., cannot verbalize meaningfully), 2. Non-ambulatory (e.g., bedbound), and 3. Incontinent of bowel and bladder. To the best of your knowledge, does this patient meet at least two of these three criteria?" Admitting providers are asked if patients met two of the three criteria in an effort to balance capturing as many patients admitted with advanced dementia as possible and the feasibility of busy hospital physicians knowing this information for patients they are only just meeting. If the admitting provider states that the patient meets at least two of the three criteria, a second pop-up appears which reads, "Patients with advanced dementia are extremely vulnerable when hospitalized. Decisions commonly arise about the use of burdensome treatments that may or may not be beneficial to or wanted by these patients. To help you optimize the care of this patient with advanced, end stage dementia, please consider obtaining an Advanced Dementia Service Consult." If the provider clicks to order the consult, they are then directed to a pop-up where they are asked to enter the reason for admission, projected discharge date, and reason for consult including assistance with defining goals of care; decision making about feeding issues; treatment options, or hospice; and other with a free text option. An automatic e-mail notifies the ADCS team of the consult request.

Pilot Testing and Data

Pilot testing of the ADCS was conducted using a pre-post design. During the 3-month control period, hospitalized patients with a prior diagnosis of dementia were screened for an advanced disease state using the first POE pop-up. Otherwise, they received usual care. During the 3-month intervention period, the second pop-up appeared which allowed admitting providers to request input from the ADCS.

Patient data, obtained from the EMR and proxy interviews, included demographic information, admitting service, comorbid health conditions, and baseline functional status using the Bedford Alzheimer's Nursing Severity Subscale (BANS-S). Data describing the hospitalization was obtained from the EMR after discharge. During the 1-month proxy interview, information about the post-discharge course and patient comfort using the Symptom Management at the End-of-Life in Dementia (SM-EOLD) scale (range 0–45 with higher score indicating greater comfort) was ascertained [11, 12].

A variety of data was collected regarding the proxies: demographic information, knowledge of advanced dementia (12 true/false questions developed by the research team based on the content of the decision-support booklet), preparedness about the course of advanced dementia, and goals of care (life-prolongation or comfort). At the 1-month follow-up, proxies were reassessed regarding knowledge, preparedness, and goals of care. They were also queried regarding advanced care planning, quality of communication with providers, and satisfaction with care during the hospitalization.

Results

Patient Identification

A total of 419 admissions generated the first POE pop-up identifying patients ≥65 years with dementia during the control period. Admitting providers initially identified 112 of these as meeting two of the three criteria for advanced dementia. Following screening by the ADCS team, the diagnosis was confirmed in 35 patients. For study purposes, 11 patients from this group were excluded as they had already been recruited or there were issues regarding proxy participation.

During the intervention period, 394 admissions generated the POE pop-up and the admitting provider indicated that 78 of these individuals met two of the three advanced dementia

criteria. A consult was requested in 30.8 % ($N=24/78$) of cases. The ADCS team confirmed the diagnosis in 11 of the referrals. Six of these patients were excluded from the study because they had already been recruited, the proxy refused enrollment, or the patient died prior to enrollment.

Baseline Characteristics

In the combined sample, the patients' mean age was 85.4 ± 6.9 (SD) years. The majority were white, female, and nursing home residents. Alzheimer's disease was the cause of dementia for 66.5 % of patients and their mean BANS-S score was 20.1 ± 1.7 (SD) which indicates severe functional disability [13]. The mean age of proxies was 58.4 ± 10.5 (SD) years. 69.0 % were the patients' children and 89.7 % were formally designated as proxies. Although the minority lived with the patient (13.8 %), 55.2 % provided over 7 h of direct care each week.

Hospital Course

The majority of patients admitted to the hospital were diagnosed with infections and, as expected, underwent potentially burdensome interventions. See Table 26.1 for characteristics of their hospitalization.

Follow-Up

At 1-month follow-up, patients in the control group were relatively less likely to have been referred to hospice and more likely to have had ER visits and rehospitalizations compared to the intervention group. In addition, three patients from the control period had feeding tube insertion post-hospitalization, compared to none in the intervention group. Proxy variables in the post-discharge interview showed a trend to more positive outcomes in the intervention versus control group including greater understanding of advanced dementia, higher recognition that the patient had <6 months to live, greater proportion stating that comfort was goal of care, lower percent reporting a problem with advance care planning, better quality of communication with hospital providers, and greater satisfaction with care scores.

Integration of Advanced Dementia Consult Service

Based on our experience, implementation of an ADCS is quite feasible and beneficial for patients and their families. Health system leaders are eager to improve patient care and

Table 26.1 Characteristics of the hospital course of patients with advanced dementia

Characteristic	Total ($N=29$)	Control ($N=24$)	Intervention ($N=5$)
Length of stay—mean days (SD)	4.6 (3.8)	4.1 (3.6)	6.6 (4.7)
Intravenous antibiotics	86.2 %	83.3 %	100 %
>5 venipuncture	44.8 %	41.7 %	60 %
Intubated	10.3 %	12.5 %	0 %
Limb restraints	13.8 %	8.3 %	40 %
Radiological exam	96.6 %	95.8 %	100 %
Goals of care discussion documented	75.9 %	70.8 %	100 %
Advance directive at admission			
Do not resuscitate	65.5 %	62.5 %	80 %
No tube feeding	3.4 %	4.2 %	0 %
Do not hospitalize	0 %	0 %	0 %
Advance directive at discharge			
Do not resuscitate	75.9 %	75 %	80 %
No tube feeding	6.9 %	4.2 %	20 %
Do not hospitalize	3.4 %	0 %	20 %

family satisfaction while reducing costs. By providing specialized care to elders with advanced dementia, these goals can be achieved while preventing often undesired aggressive interventions and rehospitalizations. Options for integration of the model into existing clinical care include folding it into a geriatric or palliative care consult service. However, the formation of a separate, interdisciplinary team focused on the special needs of this population is ideal. Electronic medical records can be extremely helpful in identifying patients who meet the criteria for advanced dementia.

Use of an ADCS is in keeping with the goals of the Affordable Care Act. At this time, consults are reimbursed under current Medicare billing regulations. However, by preventing unnecessary and unwanted aggressive interventions and hospitalizations that are not in keeping with patients' goals of care, overall cost will be reduced and elders with advanced dementia will be more likely to receive care in place, thus meeting the goals of value-based purchasing.

Conclusion

Providing optimal care for elders with advanced dementia is challenging, especially in the acute care setting. Using an ADCS, care can be improved through education of medical providers and surrogates regarding the expected disease course and common decision-making dilemmas. While accurate identification of patients is one of the primary challenges of the intervention, computerized health records can be utilized to facilitate this process. As healthcare financing evolves, programs such as the ADCS will be increasingly beneficial as preliminary findings suggest the ability to improve care for elders with advanced dementia and their families while reducing cost through elimination of unnecessary interventions and rehospitalizations.

References

1. Hebert LE, Scherr PA, Bienias JL, Bennett DA, Evans DA. Alzheimer disease in the US population: prevalence estimates using the 2000 census. Arch Neurol. 2003;60(8):1119–22.
2. Morrison RS, Siu AL. Survival in end-stage dementia following acute illness. JAMA. 2000;284(1):47–52.
3. Mitchell SL, Teno JM, Kiely DK, Shaffer ML, Jones RN, Prigerson HG, et al. The clinical course of advanced dementia. N Engl J Med. 2009;361(16):1529–38.
4. Meier DE, Ahronheim JC, Morris J, Baskin-Lyons S, Morrison RS. High short-term mortality in hospitalized patients with advanced dementia: lack of benefit of tube feeding. Arch Intern Med. 2001;161(4):594–9.
5. Givens JL, Kiely DK, Carey K, Mitchell SL. Healthcare proxies of nursing home residents with advanced dementia: decisions they confront and their satisfaction with decision-making. J Am Geriatr Soc. 2009;57(7):1149–55.
6. Sachs GA, Shega JW, Cox-Hayley D. Barriers to excellent end-of-life care for patients with dementia. J Gen Intern Med. 2004;19(10):1057–63.
7. Givens JL, Selby K, Goldfeld KS, Mitchell SL. Hospital transfers of nursing home residents with advanced dementia. J Am Geriatr Soc. 2012;60(5):905–9.
8. Gade G, Venohr I, Conner D, McGrady K, Beane J, Richardson RH, et al. Impact of an inpatient palliative care team: a randomized control trial. J Palliat Med. 2008;11(2):180–90.
9. O'Connor AM, Bennett CL, Stacey D, Barry M, Col NF, Eden KB, et al. Decision aids for people facing health treatment or screening decisions. Cochrane Database Syst Rev. 2009;3, CD001431.
10. Reisberg B, Ferris SH, de Leon MJ, Crook T. The Global Deterioration Scale for assessment of primary degenerative dementia. Am J Psychiatry. 1982;139(9):1136–9.
11. Volicer L, Hurley AC, Blasi ZV. Scales for evaluation of End-of-Life Care in Dementia. Alzheimer Dis Assoc Disord. 2001;15(4):194–200.
12. Kiely DK, Volicer L, Teno J, Jones RN, Prigerson HG, Mitchell SL. The validity and reliability of scales for the evaluation of end-of-life care in advanced dementia. Alzheimer Dis Assoc Disord. 2006;20(3):176–81.
13. Volicer L, Hurley AC, Lathi DC, Kowall NW. Measurement of severity in advanced Alzheimer's disease. J Gerontol. 1994;49(5):M223–6.

The Delirium Room: A Restraint-Free Model of Care for Older Hospitalized Patients with Delirium

27

Joseph H. Flaherty

Background and Problem Which the Delirium Room (DR) Addresses

One of the most challenging situations in the hospital is to care for a patient with delirium. Most commonly described by clinicians as "an acute change in mental status," delirium is characterized by a disturbance in consciousness and cognition, has an acute onset and fluctuating course, and is caused by an underlying medical condition or medication. Patients with delirium may have hypoactive symptoms (somnolent, drowsy), hyperactive symptoms (agitated, uncooperative with care), or a combination of these. It is common among older hospitalized patients (10–30 % of medical patients, 17–74 % of patients after coronary artery bypass graft surgery, 28–53 % of orthopedic surgical patients, and up to 80 % of patients in the intensive care unit) [1].

Delirium is considered a "dangerous diagnosis" because it is associated with increased mortality, increased length of hospital stay, loss of physical function, increased institutionalization, and increased risk of long-term cognitive impairment [1, 2]. Although these outcomes are important, most are percentages based on populations and some are only evident after the hospitalization. Thus, physicians, nurses, and many others involved in the care of older patients do not directly see these outcomes on a day-to-day basis. What health care providers often experience with older delirious patients, whether the delirium is the hypoactive, hyperactive, or mixed type, is the frustration of *caring* for these patients and the frustration of trying to diagnose and treat the underlying or concomitant medical illnesses.

The frustration is further fueled by the limitations of some of the current practices in the management of delirium: use of 1:1 sitters, antipsychotic medications, and physical restraints.

The DR model addresses all of these: the negative outcomes associated with delirium, the day-to-day frustration and challenges of managing a delirious patient, and the limitations of current management practices.

Setting, Description, and Key Principles of the Delirium Room

The DR model of care is for acute medical inpatients. It was developed in 1997 at Saint Louis University (SLU) Hospital as part of a 22-bed Acute Care of the Elderly (ACE) Unit [3], and replicated in 2003 at Des Peres Community Hospital as part of an 18-bed ACE Unit [4].

One of the most important principles of the DR is to provide a restraint-free environment with constant observation. Thus, the physical design of the DR necessitated construction of a large enough room to care for several patients so that 24-h nursing observation could be achieved without the use of 1:1 sitters and without significantly affecting nurse:patient ratios. Four beds within the DR were empirically chosen as the appropriate number that one nursing staff personnel could handle. This decision was also based on space availability within the designated wards for the DR. The SLU Hospital DR design is a two-by-two format, while the Des Peres Hospital DR design is four beds across (Fig. 27.1). Privacy is maintained by curtains; yet all patients are visible to the nursing staff in the room. The DR is the closest room to the main nursing station so that at any time, more help is close by, if needed.

The key administrative principle of the DR is that one certified nursing assistant (CNA)/nurse tech is assigned only to the DR, and a registered nurse is assigned to the DR and an additional two to three other patients on the ACE Unit. This allows for the CNA and RN to be in the DR together when

J.H. Flaherty, M.D. (✉)
Department of Internal Medicine, Division of Geriatrics, Saint Louis University School of Medicine & Geriatric Research, Education and Clinical Center (GRECC), St. Louis VA Medical Center, 1402 S Grand Blvd, Room M238, St. Louis, MO 63104, USA
e-mail: flahertyinchina@yahoo.com

M.L. Malone et al. (eds.), *Geriatrics Models of Care: Bringing 'Best Practice' to an Aging America*, DOI 10.1007/978-3-319-16068-9_27, © Springer International Publishing Switzerland 2015

281

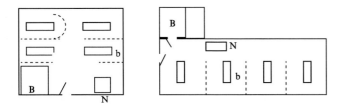

Fig. 27.1 Physical design of the Delirium Room (DR) at two hospitals. Saint Louis University Hospital DR on the *left* and Des Peres Hospital DR on the *right*. *B* bathroom; *b* bed; *N* nurse's desk. *Dashed lines* are curtains, which can wrap around beds completely

necessary, but also allows the RN to cover more than just four patients during a shift. Although nurse:patient ratios have varied over the years, in general, compared to other medical floors, there is an average of one more CNA/nurse tech for the floor, while staffing at the RN level is similar.

The DR is a nurse-driven management model. Nurses have the primary responsibility for which patients are put into the DR and who can be transferred out of the DR. However, physicians may also have input into these decisions. A strict protocol, it was decided, would delay transition in and out of the DR. Patients admitted to the hospital with delirium will need the DR immediately, but may be moved out to a typical room if the delirium improves. Other patients who develop delirium during their hospital stay can be moved into the DR at a later time. Patients without delirium may be put into the DR at the nurse's discretion, such as patients with dementia who need a higher level of observation or patients at risk of falling.

The most important principle of the DR, and perhaps the most difficult to implement, is the management of the symptoms of delirium, without the use of physical or pharmacological restraints. In order to do this, a wide array of practical management techniques is necessary. The TADA approach (Tolerate, Anticipate, and Don't Agitate) is a result of over 20 years of experience caring for delirious patients by all levels of nurses and physicians [5].

The "tolerate" principle has two mottos: "be invisibly present" and "every behavior (action) has meaning." When patients try to get out of bed by themselves or pull on oxygen tubing or telemetry monitoring systems, a health care provider's typical response is to prevent them from doing these things either because we believe that patients are about to harm themselves or the oxygen/telemetry is a necessary part of their care. However, allowing patients to respond naturally to their situation while under close observation (which often means standing or sitting very close by without the patient knowing, i.e., "being invisibly present" so as not to agitate them) gives them some semblance of control in their confused state.

In addition, tolerating behaviors allows the health care professional to get clues about what the patient needs. Oftentimes, delirious patients are unable to communicate their needs, but they can still have "actions" (which may be incorrectly interpreted as "abnormal behaviors"). For example, when a delirious patient tries to get out of bed, it might be an indication of a long list of possible needs (such as toileting, hunger, thirst, pain, or discomfort from being in bed). If care providers do not allow this action, not only could the patient become agitated, but the care provider might miss the opportunity to satisfy a basic need.

A caveat to the "tolerate" principle is that among hypoactive patients, bed rest should not be tolerated.

Anticipate, or "be prepared," is a principle that can help care providers prepare for what the delirious patient might do. Certain actions and reactions of patients with delirium are predictable and seen on a regular basis. A few of the most common ones with some options for management are described in Table 27.1.

Don't agitate is based on understanding what may be going on inside the delirious patient's brain. People who have been interviewed after their experience of delirium often describe an "inability to make sense of what is happening" and an "inability to cope with their environment." If we can understand this, and remember it when caring for delirious patients, our perception that the patient is "uncooperative" and "refuses care" will change to a view that the patient "cannot cope with our usual care" which will help us change our approach. There are numerous "agitators" in the hospital environment, some of which will agitate certain delirious patients while calming others. In other words, some agitators are predictable, and many are not.

One of the most basic care tools we have, our voice, is a great example of this unpredictability. Different voices at different times for different people can have varying effects (calming, upsetting, fear, withdrawal). Some basic tenets to keep in mind when communicating with the delirious patients are the following: a lower toned voice is better than a loud voice (older people lose their ability to detect high-pitch frequency before low pitch); one voice at a time is better than two or more voices; face-to-face level with light source behind the patient is important; and keep commands (if needed) to one step at a time. Lastly, if it seems that one voice bothers a certain patient, find someone else (i.e., a different voice), or go away and come back later.

A special comment about reorientation: it is okay to attempt it, but do not use it if it does not seem to help. When reorientation does not work, nurses are trained to use distraction techniques (change the subject) or to go along with the disorientation, as long as it is safe.

Table 27.1 Anticipate principle: Management techniques for common actions/reactions of patients with delirium

Action or reaction	Management technique
Delirious patients tend to pull on anything that is not normally present.	"Hiding" these unnatural "attachments" can help. *Example*: loosely wrapping a bandage around an IV. Using a decoy. *Example*: taping a false IV on (not in) the patient's nondominant arm.
An "attachment" is needed but delirious patients are *likely* to pull on it.	Try to use the "attachment" briefly, then get rid of it, or hide it. *Example*: give IV fluids as boluses, instead of a continuous rate. Cover up the precious IV in between the boluses. When attachments are necessary, staying flexible in their use. *Example*: telemetry for a patient with uncontrolled atrial fibrillation. Getting the patient to wear the monitor intermittently (e.g., an average of 30 min/h) might be better than agitating the patient by trying to keep it on them.
Delirious patient is pulling on an attachment that seems to be necessary or ordered by another provider.	The culture of the DR is one of asking the physicians frequently to withdraw these. *Example*: the seemingly standard telemetry monitor and oxygen tubing that most patients get are two overused attachments (also called "tethers" because of the limitation in mobility they cause). In today's hospital environment of multiple physicians per patient and fear of not doing enough for a patient, it is not easy for nurses to get physicians to discontinue certain attachments.
Delirious patients try to get out of bed.	Getting out of bed is as natural as eating and toileting. *Example*: preemptive feeding and frequent toileting *out of bed* are the culture, not asking patients *if* they are hungry or need to go to the bathroom.
Delirious patients may instinctively pull or grab things that are in their line of sight or within reach.	Dangling stethoscopes and name badges are *not* the standard in the DR.

Training and Fidelity to the DR Principles and Model of Care

Management without the use of physical and pharmacological restraints appears in textbooks, review articles, and guideline as the first approach for patients with delirium. However, in our experience, administrators and leaders in the hospital emphasize policies about the proper *use* of physical restraints instead of setting up policies that prevent them from being used. Similarly, if guidelines about pharmacological treatment of delirium are developed, there is a risk that use of drugs may actually increase. Thus, education and training in non-pharmacological management of delirium is countercultural. Recognition of the old and new culture is part of the in-services. In addition, in-services on delirium and its management need to be held frequently after a DR is opened, and then maintained on a periodic basis, as reminders to current staff and to educate new staffs. For our DRs, in-services were held approximately biweekly for a year after the DRs opened, and then monthly/bimonthly thereafter. The most effective in-services are bedside rounds with 3–5 nurses at a time, demonstrating the TADA method, and use of educational videos [6].

Fidelity to the DR principles is done through an informal monitoring system: any use of physical restraint is brought to the attention of the charge nurse, nurse manager, and/or geriatricians on the ACE Unit. Rather than developing laborious quality improvement type projects, event-related education occurs.

Further fidelity is assured because the DR is embedded within the ACE Unit, which allows patients within the DR to benefit from the principles of an ACE Unit [7]. Presence or absence of delirium for each patient is discussed at the daily ACE Unit interdisciplinary team meetings. The nurses on the ACE Unit at Des Peres Hospital report a modified Confusion Assessment Method (CAM) [8] score at the daily team meeting.

There are at least three types of delirious patients that should not be admitted to the DR: patients with delirium tremens, young adults with delirium, and young adults on suicidal precautions. Based on our experience, these types of patients need something different than the DR model of care. They also have the potential to harm older frail patients within the DR. The DR should not be mistaken as a substitute for 1:1 sitters.

Outcomes and Evidence

There are several outcomes which can be monitored in order to assure that the model is providing better care compared to usual care: change in ADL function (from admission to discharge), hospital length of stay, falls, mortality, and use of antipsychotics and other drugs intended to manage behaviors.

Outcomes data on the DR come from each of the hospitals (SLUH, Des Peres), comparing delirious patients to non-delirious patients. Some of the outcomes were chosen based on previous studies that have shown that patients with delirium, compared to patients without, have more loss of function, longer hospital stays, and increased mortality [1, 2].

Table 27.2 Outcomes data comparing delirious and non-delirious patients from two hospitals with a Delirium Room

	Saint Louis University Hospital Delirium Room		Des Peres Community Hospital Delirium Room	
	Delirious	Non-delirious	Delirious	Non-delirious
N	51	51	44	104
Age	83	82	85	83
Gender-percent female	60 %	60 %	68 %	73 %
Charlson Comorbidity score	2.2 ± 1.1	2.1 ± 1.2	2.7 ± 2.2	2.8 ± 2.0
Hospital length of stay	5.0 ± 3.3	5.2 ± 3.1	6.4 ± 3.1	5.9 ± 3.6
ADL[a]				
Admission	5.7 ± 3.6	4.9 ± 3.2	4.1 ± 4.6	7.4 ± 4.7
Discharge	5.7 ± 3.4	4.2 ± 3.0[b]	6.1 ± 3.9[c]	6.9 ± 4.5
Mortality	0/51 (0 %)	5/51 (9.8 %)[d]	2 (4.5 %)	2 (1.9 %)

[a]*ADL* activities of daily living. For the SLU hospital data, five ADLs were measured (feeding, bathing, oral care, transfer, toileting; 0=independent, 1=assist, 2=maximum assistance). Maximum dependent score was 10, so higher score was more dependent. For the Des Peres hospital data, the six ADLs (ambulation included) were measured. The scale was 0–12, and maximum dependent score was 0, so lower score was more dependent

[b]$P<0.05$ for comparison between admission and discharge of non-delirious patients

[c]$P<0.05$ for comparison between admission and discharge of delirious patients

[d]$P<0.05$ for comparison between delirious group and non-delirious group

The SLU hospital data were based on a retrospective chart review (the first 18 months of operation) which matched delirious patients with an ICD-9 diagnosis of delirium (in the DR) to non-delirious patients (in other rooms on the ACE Unit). Matching criteria included age (±3 years), gender, and major-diagnostic category-diagnostic related group (MDC-DRG).

Out of 1,121 discharges from the ACE Unit, 68/196 patients in the DR had an ICD-9 diagnosis of delirium. Based on our matching criteria, 51 of these patients were matched to non-delirious patients outside the DR.

As seen in Table 27.2 the two groups were similar in age, gender distribution, and Charlson Comorbidity scores. At SLU hospital, the delirious group had no loss of ADL function and the non-delirious group had improved ADL function. Hospital LOS was no different between the two groups and mortality was lower in the delirious group compared to the non-delirious group.

The Des Peres data were based on a prospective-retrospective observational study of 148 patients (age ≥65 years) over a 4-month period [4]. Delirium on admission (prevalence, based on physician-performed CAM) [9] was 16.2 % (24/148) and delirium during the hospital stay (incidence, based on nurse-performed CAM) was 16.1 % (20/124). As seen in Table 27.2, the delirious group showed improvement in ADL scores and the non-delirious patients showed no significant change. There were no differences in mean length of stay and mortality.

The DR has potential to decrease falls compared to other rooms on the same ward. In the calendar year 2009, there were two falls in the SLUH 4-bed DR compared to 28 falls among patients in the other 18 beds on the ward. Decreasing falls may be more than just close observation, as one study showed that a patient-sitter program did not decrease the number of falls [10].

Data on use of antipsychotics and other sedatives comes from the SLU hospital DR data: 10 % received an antipsychotic, 13 % a benzodiazepine, and 6 % received both while in the DR. This is better than what is reported in the literature [11].

Getting Buy-In from Hospital Leaders and Issues of Cost

There are four compelling reasons that hospitals would want to develop a DR: (1) delirium is not always preventable (so management models are necessary), (2) a DR is easier to implement than a hospital-wide intervention, (3) having a DR can advance the educational efforts about delirium, and (4) the DR has the potential to save costs related to 1:1 sitters.

Although the best strategy is prevention, it is unlikely that in-hospital prevention rates will get to zero. Hospital-wide programs for delirium can be successful, but are labor intensive and require unified commitment from all staffs [9]. The DR is a localized intervention (on one ward), so it is easier to get buy-in from a smaller group of staffs. The DR is also a constant educational tool: it represents to others (temporary and new staffs, families, and physicians) that delirium can be managed in a restraint-free environment.

Cohorting patients with similar diseases or illnesses has long been the standard for other specialties (oncology, stroke, orthopedics). This has allowed nursing in these areas to be better trained to the needs of these patients. Cohorting older patients with delirium allows for nurse training and skill enhancement and allows for standards (for example, no physical restraints) to be carried out.

On a practical level, cohorting patients may allow for cost savings compared to 1:1 sitters. According to one report, annual costs of sitters in three general hospitals ranged from $232,000 to $581,000 [12].

There are three main "costs" to creating Delirium Rooms in hospitals: the construction costs, additional nursing costs, and educational costs. The approximate cost to remodel two existing double-occupancy rooms into one larger four-bed room was $10,000 in 1997 (SLUH). The extra CNA per shift may be offset by use of fewer 1:1 sitters. The educational costs are either neutral (if hospitals already have ongoing educational efforts about delirium) or may be considered more cost effective than traditional educational methods (classroom) since the DR can be used as a hands-on tool for the restraint-free management of delirium. As health systems transition to value-based purchasing, these costs and cost savings will become more important.

To our knowledge there are no reports of DR-type models for hospitalized older patients in the USA. However, similar models exist in Australia [13, 14], Singapore [15], and Hong Kong (personal communication).

The DR model of care fits well with how health care will be paid for in the future for two reasons. First, the model is integrated into current hospital care. It is not an extra program that the hospital must buy and does not involve hiring outside consultants. Second, it is not based on fee for service. It is based on principles of quality care (non-pharmacological restraint-free care) and outcomes of importance (as noted in Table 27.2).

Limitations and Future Directions of the DR Model

There are several important limitations. The model has not been studied in randomized trials. It has not been used specifically for surgical patients. There are no satisfaction data available and no data available from our studies for long-term outcomes. It is also unclear which part of the intervention is helping, since the DR model includes multiple components, not just the "structure" of a room. Not having a strict protocol may also limit the ability of other hospitals to replicate this model.

It is possible that the model could be brought to scale. Although we do not have data to support use of a DR on surgical wards and general medical wards, after the opening of the DR on the ACE Unit at SLU hospital, the hospital did reconstruction on three other units for a four-bed room. Most of the time, these rooms have nursing staff in the room.

The DR model, because of its focus on delirium, should be integrated into the electronic health record (EHR). The many aspects of delirium (identification of risk for delirium, screening, and monitoring of outcomes) are appropriate points of interest that an EHR could capture.

Conclusion

For delirious patients in the acute hospital, the DR provides 24-h nursing care, emphasizes non-pharmacological approaches, and is completely free of physical restraints. The DR can lead to a culture of patient safety through nursing leadership. The DR may lessen some of the negative outcomes associated with delirium compared to patients without delirium (loss of function, falls, overuse of antipsychotics, increased hospital lengths of stay, and increased mortality). While limitations exist, a DR may be a cost-effective way to safely manage patients with delirium.

References

1. Flaherty JH. The evaluation and management of delirium among older persons. Med Clin North Am. 2011;95(3):555–77.
2. Siddiqi N, House AO, Holmes JD. Occurrence and outcome of delirium in medical in-patients: a systematic literature review. Age Ageing. 2006;35(4):350–64.
3. Flaherty JH, Tariq S, Raghavan S, et al. A model for managing delirious older inpatients. J Am Geriatr Soc. 2003;51(6):1031–5.
4. Flaherty JH, Steele DK, Chibnall JT, Vasudevan VN, Bassil N, Vegi S. An ACE Unit with a delirium room may improve function and equalize length of stay among older delirious medical inpatients. J Gerontol A Biol Sci Med Sci. 2010;65(12):1387–92.
5. Flaherty JH, Little MO. Matching the environment to patients with delirium: lessons learned from the delirium room, a restraint-free environment for older hospitalized adults with delirium. J Am Geriatr Soc. 2011;59:S295–300.
6. https://www.americandeliriumsociety.org/resources/videos. Accessed 1 Sep 2014.
7. Palmer RM, Counsell S, Landefeld CS. Clinical intervention trials: the ACE unit. Clin Geriatr Med. 1998;14(4):831–49.
8. Inouye SK, van Dyck CH, Alessi CA, et al. Clarifying confusion: the confusion assessment method. A new method for detection of delirium. Ann Intern Med. 1990;113(12):941–8.
9. Rizzo JA, Bogardus Jr ST, Leo-Summers L, Williams CS, Acampora D, Inouye SK. Multicomponent targeted intervention to prevent delirium in hospitalized older patients: what is the economic value? Med Care. 2001;39:740–52.
10. Boswell D, Ramsey J, Smith MA, Wagers B. The cost-effectiveness of a patient-sitter program in an acute care hospital: a test of the impact of sitters on the incidence of falls and patient satisfaction. Qual Manag Health Care. 2001;10(1):10–6.
11. Elie M, Boss K, Cole MG, McCusker J, Belzile E, Ciampi A. A retrospective, exploratory, secondary analysis of the association between antipsychotic use and mortality in elderly patients with delirium. Int Psychogeriatr. 2009;21(3):588–92.
12. Moore P, Berman K, Knight M, Devine J. Constant observation: implications for nursing practice. J Psychosoc Nurs Ment Health Serv. 1995;33(3):46–50.
13. Eeles E, Thompson L, McCrow J, Pandy S. Management of delirium in medicine: experience of a Close Observation Unit. Australas J Ageing. 2013;32(1):60–3.
14. Mudge AM, Maussen C, Duncan J, Denaro CP. Improving quality of delirium care in a general medical service with established interdisciplinary care: a controlled trial. Intern Med J. 2013;43(3):270–7.
15. Chong MS, Chan M, Tay L, Ding YY. Outcomes of an innovative model of acute delirium care: the Geriatric Monitoring Unit (GMU). Clin Interv Aging. 2014;9:603–12.

OPTIMISTIC: A Program to Improve Nursing Home Care and Reduce Avoidable Hospitalizations

Laura R. Holtz, Helen Maurer, Arif Nazir, Greg A. Sachs, and Kathleen T. Unroe

Background

Mrs. A. is an 84-year-old nursing facility resident. She has been living in the facility for 2 years; her primary issues are advanced dementia and congestive heart failure. She has been medically stable and has few behaviors related to her dementia. One evening when the certified nursing assistant (CNA) came to help Mrs. A to bed, she found her laboring to breathe. The unit nurse assessed her and found that her respirations were 30 breaths per minute, oxygen saturation 82 %, pulse 110, blood pressure 86/50. The nurse called the physician covering that evening who agreed with the plan to transfer Mrs. A to the emergency room. The following day, the Director of Nursing asked the nurse who sent the patient out, "Could this transfer have been avoided?" The nurse answered emphatically, "No, Mrs. A was unstable." After several days at the hospital, the resident returned to the nursing facility. Her daughter reported the hospitalization was very stressful and is upset that her mother seems so much weaker.

Similar situations frequently play out at nursing facilities across the country. A body of research has demonstrated that many hospitalizations of nursing facility residents are potentially avoidable [1–5]. The nurse's reaction in the vignette above is indignant—this was an unstable patient—of course transfer was necessary! Digging deeper, however, reveals a complexity to decisions to transfer frail nursing home residents that involve both clinical and non-clinical factors. Residents with dementia may have difficulty communicating new symptoms. Multiple medical issues may complicate the clinical picture. Availability of medical providers, communication among staff, staff to provider communication, family involvement and comfort with care in the facility, liability concerns, financial incentives, and resident preferences all may play a role [6].

Unnecessary transitions are costly, as well as burdensome for vulnerable residents and their families. Centers for Medicare and Medicaid Services research on dual eligible enrollees in nursing facilities found that approximately 45 % of hospital admissions could have been avoided, accounting for 314,000 potentially avoidable hospitalizations and $2.6 billion in Medicare expenditures in 2005 [7].

Centers for Medicare and Medicaid Services (CMS) Innovations Center and the Office of Medicare and Medicaid Coordination are running an initiative focused on this burdensome and costly problem. The "Initiative to Reduce Avoidable Hospitalizations Among Nursing Facility Residents" [7] is a 4-year demonstration project (2012–2016) focused on long-stay nursing facility residents aimed at reducing avoidable hospitalizations. For this demonstration project, eligibility is defined as long-stay nursing home residents with stays greater than 100 days in the facility or with no plan for discharge from the facility.

The OPTIMISTIC—Optimizing Patient Transfers, Impacting Medical Quality, and Improving Symptoms: Transforming Institutional Care—model, developed by clinicians and researchers at Indiana University, was built on experiences with successful research for care for frail elders [8, 9], clinical expertise in nursing home medicine, research infrastructure, and strong community partnerships. Strategies for reducing avoidable hospitalizations include

L.R. Holtz, B.S. • H. Maurer, M.A., C.H.E.S.
IU Center for Aging Research, Regenstrief Institute,
410 W. 10th Street, HITS Suite 2000, Indianapolis,
IN 46202, USA
e-mail: holtzl@iupui.edu; maurerh@iupui.edu

A. Nazir, M.D. • G.A. Sachs, M.D.
Division of General Internal Medicine and Geriatrics,
Indiana University School of Medicine, 720 Eskenazi Ave.,
Faculty 5/3 Bldg, Indianapolis, IN 46202, USA
e-mail: anazir@iu.edu; sachsg@iu.edu

K.T. Unroe, M.D., M.H.A. (✉)
Division of General Internal Medicine and Geriatrics,
Indiana University School of Medicine, 410 W. 10th Street,
HITS Suite 2000, Indianapolis, IN 46202, USA
e-mail: kunroe@iu.edu

M.L. Malone et al. (eds.), *Geriatrics Models of Care: Bringing 'Best Practice' to an Aging America*,
DOI 10.1007/978-3-319-16068-9_28, © Springer International Publishing Switzerland 2015

(1) preventing conditions from occurring (e.g. preventing falls by managing polypharmacy), (2) early detection and intervention for changes in condition (e.g. observing subtle changes in behavior that could represent an infection), (3) ensuring resources are available to manage conditions in the nursing facility, and (4) advance care planning to allow residents to receive care consistent with their preferences [6]. Thus, the OPTIMISTIC model incorporates these evidence-based strategies with the aim to reduce avoidable hospitalizations for the long-stay nursing home resident.

Circling back to the vignette, if a root-cause analysis was done for Mrs. A's transfer, multiple opportunities for quality improvement and perhaps preventing the transfer may be identified. In this case, the Certified Nursing Assistant (CNA) had noticed that Mrs. A's shoes were harder to put on and so had placed her slippers on her for the past 3 days. If she had reported this finding as a change in condition to the nurse, who then followed up with an assessment, signs of heart failure exacerbation may have been detected sooner. If this was communicated in a clear and timely manner to the medical providers, Mrs. A could have been treated safely in the facility. Further, had the facility proactively engaged the patient's daughter in a discussion regarding pros and cons of hospitalizations in a patient with advanced dementia and heart failure, before this crisis, it is possible that she may have opted for comfort care at the facility and hence preventing a burdensome transfer.

Optimistic Model Overview

The OPTIMISTIC model entails interventions in three domains: medical care; palliative care; and transitional care. To monitor the implementation of the intervention, data collection and management support are included; and to ensure systematic deployment of the intervention across the project sites, education and training of the clinical staff are critical (Fig. 28.1).

The program is administered by specially trained Registered Nurses (RNs) stationed full time at the nursing facility to provide direct clinical support, and education and training to the staff, assist with review of medications, and facilitate goals of care discussions with the family. They also utilize the results of the root-cause analyses to suggest areas of quality improvement in the facility. Nurse Practitioners (NPs), with late morning to evening and weekend availability for in-person evaluations, work with 3–4 facilities to respond to urgent resident care needs. Moreover, they evaluate residents returning to the facility after a hospital or an emergency department visit to assure best practices in transitional care, and lead collaborative care management reviews to optimize chronic disease management. For the latter, the NPs lead collaborative care planning by engaging the resident and family, the staff and clinical providers in management discussions. The clinical staff is supported by a project team with extensive expertise in geriatrics, palliative care, and project management.

Medical Care

Early identification and assessment of changes in condition is a strategy identified to decrease potentially avoidable hospitalizations. OPTIMISTIC utilizes the Interventions to Reduce Acute Care Transfers (INTERACT) [10] tools to educate and mentor nursing facility staff to improve early recognition and management of acute conditions. The INTERACT tools also provide guided, systematic protocols to help nursing facility staff collect and relay critical clinical information to the medical providers. OPTIMISTIC nurses serve as INTERACT champions for the facilities by implementing care pathways and INTERACT tools designed to improve communication and integrate them into the work flow.

In addition to interventions for acute care, the OPTIMISTIC intervention also includes the collaborative, proactive review and management of the residents to promote care that is patient-centered and evidence-based. The RNs and NPs work together to conduct the Collaborative Care Reviews (CCRs) for medically complex resident. The CCR process is based on the principles of the Chronic Care Delivery model that emphasize the use of: (1) a proactive team; (2) engaged resident/family; and (3) systems for effective communication among team members and the residents, and is consistent with prior work done at Indiana University which demonstrated the effectiveness of collaborative care models targeting frail elders [8, 9]. CCRs employ principles of geriatric assessment to review the residents' diagnoses, recent hospitalizations, medications and their related diagnoses, function, cognition, mood, life-quality and satisfaction with care, chronic and acute symptoms, weights and nutrition, skin assessments, fall risks, vaccination status, advance directives, and overall goals of care. Recommendations, including medication adjustments, symptom management and quality of life items, generated from the CCR are discussed with a project geriatrician. The NP discusses the recommendations with the primary care provider and final recommendations are implemented as orders and communicated by the RN to the family and the facility. A summary of the CCR—the CCR consult—is placed in the resident's chart.

Palliative Care

Advance care planning and a focus on palliation is an integral component of the OPTIMISTIC model. Advance

Fig. 28.1 The OPTIMISTIC model

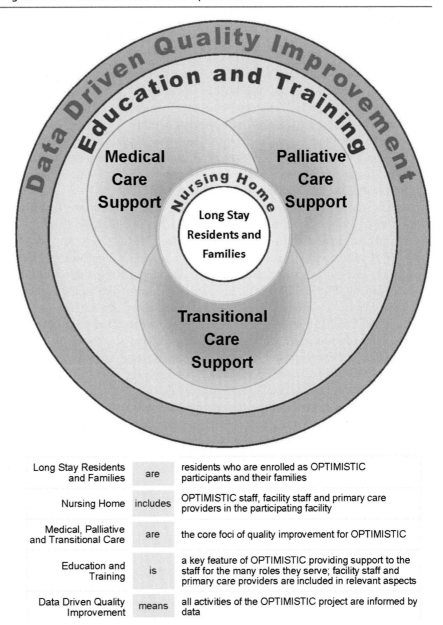

Long Stay Residents and Families	are	residents who are enrolled as OPTIMISTIC participants and their families
Nursing Home	includes	OPTIMISTIC staff, facility staff and primary care providers in the participating facility
Medical, Palliative and Transitional Care	are	the core foci of quality improvement for OPTIMISTIC
Education and Training	is	a key feature of OPTIMISTIC providing support to the staff for the many roles they serve; facility staff and primary care providers are included in relevant aspects
Data Driven Quality Improvement	means	all activities of the OPTIMISTIC project are informed by data

care planning with adequate documentation of such planning allows residents to receive care consistent with their preferences.

OPTIMISTIC staff completed the Respecting Choices® Last Steps [11] POLST facilitators training program. The training provides evidence-based standardized scripting and guidance for the conversations with patients and their families about medical decisions and offers the opportunity to appoint a health care representative. The treatment preferences decided by the resident and families are documented and translated into actionable medical orders with the utilization of the Physician Orders for Scope of Treatment (POST) form. POST is the Indiana version of the Physician Orders for Life Sustaining Treatment (POLST) paradigm, passed into law in July 2013.

In addition to conducting advance care planning conversations with residents, the OPTIMISTIC staff completed certification as End-of-Life Nursing Education Consortium (ELNEC)-Geriatric trainers [12]. This train-the-trainers educational program was designed to improve palliative care knowledge for staff in the long-term care setting. ELNEC-Geriatric content includes pain and symptom management, cultural considerations, ethical and legal issues, communication, grief, loss, and bereavement, and preparation and care at the time of death.

Educational materials have been created for facility staff and residents and their families to improve palliative care understanding and implementation. Topics include comfort care, palliative care and hospice, artificial nutrition and hydration, pain management, antibiotic use, and symptom management.

Transitional Care

When a transfer to the hospital is necessary, OPTIMISTIC interventions seek to minimize harm and disruption of care that may occur with transitions. Research in this area has identified best practices in transitional care that includes timely transfer of records, medication reconciliation, advance care planning and patient and family education [13]. As described above, the OPTIMISTIC NPs make timely "transition visits" to assure that transitions are high quality by focusing on detailed medication reconciliation, evaluation of the recent hospitalization, and review of the resident's goals of care. These visits are meant to supplement and not replace the visits that are required from the primary care teams. The OPTIMISTIC team reviewed transfer procedures at the nursing facility to assess if they met standards of care and offered recommendations. The OPTIMISTIC program also introduced and helped to integrate into facility processes a Transition Cue Card tool, developed by the regional patient safety coalition. The cue card has prompts for the accepting nurse to request and document key information from the hospital visit at the time of hospital to facility discharge to increase the quality of the hospital to facility transitions.

Finally, to better understand the reasons for facility to hospital transfer and to identify areas for quality improvement, the OPTIMISTIC RNs conduct a root-cause analysis on every resident transfer to the hospital.

Staff Education and Training

All OPTIMISTIC staff received a 2 week "boot camp" training designed to introduce them to the overall project and their facilities. They also attended a day-long INTERACT training session accompanied by the leadership from all of the project facilities. The OPTIMISTIC staff spent their first weeks in the facilities going through orientation to the facility and introducing the program to the staff. The OPTIMISTIC clinical staff received training in the following domains and training session:

- Communications and interpersonal relationships: Building Effective Working Relationships, Communication and Information Sharing Among the Team, Practical Application of Communication Skills, Delivering Effective Adult Education;
- Nursing Home clinical setting: Consistent Assignment, Critical Thinking in the Nursing Home, Origin and Intent of Nursing Home Regulation, Quality Assurance (QA) and Performance Improvement (PI) Approach to Staff Stability, Nursing Home Capabilities, Resources and Expectations;
- Clinical topics: Respecting Choices® Last Steps POLST facilitators training program, Link Between Quality of Life and Quality of Care, Reducing Distress and the Use

of Anti-Psychotics: Case Studies, INTERACT Implementation, End-of-Life Nursing Education Consortium (ELNEC)-Geriatric, Dementia—What do I Really Need to Know?, Infections and Antibiotics, Geriatric Nursing Sessions, Root Cause Analysis, Transitional Care: Case Studies.

The clinical staff received ongoing training for one half day per week for the first year of the project and now spend about two half days per month in training sessions.

Lessons Learned from the Implementation Experience

Nursing facilities represent a complex adaptive system and resist attempts to change [14]. The challenges that emerged during the implementation of the OPTIMISTIC project validated this notion and provided the project team with key lessons regarding implementing change in the nursing home environment.

1. Engagement of the facility leadership: OPTIMISTIC clinical staff are employed by the project team but embedded in individual nursing facilities with unique cultures and varying degrees of engagement in quality improvement efforts. Characteristics of facilities with successful integration of the OPTIMSITC program have direct engagement from the facility leadership, particularly in nominating a "point person" who will meet regularly with the OPTIMISTIC RN and serve as an internal champion for the project—this has been the Director of Nursing (DoN) in nearly every facility.

2. Role clarification: For an effective partnership between the nursing facility and the OPTIMISTIC program, clear definitions of the OPTIMISTIC RN and NP roles were necessary. Further clarification was required of how these roles differed from the responsibilities of other RNs and NPs in the building.

3. Ongoing education and feedback from stakeholders: Before each component of the intervention was launched, several key stakeholders were engaged. These included corporate leadership and facility administrators, medical directors and affiliated physicians, and facility champions and frontline nursing facility staff. The implementation approach started with an introduction to the concept—by email or in-person meetings. Model policies, frequently asked questions, sample forms, intervention materials, and background materials were provided. Pilot periods for rollout were established and feedback was solicited following pilots. After reviewing feedback, the project team revised interventions and dissemination strategies to respond to concerns. To fully integrate these concepts into the facility work flow, refresher or "booster" sessions were presented by the OPTIMISTIC RNs after the initial rollout.

Implementation for the advance care planning and POST form implementation was the most intensive. Due to the newly legalized POST form in Indiana, which coincided with the roll out of the project intervention, there was extensive need for education with additional stakeholders including hospitals, EMS, social workers, primary care providers and patients and families.

4. Individualized problem-solving: Concerns about implementation have been addressed on a case-by-case basis. When confronted with barriers, facility-specific action plans have been developed with the facility and project leadership to resolve issues, including promotion of clear communication and time management.

5. Systems for ongoing monitoring: Data collected for the project have been used to evaluate the level of impact or "dose" at the individual facility. A quarterly check-in survey completed by the facility executive directors and DoNs assesses the level of engagement and stage of implementation of components of the project.

6. Sharing of results with our partners: Data collection by the OPTIMISTIC clinical staff is entered into a data system which is merged with resident information from the nursing facilities electronic medical records (EMRs), and a weekly Minimum Data Set (MDS) data feed. Transfer tracking and quality improvement reports from this data system are disseminated to the facilities to inform decision making and quality improvement efforts.

In summary, effective implementation has required frequent communication with the many external stakeholders including the diverse facility partners, corporate leadership, administrators, DoNs, medical directors and primary care providers, nursing facility staff and residents and families. Program protocols, materials and tools are reviewed and feedback provided by the project's Advisory Board and a Clinician Advisory Council. The Advisory Board's membership is comprised of representation from the state Medicaid office, trade associations, Ombudsman, Emergency Medical Services providers, and the Quality Improvement Organization. A quarterly meeting with partnering physicians and NPs (Clinician Advisory Council) has also helped disseminate the intervention strategies and also to gain feedback from this group of key stakeholders.

Outcomes

The primary outcome will be reduction in avoidable hospitalizations of long-stay nursing facility residents. The outcomes of OPTIMISTIC and the other related demonstration projects are undergoing an external evaluation by a third-party evaluator. The evaluator is collecting qualitative data through interviews with facility stakeholders and project team members. A quantitative analysis using claims data for enrolled residents and matched facility controls is also planned.

We anticipate reduction in hospitalizations will occur based on the success the components of the OPTIMISTIC intervention have had in other studies, in particular INTERACT [10] and POLST [15]. In addition, the OPTIMISTIC RNs and NPs represent true added resources to support clinical care of residents who have a change in status.

Interim measures of success include: (1) the numbers of residents who do have a transfer out who are seen by our NPs soon after return for a comprehensive transfer visit, (2) the number of residents and families who participate in advance care planning conversations, (3) the number of residents who have completed Collaborative Care Reviews, and (4) the extent of implementation of INTERACT tools [10].

Policy Implications

Expanding the demonstration project OPTIMISTIC into a scalable model entails multiple considerations, including a review of the other six similar models that are being tested through this mechanism. All OPTIMISTIC facilities were located within 45 min of central Indianapolis, allowing project NPs to cover multiple facilities and respond to acute clinical issues. This geographic closeness has also enabled visits by the project team leadership to the nursing facilities to maintain relationships and problem solve when barriers are encountered. The model will need to be adapted in areas where facilities are spread over a wider area.

Infrastructure to support a clinical staff providing direct care is needed, including salary, benefits, and malpractice coverage, as well as dedicated FTE for the specialized supervision and coordination involved. The clinical staff practices at multiple different sites, integrating into the practices and culture of a given facility. Supervisors need to navigate potentially multiple different organizations to address issues an OPTIMISTIC nurse may be experiencing at a site.

The role of the OPTIMISTIC RNs differs from traditional nursing roles and has been defined and refined throughout the project, based on feedback from the RNs themselves, as well as facility stakeholders. As described, extensive training covering both content and skill development is needed to perform in this role.

In OPTIMISTIC, the project leadership team guided the roll-out of the implementation of the pieces of the intervention, working with clinical staff to tailor the timing as needed based on the facility. There were key physician leaders on the project team who spent considerable time in outreach to medical providers in the community, garnering this key support for collaborative practice.

Data collection has required significant resources of the clinical staff and project team. Data are centrally managed and reports, based on data gathered by the project clinical staff, were generated and provided back to facilities to support quality improvement efforts. Data reports were also produced regularly to monitor clinical staff activities and overall implementation of the project from multiple viewpoints.

Finally, another driver of avoidable hospitalizations of nursing home residents is a flawed incentive structure where nursing facilities and providers are often not reimbursed for additional resources needed to care for a sick resident in place, but will be reimbursed at higher rates if the resident is hospitalized and later returns to the facility [6]. These financial incentives are recognized by policymakers. Financial reform is an important complement to efforts to enhance care delivery for nursing home residents.

References

1. Brownell J, Wang J, Smith A, Stephens C, Hsia RY. Trends in emergency department visits for ambulatory care sensitive conditions by elderly nursing home residents, 2001 to 2010. JAMA Intern Med. 2014;174(1):156–8.
2. Kramer A, Eilertsen T, Goodrich G, Min S. Understanding temporal changes in and factors associated with SNF rates of community discharge and rehospitalization. Washington, DC: Medicare Payment Advisory Commission; 2007.
3. Ouslander JG, Lamb G, Perloe M, Givens JH, Kluge L, Rutland T, et al. Potentially avoidable hospitalizations of nursing home residents: frequency, causes, and costs: [see editorial comments by Drs. Jean F. Wyman and William R. Hazzard, pp 760-761]. J Am Geriatr Soc. 2010;58(4):627–35.
4. Saliba D, Kington R, Buchanan J, Bell R, Wang M, Lee M, et al. Appropriateness of the decision to transfer nursing facility residents to the hospital. J Am Geriatr Soc. 2000;48(2):154–63.
5. Walsh EG, Freiman M, Haber S, Bragg A, Ouslander J, Wiener J M. Cost drivers for dually eligible beneficiaries: potentially avoidable hospitalizations for nursing facility, skilled nursing facility, and home and community-based services waiver programs: centers for medicare and medicaid services; 2010. http://www.cms.gov/Research-Statistics-Data-and-Systems/Statistics-Trends-and-Reports/Reports/downloads/costdriverstask2.pdf. Accessed 23 Feb 2014.
6. Polniaszek S WE, Wiener JM. Hospitalizations for Nursing Home Residents: Background and Options: Health and Human Services; June 2011 http://aspe.hhs.gov/daltcp/reports/2011/NHResHosp.pdf. Accessed 12 Sept 2014.
7. Center for Medicare and Medicaid Services. Initiative to reduce avoidable hospitalization among nursing facility residents 2014. http://innovation.cms.gov/initiatives/rahnfr/. Accessed 7 Feb 2014.
8. Callahan CM, Boustani MA, Unverzagt FW, Austrom MG, Damush TM, Perkins AJ, et al. Effectiveness of collaborative care for older adults with Alzheimer disease in primary care: a randomized controlled trial. JAMA. 2006;295(18):2148–57.
9. Counsell SR, Callahan CM, Clark DO, Tu W, Buttar AB, Stump TE, et al. Geriatric care management for low-income seniors: a randomized controlled trial. JAMA. 2007;298(22):2623–33.
10. Ouslander JG, Lamb G, Tappen R, Herndon L, Diaz S, Roos BA, et al. Interventions to reduce hospitalizations from nursing homes: evaluation of the INTERACT II collaborative quality improvement project. J Am Geriatr Soc. 2011;59(4):745–53.
11. Gundersen Health System. Respecting choices: advance care planning. 2014.
12. Kelly K, Ersek M, Virani R, Malloy P, Ferrell B. End-of-Life Nursing Education Consortium Geriatric Training Program: improving palliative care in community geriatric care settings. J Gerontol Nurs. 2008;34(5):28–35.
13. LaMantia MA, Scheunemann LP, Viera AJ, Busby-Whitehead J, Hanson LC. Interventions to improve transitional care between nursing homes and hospitals: a systematic review. J Am Geriatr Soc. 2010;58(4):777–82.
14. Boustani MA, Munger S, Gulati R, Vogel M, Beck RA, Callahan CM. Selecting a change and evaluating its impact on the performance of a complex adaptive health care delivery system. Clin Interv Aging. 2010;5:141–8.
15. Hickman SE, Tolle SW, Brummel-Smith K, Carley MM. Use of the Physician Orders for Life-Sustaining Treatment program in Oregon nursing facilities: beyond resuscitation status. J Am Geriatr Soc. 2004;52(9):1424–9.

High-Intensity Telemedicine-Enhanced Acute Care for Elders Model

Nancy E. Wood and Manish N. Shah

Background and Setting

"Telemedicine" is most simply defined as the use of health information technology for clinical care when distance and time separate the patient and healthcare provider. Telemedicine care can range from low-intensity, which includes only video conferencing, to high-intensity, which includes broader functions such as capture of diagnostic quality sound, images, and video, as well as point of care testing. This high-intensity, telemedicine-enhanced, acute care model was implemented in Rochester, NY in November 2010 with funding from the Agency for Healthcare Research and Quality, with a primary goal of reducing emergency department use while providing quality care in a more patient-centered environment.

This care model could apply to older adults in many settings, but we focused on adults living in senior-living communities (SLCs), which consist of independent or assisted living. SLCs provide a wide range of support services from basic housekeeping or social activities with no onsite medical staff to meal service and medication management with varying levels of nursing staff. Due to the relatively low level of medical support in SLCs and previous studies showing high levels of ED use among SLC residents, we felt that telemedicine could have a significant impact in this setting. We did not focus on skilled nursing facilities because: (1) studies have already shown that telemedicine-enhanced acute care is feasible and acceptable in nursing homes, (2) local nursing home patients use ED care at a rate less than one-half of SLC residents, and (3) within the next 20 years, both settings will have similar numbers of residents [1–4]. Furthermore, we believe our results will be generalizable to other settings similar to SLCs that are growing rapidly, such as naturally occurring retirement communities.

The Problem

By 2030, the United States older adult (age ≥65) population will double to over 70 million individuals, thus requiring increasing quantity and intensity of acute, unscheduled care. Inadequate access to acute, unscheduled care already exists among older adults and will only worsen as the population grows [5]. Manpower projections indicate that the number of primary care physicians (PCPs) will continue to be insufficient, and access is particularly problematic when older adults seek timely care for acute illnesses [6]. Difficulties in obtaining same-day visits require patients to delay care or obtain care at an ED, forcing older adults to decide which of these alternatives is least detrimental as both are associated with significant health risks and costs.

When an SLC resident requires acute illness care, the patient or a formal or informal caregiver calls the PCP for advice. The PCP relies on symptoms described by phone to decide if the patient requires immediate evaluation. Information from the patient or caregiver may be inaccurate because of limited medical understanding, illness effects, or cognitive impairment, and because the observation skills and training of family and staff is variable. These challenges may lead the on-call PCP to recommend an in-person evaluation in an ED because same-day PCP care is often unavailable or not practical [5].

While older adults are highly dependent upon the ED for acute, unscheduled illness care, the emergency care system is not an ideal location for their care. Taking an older adult to an unfamiliar location like an ED can be stressful and confusing. EDs are generally windowless, have poor lighting,

N.E. Wood, M.S.
Department of Emergency Medicine, University of Rochester Medical Center, 265 Crittenden Blvd., Box 655C, Rochester, NY 14642, USA
e-mail: Nancy_Wood@urmc.rochester.edu

M.N. Shah, M.D., M.P.H. (✉)
Departments of Emergency Medicine, Public Health Sciences, and Geriatrics, University of Rochester School of Medicine and Dentistry, 265 Crittenden Blvd., Box 655C, Rochester, NY 14642, USA
e-mail: Manish_Shah@urmc.rochester.edu

M.L. Malone et al. (eds.), *Geriatrics Models of Care: Bringing 'Best Practice' to an Aging America*, DOI 10.1007/978-3-319-16068-9_29, © Springer International Publishing Switzerland 2015

and are noisy—all factors that can lead to delirium and other poor outcomes. Usually, little medical history is communicated to the ED and, consequently, the transition to the ED often results in fragmented and inefficient care and places the patient at high risk for adverse events [5]. Older adults in the ED can also experience infections, delirium, falls, and other adverse events [7–11]. Finally, some SLC residents have chosen care focused on quality of life, with limited medical interventions, but these important decisions often are not communicated to ED staff. The Rochester high-intensity, telemedicine-enhanced model of care was specifically designed to address older adult's acute care needs while maximizing their health, comfort, and satisfaction, respecting their wishes, and minimizing cost.

The Solution: An Overview of the Model

This older-adult telemedicine model is an adaptation of a validated and well-established pediatric acute care telemedicine program, Health-e-Access, which provides pediatric care for children in school and daycare settings for common acute childhood illnesses and management of common chronic conditions [12–14]. There are many commonalities between the older adult and pediatric populations relating to the need for acute illness care and barriers to transportation, which we believe makes the pediatric model valuable for adaptation to older adults.

In our model, the participating primary care office is a geriatrics practice comprised of geriatric board-certified medical doctors, nurse practitioners, and physician assistants serving patients in skilled nursing facilities and senior living communities. The providers travel to the SLCs at fixed times to deliver care, generally once or twice each week. Due to the size of the practice, nurse practitioners or physician assistants are based in a central administrative office to address acute illness calls and manage paperwork. Following the general protocol in Fig. 29.1, when an SLC patient or caregiver calls the practice regarding an acute illness, the triage nurse determines the needed care based on the information available. If the patient needs to be seen by a provider, but is not considered sick enough to refer to the ED, the patient is given the option to be scheduled with an in-person provider within a few days when the provider will be seeing patients at that SLC location, or to schedule a telemedicine visit. The telemedicine visit could be completed within 1–2 h the same day, or scheduled the following day based on urgency, provider preference, and convenience to the patient. When a patient chooses a telemedicine visit, the triage nurse coordinates with the available providers to determine which clinician will complete the visit, when they would like the visit to be ready for review, what protocol should be followed, and any additional instructions for the telehealth

assistant. The triage nurse also coordinates with the telehealth assistant to schedule when he or she should arrive at the patient's home and what equipment or supplies will be necessary for the visit.

We established predefined protocols for common chief complaints, including altered mental status, fever, pain, skin changes, and shortness of breath, as well as a general "other" protocol. Each protocol requires the telehealth assistant to collect historical elements relevant to that chief complaint using drop-down menus (e.g., Fever—"Pattern of fever: continuous, intermittent, other (specify)" or Skin—"Describe distribution of skin change: face, trunk, extremities, other (specify)"). The protocols also require medication reconciliation, collection of vital signs, and obtaining specified sounds, images, and videos. The protocols also may request specific point of care testing or specimen collection, such as throat cultures, skin cultures, urine specimens, influenza swabs, and blood.

Our telehealth assistants are individuals typically with little or no medical background who have been trained specifically to drive to the patient's SLC and facilitate telemedicine visits. They complete a curriculum that we developed, which includes approximately 10 h of classroom instruction and 20–30 h of shadowing and field training. Topics include technical training on use of the equipment and software, as well as clinical training to master skills such as capturing vital signs, procedures for obtaining good quality heart, lung and bowel sounds, and communicating with older patients (e.g., with cognitive and functional deficiencies). Telehealth assistants also complete the standard hospital phlebotomy course so they can collect blood samples. We have frequently utilized recent college graduates who are taking time out before entering medical school to fill this role with success, and have found that they generally require a shorter mentoring period to demonstrate competency.

The equipment used for these visits includes a laptop computer in a rugged travel case with an electronic stethoscope, digital camera, video otoscope, temporal thermometer, pulse oximeter, 12-lead portable ECG, acoustic reflectometer, and a USB scanner and printer. At the time of implementation, the practice was not using an electronic medical record (EMR), so a stand-alone telemedicine software was used to gather data and document results with a printed copy of the provider note going into the paper chart after each visit. Software on the laptop manages the capture and upload of images, video, sound and PDF files as well as videoconferencing. It is important to note that, in this model, videoconferencing is used only as a communication tool and not to transmit diagnostic images or video. Video used for diagnostic purposes (e.g., gait) is gathered and uploaded to the record via a secure connection so that it can be retained for future needs (e.g., quality assurance, future care).

Fig. 29.1 High-intensity telemedicine-enhanced acute care for elders model

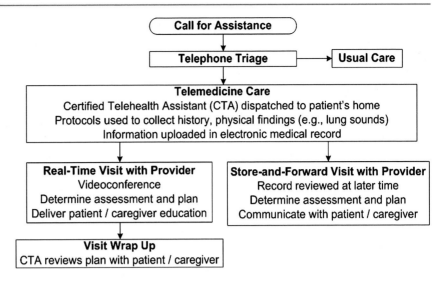

The telemedicine visits could be completed either "real-time," where live interaction occurs with the patient, or "store and forward," where clinical information is collected and viewed by a provider later. In a typical visit, when the telehealth assistant completes all data gathering, he or she calls the designated provider to report that the record is ready for review. The provider may review the record immediately and then connect by videoconference to complete the visit in real-time, or the provider may talk with the teleheath assistant and the patient by phone and elect to review the completed visit later, often after key lab results are available. For a store and forward visit, the provider will arrange to contact the patient at a later time to discuss findings and any recommended treatment or follow-up. If the provider elects to connect with the patient by videoconference and complete the visit in real-time, the telehealth assistant facilitates establishing the videoconference, prints the provider letter for the patient at the end of the visit, and ensures that the patient understands the written instructions and is comfortable with any recommendations before the telehealth assistant leaves. For store and forward visits the visit documentation is usually mailed to the patient and/or faxed to the facility.

Patient Inclusion/Exclusion

We included all consenting individuals residing at SLCs in this program. Based on our experience, no particular subgroup of residents should be automatically excluded. However, individuals wishing to replicate this program must realize that patients frequently have cognitive impairment (48 % in our population) and family members are frequently involved in the care of these patients. Thus, program staff members must undergo specific training related to working with this patient population and working effectively with family members and facility staff members. The appropriate-

ness of each telemedicine visit was determined on a case-by-case basis during triage for those patients who had elected to participate in the program, and individual clinical cases will depend on each patient's illness severity. Conditions that can safely be handled on the phone should still be managed in that manner, while conditions requiring the resources of an ED should continue to be referred to the ED.

Monitoring Outcomes

Our primary research goal in testing this model was to reduce ED visits and healthcare costs and these analyses are underway. For those replicating this program, a number of process metrics are critical to monitor successful implementation. Because we aimed to provide care within 1–2 h unless a delayed visit (e.g., for the next day) was requested by the practice or the patient, we monitored time to deliver care from initial phone call to telemedicine assistant arriving at the home to facilitate the visit. We also monitored successful visit completion, defined as completing the requested visit with a plan for care and without the patient needing to also seek out of home care (e.g., ED, immediate PCP visit) or diagnostic testing. We observed a 94 % successful completion rate (Table 29.1) for telemedicine-enhanced visits using this model [15]. A third important metric is satisfaction. Satisfaction of all stakeholders including providers, patients, families, and facility staff is critical to sustainability. If providers consider the system cumbersome or challenging to use, they will not engage with the technology. If families or facility staff do not trust the technology, they will discourage the patient from using it, and, if patients are not completely comfortable using telemedicine-enhanced care, they will continue to opt for ED care or wait for the next available in-person visit. Patients and their families in this model overwhelmingly reported satisfaction with their telemedicine-enhanced care,

Table 29.1 Characteristics of initiated telemedicine visit (*N*=539)

Characteristic	N (%)
CTA sent to patient's home	523 (97.0)
CTA successfully collected patient information	511 (94.8)
Visits completed with care plan	509 (94.4)
Location of visit	
Independent living	330 (61.2)
Assisted living	209 (38.8)
Testing ordered for completed visits	
Radiology (including ultrasound)	152 (29.9)
Laboratory	293 (57.6)
New medication prescribed	79 (15.5)
Disposition of completed visits	
Sent to emergency department	17 (3.3)
Appointment in the next 24 h	34 (6.7)
Follow up as needed	458 (90.0)
Provider time to evaluate completed visits (median, IQR)	20 (15, 30)
Diagnosis category of completed visits	
Respiratory	101 (19.8)
Circulatory	79 (15.5)
Skin	60 (11.8)
Musculoskeletal	49 (9.6)
Digestive	36 (7.1)
Infectious	30 (5.9)
Injury	27 (5.3)
Mental	24 (4.7)
Other (senses, GU, nervous, symptom, endocrine)	103 (20.2)
Domiciliary/home CPT coding, established patients	
Straightforward (99,334)	73 (14.3)
Low (99,335)	273 (53.6)
Moderate (99,336)	139 (27.3)
Complex (99,337)	15 (3.0)
Insufficient documentation to code	9 (1.8)

CTA certified telehealth assistant

particularly in terms of convenience, speed, and completeness of the evaluation, and providers thought telemedicine made them more efficient [16].

Buy-in and Scale-up

Telemedicine is a disruptive innovation that changes the way providers manage their practice, their patients, and their office processes [17]. An upfront process of meeting interactively with stakeholders as opposed to presenting them with a ready-to-execute program helped us to achieve the necessary level of buy-in to make implementation of the program highly successful despite its disruptive nature.

Patients and family members may have limited experience with technology, much less telemedicine care. Therefore, prior to program implementation we held meetings at each SLC to demonstrate the technology, highlight its

benefits to patients, and emphasize the support of the PCP. We also directly approached new patients and their family members during their initial visit with the geriatrics practice, allowing the PCP to introduce the program and express their support. Because caregivers often participate in initial visits with the practice, this also allowed us to leverage the opportunity to speak to both the patient and caregivers together.

To ensure provider buy-in, a program should start with at least one strong clinical champion who is respected, highly invested, and will work to adapt the model to fit local needs. When establishing this program, the practice medical director was our clinical champion and provided critical insight into the needs and expectations of the providers. We also met individually with each PCP who had patients eligible for telemedicine care to further ensure all concerns could be addressed prior to implementation.

Although the SLC staff have limited direct healthcare roles, they are important stakeholders and can influence patient and caregiver decision-making. In acknowledgement of this, we met with administrative staff at each SLC to discuss how the model might be best operationalized at that SLC, and to address any questions or concerns they had regarding the program. In addition, we met separately with staff who routinely interacted with residents at the SLC, including any clinical staff and any social programming staff (e.g., activities directors) to introduce the program and solicit advice and recommendations about best practices for implementation. This was successful at all but one site. At that site, the staff made it evident that they did not support the program and we had to end telemedicine research there.

Buy-in also requires consideration of financial incentives. Research may show overall cost-effectiveness, but the healthcare providers, health systems, and insurers must accrue recognizable benefits. If services can be delivered that increase patient satisfaction at no additional cost, the model is desirable. The model becomes even more desirable if it allows care to be delivered at a lower cost. The actual costs of operating a high-intensity acute care telemedicine program can vary widely based on the costs of equipment (purchased or leased), software, data storage, and the staffing model used. Each new program should carefully consider what equipment and software is needed to accommodate the needs of that patient population, and what level of training is required for the telehealth assistants to meet those needs. We elected to train lay staff with no formal medical background and this was effective for our needs, but some programs may require that the telehealth assistants have other credentialing (e.g., using registered nurses to allow for activities such as wound care). The primary care practice we worked with in this program also had a mixed staffing model with experienced geriatricians, nurse practitioners, and physician assistants. Telemedicine provides an ideal opportunity to maximize the use of mid-level providers because physician back-up can be easily provided as-needed from wherever the physician is located. All clinical data are stored on a secure server and are available for simultaneous review to enhance collaboration between two providers when there are questions or concerns. All of these factors must be considered in comparison to the cost of routine acute care in the absence of telemedicine to determine cost-effectiveness for a given patient population.

This model is also easily scalable to accommodate a larger volume of patients within a defined region. Each telemedicine unit is mobile and can be paired with a trained telehealth assistant to travel as needed to SLCs. There are economies of scale in terms of equipment and software licensing. A larger patient population might also allow for a mixed staffing model for telehealth assistants where most are lay-trained but registered nurses float into the field as needed to perform tasks that require nursing expertise such as wound care, difficult blood draws, or administering IV medications. Time management and careful titration of resources is critical in that you need to determine the correct staffing level so that patients are not waiting extended periods for a visit, but telehealth assistants are also not spending large amounts of idle time waiting for visits to be requested. A case mix of higher and lower acuity as you might find in a larger volume of patients is ideal because less acute visits can often be scheduled at a later time or the following day to accommodate more urgent acute visits.

The Future

The Institute of Medicine has stated that innovative solutions must be developed to provide safe, high-quality, cost-effective care for acute illness, and that these solutions must satisfy patients, families, and healthcare providers; must promote safe, high-quality care; must improve continuity of care; must be efficient; and must be cost-effective [18]. These solutions must take place in the setting of a system that is moving from a fee-for-service to a value-driven system.

First, research is critical to evaluate the feasibility, acceptability, effectiveness, and cost-effectiveness of telemedicine services. Through high-quality research, we can discover how to structure the healthcare system under the Affordable Care Act and what value stems from this model of care.

Second, policy changes will be necessary. Licensing and credentialing issues are faced in many telemedicine organizations, and may require legislative changes. Reimbursement for the cost of telemedicine services exists from many insurance providers. In fact, many states require insurance providers to reimburse for telemedicine visits for conditions that would have been covered if seen in-person. However, Medicare reimbursement for telehealth services is severely limited, allowable only when the originating site (where the patient is) is in a Health Professional Shortage Area or in a county that is outside of any Metropolitan Statistical Area. In addition, the originating site must also be a medical facility and not the patient's home [19]. The Affordable Care Act, however, gives Medicare the ability to participate in transitional payment reforms through Accountable Care Organizations which accept accountability for the quality, cost, and overall care of the Medicare beneficiaries assigned to it [20]. With its potential to reduce cost while increasing patient satisfaction, acute care telemedicine models such as this should be ideally situated for expansion under the rapidly approaching Accountable Care Organization system of healthcare.

References

1. Hui E, et al. Telemedicine: a pilot study in nursing home residents. Gerontology. 2001;47(2):82–7.
2. Lyketsos CG, et al. Telemedicine use and the reduction of psychiatric admissions from a long-term care facility. J Geriatr Psychiatry Neurol. 2001;14(2):76–9.
3. Wakefield BJ, et al. Interactive video specialty consultations in long-term care. J Am Geriatr Soc. 2004;52(5):789–93.
4. Gray LC, et al. Telehealth for nursing homes: the utilization of specialist services for residential care. J Telemed Telecare. 2012;18(3): 142–6.
5. Morganti K, Bauhoff S, Blanchard JC, et al. The Evolving Role of Emergency Departments in the United States, in RAND Corporation research report series. Santa Monica, CA: The RAND Corporation; 2013.
6. Cooper RA, Getzen TE, McKee HJ, Laud P. Economic and demographic trends signal an impending physician shortage. Health Aff. 2002;21:140–54.
7. Caterino JM, Emond JA, Camargo CA. Inappropriate medication administration to the acutely ill elderly: a nationwide emergency department study. J Am Geriatr Soc. 2004;52(11):1847–55.
8. Elie M, Rousseau F, Cole M. Prevalence and detection of delirium in elderly emergency department patients. CMA. 2000;163(8): 977–81.
9. Hastings SN, Schmader KE, Sloane RJ, Weinberger M, Goldberg KC, Oddone EZ. Adverse health outcomes after discharge from the emergency department—incidence and risk factors in a veteran population. Med Care. 2007;46:771–7.
10. Hwang U, Morrison RS. The geriatric emergency department. J Am Geriatr Soc. 2007;55(11):1873–6.
11. Leape LL, Brennan TA, et al. The nature of adverse events in hospitalized patients. Results of the Harvard Medical Practice Study II. N Engl J Med. 1991;324(6):377–84.
12. McConnochie KM, Wood NE, Herendeen NE, et al. Acute illness care patterns change with use of telemedicine. Pediatrics. 2009;123: e989–95.
13. McConnochie KM, Wood NE, Kitzman HJ, Herendeen NE, Roy J, Roghmann KJ. Telemedicine reduces absence resulting from illness in urban child care: evaluation of an innovation. Pediatrics. 2005;115:1273–82.
14. McConnochie KM, Wood NE, Herendeen NE, ten Hoopen CB, Roghmann KJ. Telemedicine in urban and suburban childcare and elementary schools lightens family burdens. Telemed J E Health. 2010;16:533–42.

15. Shah MN, Gillespie SM, Wood N, Wasserman EB, Nelson DL, Dozier A, McConnochie KM. High-intensity telemedicine-enhanced acute care for older adults: an innovative health care delivery model. J Am Geriatr Soc. 2013;61:2000–7.

16. Shah MN, Morris D, Jones CMC, Gillespie SM, Nelson DL, McConnochie KM, Dozier A. A qualitative evaluation of a telemedicine-enhanced emergency care program for older adults. J Am Geriatr Soc. 2013;61:571–6.

17. Christensen CM, Grossmann JH, Hwang MD. The innovator's prescription: a disruptive solution for health care. New York: McGraw Hill; 2009.

18. Medicine I. Retooling for an Aging America. Washington, DC: The National Academies Press; 2008.

19. HRSA. What are the reimbursement issues for telehealth? 2014 http://www.hrsa.gov/healthit/toolbox/RuralHealthITtoolbox/Telehealth/whatarethereimbursement.html. Accessed 21 Jul 2014.

20. Miller HD. Transitioning to accountable care: incremental payment reforms to support higher quality, more affordable health care. Pittsburgh, PA: Center for Healthcare Quality and Payment reform; 2011.

Comfort Care for People with Dementia: The Beatitudes Campus Model

30

Tena M. Alonzo, Karen M. Mitchell, and Cheryl E. Knupp

Today millions of Americans are experiencing some form of dementia and by 2050 the number of people with Alzheimer's disease and other dementias is expected to increase to 16 million [1]. Dementia is a fatal condition with no known cure or appreciable treatments. Historically, traditional models of care are curative-based and do not address the specific needs of people with moderate to advanced dementia. Recognizing a gap in service, Beatitudes Campus transformed a traditional care model to a comfort-focused model by changing personal practice for all interprofessional team members and renovating organizational systems. Once the Beatitudes Campus model was implemented, people living with dementia in the health care center experienced several positive outcomes including reduction in unnecessary medications, fewer emergency department and hospital visits and an elimination of Sundown syndrome symptoms.

The Beatitudes Campus

Founded in 1964, Beatitudes Campus is a faith-based not-for-profit continuing care retirement community in Phoenix, Arizona offering a wide spectrum of services for older people including independent living, assisted living, skilled nursing, memory support, and home care services. The campus, which serves more than 700 people, offers a model of wellness that promotes soundness of mind, spirit, and body.

T.M. Alonzo, M.A. (✉)
Department of Education and Research, Beatitudes Campus, 1610 West Glendale Avenue, Phoenix, AZ 85021, USA
e-mail: talonzo@beatitudescampus.org

K.M. Mitchell, B.S.N.
Health Care Center, Beatitudes Campus, 1712 W. Glendale Avenue, Phoenix, AZ 85021, USA
e-mail: kmitchell@beatitudescampus.org

C.E. Knupp, B.S.
Beatitudes Campus, 1601 W. Glendale Avenue, Phoenix, AZ 85021, USA
e-mail: cknupp@beatitudescampus.org

In 1998, Beatitudes Campus adopted a comfort-focused, person-directed approach to address the needs of people living in the skilled nursing neighborhood known as Vermilion Cliffs. The Vermilion Cliffs serves a maximum of 37 people at a time with moderate to advanced dementia and is named for the national monument located in Northeast Arizona. This national monument features majestic red rock cliffs that stand 3,000 ft tall. Choosing this name was simple. The Vermilion Cliffs are much like people with dementia: both have been challenged and are resilient and beautiful (Fig. 30.1).

Changing the model of care from traditional to comfort-focused began with the realization that quality of life for people living in Vermilion Cliffs was less than desirable. Discomfort was evident. Often people rejected care, experienced routine weight loss and were physically and chemically restrained. Family members were dissatisfied with care and considerable staff time was used to address complaints. Strong evidence suggested that staff across all departments, although very caring, did not have an adequate knowledge and understanding of dementing illnesses. This lack of knowledge and understanding fueled poor outcomes and the Vermilion Cliff's team understood that staff practice and organizational systems on neighborhood were out-of-date, not dementia-friendly and change was essential.

Three areas of concern were identified: organizational routines, medical management and a milieu which did not support people with dementia. Regimented institutional policy regarding caregiving tasks and work assignments were structured according to staff expediency and dictated when people with dementia were expected to sleep, eat, toilet, bathe, and socialize. Medical management was focused on curative measures rather than acknowledging the terminal nature of dementia. The milieu suffered from an abundance of commotion which included overhead paging, loud television and radio, and hurried staff.

In response to these challenges, the Vermilion Cliffs team developed five key concepts which became the foundation for a comfort-focused model of care (Table 30.1).

M.L. Malone et al. (eds.), *Geriatrics Models of Care: Bringing 'Best Practice' to an Aging America*,
DOI 10.1007/978-3-319-16068-9_30, © Springer International Publishing Switzerland 2015

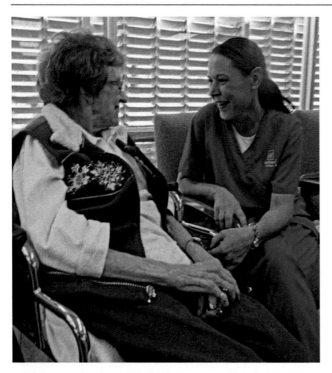

Fig. 30.1 "Knowing the person makes comfort for everyone possible."—Doris Olson, resident Beatitudes Campus and Christine Parish, BSN Charge Nurse for Vermilion Cliffs, Beatitudes Campus

Table 30.1 Key concepts for comfort care

Comfort Care refers to the care required to meet a broad spectrum of needs for persons with dementia. This spectrum includes not only medical and physical needs of individuals, but also social, spiritual and emotional needs as well. Comfort care is NOT just for end-of-life [2].

Anticipation of Needs is an approach for meeting basic needs of persons with dementia. In simplest terms, anticipation of needs means feeding people before they are hungry, give them fluids before they are thirsty, helping them lie down before they fall asleep, providing comfort measures as soon as pain is recognized, and helping them occupy their time before they become bored.

Know the Person refers to being knowledgeable about an individual's important life events, past daily routines and vocation, as well as knowing the person's family members and friends. To know the person also means that caregivers are knowledgeable about what makes an individual comfortable and happy given the challenges of dementia.

Person-directed Practice describes caregiving that focuses on the individual needs and life patterns of a person with dementia. This approach to care addresses an individual's physical, social, spiritual, medical, and emotional needs. Person-directed Practice is concerned with evaluating individual needs by observing and interpreting a person's behavior. In other words, all human behavior is communication [3].

Staff Empowerment means giving all staff members the "go ahead" to do what is best for individuals with dementia—within the policies and procedures of the organization. Empowerment is not limited to a particular department or job role; but involves all staff working together on the interprofessional team. Staff members who are empowered become the voice of the person with dementia [4].

Using these key concepts as a foundation, change in staff practice and organizational systems began. Early on it was discovered staff had limited factual knowledge about people with dementia and there was widespread misunderstanding regarding caregiving practices. To meet the needs of staff an education program was developed. The education program taught realistic expectations for people with dementia allowing for a quick adoption of comfort-focused care philosophy. The education program consists of five courses in which all members of the interprofessional team participate.

- *Key Concepts in Dementia Care Education* elaborates on the definitions of the five concepts and provides a rationale for their importance in the care of persons with dementia.
- *What Caregivers Need to Know about Comfort Care* expands the inter-professional team's knowledge of key concepts and broadens them into competencies tailor-made for staff according to their job roles.
- *Comfort-Focused Approaches to Dementia-Related Behaviors* teaches the inter-professional team not only to detect behaviors associated with dementia in individuals and groups of persons, but also to interpret those behaviors as communications about unmet needs. In addition, staff become acquainted with a variety of comfort-focused approaches to improve life situations, including anticipation of needs.
- *Assessing and Addressing Pain in Persons with Dementia* educates the inter-professional team about physical pain for persons and what to do when pain is detected.
- *The Magic of Making Connections* assists the interprofessional team in helping persons with dementia make connections with others and with the environment in which they live.

Once the education process was implemented, the team began to change staff practice and organization to a comfort-focused model of care that was named the Beatitudes Campus Model now known at Comfort Matters™.

The Beatitudes Campus Model and the Role of the Vermilion Cliffs Interprofessional Team

Because many staff impact the lives of people with dementia, the campus learned to think broadly about who should be included in the interprofessional team. Traditionally, this team was limited to a few roles such as the geriatrician and nurse. Through the education experience. the Vermilion Cliffs interprofessional team learned that any staff member who came in contact with people with dementia could contribute to their comfort or discomfort. Consequently, the team was expanded to represent staff from all shifts and departments including certified nursing assistants, social workers, nurses, environmental and food service staff, and activity professionals. While all staff had a responsibility to create comfort, it was quickly determined that frontline staff certified nursing assistants, social workers, environmental and food service staff, and activity professionals were often the most knowledgeable and successful in accomplishing comfort for people with dementia.

As the Vermilion Cliffs interprofessional team came together, the members met weekly to review organizational systems to determine how to adapt systems to a comfort-focused model of care. These meetings, which were facilitated by a social worker, followed a quality assurance, performance improvement method for change. The meetings examined each organizational system to identify what was dementia-friendly and comfortable and what was not. The team changed organizational systems such as dining and sleep/wake patterns and within 2 years people living in the Vermilion Cliffs experienced daily routines that were entirely individualized. People slept when they were tired, activities of daily living were delivered on each person's terms and they ate what they enjoyed day or night.

The Beatitudes Campus and the Role of the Geriatrician

Initially, people with dementia experienced uncomfortable medications, treatments, and diagnostic tests that did not improve their overall quality of life. For each person with dementia, the geriatrician conducted a risk/benefit analysis to discontinue unnecessary medications, treatments, and diagnostic tests. Additionally, therapeutic diets were eliminated and the geriatrician collaborated with the team to address and treat physical pain. Throughout the process, the geriatrician taught the Vermilion Cliffs interprofession team why changes in medical management were needed and supported the wellbeing of people with dementia.

In addition to staff education, the geriatrician met with families about the meaning of comfort for people with dementia and how diagnostic tests, medications, and treatments could be used or not used. These meetings included a discussion of care goals and advanced care planning. Families generally identified comfort as the goal and a comfort-focused care plan was created for each person with dementia. Frequently, families were relieved to discover that comfort-focused care was an option and many were surprised when the person with dementia experienced positive outcomes such as an elimination of dementia-related behavior.

Obstacles to Implementation of the Beatitudes Campus Model

During the implementation of the Beatitudes Campus Model, two primary barriers surfaced. First, the organization followed a traditional model of care anchored in staff efficiency, based on nursing hierarchy and driven by state and federal regulations. Secondly, staff had limited knowledge and success in dementia caregiving practices.

Stepping away from the traditional model of care was difficult for obvious reasons. The traditional model, although not effective, was safe, the state/federal regulations were well known and the traditional routines and systems were sanctioned by the campus. Deciding to adopt a different model of care required a thorough assessment of process, practice, and a belief that change was both necessary and possible. Quality improvement strategies helped in this process as did thoughtful reflection of the patients' and caregivers' needs.

Staff could not see beyond the confusion and debility of people with dementia and misunderstandings were prevalent. A common misunderstanding was that people with dementia demonstrate dementia-related behavior and there is nothing that can be done to help. In time, the Vermilion Cliffs interprofessional team learned that people with dementia are experts on their personal comfort and although verbal communication is often impaired they can communicate whether or not they feel comfortable through their actions [5]. Once the team understood the connection between communication and dementia-related behavior, they changed their approach and dementia-related behavior was reduced significantly.

A Case Study: Edna's Story

Edna, an 89-year-old woman with moderate Alzheimer's disease, relocated to the Beatitudes Campus after being asked to leave several other long-term care organizations. Edna's son, John explained that his mother frequently rejected care and the other organizations had found it impossible to care of her. Upon admission, the interprofessional team worked with Edna and her family to identify what created comfort for her. The team learned Edna was a Sunday school teacher for 45 years and she loved small children, listening to folk music and dancing.

During Edna's admission assessment, the geriatrician and charge nurse identified that Edna had knee and shoulder pain. As the team cared for Edna, it became clear that Edna was communicating her pain by rejecting care. The geriatrician prescribed routine pain medication given around-the-clock and the staff adjusted their caregiving approach to

Table 30.2 Improvements in care for people with dementia at the beatitudes campus Comfort Matters™ model

Beatitudes campus traditional model outcomes	Beatitudes campus Comfort Matters™ model outcomes
All people with dementia use physical restraints.	No people with dementia use physical restraints.
All people with dementia receive an antipsychotic and anxiolytic medications.	People with dementia receive only minimal antipsychotic and anxiolytic medications.
25–40 % of people with dementia lose weight every month.	Weight loss is rare for people with dementia.
Strict adherence to therapeutic diets for all people with dementia.	No therapeutic diets used for people with dementia.
Spent $30,000 annually on supplements.	Spend $0 on supplements annually.
People with dementia often reject care.	People with dementia rarely reject care.
Sleep/wake routine was staff-driven.	People sleep, wake, and eat as they desire.
People with dementia often demonstrate Sundown symptoms.	No people with dementia demonstrate Sundown symptoms.
Widespread poly-pharmacy for people with dementia.	Fewer than 5 medications prescribed per person.
Frequent use of hospital and emergency department.	Less than 3 % of people with dementia use hospital and emergency department.
Most families were dissatisfied.	Families are highly satisfied and part of the team.
Total focus on medical needs for people with dementia.	Total focus on mind, body, spirit for people with dementia.

minimize Edna's discomfort by creating an experience which incorporated Edna's love of children, folk music and dancing during all caregiving tasks and within a few days Edna no longer rejected care.

The Evolution of Care Models at the Beatitudes Campus

After adopting the Beatitudes Campus Model there have been numerous improvements in care that resulted in positive outcomes for people with dementia. Several of these outcomes are listed in Table 30.2 [6].

The Beatitudes Campus Model and Health System Acceptance

Creating quality of life and comfort for people with dementia has always been the focus of the Beatitudes Campus Model, however the campus also had cost-saving benefits as well. These cost-saving benefits were the result of reduced caregiving costs, such as substituting nutritional supplements with snacks people enjoyed. Further cost saving was attained from improved staff retention. Recognizing the Beatitudes Campus Model as a cost-effective approach to caring for people with dementia is consistent with the Affordable Care Act and opens the door to dissemination of comfort for people with dementia living in long-term care settings.

Over the past several years, the Beatitudes Campus has shared the benefits of comfort for people with dementia by helping other long-term organizations across the country replicate the model. To enhance the educational experience, Beatitudes Campus has designed an educational program which teaches staff at all levels of an organization how to change their practice and organizational systems to create comfort for people with dementia. Replicating the Beatitudes Campus Model across the country has drawn overwhelming support from families and consumer advocacy groups. As the prevalence of dementia increases over the next several decades in the United States, the Beatitudes Campus Model has widespread application in all settings that serve people with dementia.

References

1. Alzheimer's Association Facts & Figures 2014
2. Kolcaba K. A theory of holistic comfort for nursing. J Adv Nurs. 1994;19(6):1178–84.
3. Kitwood T. The experience of dementia. Aging Ment Health. 1997; 1(1):13–22.
4. March A, McCormack D. Nursing theory-directed healthcare: modifying Kolcaba's comfort theory as an institution-wide approach. Holist Nurs Pract. 2009;23(2):75–80.
5. Hubbard G, Cook A, Tester S, Downs M. Beyond words: older people with dementia using and interpreting nonverbal behavior. J Aging Stud. 2002;16(2):155–67.
6. Long CO, Alonzo TR. Palliative care for advanced dementia: a model teaching unit-practical approaches and results. Ariz Geriatr Soc. 2008;13(2):14–7.

Path Clinic: Palliative and Therapeutic Harmonization

Laurie Mallery and Paige Moorhouse

Case Example

Mr. PN (pulmonary nodule) is an 85-year-old man with moderate-stage dementia, congestive heart failure, hypertension, diabetes, and chronic kidney disease (creatinine value of 1.98 mg/dL or 175 μmol/L, with a calculated creatinine clearance of 27 mL/min). Mr. PN lives alone and despite his multiple medical conditions, his family indicates that he has a relatively good quality of life due to close family relationships and enduring friendships. A chest x-ray, performed when Mr. PN had pneumonia, revealed a solitary pulmonary nodule. Further evaluation determined that the nodule was consistent with non-small cell lung cancer.

Mr. PN underwent surgical resection of the nodule as curative treatment. Following surgery, cognition, mobility, kidney function, and heart failure worsened. Despite a valiant attempt at rehabilitation, Mr. PN could not return to independent living. In the course of his postoperative care, Mr. PN was assessed by a cardiologist, nephrologist, internist, dietician, social worker, physical therapist, occupational therapist, and home care staff. These health professionals completed at least ten separate assessments, yet none generated a full understanding of the implications of Mr. PN's new health status.

Is there a process by which health professionals, patients, and families can better understand whether Mr. PN should have undergone resection of the pulmonary nodule for cure?

L. Mallery, M.D. (✉)
Department of Medicine, Faculty of Medicine, Dalhousie University, 5955 Veterans Memorial Lane, Halifax, NS, Canada B3H2P1
e-mail: laurie.mallery@cdha.nshealth.ca

P. Moorhouse, M.D., M.P.H.
Faculty of Medicine, Dalhousie University, 5955 Veterans Memorial Lane, Halifax, NS, Canada B3H2P1
e-mail: paige.moorehouse@cdha.nshealth.ca

Introduction

Frail older adults have complex medical illnesses severe enough to compromise their ability to live independently. In addition to multi-morbidity, many frail individuals also have dementia, impaired mobility, compromised functional ability, and uncontrolled symptoms. Frailty brings vulnerability; it increases the risk of adverse events from medical and surgical procedures, complicates drug therapy, prolongs length of stay in hospital, leads to functional and cognitive decline, increases the risk of institutionalization, and reduces life expectancy [1]. When frailty is present, high-level care planning is crucial in order to understand whether standard of care interventions align with the individual's overall goals of care and prognosis.

The Palliative and Therapeutic Harmonization (PATH) model is a frailty-specific model that puts frailty at the forefront of evidence-informed decision-making [2, 3]. The program to advocates for potentially beneficial interventions in less frail older adults, avoids interventions that will be harmful or ineffective, and palliates irreversible symptoms. The end result is that (1) specialists and health professionals are better able to assess and consider frailty when making important clinical decisions; (2) team-based care becomes more collaborative and efficient; (3) patients/families are empowered to make relevant decisions about surgical and medical interventions; and (4) end-of-life care is administered in a timely way. The PATH model has been translated into clinical programs that have been successfully implemented in community care, home care, long-term care, and tertiary care environments in Nova Scotia and other jurisdictions across Canada.

The use of the PATH process appears to result in more appropriate care. Analysis of the first 150 patients who completed the PATH program in a tertiary care centre demonstrated a patient or family-led 75 % reduction in the demand for interventional treatments for those who were significantly frail and were being considered for surgery or other interventional therapies [2]. Decisions to proceed with scheduled medical or surgical interventions correlated with baseline frailty and dementia stage, such that those participants who had a greater degree of frailty or more advanced dementia were less likely to choose aggressive treatment options. The PATH model enabled 10 % of this cohort, many of whom had multiple hospitalizations prior to PATH, to receive end-of-life care at home [2]. This chapter describes the process of developing the PATH model, the structure of the program, and the adaptation of the PATH model into clinical programs.

Geriatric Medicine as an Impetus for Program Development

In the 1930s, infirm older adults residing in "workhouse wards" in the United Kingdom were gravely neglected. At that time, Dr. Marjory Warren and other founders of geriatric medicine showed that simple medical interventions, rehabilitative therapies, and proper equipment could improve the health of many frail older adults [4]. But 70 years later, the landscape has shifted. The cultural pendulum in geriatrics has swung so far in the direction of restorative interventions that we have neglected those who, due to overwhelming frailty, will not benefit from the traditional rehabilitative model. The PATH program aims to address this gap in the care of people who are not actively dying—those who do not necessarily fit under the auspices of hospice care—but for whom interventions aimed at prevention or life extension may not benefit or may carry very high risk.

Problems the PATH Model Addresses

These recognized challenges became the framework for a new model that could respond to the needs of those frail adults who were facing decisions about medical or surgical interventions, as well as severely frail individuals whose health was declining despite the best efforts of modern medical health care. The model began as a grassroots movement that quickly evolved into distinct programs.

From our perspective, the foundational obstacles to optimal care for frail older adults include the following:

The Prognostic Significance of Frailty Is Under-Appreciated

Frailty is under-diagnosed and therefore insufficiently considered when making treatment choices. For instance, although dementia is a key determinant of frailty, studies find that between 29 to 76 % of people with dementia or probable dementia are not diagnosed by primary care physicians [5],

let alone by specialist physicians who routinely make decisions about complex treatments such as surgical procedures. Likewise, other health professionals and multidisciplinary teams may devote little attention or rigor to the prognostic significance of cognitive impairment.

When frailty is not identified, older individuals with advanced and incurable diseases can assent to interventions and treatments that may have limited chance of success and result in poorly controlled physical symptoms and psychological distress [6].

The Case of Mr. PN

In addition to lung cancer, Mr. PN had three other progressive medical conditions—dementia, heart failure, and kidney disease—that could shorten life and increase the risk of surgery. Despite the presence of frailty, there was little consideration of how moderate-stage dementia and Mr. PN's other comorbidities would impact surgical outcomes. Many would cite Mr. PN's good quality of life as a reason to pursue surgery. However, due to the vulnerability of frailty, it is more likely that surgery could upset this man's fragile good quality of life rather than preserve it.

Frailty Typically Culminates in an Epidemic of Assessments That Often Fail to Adequately Assess Cognition

Even when teams and physicians acknowledge frailty, they typically evaluate patients from the limited perspective of their specific discipline. The end result of this approach is multiple, redundant, and fragmented pieces of information about mobility, function, and social circumstances. In many cases, dementia is present but not properly diagnosed or staged. Consequently, the team may develop care plans derived from inaccurate information based on inquiries made directly to the patient. These practices fail to integrate information into a high-level understanding of patient prognosis.

The Case of Mr. PN

When we ask audiences at rounds and seminars how they would approach the question of whether Mr. PN should have surgery, the majority of respondents indicate that Mr. PN should decide for himself, based on his values and goals. However, it is unlikely that an individual with moderate-stage dementia has the capacity to make this kind of complicated medical decision. Asking individuals with dementia to make treatment choices is common and in one estimate, physicians misidentify incapacity 58 % of the time [7]. Patients with executive dysfunction related to dementia may have difficulty imagining future circumstances [8] and may, therefore, struggle with the nuances of advance directives. Notably, studies show that even those with mild cognitive impairment have difficulty with some aspects of the consent process [9, 10]. As cognitive impairment progresses, and capacity to participate in care planning declines, patients are more likely to select life-sustaining treatments [11].

Existing Communication Strategies Do Not Adequately Disclose the Impact of Chronic Medical Conditions on Life Expectancy and Quality of Life

Patients and families can only plan appropriately if they are aware of illness severity and prognosis. Yet frail individuals and their families are not always informed about prognosis and are often unaware of the limited life expectancy associated with frailty [12]. Moreover, physicians themselves may not appreciate the severity of a patient's complex illnesses [13]. The lack of awareness about the prognosis of frailty leads to poorly informed decision-making. In these cases, patients and their families may walk blindly into adverse outcomes and protracted suffering.

The Case of Mr. PN

The increased surgical risks associated with frailty were not considered. As such, Mr. PN's family was not prepared for the deterioration in function, cognition, and mobility that followed surgery. In addition, although information about the prognosis of dementia significantly influences care decisions [14, 15], Mr. PN's family was not provided information about the expected progression of dementia when considering whether to go ahead with surgery.

Clinicians Apply Conventional Standards of Care Without Specific Analysis of the Risks and Benefits Associated with Frailty

Due to the vulnerability and shortened life expectancy associated with frailty, treatment outcomes for the frail are different than those achieved by healthier populations. In fact, frailty has been associated with poor health outcomes across populations and healthcare settings [16]. Yet evidence-based guidelines created for patients with single-system disease are often indiscriminately applied to those with frailty, despite the systematic exclusion of frail patients from the scientific studies upon which guidelines are based [17]. This practice can lead to harm, unnecessary cost, and overprescribing [18–20].

The Case of Mr. PN

Despite Mr. PN's moderate-stage frailty, his medications keep his blood pressure below 140 mmHg and his HbA1C at 7.5 %. These targets are based on clinical practice guidelines

that have little evidence to support them, especially in those with limited life expectancy [21].

Due to the Multiple Conditions Associated with Frailty, Frailty Care Is Often Uncoordinated

Most healthcare systems have evolved using a specialty-based, single-system illness model that aims to fix one thing at a time. As such, care tends to be fragmented (even chaotic) and falls short of expected outcomes as the frail person with multiple medical conditions moves from one singularly focused clinician to another, without recognizing the impact of each illness on other illnesses. For example, the presence of a chronic health issue associated with shortened life expectancy, such as chronic obstructive pulmonary disease (COPD) or congestive heart failure (CHF), may affect care-planning decisions for patients with dementia at the end of life. Further, with severe stage frailty, successful treatment of curable health issues may increase the likelihood of survival to progress through the stages of dementia. Some patient goals and values may be more aligned with a care plan that allows natural death from acute exacerbation of concurrent chronic illness rather than experiencing the progressive stages of dementia or another terminal disease.

Frailty Symptoms May Not Be Adequately Ameliorated at the End of Life

Reminiscent of the situation in the pre-palliative era of the 1960s, when symptoms related to cancer were not always adequately treated, currently, symptoms related to frailty may not be sufficiently ameliorated at the end of life [22].

The Effectiveness of Traditional Advance Care Planning Is Overestimated

Although advance care planning (ACP) may offer individuals the opportunity to make decisions about future health, the central assumptions of ACP may fail in frailty. Problems arise because frailty is dynamic—treatments that may be appropriate today may not be appropriate tomorrow. The very complexity of the medical comorbidities that create frailty makes it difficult for patients to make specific statements about how to manage the multiple components of frailty or the limitless combinations of health crises. Further, the prevalence of (often unrecognized) cognitive impairment in frailty means that individuals may be called upon to make advance care plans without fully appreciating their health issues, including the progressive deterioration that is associated with dementia.

We Fail to Achieve Cost-Effective Care During Transition from Severe Frailty to End of Life

More healthcare dollars are spent on seniors than any other age group, largely a consequence of the cost of care in the final few months of life, as well as the costs associated with treating the complex chronic conditions associated with frailty [23]. Dementia is a common driver of frailty, affecting 30 % of the population over the age of 80 [24]. Canada's total direct and indirect cost of dementia alone was $33 billion in 2011 [25]. When the cost of managing other common chronic conditions, such as cardiovascular disease and diabetes included, the potential expenditure required to manage elderly patients becomes staggering.

How Does PATH Meet System Challenges?

The Structure of the PATH Model

With major barriers identified, PATH set out to remediate them through new services and protocols that guide health professionals, frail older adults, and families toward appropriate decision-making with frailty, while at the same time restructuring healthcare teams and systems to build efficiency.

The basic infrastructure of the PATH model is a standardized methodology that prioritizes the consideration of frailty when making treatment decisions. The program proceeds in four steps: (1) adeptly assemble pertinent health information to inform and refine an understanding of frailty; (2) ensure that patients and/or families understand the vulnerability and shortened life expectancy associated with frailty; (3) help patients/families and health professionals make healthcare decisions that consider frailty; and (4) improve the ability of physicians to respond to health urgencies/emergencies (i.e., the health crisis). These steps called *understand, communicate, plan,* and *respond* remediate many of the problems identified above and include the following methodology:

1. *Identify and respond to frailty as a standard of care.* To help specialists and others routinely take frailty into account, the PATH has developed several assessments and protocols, as follows:
   (a) Frailty screen. The Frailty Assessment for Care-planning Tool (FACT) quickly identifies frailty by assessing cognition, mobility, social circumstances, and function using a combination of caregiver report and objective measures [26]. The FACT assessment can be completed in busy clinical settings and takes about 5 min to complete once a caregiver is identified. The FACT can be routinely used on services with a high prevalence of frailty and a disposition to recommend interventional treatments, such as the

cardiology inpatient service or in outpatient surgical clinics.
   (b) Standardized tools for team assessment of frailty (see below).
   (c) Designated PATH services for specialists. Once suspicion arises that an individual may be frail, they can be referred for a specialized PATH assessment, which comprehensively assesses cognition and other domains of frailty, followed by the second and third steps of PATH: communicate and care-planning.

The Case of Mr. PN

If the FACT screen was used during Mr. PN's pre-surgical assessment, it would have identified that Mr. PN had moderate impairment of cognition and function. He subsequently could have been referred to the outpatient PATH clinic for a more comprehensive assessment of health and informed decision-making.

2. *Improve the team assessment of frailty to reduce the epidemic of assessments.* The opportunity for team-based care has never been greater, but we need to improve team effectiveness and efficiency. We accomplish this through:
   (a) Team training. PATH training aims for a common understanding of frailty and its clinical drivers, including dementia. The Standardized Team Education Program (STEP) is a hands-on program of team reorganization and capacity building that seeks to: (1) eliminate repetitive assessments; (2) improve the relevance of the patient assessment; (3) optimize team communication; (4) make better use of the assessment for care planning; and (5) improve system navigation for patients and families. The approach is founded on the premise that a shared skill-set for understanding frailty provides the ideal foundation for optimal collaborative care.
   (b) Specialized assessment tools for the entire team. The PLAN tool (Plan for Appropriateness Now) is a standardized approach to comprehensive geriatric assessment for the entire team and is central to STEP training. PLAN replaces parallel (and often redundant) discipline-based evaluations, thereby bringing frailty and cognitive status into focus for the entire team. The shared tool is meant to enhance the collective and longitudinal understanding of the patient's issues throughout the healthcare continuum. Equipped with an appreciation of the clinical hallmarks and implications of frailty, the team can:
      • develop high-level realistic care plans,
      • decide whether and when additional resources are needed,
      • transition patients through palliative care when appropriate.

3. *Improve communication strategies.* The second step of PATH aims to comprehensively communicate information about expected health trajectory and prognosis. Semi-structured scripts and deliberate communication strategies provide a common understanding from which informed decisions can be made. This transfer of knowledge puts decision-makers in an informed and autonomous position from which to apply their values and goals to reach appropriate decisions.

4. *Improve care planning and decision-making with frailty.* The third step of PATH, "*Empower* and *Plan*," provides decision-makers with the necessary skills to make informed decisions by applying framing questions that help patients and families gather relevant information from physicians and health professionals to make decisions during any health crisis. The framing questions include:

   (a) Which health conditions are easily treatable? Which are not?

   (b) How will frailty make treatment risky?

   (c) How can symptoms be safely and effectively managed?

   (d) Will the proposed treatment improve or worsen function and memory?

   (e) Will the proposed treatment require time in hospital? If so, for how long?

   (f) Will the treatment increase good quality years, especially at home?

   (g) What can we do to promote comfort and dignity in the time left?

The framework questions are also used to help patients and families make specific decisions in advance (where appropriate) about possible future treatments, such as whether or not to undergo surgery or use antibiotics.

The Case of Mr. PN

In an alternate scenario, after completing the PATH process, Mr. PN's family (his substitute decision-maker) more fully understands his medical conditions, as well as the probability of worsening health over time due to the expected progression of dementia and other health issues. The framing questions, described above, help the family recognize that surgery could worsen functional and cognitive abilities. As such, the family decides not to proceed with surgery. Mr. PN retains a good quality of life for one year, at which time his health deteriorates due to progression of dementia and heart failure.

5. *Develop new guidelines specific to frailty.* In collaboration with other groups, such as the Dalhousie Academic Detailing Service and the Diabetes Care Program of Nova Scotia, PATH has developed and disseminated frailty-relevant, evidence-informed treatment recommendations for common conditions that occur in frailty, such as diabetes, hypertension, and hyperlipidemia [26–28]. The guidelines recommend liberalized treatment targets.

6. *Improve system coordination across the healthcare continuum.* Since frail patients have multiple health issues, they benefit from organizational structures that can coordinate the issues related to frailty. When PATH is applied throughout the healthcare continuum, it provides a common language, approach, and communication strategy. We provide patients and families with expert advice and system navigation and encourage decision-makers to contact the program when faced with difficult decisions or a health crisis.

7. *Identify and respond to end-of-life issues.* By acknowledging a shortened life expectancy and the expected health trajectory associated with frailty, healthcare providers open the door to a shift in medical decision-making toward more holistic and realistic approaches to care.

8. *Create a cost-effective program for frail older adults.* PATH's family-led care planning processes aim to achieve better management of health-related costs by avoiding harmful or unnecessary surgeries/interventions, reducing redundant assessment, improving multi-disciplinary team effectiveness, making communication processes within and between care facilities more efficient, and minimizing polypharmacy.

Implementation of the PATH model across the continuum of care would result in benefits to patients, their families, and service providers, while having a profound impact on the health system as a whole. An early assessment by Deloitte conducted in Nova Scotia, Canada estimated a potential "savings" of 2.5 to 3.8 % of total provincial health expenditures from inappropriate medical and surgical treatments for frail seniors alone, if the PATH model were fully deployed in community care, long-term care, and tertiary care environments. At a national level, the model indicated savings of up to 3.1 % of Canadian provincial health expenditures, accounting for $4.2 billion in savings. Although these metrics are profound, those exposed to the PATH model understand that reduced costs associated with a reduction in medical and surgical procedures is just the tip of the iceberg in terms of medical and economical efficiencies. Arguably, the largest savings are not yet measurable, and will be the "effect" of initial procedure avoidance. A 76 % reduction in the demand for interventional treatments for those who are significantly frail will also lead to a corresponding decrease in adverse medical events, time in specialty care, transfer costs from home to emergency care, and medication cost for the system and patients. This in turn will improve hospital flow, wait times, health professional availability through improved resource allocation, and care sustainability. Economic benefit estimates are expected to be equally optimistic amongst other national jurisdictions with similar care standards (such as the United States), where savings would grow proportional to the number of frail seniors in the population and the cost of healthcare provision.

PATH Programs

PATH was developed in Canada and has been adopted in several provinces. It has been designated as a leading practice by Accreditation Canada.

PATH Home Care

The hours designated for home care assessment present a major opportunity to understand frailty—one that is frequently missed. The *PATH Home Care Assessment Tool* brings frailty into focus for improved navigation and planning across the healthcare continuum to achieve a better understanding of health for improved care planning. If appropriate, a PATH clinic referral can help with decision-making.

PATH Outpatient Services

Clinic and home-based PATH consultation services help community-dwelling older adults receive assistance with: general care planning; decision-making about specific health interventions such as surgery or chemotherapy; care planning to avoid hospitalization; and end-of-life care.

PATH Tertiary Care

PATH inpatient consultation services help specialists in tertiary care hospitals receive high-level assistance with treatment planning that takes frailty and its impact upon outcomes into account. In addition to general consultation services, specialized applications include:

Renal-PATH

Patients with chronic kidney disease are at risk for cardiovascular disease culminating in frailty. Therefore, all patients over the age of 75 who attend the nephrology clinic are screened for frailty using the FACT. Patients who screen positive for frailty are seen by a PATH-trained nurse practitioner for a more in-depth assessment of frailty. Patients and families also receive individualized assistance with decision-making regarding dialysis.

Cardiac-PATH

Over the past several years, there has been a seismic shift in the age distribution of cardiology inpatients at the Queen Elizabeth Health Sciences Centre, the hospital where we work, with more than 60 % of admitted patients over the age of 65. Since frail older adults commonly face complex decisions, the FACT screen for frailty can identify those patients who would benefit from an in-depth assessment of frailty for responsive care planning.

Pre-surgical PATH

Routine screening for frailty using the FACT alerts surgeons and anesthesiologists to the risks associated with frailty and offers the opportunity for focused decision-making prior to surgical interventions.

PATH Long-Term Care (PATH-LTC)

PATH-LTC brings PATH organization, tools, guidelines, and team-based education into the nursing home to highlight the significance of frailty and improve care planning. In this setting, staff engages in a longitudinal assessment of health, which informs the team about how to help this most frail and vulnerable population (or their surrogates) engage in individualized discussions of prognosis and develop transformational care plans designed to optimize appropriateness and avoid suffering. Polypharmacy is addressed through evidence-informed guidelines specifically developed for frailty [26–28].

Standardized Team Education Program (STEP)

In addition to our clinical programs, PATH identifies the need to build capacity and change the culture of how we deliver care to frail older adults by restructuring team-based care.

As described above, the promulgation of PATH principles is made possible through the training program and instructional manual, which helps individual practitioners and health teams from all sectors and disciplines build efficiency and capacity for appropriate care through the delivery of PATH programs.

Conclusion

PATH presents a tested and validated model to provide optimal, appropriate, and fiscally responsible care. Our goal is to build an effective healthcare system and assemble teams that have a sense of clarity and confidence so that:
- there is better recognition and responsiveness to frailty across disciplines and health settings;
- a shared language is used by all health professionals (physicians and non-physicians) to build a common understanding across disciplines and settings;
- team-based care is more effective and efficient;
- frailty is at the forefront of evidence-informed decision-making in a way that encourages health professionals, patients, and families to understand and consider frailty when making treatment decisions;

- patients and families feel empowered by information;
- more attention is paid to end-of-life experiences for frail older adults with limited life expectancy or debilitating symptoms;
- evidence-based clinical practice guidelines, created for patients with single-system disease, are not indiscriminately applied to frail patients;
- care is continuous so that there is appropriate navigation across all health care services and responsiveness to severe illness is optimized;
- we can provide better care with fewer (re-organized) resources.

PATH continues to grow within Nova Scotia and nationally. PATH is now set up for large-scale implementation of the full model. The creators of the program would like to work with healthcare leaders to implement PATH in a way that integrates the program across the healthcare continuum—from home care to hospital, community, pre-surgical decision-making, and long-term care. The future of health care will be contingent upon how healthcare systems adapt to meet the challenges of frailty.

References

1. Theou O, Rockwood K. Should frailty status always be considered when treating the elderly patient? J Aging Health. 2012;8:261–71.
2. Moorhouse P, Mallery LH. Palliative and therapeutic harmonization: a model for appropriate decision-making in frail older adults. J Am Geriatr Soc. 2012;60:2326–32.
3. www.pathclinic.ca
4. Matthews DA. Dr. Marjory Warren and the origin of British geriatrics. J Am Geriatr Soc. 1984;32:253–8.
5. Holsinger T, Boustani M, Abbot D, Williams JW. Acceptability of dementia screening in primary care patients. Int J Geriatr Psychiatry. 2011;26:373–9.
6. Travis SS, Bernard M, Dixon S, McAuley WJ, Loving G, McClanahan L. Obstacles to palliation and end-of-life care in a long-term care facility. Gerontologist. 2002;42:342–9.
7. Sessums LL, Zembrzuska H, Jackson JL. Does this patient have medical decision-making capacity? JAMA. 2011;306:420–7.
8. Dening KH, Jones L, Sampson EL. Advance care planning for people with dementia: a review. Int Psychogeriatr. 2011;23:1535–51.
9. Okonkwo O, Griffith HR, Belue K, et al. Medical decision-making capacity in patients with mild cognitive impairment. Neurology. 2007;69:1528–35.
10. Okonkwo OC, Griffith HR, Copeland JN, et al. Medical decision-making capacity in mild cognitive impairment: a 3-year longitudinal study. Neurology. 2008;71:1474–80.
11. Fazel S, Hope T, Jacoby R. Effect of cognitive impairment and premorbid intelligence on treatment preferences for life-sustaining medical therapy. Am J Psychiatry. 2000;157:1009–11.
12. Zapka JG, Carter R, Carter CL, Hennessy W, Kurent JE, DesHarnais S. Care at the end of life: focus on communication and race. J Aging Health. 2006;18:791–813.
13. Mitchell SL, Kiely DK, Hamel MB. Dying with advanced dementia in the nursing home. Arch Intern Med. 2004;164:321–6.
14. Murphy DJ, Burrows D, Santilli S, et al. The influence of the probability of survival on patients' preferences regarding cardiopulmonary resuscitation. N Engl J Med. 1994;330:545–9.
15. Volandes AE, Paasche-Orlow MK, Barry MJ, et al. Video decision support tool for advance care planning in dementia: randomised controlled trial. BMJ. 2009;338:b2159.
16. Ekerstad N, Swahn E, Janzon M, et al. Frailty is independently associated with short-term outcomes for elderly patients with non-ST-segment elevation myocardial infarction. Circulation. 2011;124:2397–404.
17. Van Spall HG, Toren A, Kiss A, Fowler RA. Eligibility criteria of randomized controlled trials published in high-impact general medical journals: a systematic sampling review. JAMA. 2007;297:1233–40.
18. Hanlon JT, Schmader KE, Samsa GP, et al. A method for assessing drug therapy appropriateness. J Clin Epidemiol. 1992;45:1045–51.
19. Holmes HM, Hayley DC, Alexander GC, Sachs GA. Reconsidering medication appropriateness for patients late in life. Arch Intern Med. 2006;166:605–9.
20. Tinetti ME, Bogardus STJ, Agostini JV. Potential pitfalls of disease-specific guidelines for patients with multiple conditions. N Engl J Med. 2004;351:2870–4.
21. Braithwaite RS, Fiellin D, Justice AC. The payoff time: a flexible framework to help clinicians decide when patients with comorbid disease are not likely to benefit from practice guidelines. Med Care. 2009;47:610–7.
22. Hanson LC, Eckert JK, Dobbs D, et al. Symptom experience of dying long-term care residents. J Am Geriatr Soc. 2008;56:91–8.
23. CIHI (2013) National Health Expenditure Trends, 1975 to 2013. https://secure.cihi.ca/free_products/NHEXTrendsReport_EN.pdf
24. Canadian study of health and aging: study methods and prevalence of dementia. CMAJ. 1994;150:899–913.
25. A new way of looking at the impact of dementia in Canada. Alzheimer Society of Canada. (2012). http://www.alzheimer.ca/~/media/Files/national/Mediareleases/asc_factsheet_new_data_09272012_en.pdf
26. Mallery LH, Allen M, Fleming I, et al. Promoting higher blood pressure targets for frail older adults: a consensus guideline from Canada. Cleve Clin J Med. 2014;81(7):427–37.
27. Lipids in primary prevention. http://www.medicine.dal.ca/content/dam/dalhousie/pdf/faculty/medicine/departments/core-units/cpd/statins_2013.pdf
28. Mallery LH, Ransom T, Steeves B, Cook B, Dunbar P, Moorhouse P. Evidence-informed guidelines for treating frail older adults with type 2 diabetes: from the Diabetes Care Program of Nova Scotia (DCPNS) and the Palliative and Therapeutic Harmonization (PATH) program. J Am Med Dir Assoc. 2013;14:801–8.

Index